D1629186

Edited by János Fischer,
C. Robin Ganellin and
David P. Rotella

Analogue-based Drug Discovery III

Related Titles

Fischer, J., Ganellin, C. R. (Eds.)

Analogue-based Drug Discovery II

2010

ISBN: 978-3-527-32549-8

IUPAC, Fischer, J., Ganellin, C. R. (Eds.)

Analogue-based Drug Discovery

2006

ISBN: 978-3-527-31257-3

Abraham, D. J., Rotella, D. P.

Burger's Medicinal Chemistry, Drug Discovery and Development

8 Volume Set

2010

ISBN: 978-0-470-27815-4

Li, J. J., Johnson, D. S. (eds.)

Modern Drug Synthesis

2010

ISBN: 978-0-470-52583-8

Lednicer, D.

Strategies for Organic Drug Synthesis and Design

2008

ISBN: 978-0-470-19039-5

Chorghade, M. S. (ed.)

Drug Discovery and Development

2 Volume Set

2007

ISBN: 978-0-471-39846-2

Edited by János Fischer, C. Robin Ganellin and David P. Rotella

Analogue-based Drug Discovery III

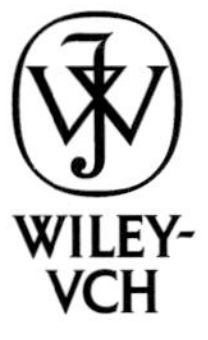

WILEY-VCH Verlag GmbH & Co. KGaA

The Editors

Prof. Dr. János Fischer
Gedeon Richter Plc.
Gyömröi ut 30
1103 Budapest
Hungary

Prof. Dr. C. Robin Ganellin
University College London
Department of Chemistry
20 Gordon Street
London WC1H 0AJ
United Kingdom

Prof. Dr. David P. Rotella
Montclair State University
Department of Chemistry & Biochemistry
Montclair, NJ 07043
USA

Supported by the international Union of Pure and Applied Chemistry (IUPAC)
Chemistry and Human Health Division
PO Box 13757
Research Triangle Park, NC 2770-3757
USA

All books published by **Wiley-VCH** are carefully produced. Nevertheless, authors, editors, and publisher do not warrant the information contained in these books, including this book, to be free of errors. Readers are advised to keep in mind that statements, data, illustrations, procedural details or other items may inadvertently be inaccurate.

Library of Congress Card No.: applied for

British Library Cataloguing-in-Publication Data
A catalogue record for this book is available from the British Library.

Bibliographic information published by the Deutsche Nationalbibliothek
The Deutsche Nationalbibliothek lists this publication in the Deutsche Nationalbibliografie; detailed bibliographic data are available on the Internet at http://dnb.d-nb.de.

© 2013 Wiley-VCH Verlag & Co. KGaA, Boschstr. 12, 69469 Weinheim, Germany

All rights reserved (including those of translation into other languages). No part of this book may be reproduced in any form – by photoprinting, microfilm, or any other means – nor transmitted or translated into a machine language without written permission from the publishers. Registered names, trademarks, etc. used in this book, even when not specifically marked as such, are not to be considered unprotected by law.

Print ISBN: 978-3-527-33073-7
ePDF ISBN: 978-3-527-65111-5
ePub ISBN: 978-3-527-65110-8
mobi ISBN: 978-3-527-65109-2
oBook ISBN: 978-3-527-65108-5

Cover Design Grafik-Design Schulz, Fußgönheim

Typesetting Thomson Digital, Noida, India

Printing and Binding Markono Print Media Pte Ltd, Singapore

Printed on acid-free paper

Contents

Preface

The editors of the third volume of the book series "Analogue-Based Drug Discovery" thank the International Union of Pure and Applied Chemistry (IUPAC) for supporting this book project. We also thank the coworkers at Wiley-VCH, Dr. Frank Weinreich and Waltraud Wüst, for their excellent help, and last but not least we are grateful to all the contributors of this book. Special thanks are due to the following reviewers who helped both the authors and the editors: Klaus Peter Bøgesø, Helmut Buschmann, Paul W. Erhardt, Staffan Erickson, Susan B. Horwitz, Manfred Jung, Amit Kalgutkar, Danijel Kikelj, Andrew MacMillan, Eckhard Ottow, Jens-Uwe Peters, Henning Priepke, John Proudfoot, Stephen C. Smith, Bernard Testa, and Han van de Waterbeemd.

Analogue-based drug discovery is a basic principle of drug research. In this book series, we focused on analogues of existing drugs. In the first volume (2006), we discussed structural and pharmacological analogues, whereas the second volume (2010) also included analogues with pharmacological similarities.

In this volume, we continued the same concept, recognizing that in several cases there is only a narrow gap between a pioneer and an analogue drug because of the strong competitive environment in the industry. A new promising molecular biological target inspires parallel research efforts at several companies. It can happen that the first discovery does not lead to a marketed drug; instead, a molecule discovered later proves to be the first to be launched. As a result of the strong competition, it can also happen that two pioneer drugs are introduced nearly simultaneously in the market, and these drugs often have chemical and pharmacological similarities.

The third volume of Analogue-Based Drug Discovery consists of three parts.

Part I (General Aspects)

The introductory chapter discusses the relationship between the pioneer and analogue drugs, where their overlapping character can be observed. A chapter by Christian Tyrchan and Fabrizio Giordanetto (AstraZeneca) analyzes competition in pharmaceutical drug development. Amit S. Kalgutkar and Antonia F. Stepan (Pfizer) study the important role of metabolic stability in drug research. Mark L. Peterson, Hamit Hoveyda, Graeme Fraser, Éric Marsault, and René Gagnon

(Tranzyme Pharma Inc.) write on the use of peptide-based macrocycles in drug design exemplified with the discovery of ulimorelin.

Part II (Drug Classes)

A. Ganesan (University of East Anglia) gives an overview of discovery research into anticancer epigenetic drugs. Joseph A. Jakubowski (Lilly) and Atsushiro Sugidachi (Daiichi Sankyo) evaluate the structurally diverse drug class of the antithrombotic $P2Y_{12}$ receptor antagonists. Paul Erhardt, Amarjit Luniwal, and Rachael Jetson (University of Toledo, USA) summarize the medicinal chemistry of selective estrogen receptor modulators. Kazumi Kondo and Hidenori Ogawa (Otsuka Phramaceutical Co., Japan) describe the discovery of aquaretics that are vasopressin V2 receptor antagonists. Peter R. Bernstein (PhaRmaB LLC) evokes the discovery of cysteinyl leukotriene receptor antagonists that are important in the treatment of asthma.

Part III (Case Histories)

Norbert Hauel, Andreas Clemens, Herbert Nar, Henning Priepke, Joanne van Ryn, and Wolfgang Wienen (Boehringer Ingelheim, Biberach, Germany) report on the discovery of dabigatran etexilate, an oral direct thrombin inhibitor approved for use in the treatment of acute thrombosis. Klaus P. Bøgesø and Connie Sánchez (Lundbeck) describe the discovery of escitalopram, which is one of the most successful selective serotonin reuptake inhibitors in the treatment of depressive disorders. Helmut Buschmann (Pharma-Consulting, Aachen, Germany) analyzes the discovery of tapentadol, a novel centrally acting synthetic analgesic with a dual mechanism of action. Hervé Bouchard, Drothée Semiond, Marie-Laure Risse, and Patricia Vrignaud (Sanofi) describe the discovery of cabazitaxel, a novel semisynthetic taxane, a new anticancer drug. Srikanth Venkatraman, Andrew Prongay, and George F. Njoroge (Merck) summarize the discovery of boceprevir and narlaprevir, hepatitis C protease inhibitors. Ken Okamoto, Shiro Kondo, and Takeshi Nishino (Nippon Medical School, Teijin Ltd, and University of Tokyo) describe the discovery of febuxostat, a new uric acid production inhibitor.

The above 15 chapters of the book with 40 authors from 9 countries bring important and successful drug discoveries closer to the medicinal chemists and to all who are interested in the complicated history of drug discoveries.

The major parts of the chapters are written by key inventors.

We hope that also the third volume of this book series will be well received by people interested in medicinal chemistry.

May 2012
Budapest, Hungary — *János Fischer*
London, UK — *C. Robin Ganellin*
Montclair, NJ, USA — *David P. Rotella*

List of Contributors

Peter R. Bernstein
PhaRmaB LLC
14 Forest View Road
Rose Valley, PA 1908-6721
USA

Klaus P. Bøgesø
H. Lundbeck A/S
Lundbeck Research Denmark
9 Ottiliavej
2500 Valby
Denmark

Hervé Bouchard
Sanofi
LGCR/Natural Product & Protein
Chemistry (NPPC)
13 quai Jules Guesde
94400 Vitry-sur-Seine
France

Helmut Buschmann
Sperberweg 15
52076 Aachen
Germany

Andreas Clemens
Boehringer Ingelheim Pharma
GmbH & Co. KG
Department of Medicinal Chemistry
Birkendorfer Straße 65
88400 Biberach an der Riß
Germany

Paul Erhardt
The University of Toledo
College of Pharmacy
2801 West Bancroft Street
Toledo, OH 43606-3390
USA

János Fischer
Gedeon Richter Plc.
Department of Medicinal Chemistry
Gyömröi ut 19/21
1103 Budapest
Hungary

Graeme Fraser
Tranzyme Pharma, Inc.
3001, 12th Avenue Nord
Sherbrooke, Quebec J1H 5N4
Canada

René Gagnon
Tranzyme Pharma, Inc.
3001, 12th Avenue Nord
Sherbrooke, Quebec J1H 5N4
Canada

C. Robin Ganellin
University College London
Department of Chemistry
20 Gordon Street
London WC1H 0AJ
UK

A. Ganesan
School of Pharmacy
University of East Anglia
Norwich NR4 7TJ
United Kingdom

Fabrizio Giordanetto
AstraZeneca CV/GI
Lead Generation Department
Pepparedsleden 1
43150 Mölndal
Sweden

Norbert Hauel
Boehringer Ingelheim Pharma
GmbH & Co. KG
Department of Medicinal Chemistry
Birkendorfer Straße 65
88400 Biberach an der Riß
Germany

Hamid Hoveyda
Tranzyme Pharma, Inc.
3001, 12th Avenue Nord
Sherbrooke, Quebec J1H 5N4
Canada

Joseph A. Jakubowski
Eli Lilly and Company
Lilly Research Laboratories
Indianapolis, IN 46285
USA

Rachael Jetson
The University of Toledo
College of Pharmacy
2801 West Bancroft Street
Toledo, OH 43606-3390
USA

Amit S. Kalgutkar
Pfizer Worldwide Research and Development
Department of Pharmacokinetics, Dynamics, and Metabolism
MS 8220-3529
Groton CT 06340
USA

Kazumi Kondo
Otsuka Pharmaceutical Co. Ltd.
Qs' Research Institute
463-10 Kagasuno, Kawauchicho
Tokushima 771-0192
Japan

Shiro Kondo
Teijin Ltd.
Kondo Laboratory
4-3-2 Asahigaoka, Hino
Tokyo 191–8512
Japan

Amarjit Luniwal
The University of Toledo
College of Pharmacy
2801 West Bancroft Street
Toledo, OH 43606-3390
USA

Éric Marsault
Tranzyme Pharma, Inc.
3001, 12th Avenue Nord
Sherbrooke, Quebec J1H 5N4
Canada

Herbert Nar
Boehringer Ingelheim Pharma
GmbH & Co. KG
Department of Medicinal Chemistry
Birkendorfer Straße 65
88400 Biberach an der Riß
Germany

Takeshi Nishino
The University of Tokyo
Graduate School of Agricultural and Life Sciences
Department of Applied Biological Chemistry
1-1-1 Yayoi, Bunkyo-Ku
Tokyo 113–8657
Japan

George F. Njoroge
Eli Lilly and Company
Lilly Research Laboratories
Indianapolis, IN 46285
USA

Hidenori Ogawa
Otsuka Pharmaceutical Co. Ltd.
Qs' Research Institute
463-10 Kagasuno, Kawauchicho
Tokushima 771-0192
Japan

Ken Okamoto
Nippon Medical School
Department of Biochemistry
1-1-5 Sendagi, Bunkyo-ku
Tokyo 113-8602
Japan

Mark L. Peterson
Tranzyme Pharma, Inc.
3001, 12th Avenue Nord
Sherbrooke, Quebec J1H 5N4
Canada

Henning Priepke
Boehringer Ingelheim Pharma
GmbH & Co. KG
Department of Medicinal Chemistry
Birkendorfer Straße 65
88400 Biberach an der Riß
Germany

Andrew Prongay
Merck Research Laboratories
Chemical Research
2015 Galloping Hill Road
Kenilworth, NJ 07033
USA

Marie-Laure Risse
Sanofi Oncology
Centre de Recherche de
Vitry-Alfortville
13 quai Jules Guesde
94400 Vitry-sur-Seine
France

David P. Rotella
Montclair State University
Department of Chemistry &
Biochemistry
1 Normal Ave
Montclair, NJ 07043
USA

Connie Sánchez
Lundbeck Research USA
Department of Neuroscience
215 College Road
Paramus, NJ 07652
USA

Dorothée Semiond
Sanofi
Centre de Recherche de
Vitry-Alfortville
Department of Disposition, Safety
and Animal Research (DSAR)
13 quai Jules Guesde
94400 Vitry-sur-Seine
France

Antonia F. Stepan
Pfizer Worldwide Research and
Development
Neuroscience Medicinal Chemistry
700 Main Street
Cambridge, MA 02139
USA

Atsuhiro Sugidachi
Daiichi Sankyo Co., Ltd.
Biological Research Laboratories
1-2-58 Hiromachi, Shinagawa-ku
Tokyo 140-8710
Japan

Christian Tyrchan
AstraZeneca CV/GI
Lead Generation Department
Pepparedsleden 1
43150 Mölndal
Sweden

Joanne van Ryn
Boehringer Ingelheim Pharma
GmbH & Co. KG
Department of Medicinal Chemistry
Birkendorfer Straße 65
88400 Biberach an der Riß
Germany

Srikanth Venkatraman
Schering-Plough Research Institute
Department of Medicinal Chemistry
2015 Galloping Hill Road
Kenilworth, NJ 07033-1335
USA

Patricia Vrignaud
Sanofi Oncology
Centre de Recherche de
Vitry-Alfortville
13 quai Jules Guesde
94400 Vitry-sur-Seine
France

Wolfgang Wienen
Boehringer Ingelheim Pharma
GmbH & Co. KG
Department of Medicinal Chemistry
Birkendorfer Straße 65
88400 Biberach an der Riß
Germany

Part I
General Aspects

Analogue-based Drug Discovery III, First Edition. Edited by János Fischer, C. Robin Ganellin, and David P. Rotella.
© 2013 Wiley-VCH Verlag GmbH & Co. KGaA. Published 2013 by Wiley-VCH Verlag GmbH & Co. KGaA.

1
Pioneer and Analogue Drugs

János Fischer, C. Robin Ganellin, and David P. Rotella

A *pioneer drug* ("first in class") represents a breakthrough invention that affords a marketed drug where no structurally and/or pharmacologically similar drug was known before its introduction. The majority of drugs, however, are *analogue drugs*, which have structural and/or pharmacological similarities to a pioneer drug or, as in some cases, to other analogue drugs.

The aim of this chapter is to discuss these two drug types [1].

The term "pioneer drug" is not used very often, because only a small fraction of drugs belongs to this type and in many cases the pioneer drugs lose their importance when similar but better drugs are discovered. A pioneer drug and its analogues form a drug class in which subsequent optimization may be observed. Analogue drugs typically offer benefits such as improved efficacy and/or side effect profiles or dose frequency than a pioneer drug to be successful on the market.

The discovery of both *pioneer* and *analogue drugs* needs some serendipity. A pioneer drug must clinically validate the safety and efficacy of a new molecular target and mechanism of action based on a novel chemical structure. In the case of an analogue drug, it is helpful that a pioneer or an analogue exists; nevertheless, some serendipity is needed to discover a new and better drug analogue, because there are no general guidelines on how such molecules can be identified preclinically. The analogue approach is very fruitful in new drug research, because there is a higher probability of finding a better drug than to discover a pioneer one. A significant risk with this approach is based on the potential for one of the many competitors in the drug discovery area to succeed prior to others.

The similarity between two drugs cannot be simply defined. Even a minor modification of a drug structure can completely modify the properties of a molecule. Levodopa (**1**) and methyldopa (**2**) are applied in different therapeutic fields; however, their structures differ only in a methyl group. Both molecules have the same stereochemistry as derivatives of L-tyrosine. Levodopa [2] is used for the treatment of Parkinson's disease as a dopamine precursor, whereas methyldopa [3] was an important antihypertensive agent before safer and more efficacious molecules (e.g., ACE inhibitors) appeared on the market.

Analogue-based Drug Discovery III, First Edition. Edited by János Fischer, C. Robin Ganellin, and David P. Rotella.
© 2013 Wiley-VCH Verlag GmbH & Co. KGaA. Published 2013 by Wiley-VCH Verlag GmbH & Co. KGaA.

Methyldopa (first synthesized at Merck Sharp & Dohme) has a dual mechanism of action: it is a competitive inhibitor of the enzyme DOPA decarboxylase and its metabolite acts as an α-adrenergic agonist.

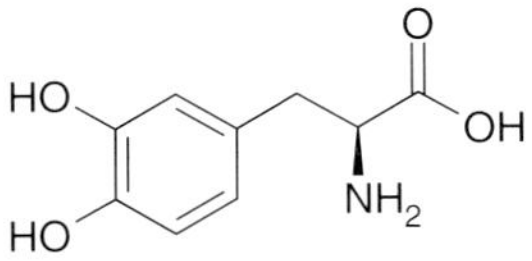

levodopa
1

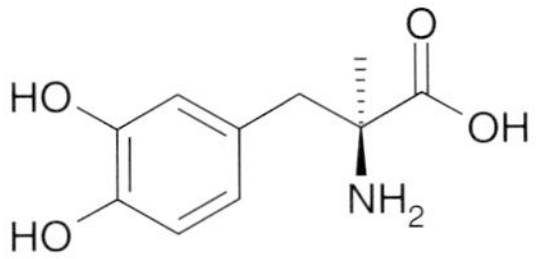

methyldopa
2

Levodopa and methyldopa are not analogues from the viewpoint of medicinal chemistry. Both are pioneer drugs in their respective therapeutic fields and can be considered as stand-alone drugs, because they have no successful analogues.

There are several examples, and it is a usual case that a minor modification of a drug molecule affords a much more active drug in the same therapeutic field. The pioneer drug chlorothiazide (**3**) and its analogue hydrochlorothiazide (**4**) from Merck Sharp & Dohme differ only by two hydrogen atoms; however, the diuretic effect of hydrochlorothiazide [4] is 10 times higher than that of the original drug. The pioneer drug chlorothiazide is rarely used, but its analogue, hydrochlorothiazide, is an important first-line component in current antihypertensive therapy as a single agent and in combination with other compounds.

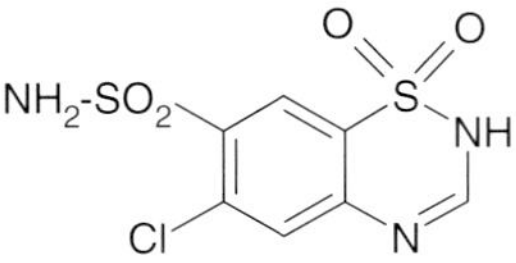

chlorothiazide
3

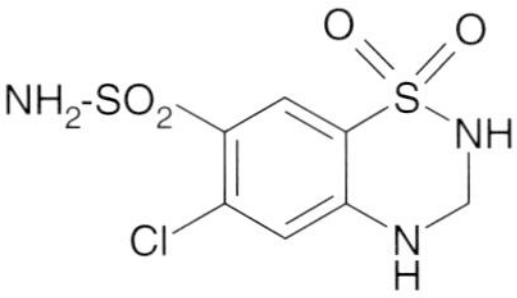

hydrochlorothiazide
4

Chlorothiazide and hydrochlorothiazide are *direct analogues*, which term emphasizes their close relationship.

The terms “pioneer drugs” and “analogue drugs” will be discussed in the following sections.

1.1 Monotarget Drugs

1.1.1 H_2 Receptor Histamine Antagonists

Before the launch of cimetidine (1976), only short-acting neutralization of gastric acid was possible by administration of various antacids (e.g., sodium bicarbonate, magnesium hydroxide, aluminum hydroxide, etc.) that did not affect gastric acid secretion. Cimetidine [5], the first successful H_2 receptor histamine antagonist, a pioneer drug for the treatment of gastric hyperacidity and peptic ulcer disease, was discovered by researchers at Smith, Kline & French. The inhibition of histamine-stimulated gastric acid secretion was first studied in rats. Burimamide (**5**) was the first lead compound, a prototype drug, that also served as a proof of concept for inhibition of acid secretion in human subjects when administered intravenously, but its oral activity was insufficient. Its analogue, metiamide (**6**), was orally active, but its clinical studies had to be discontinued because of a low incidence of granulocytopenia. Replacing the thiourea moiety in metiamide with a cyanoguanidino moiety afforded cimetidine (**7**). Its use provided clinical proof for inhibition of gastric acid secretion and ulcer healing and was a great commercial and clinical success in the treatment of peptic ulcer disease.

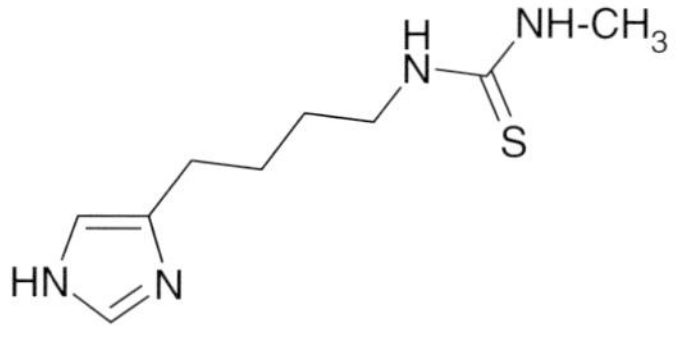

burimamide
5

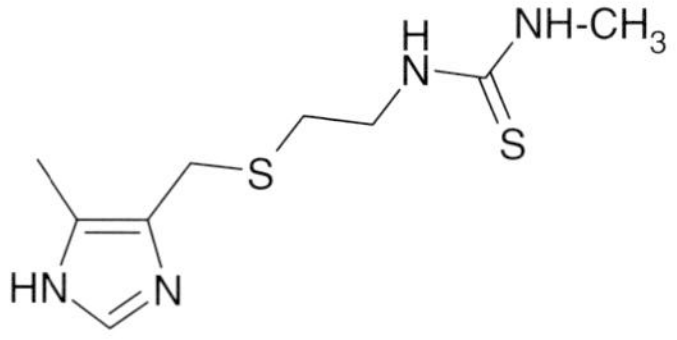

metiamide
6

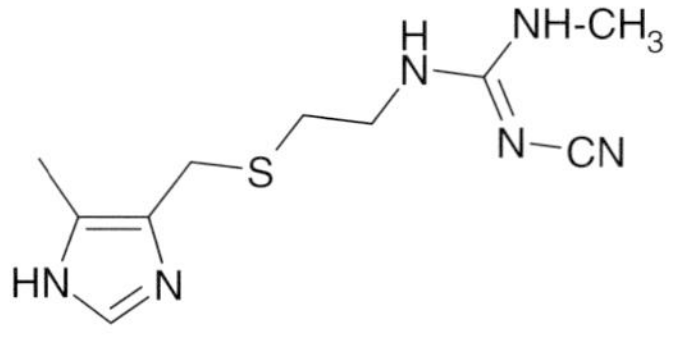

cimetidine
7

Although cimetidine was very effective for the treatment of peptic ulcer disease and related problems of acid hypersecretion, there were some side effects associated with its use, albeit at a very low level. A low incidence of gynecomastia in men can occur at high doses of cimetidine due to its antiandrogen effect. Cimetidine also inhibits cytochrome P450, an important drug metabolizing enzyme. It is therefore advisable to avoid coadministration of cimetidine with certain drugs such as propranolol, warfarin, diazepam, and theophylline.

Cimetidine led to the initiation of analogue-based drug research affording more potent analogue drugs such as ranitidine (**8**) and famotidine (**9**) that lack the above side effects of cimetidine.

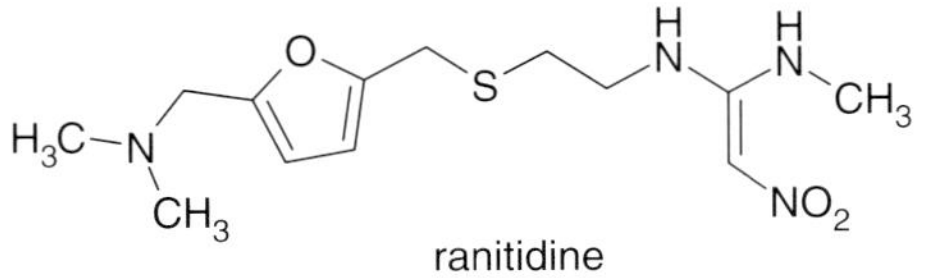

ranitidine
8

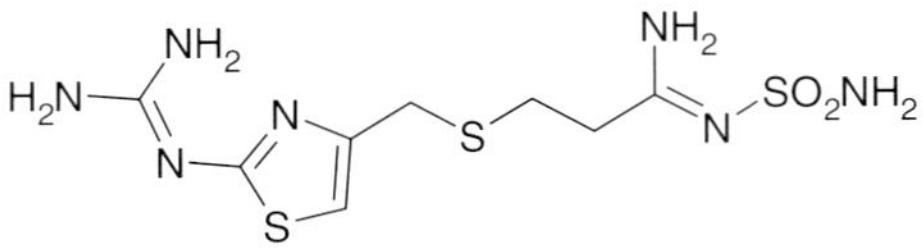

famotidine
9

Ranitidine [6] also has a pioneer character, because ranitidine is the first H_2 receptor histamine antagonist that has no antiandrogen adverse effect and does not inhibit the cytochrome CYP450 enzymes. Famotidine is the most potent member of this drug class, which has been discussed in Volume I of this series [7].

Summary:

Pioneer H_2 receptor histamine antagonist: cimetidine.
First H_2 receptor histamine antagonist with no antiandrogen adverse effects and without inhibition of P450 enzymes: ranitidine.

1.1.2 ACE Inhibitors

A natural product, the nonapeptide teprotide (**10**), was the pioneer drug for angiotensin-converting enzyme (ACE) inhibitors. Teprotide [8] was used as an active antihypertensive drug in patients with essential hypertension. It could only be administered parenterally, which is a great drawback for chronic use of a drug. A breakthrough occurred with the approval of the first orally active ACE inhibitor captopril (**11**) in 1980 by Squibb. Captopril [9] has a short onset time (0.5–1 h), and its duration of action is also relatively short (6–12 h); as a result, two to three daily doses are necessary. Captopril can be regarded as a pharmacological analogue of teprotide, but it is also the pioneer orally active ACE inhibitor. Captopril's discovery initiated intensive research by several other drug companies to discover longer acting ACE inhibitors. Enalapril (**12**) was introduced by Merck in 1984. Enalapril [10] can be regarded as the first long-acting oral ACE inhibitor. The long-acting ACE inhibitors are once-daily antihypertensive drugs. There are several long-acting ACE inhibitors, whose differences have been discussed in the first volume of this book series [11].

pyro-Glu - Trp - Pro - Arg - Pro - Gln - Ile - Pro - Pro -OH

teprotide
10

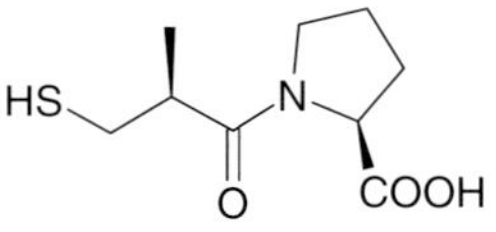

captopril
11

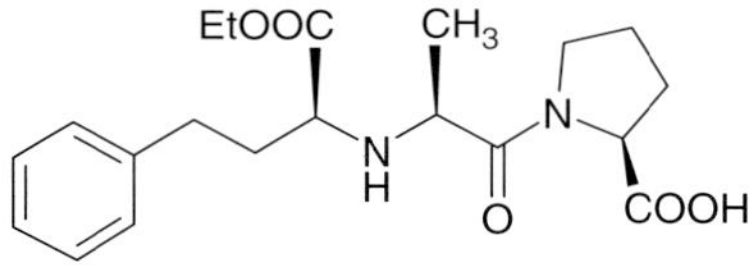

enalapril
12

Summary:

Pioneer ACE inhibitor drug: teprotide.
First orally active ACE inhibitor drug: captopril.
First orally long-acting ACE inhibitor drug: enalapril.

1.1.3
DPP IV Inhibitors

Sitagliptin (**13**) [12], a pioneer dipeptidyl peptidase IV (DPP IV) inhibitor, was launched in 2006 by Merck for the treatment of type 2 diabetes. The medicinal chemistry team began its research in 1999 when some DPP IV inhibitor molecules were known as substrate-based analogues. The lead molecule derived from this research was vildagliptin (**14**) [13]; discovered at Novartis in 1998, it was the second compound to be introduced to the market.

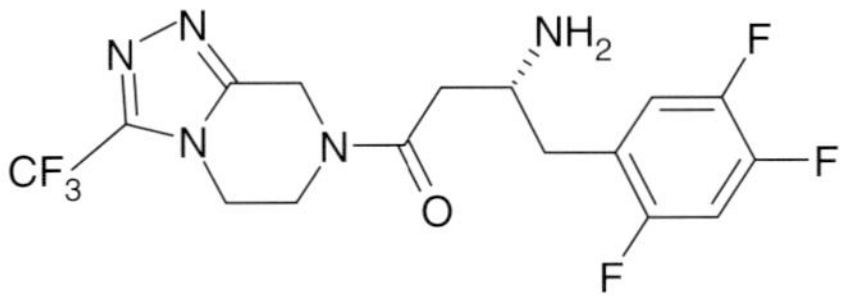

sitagliptin
13

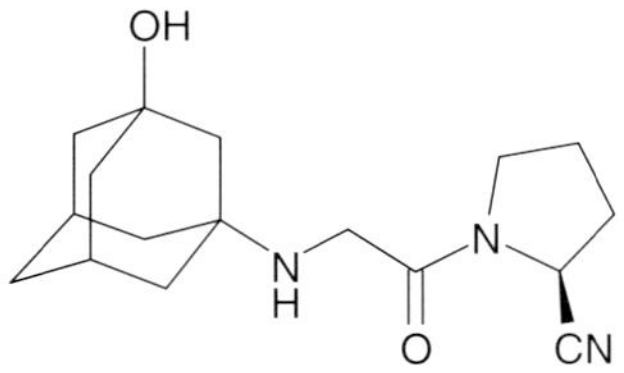

vildagliptin
14

The pioneer drug sitagliptin is a commercial success with 2010 sales greater than USD 3 billion. Vildagliptin was the first successful discovery in this drug class, but its development time was longer and it was introduced in 2007, after sitagliptin. Vildagliptin is only moderately selective over DPP-8 and DPP-9 compared to sitagliptin that is a highly selective DPP IV inhibitor. Based on long-term safety studies, these selectivity differences do not influence the toxicity of vildagliptin. Sitagliptin and vildagliptin show similar clinical efficacies. Vildagliptin has a short half-life (3 h) and its dosing regimen is twice a day, whereas sitagliptin has a long half-life (12 h) and once-daily dosing is used. DPP IV inhibitors are typical early-phase analogues that result from a highly competitive industry, and not the first candidate (vildagliptin) but a follow-on drug (sitagliptin) became the pioneer drug on the market ("first-in-class drug"). Further DPP IV inhibitors are available (alogliptin, saxagliptin, and linagliptin) and the individual compounds differ significantly in their mode of metabolism and excretion and these differences help the treatment of patients with type 2 diabetes in an individual way [14] (see Chapter 5 of Volume II of this book series).

Summary:

Pioneer DPP IV inhibitor drug: sitagliptin (long-acting inhibitor).
First DPP IV inhibitor analogue drug: vildagliptin (short-acting inhibitor).

1.1.4
Univalent Direct Thrombin Inhibitors

Thrombin is a serine protease enzyme whose inhibition plays an important role in the mechanism of several anticoagulants. Univalent direct thrombin inhibitors bind only to the active site of the enzyme, whereas bivalent direct thrombin inhibitors (e.g., hirudin and bivalirudin) block thrombin at both the active site and exosite 1.

The pioneer univalent direct thrombin inhibitor is argatroban monohydrate (**15**) [15] that was launched by Daiichi Pharmaceutical and Mitsubishi Pharma in 1990. Argatroban was approved by the FDA for prophylactic anticoagulation in the treatment of thrombosis in patients with heparin-induced thrombocytopenia. Argatroban is a rather selective reversible inhibitor for human thrombin. Despite its low molecular weight, argatroban is administered parenterally due to the presence of the highly basic guanidine moiety that prevents absorption from the gastrointestinal tract. This characteristic limits the clinical use of the compound. The first oral direct thrombin inhibitor was ximelagatran (**17**) [16], which was introduced in 2004 by AstraZeneca. Ximelagatran is a double prodrug derivative of melagatran (**16**) with a bioavailability of about 20%, a measurable improvement compared to melagatran with oral bioavailability of 5.8%. Ximelagatran was withdrawn from the market in 2006 because of unacceptable hepatic side effects (alanine aminotransferase increased threefold and bilirubin level increased twofold above the normal upper limit) [17]. In this drug class, dabigatran etexilate (**18**) [18] was discovered by Boehringer Ingelheim as a new direct thrombin inhibitor without adverse liver effects [19] (see Chapter 10)

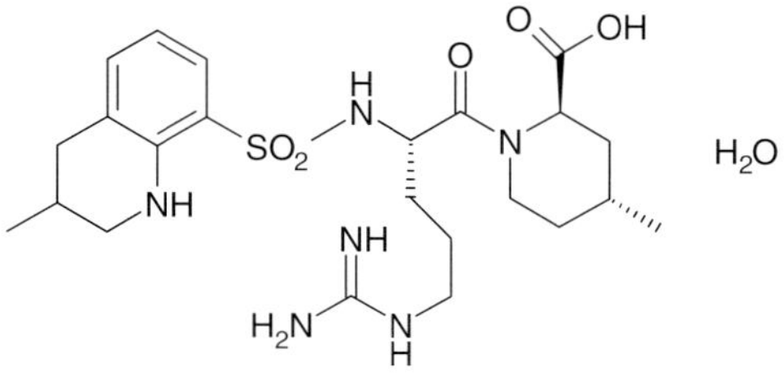

argatroban monohydrate
15

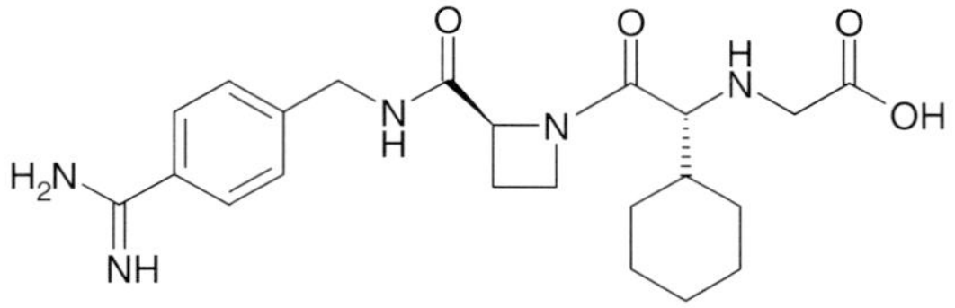

melagatran
16

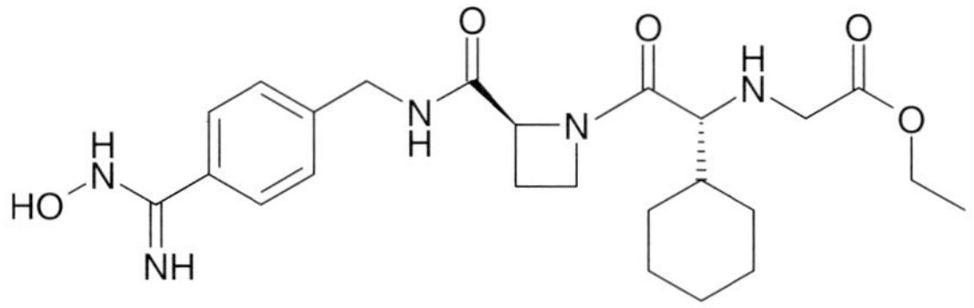

ximelagatran
17

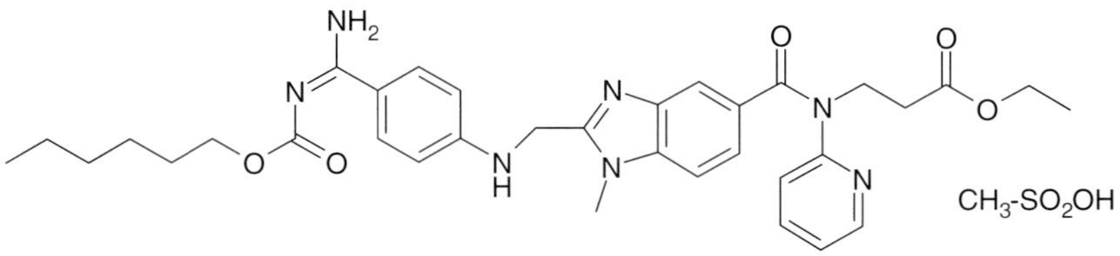

dabigatran etexilate mesylate
18

Summary:

Pioneer univalent direct thrombin inhibitor drug: argatroban.
First orally active univalent thrombin inhibitor: ximelagatran.
First orally active univalent thrombin inhibitor without adverse liver affects: dabigatran etexilate.

1.2
Dual-Acting Drugs

1.2.1
Monotarget Drugs from Dual-Acting Drugs

1.2.1.1 Optimization of Beta-Adrenergic Receptor Blockers

James W. Black and coworkers at ICI invented propranolol as a product of analogue-based drug discovery (ABDD) using their prototype drug, pronethalol (**19**), as a lead compound. Pronethalol [20] was an active drug for the treatment of angina pectoris in humans, but its development was discontinued because it proved to be carcinogenic in mice in long-term toxicology studies. Continuation of the analogue-based drug discovery afforded propranolol (**20**), where an oxymethylene link was inserted between the 1-napthyl group and the secondary alcohol moiety of pronethalol. Propranolol [21] was more potent than pronethalol. Propranolol became the pioneer nonselective β-adrenergic receptor antagonist, a true antagonist without partial agonist properties (intrinsic sympathomimetic activity). It was a breakthrough discovery for the treatment of arrhythmias, angina pectoris, and hypertension.

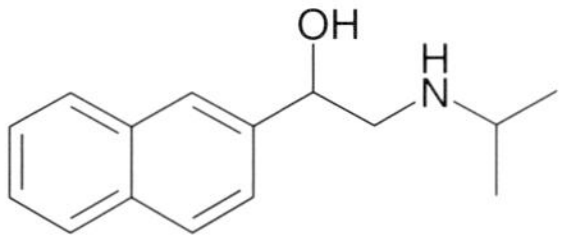

pronethalol
19

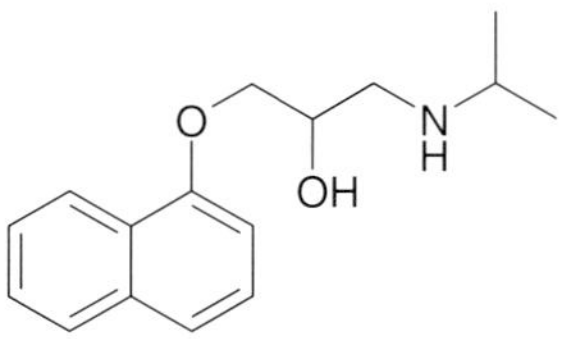

propranolol
20

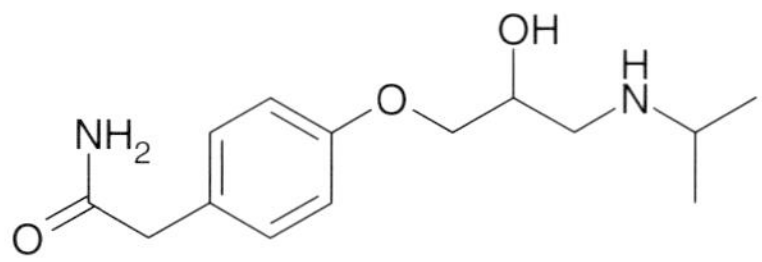

atenolol
21

The pioneer drug propranolol has equal antagonist affinity for β_1 and β_2 adrenergic receptors; however, β_1 receptors are located only in the heart and the non-selective propranolol also blocks β_2 receptors in bronchial smooth muscle. Therefore, propranolol is not used in patients with bronchial asthma. Several analogues have been tested in a battery of *in vivo* pharmacological tests resulting in the discovery of atenolol (**21**) [22]. A guinea pig bronchospasm test served for investigation and demonstration of β_1 selectivity. Atenolol had no intrinsic sympathomimetic effect (partial agonism), similar to propranolol (see Chapter 8 of Volume I (Part II) of this book series).

Summary:

Pioneer dual-acting (β_1 and β_2) beta-adrenergic receptor antagonist: propranolol.
First β_1 selective antagonist drug without intrinsic sympathomimetic activity: atenolol.

1.2.2 Dual-Acting Drugs from Monotarget Drugs

1.2.2.1 Dual-Acting Opioid Drugs

Most ligands designed from the morphine template are mu (μ) opioid receptor (MOP) agonists. A simplified version of the morphine skeleton afforded tramadol that is marketed in its racemic form. The (+)-isomer is a weak MOP agonist, whereas the (−)-isomer inhibits neurotransmitter reuptake. Tramadol (**22**) [23] was discovered by Grünenthal and was introduced in 1977 for the treatment of moderate to severe pain.

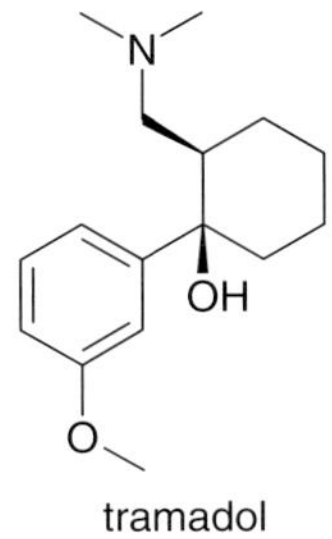

N OH O

tramadol
22

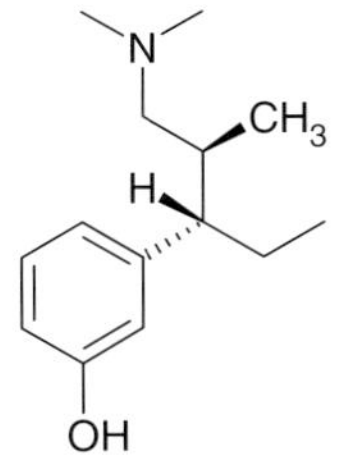

N CH_3 H OH

tapentadol
23

Grünenthal continued analogue-based drug research using tramadol as a starting compound, and out of several analogues, tapentadol (**23**) [24] was selected and developed. It was introduced in 2009 to the market as a new opioid analgesic drug with dual activity: a MOP agonist and an inhibitor of norepinephrine reuptake. Tramadol is thousands of times less potent than morphine on the mu opioid receptor, whereas tapentadol's analgesic activity is comparable to that of oxycodone with reduced constipation and respiratory depression (see Chapter 12).

Summary:

Pioneer dual-acting (MOP agonist and norepinephrine reuptake inhibitor) opioid drug racemate: tramadol.
First dual-acting (MOP agonist and norepinephrine reuptake inhibitor) opioid drug in a single molecule: tapentadol.

1.3 Multitarget Drugs

1.3.1 Multitarget Drug Analogue to Eliminate a Side Effect

1.3.1.1 Clozapine and Olanzapine

Clozapine (**24**) [25] is the pioneer drug in the class of atypical antipsychotic agents. It was a serendipitous discovery by researchers at Wander in Switzerland in 1960 from the structural analogue antidepressant amoxapine (**25**). Its discovery was unexpected from the structurally very close analogue and therapeutically it had a great advantage over the typical antipsychotic drugs such as chlorpromazine and haloperidol because clozapine produced no extrapyramidal side effects (EPS). Clozapine causes agranulocytosis in about 1% of the patients, and this side effect limited its application. Analogue-based drug design afforded quetiapine (**26**) [26], a clozapine analogue without this side effect. It was discovered at ICI in 1986 and it became one of the main products of AstraZeneca. Instead of the dibenzodiazepine nucleus of clozapine, the analogue quetiapine has a dibenzothiazepine scaffold. Both clozapine and quetiapine have affinity for a number of receptors. The antipsychotic activity is believed to be associated primarily by virtue of affinity for D_2 and 5-HT_{2A} receptors. Chapter 3 discusses metabolic aspects that may contribute to the distinct adverse event profiles of these two drugs (see the chapter of Volume I on clozapine analogues).

Summary:

Pioneer atypical antipsychotic drug: clozapine.
First atypical clozapine-like antipsychotic drug without the side effect of agranulocytosis: quetiapine.

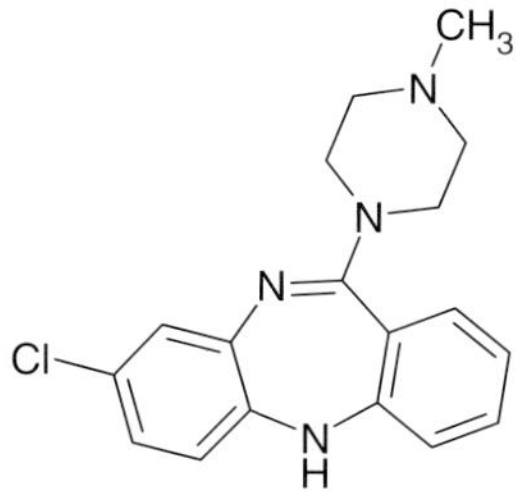

clozapine
24

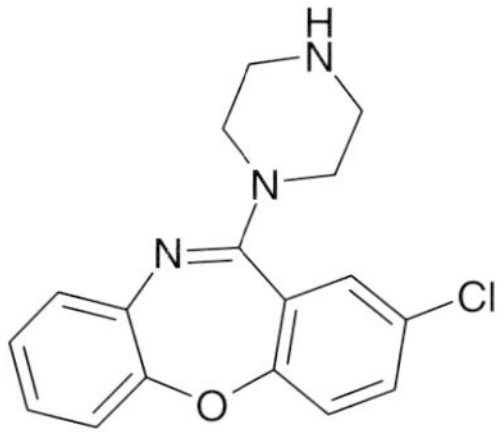

amoxapine
25

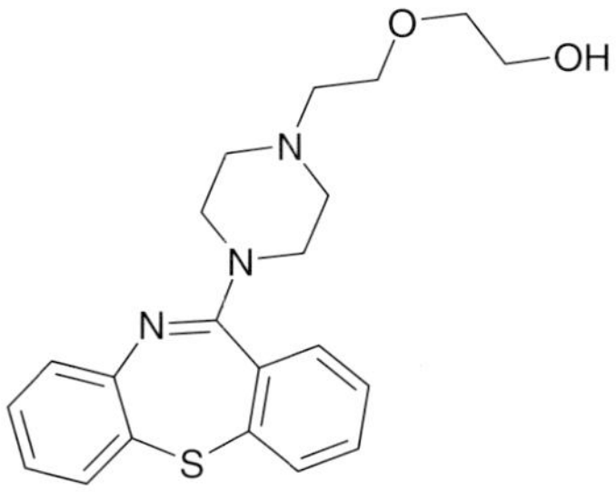

quetiapine
26

1.3.2 Selective Drug Analogue from a Pioneer Multitarget Drug

1.3.2.1 Selective Serotonin Reuptake Inhibitors

From a retrospective viewpoint, imipramine (**27**) was the pioneer antidepressant drug with a multitarget receptor profile, where serotonin and norepinephrine reuptake inhibition played an important role, but no *in vitro* activities were known at the time of its serendipitous discovery. Researchers at Geigy first synthesized the molecule in 1948. It was an analogue of the antipsychotic chlorpromazine (**28**), but the Swiss psychiatrist Roland Kuhn [27] found imipramine to be an effective antidepressant drug. It was launched by Geigy in 1959.

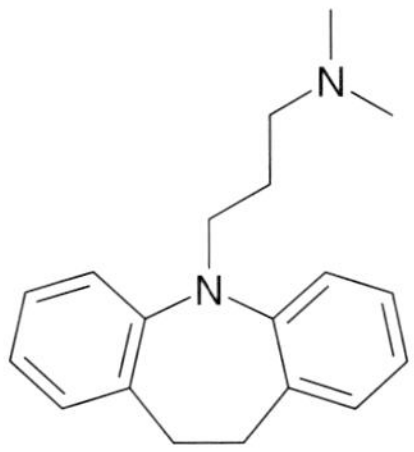

imipramine
antidepressant
27

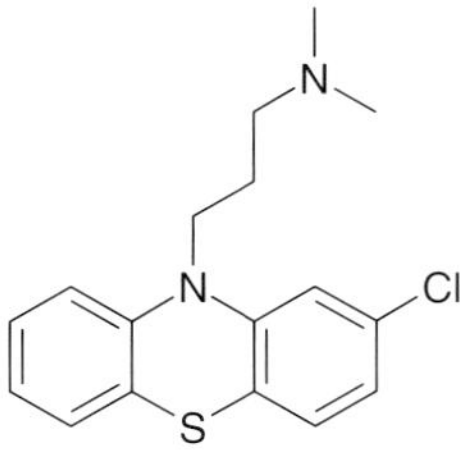

chlorpromazine
antipsychotic
28

Imipramine and the analogue tricyclic antidepressants inhibit the reuptake of serotonin and norepinephrine but they also exhibit a variety of side effects. The anticholinergic side effects include dry mouth, blurred vision, and sinus tachycardia. The histamine H_1 receptor antagonist activity likely contributes to the sedative effects associated with the compound.

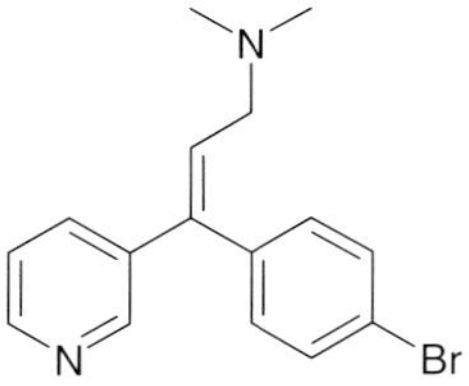

zimelidine
29

Arvid Carlsson initiated research on selective serotonin reuptake inhibitors (SSRIs) in order to get new antidepressants with less side effects. The first SSRI was zimelidine (**29**) [28]. It was launched by Astra in 1982, but it had to be withdrawn shortly afterward because of serious peripheral nerve side effects. Further research was continued at several pharmaceutical companies. The first successful SSRIs were fluoxetine (**30**) [29] (Lilly, 1988) and citalopram (**31**) [30] (Lundbeck, 1989). The antihistamine diphenhydramine (**32**) served as a lead compound for fluoxetine, whereas talopram (**33**) was the lead structure for citalopram. The discovery of citalopram and its refinement to escitalopram is discussed in Chapter 11.

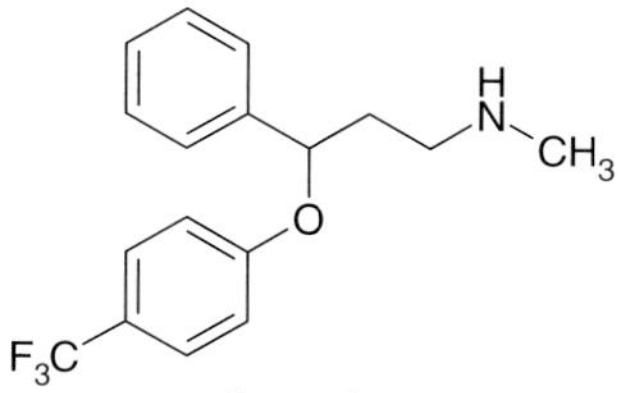

fluoxetine
30

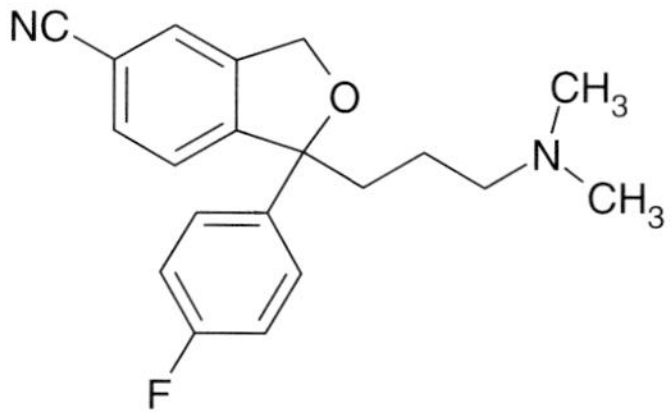

citalopram
31

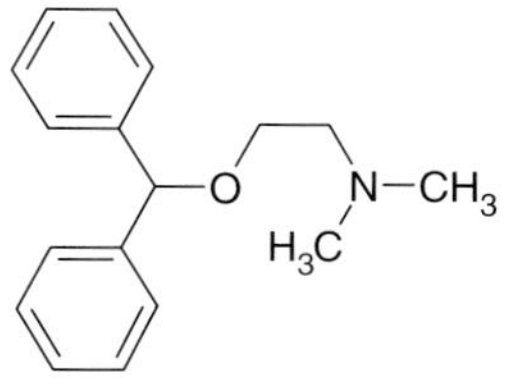

diphenhydramine
(lead for fluoxetine)
32

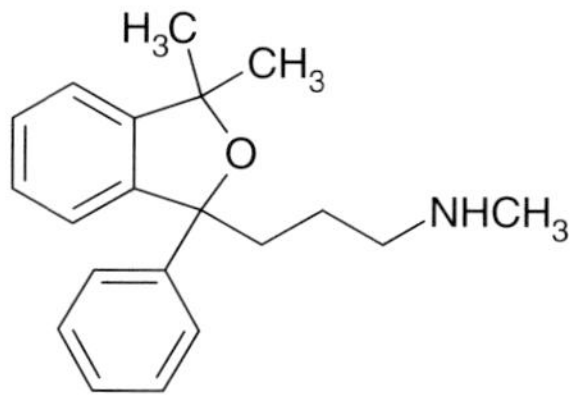

talopram
(lead for citalopram)
33

Summary:

Pioneer multitarget nonselective serotonin/norepinephrine reuptake inhibitor antidepressant drug: imipramine.
First (but unsuccessful) selective serotonin reuptake inhibitor: zimelidine.
First selective serotonin reuptake inhibitors: fluoxetine and citalopram.

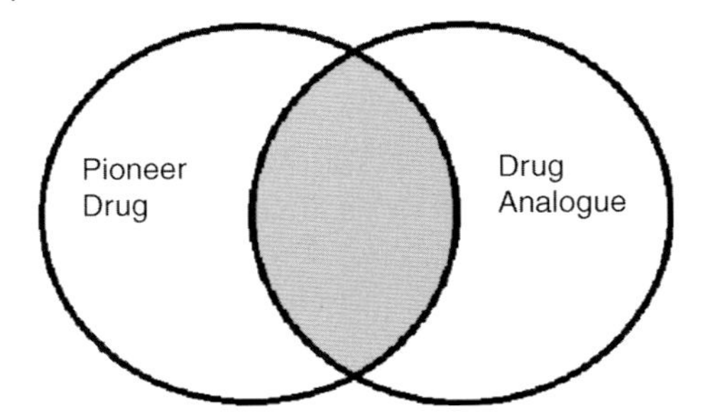

Figure 1.1 Pioneer drugs and drug analogues have overlapping properties.

1.4 Summary

Pioneer drugs open up new therapeutic treatments. They are also called "first-in-class" drugs.

Analogue-based drug discovery is a very important part of medicinal chemistry, because the analogues frequently are intended to optimize drug therapy. There is a continuous development in a drug class and in several cases the pioneer drugs disappear from the market and analogue drugs achieve a dominant role. It is the main reason why so many successful drugs are among the analogue drugs. The above examples focused on some cases where these drugs have a unique character in a drug class.

For early-phase analogues, it is possible that a pioneer drug derives from the analogue-based drug discovery for different reasons; for example, a more convenient lead compound or a more successful optimization can strongly influence which drug will be introduced to the market as a pioneer drug.

There are several examples where a new prototype drug candidate was discontinued at the late phase of drug research and then an analogue was introduced to the market as a successful pioneer drug.

The properties of pioneer and analogue drugs overlap (Figure 1.1). The drug analogues preserve some properties of the pioneer drug and they have to achieve some new and better properties in order to be successful on the market.

Acknowledgments

We thank Klaus Peter Bøgesø, Helmut Buschmann, Jens-Uwe Peters, and Henning Priepke for carefully reading and reviewing the manuscript.

References

1 Fischer, J. (2011) Pioneer and analogue drugs. 43rd IUPAC World Chemistry Congress, August 3, 2011, San Juan, Puerto Rico, Abstract No. 848.

2 Carlson, A. (1971) *Recent Advances in Parkinson's Disease* (eds F.H. McDowett and C.H. Markham), Davis, Philadelphia, PA, pp. 1–10.

3 Oates, J.A., Gillespie, S., Udenfriend, S., and Sjoerdsma, A. (1960) Decarboxylase inhibition and blood pressure reduction of alpha methyl-3,4-dihydroxy-DL-phenylalanine. *Science*, **131**, 1890–1891.
4 DeStevens, G., Werner, L.H., Holamandris, A., and Ricca, S., Jr. (1958) Dihydrobenzothiazine dioxides with potent diuretic effect. *Experientia*, **14**, 463.
5 Ganellin, C.R. (1982) Cimetidine, in *Chronicles of Drug Discovery*, vol. 1 (eds J.S. Nindra and D. Lednicer), John Wiley and Sons, Inc., New York, pp. 1–38.
6 Pearce, P. and Funder, J.W. (1980) Histamine H_2-receptor antagonist: radioreceptor assay for antiandrogenic side effects. *Clin. Exp. Pharmacol. Physiol.*, **7**, 442.
7 Ganellin, C.R. (2006) Development of antiulcer H_2-receptor histamine antagonists, in *Analogue-Based Drug Discovery* (eds J. Fischer and C.R. Ganellin), Wiley-VCH Verlag GmbH, Weinheim, pp. 71–80.
8 Bakhle, Y.S. (1972) Inhibition of converting enzyme by venom peptides, in *Hypertension* (eds J. Genest and E. Koiw), Springer, Berlin, pp. 541–547.
9 Ondetti, M.A., Rubin, B., and Cushman, D.W. (1977) Design of specific inhibitors of angiotensin-converting enzyme: new class of orally active antihypertensive agents. *Science*, **196**, 441–444.
10 Patchett, A.A., Harris, E., Tristram, E.W., Wyvratt, M.J., Wu, M.T., Taub, D., Peterson, E.R., Ikeler, T.J., Ten Broeke, J., Payne, G., Ondeyka, D.L., Thorsett, E.D., Greenlee, W.J., Lohr, N.S., Hoffsommer, R.D., Joshua, H., Ruyle, J., Rothrock, W., Aster, S.D., Maycock, A.L., Robinson, F.M., Hirschmann, R., Sweet, C.S., Ulm, E.H., Gross, D.M., Vassil, C., and Stone, C.A. (1980) A new class of angiotensin-converting enzyme inhibitors. *Nature*, **288**, 280–283.
11 Alföldi, S. and Fischer, J. (2006) Optimizing antihypertensive therapy by angiotensin converting enzyme inhibitors, in *Analogue-Based Drug Discovery* (eds J. Fischer and C.R. Ganellin), Wiley-VCH Verlag GmbH, Weinheim, pp. 169–179.
12 Biftu, T., Scapin, G., Singh, S., Feng, D., Becker, J.W., Eiermann, G., He, H., Lyons, K., Patel, S., Petrvov, A., Sinha-Roy, R., Zhang, B., Wu, J., Zhang, X., Doss, G.A., Thornberry, N.A., and Weber, A.E. (2007) Rational design of a novel, potent and orally bioavailable cyclohexylamine DPP-4 inhibitor by application of molecular modeling and X-ray crystallography of sitagliptin. *Bioorg. Med. Chem. Lett.*, **17**, 3384–3387.
13 Villhauer, E.B., Brinkmann, J.A., Naderi, G.B., Burkey, B.F., Dunning, B.E., Prasad, K., Mangold, B.L., Russell, M.E., and Hughes, T.E. (2003) 1-[[(3-Hydroxy-1-adamantyl)amino]acetyl]-2-cyano-(*S*)-pyrrolidine: a potent, selective, and orally bioavailable dipeptidyl peptidase IV inhibitor with antihyperglycemic properties. *J. Med. Chem.*, **46**, 2774–2789.
14 Peters, J.-U. and Mattei, P. (2010) Dipeptidyl peptidase IV inhibitors for the treatment of type 2 diabetes, in *Analogue-Based Drug Discovery II* (eds J. Fischer and C.R. Ganellin), Wiley-VCH Verlag GmbH, Weinheim, pp. 109–134.
15 Jeske, W., Walenga, J.M., Lewis, B.E., and Fareed, J. (1999) Pharmacology of argatroban. *Expert Opin. Invest. Drugs*, **8** (5), 625–654.
16 Gustafsson, D. and Elg, M. (2003) The pharmacodynamics and pharmacokinetics of the oral direct thrombin inhibitor ximelagatran and its active metabolite melagatran: a mini-review. *Thromb. Res.*, **109** (Suppl. 1), S9–S15.
17 Lee, W.M., Larrey, D., Olsson, R., Lewis, J. H., Keisu, M., Auclert, L., and Shet, S. (2005) Hepatic findings in long-term clinical trials of ximelagatran. *Drug Saf.*, **28** (4), 351–370.
18 Hauel, N.H., Nar, H., Priepke, H., Ries, U., Stassen, J.M., and Wienen, W. (2002) Structure-based design of novel potent nonpeptide thrombin inhibitors. *J. Med. Chem.*, **45**, 1757–1766.
19 Eikelboom, J.W. and Weitz, J.I. (2010) Update on antithrombotic therapy. New anticoagulants. *Circulation*, **121**, 1523–1532.
20 Black, J.W. and Stephenson, J.S. (1962) Pharmacology of a new adrenergic beta-receptor-blocking compound. *Lancet*, **2** (7251), 311–314.

21 Black, J.W., Crowther, A.F., Shanks, R.G., Smith, L.H., and Dornhorst, A.C. (1964) A new adrenergic beta-receptor antagonist. *Lancet*, **1** (7342), 1080–1081.
22 Barrett, A.M., Carter, J., Fitzgerald, J.D., Hull, R., and Le Count, D. (1973) A new type of cardioselective adrenoceptive blocking drug. *Br. J. Pharmacol.*, **48**, 3408.
23 Flick, K., Frankus, E., and Friderichs, E. (1978) Studies of chemical structure and analgetic activity of phenyl substituted aminomethylcyclohexanoles. *Arzneim.-Forsch./Drug Res.*, **28** (I), 107–113.
24 Buschmann, H., Strassburger, W., and Friderichs, F. (2001) 1-Phenyl-3-dimethylaminopropane compounds with a pharmacological effect. EP 693 475.
25 Schmutz, J. and Eichenberger, E. (1982) Clozapine, in *Chronicles of Drug Discoveries*, vol. 1 (eds J.S. Bindra and D. Lednicer), John Wiley & Sons, Inc., New York, pp. 39–60.
26 Szegedi, A., Wiesner, J., Hillert, A., Hammes, E., Wetzel, H., and Benkert, O. (1993) ICI 204,636, a putative "atypical" antipsychotic, in the treatment of schizophrenia with positive symptomology: an open clinical trial. *Pharmacopsychiatry*, **26**, 197.
27 Kuhn, R. (1957) Über die Behandlung depressiver Zustände mit einem Iminodibenzyl Derivat (G 22355). *Schweiz. Med. Wochensch.*, **87**, 1135.
28 Montgomery, S.A., McAuley, R., Rani, S.J., Roy, D., and Montgomery, D.B. (1981) A double blind comparison of zimelidine and amitriptyline in endogenous depression. *Acta Psychiatr. Scand. Suppl.*, **290**, 314–327.
29 Wong, D.T., Horng, J.S., Bymaster, F.P., Hauser, K.L., and Malloy, B.B. (1974) A selective inhibitor of serotonin uptake: Lilly 110140, 3-(*p*-trifluoromethylphenoxy)-*N*-methyl-3-phenylpropylamine. *Life Sci.*, **15**, 471–479.
30 Bigler, A.J., Bùgesù, K.P., Toft, A., and Hansen, V. (1977) Quantitative structure–activity relationships in a series of selective 5-HT uptake inhibitors. *Eur. J. Med. Chem.*, **12**, 289–295.

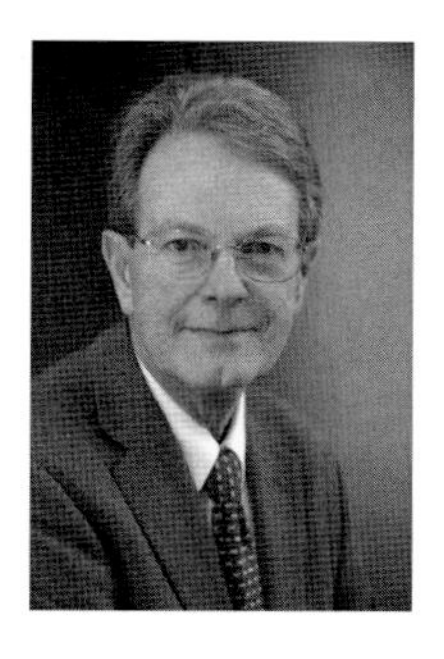

János Fischer is Senior Research Scientist at Richter Plc. (Budapest, Hungary). He received his education in Hungary with M.Sc. and Ph.D. degrees in Organic Chemistry from Eotvos University of Budapest with Professor A. Kucsman. Between 1976 and 1978, he was a Humboldt Fellow at the University of Bonn with Professor W. Steglich. He has worked at Richter Plc. since 1981, where he participated in the research and development of leading cardiovascular drugs in Hungary. His main current interest is analogue-based drug discovery. He is author of some 100 patents and scientific publications. In 2012, he was reelected Titular Member of the Chemistry and Human Health Division of IUPAC. He received an honorary professorship at the Technical University of Budapest.

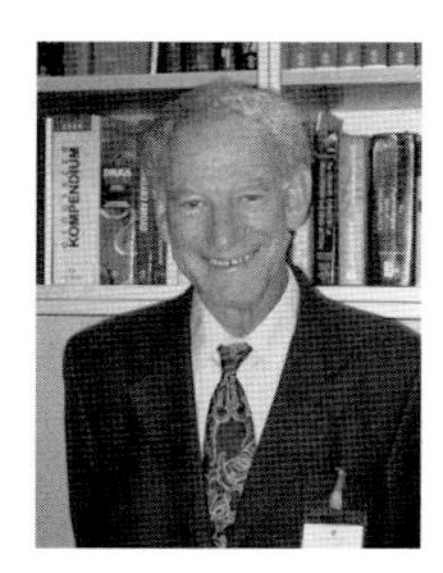

C. Robin Ganellin studied chemistry at London University, receiving a Ph.D. in 1958 under Professor Michael Dewar, and was a Research Associate at MIT with Arthur Cope in 1960. He then joined Smith, Kline & French Laboratories in the United Kingdom and was one of the co-inventors of the revolutionary drug cimetidine (also known as Tagamet®), eventually becoming Vice President for Research. In 1986, he was made a Fellow of the Royal Society and appointed to the SK&F Chair of Medicinal Chemistry at University College London, where he is now Professor Emeritus of Medicinal Chemistry. Professor Ganellin is co-inventor on over 160 patents and has authored over 250 scientific publications. He was President of the Medicinal Chemistry Section of IUPAC and is currently Chairman of the IUPAC Subcommittee on Medicinal Chemistry and Drug Development.

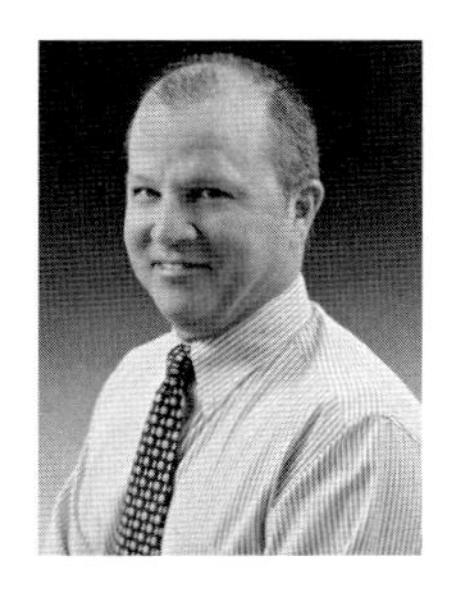

David P. Rotella is the Margaret and Herman Sokol Professor of Medicinal Chemistry at Montclair State University. He earned a B.S. Pharm. degree at the University of Pittsburgh (1981) and a Ph.D. (1985) at The Ohio State University with Donald. T. Witiak. After postdoctoral studies in organic chemistry at Penn State University with Ken S. Feldman, he worked as an Assistant Professor at the University of Mississippi. David worked at Cephalon, Bristol-Myers, Lexicon, and Wyeth, where he was involved in neurodegeneration, schizophrenia, cardiovascular, and metabolic disease drug discovery projects.

2
Competition in the Pharmaceutical Drug Development

Christian Tyrchan and Fabrizio Giordanetto

2.1
Introduction

Granted patents give the right to exclude others from making, using, selling, offering for sale, or importing the claimed invention for a given time period that can vary between countries. A filed patent in the United States, in principle, expires 20 years after the filing date. In the European Union (EU), applicants are required to disclose their inventions in a sufficiently clear and complete way so that the innovative step can be carried out by a person skilled in the art. In the United States, inventors are additionally required to include the "best mode" of making or practicing the invention. Failure to include such "best mode," which is the best available at the time of filing of the application, has been a potential ground for invalidation of the patent.

In such encouraged competitive environment, innovation is more likely to stem from small, incremental cycles, following an evolutionary rather than revolutionary path. Indeed, the patent system stimulates innovation by rewarding improvements to be published, and by this recognizing the reality of incremental innovation [1]. Consequently, in the pharmaceutical field, patents that claim similar structural spaces normally occur. This is because of different interpretations of commonly available knowledge, or because of convergence from different starting points as key scientific publications.

In this respect, it is important to recognize that what is normally referred to as pioneer, first-in-class, or breakthrough drug is the first compound reaching the market following the approval of the regulatory offices and not the first filed in a patent specification (the term "patent specification" is used throughout the chapter as a general reference to a patent text be it application or granted patent). These compounds then constitute a new class of drugs in that they introduce a novel mode of action (MoA) or provide a significant improvement over the standard therapy, if not directly enabling a therapy, in terms of efficacy and safety. An analogue-based drug (also termed follow-on drug) is normally a chemical entity that has the same pharmacological MoA as the pioneer drug but it is registered afterward [2], regardless of its patent publication date.

Analogue-based Drug Discovery III, First Edition. Edited by János Fischer, C. Robin Ganellin, and David P. Rotella.
© 2013 Wiley-VCH Verlag GmbH & Co. KGaA. Published 2013 by Wiley-VCH Verlag GmbH & Co. KGaA.

The ever-changing and demanding health economic environment and the increasing costs and attrition of drug development have pressed pharmaceutical companies to constantly look for opportunities to de-risk their programs [2–7]. Here, the aim toward developing "lower risk" analogues rather than "high-risk" pioneer drugs has been fueled by the steady increase in external and internal knowledge around a specific MoA, as from publications such as peer-reviewed journals, patents, and clinical trial results' analyses. However, because the information is publicly available, the ability to differentiate the final products against the expected competitors becomes key to success. Accordingly, any analogous drug is sought to become a best-in-class drug.

2.2
Analogue-Based Drugs: Just Copies?

The approach to analogue-based drug design is controversially discussed in the literature, most notably in terms of different value propositions such as innovation, risk of failure, marketing costs, and price competition, among others [2, 8, 9]. In two seminal publications, DiMasi *et al.*, from the Tufts Center for the Study of Drug Development, discussed the economics of first-in-class and follow-on drugs and the kind of competitiveness in pharmaceutical R&D from a marketed drug space perspective [2, 10]. Two important questions are raised and answered:

- Are pioneer drugs best in class, in terms of treatment value?
- Can analogue-based drugs deliver therapeutic benefit?

First, they report that the period of marketing exclusivity until an analogous drug reaches the market has fallen in the United States (from time of launch) for the pioneer drug from a median of 10.2 years in the 1970s to 1.2 years in the late 1990s. Furthermore, they find that approximately one-third of the overall analogue-based drugs have received a priority rating from the FDA. This priority rating is granted by the FDA for compounds that are considered to add significant value compared to the standard therapy. These findings are reported for 57% of the defined drug classes and clearly point toward the continuous evolution in a drug class. Consequently, analogous drugs can provide true therapeutic benefit, although this will only be apparent after substantial investigation in a clinical setting [2, 10].

In some cases, an analogue drug appears later on the US market than the first-in-class compound of the same drug class. Its reasons were discussed by Agarwal and Gort [11]. The authors conclude that the main factors are increased mobility of skilled labor, rapid diffusion of scientific and technical information (information age), increased competition, and expansion of emerging markets [2, 11]. Taken together, these data reflect a highly dynamic race among competitors rather than a simple imitation exercise. The following examples, supported by the original patent publication dates, further reinforce this notion.

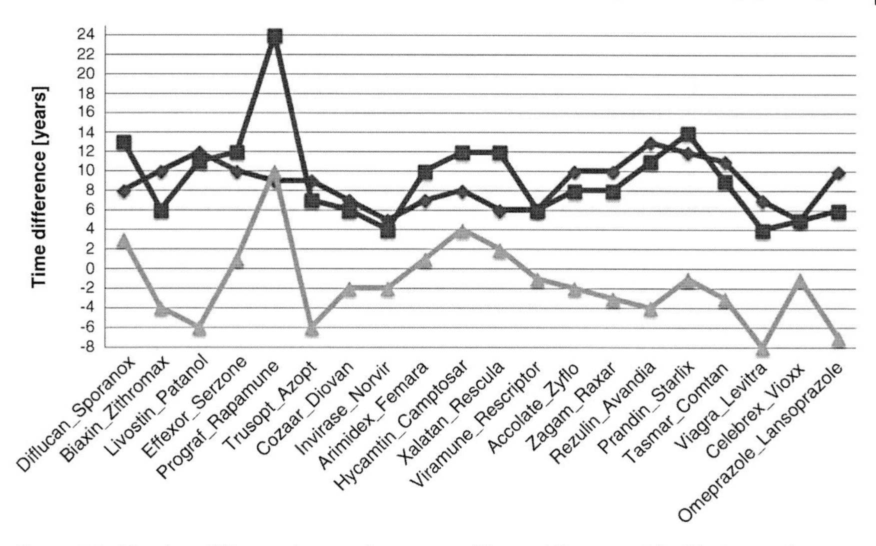

Figure 2.1 The time difference in years from patent filing to US approval for 20 pioneer drugs (diamond) with their second entrant (square). The triangles denote the time difference in years between the patent filing date of the first-in-class and second-entry drug.

An interesting molecular pair is provided by the prostaglandin (PG) analogues latanoprost and unoprostone. Latanoprost (Xalatan^{TM}) was approved as a first-in-class treatment for elevated intraocular pressure (IOP) in 1996, while unoprostone (Rescula^{TM}) received approval in 1994 as a follow-on PG analogue. Nevertheless, unoprostone was actually disclosed in the patent literature prior to latanoprost: 1988 and 1990, respectively [12, 13]. While the reasons for the faster development-to-launch course of latanoprost are not known (cf. 6 and 12 years, Figure 2.1), its structural similarity to unoprostone is striking (Figure 2.2). Both latanoprost and unoprostone are prostaglandin $F_{2\alpha}$ ($PGF_{2\alpha}$) derivatives, where the omega chain of $PGF_{2\alpha}$ has been the subject of chemical modifications, as shown in Figure 2.2. Interestingly, researchers at R-Tech Ueno Ltd modified $PGF_{2\alpha}$ to mimic existing $PGF_{2\alpha}$ metabolites where the hydroxyl group at position 15 is oxidized to the

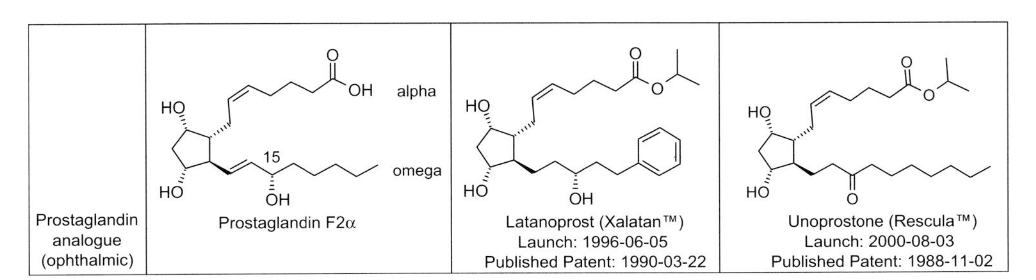

Figure 2.2 First-in-class and follow-on prostaglandin analogue drug pair and the natural agonist $PGF_{2\alpha}$.

corresponding ketone [12]. Scientists at Pharmacia AB resolved to introduce an aromatic ring as a way to circumvent the irritative effects of the naturally occurring $PGF_{2\alpha}$. Although both groups started from the same chemical matter and opted for the same prodrug approach, the medicinal chemistry strategies to modify the omega chain of $PGF_{2\alpha}$ were different and resulted in two safe and well-tolerated drugs. Despite the largely similar chemical structures and safety profiles, several differences in terms of metabolic fate and pharmacokinetics [14, 15], and more importantly therapeutic effects, discriminate unoprostone from latanoprost, the latter being more efficacious in a clinical setting [16].

Even though anastrozole (Arimidex™) was patented later than letrozole, it won the race to be the first-in-class third-generation aromatase inhibitor (AI) to be launched in the United States by merely 1 year, as depicted in Figure 2.3. Anastrozole was launched in 1996 for the treatment of advanced breast cancer in postmenopausal women. Previous first- and second-generation AIs suffered from limited enzyme selectivity and clinical efficacy. Letrozole was then launched in 1997 despite being patented earlier than anastrozole: 1987 and 1988, respectively [17, 18]. Scientists at Ciba-Geigy discovered letrozole through the iterative optimization of fadrozole [19], a second-generation AI originated in the same laboratories [20, 21]. Here, the original innovation step revolved around the mechanistic hypothesis that imidazole-containing compounds could be selective P450 inhibitors [20], analogously to what was observed in a parallel discovery program against thromboxane A2 synthetase [22]. In an effort to further improve upon fadrozole selectivity, simplification of fadrozole's structure through ring opening and chiral center removal, followed by the subsequent azaheterocycle optimization, resulted in the discovery of letrozole [19], a totally selective aromatase inhibitor. Simultaneous research activities by medicinal chemists at ICI resulted in anastrozole, another safe and effective 1,2,4-triazole-based AI with similar structure to letrozole [23]. Interestingly though, the chemical starting point that led to the

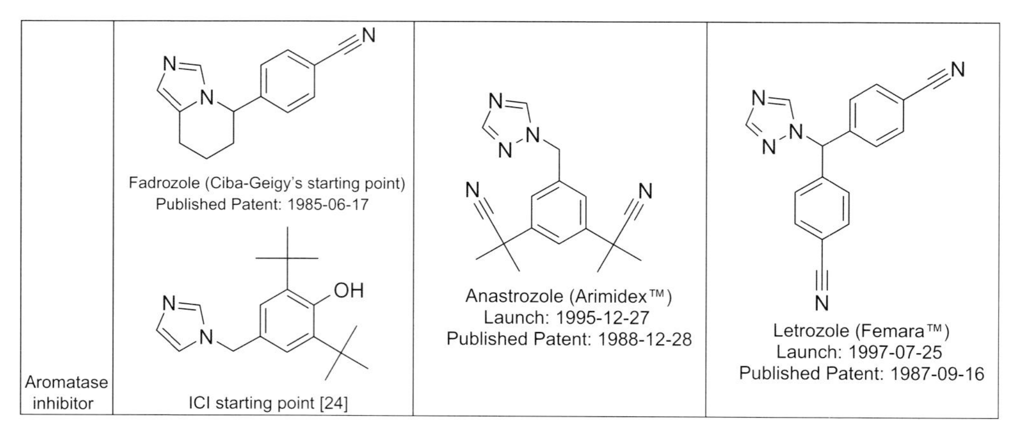

Figure 2.3 First-in-class and follow-on third-generation AI pair. Fadrozole, a second-generation AI and the initial starting point for AI discovery at ICI [24] are shown as a reference.

discovery of anastrozole was already identified in late 1970s through random screening of the ICI collection [24].

Moreover, design principles aimed at increasing selectivity over other P450 enzymes led to the final selection of anastrozole for subsequent development in a very "intense competitive situation," in the author's own words [24]. While anastrozole and letrozole are classified as first-in-class and follow-on third-generation AIs, their discoveries originated and followed fairly different tracks [19, 20, 24]. The timings of initial discoveries, program sanctions, patent publications, and market launch further reflect a highly competitive race rather than imitation [10]. In these settings, their structural similarity is even more remarkable and could only serve as inspiration to medicinal chemists in their next design round. Nevertheless, those limited structural differences are still responsible for the different pharmacokinetic profiles of the two AIs, as well as the superior preclinical pharmacodynamic properties of letrozole [25]. The currently ongoing, randomized head-to-head trial in early breast cancer (id: NCT00248170) will hopefully set the dispute over which one is the best AI.

In a similar fashion, "best in class" represents the ultimate goal. As market exclusivity is no longer an advantage due to increased competition, and different groups have faster access to increasing amounts of information, even the smallest chemical variations over existing chemotypes need to demonstrate tangible experimental advantages. The fact that 70% of the first-in-class drug–analogous drug pairs analyzed by Giordanetto *et al.* [26] differed minimally from a structural perspective, yet diverged in their experimental properties, further highlights such opportunities.

2.3 How Often Does Analogue-Based Activity Occur? Insights from the GPCR Patent Space

Considering the highly competitive environment, follow-on of external information remains a vital activity for any drug researcher. As outlined above, this is simply the result of the incremental nature of research, where knowledge and insight evolve with time. Indeed, the chemical information landscape is changing rapidly with a yearly increase of over 1 million new compounds and more than 700 000 publications related to chemistry [27].

Accordingly, the chemical space claimed by patent specifications is becoming more crowded and competitive, especially for target classes such as protein kinases and G-protein-coupled receptors (GPCRs). Exploring the chemical space covered by relevant journals and patent specifications is an important activity in medicinal chemistry projects due to the constant need to convert information into knowledge to support business decisions. This is also greatly aided by the unprecedented access to large quantities of data. A variety of commercial institutions now supply databases with high-quality, manually extracted structures of patent examples [28]. Following the advances in text mining technologies and improvements of the chemical named entity recognition (NER) process, several databases containing automatically extracted chemical entities from patent specifications are also available [29–32]. Consequently, computational methods developed in the fields of chemoinformatics or patent informatics [33] can be applied for data analysis and visualization to support medicinal chemistry teams in evaluating and exploiting the available information.

To investigate the occurrence of drug discovery follow-on activities as captured by the pharmaceutical patent space (in contrast to the marketed drug space), we abstracted 11 827 patent specifications that are linked to a GPCR target with a defined Entrez Gene ID from the GVKBIO databases (as of November 2010) [28]. The GVKBIO Medicinal Chemistry and Target Class databases capture explicit relationships between published documents, compounds, assay results, and targets extracted by manual curation. In a next step, we focused on small molecules by removing all peptides, based on substructural and physicochemical properties' analysis. By focusing on the top 100 companies, in terms of number of published patent specifications, this resulted in a total of 10 253 patents. The set was further consolidated by associating patent specifications based on known mergers and acquisitions until 2008. Subsequently, all possible patent specification combinations were created and a competitive activity was recorded if two patent specifications shared the same gene name and were published by different companies within a 6-year interval.

Similarity descriptors such as the Shannon entropy (SE, based on the number of atoms of the joined substructures, using 26 bins) and corresponding scores could be generated for 1 570 381 out of a total of 1 608 368 patent specification pairs (97.6%) [34]. All calculations were performed with Pipeline Pilot 7.5.2 and Python scripts [35].

Using a conservative cutoff ($SE \geq 4$) to identify patent specifications sharing at least one compound with high structural similarity, we found 6516 (64%) patents linked to analogue-based activities (from 49 638 patent pairs over 28 years and 433 different gene ids). These patent specifications were further classified as follows:

- **Originator:** a patent specification that is linked to a later patent specification by structural similarity.
- **Follower:** a patent specification that is linked by structural similarity to an earlier patent specification and is published between 2 and 6 years of the earlier patent specification.
- **Competitor:** a patent specification that is linked by structural similarity and is published in the same year.

The results shown in Figures 2.4 and 2.5 demonstrate that pharmaceutical research is indeed highly competitive and dynamic. Sixty-four percent of the published patent specifications targeting a specific GPCR are linked by significant structural similarity to other patent specifications for the same GPCR. Most of the follow-on patent specifications (74%) are published within the first 2 years of the originator. This stresses the importance of speed (and commitment) when reacting to an external patent specification. Strategically, this would translate in a maximum

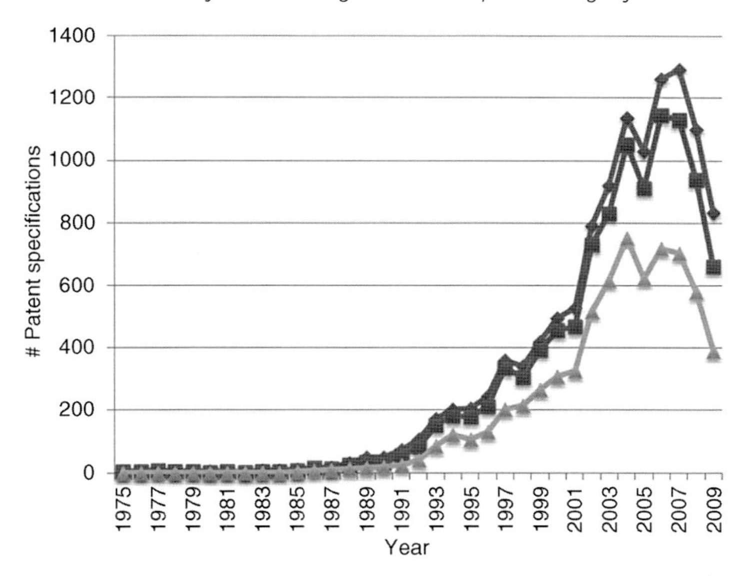

Figure 2.4 Number of patent specifications published in the GPCR field: overall (diamond), top 100 companies (square), and linked to follow-on activities (triangle).

period of 6 months from the publication date of the originator patent specification to the follow-on's patent specification submission.

It is interesting to note that, overall, out of the final set of 6561 patent specifications involved in follow-on activities, only 1705 patent specifications (26%) are classified as originator or competitor or combination thereof, whereas 4811 (74%)

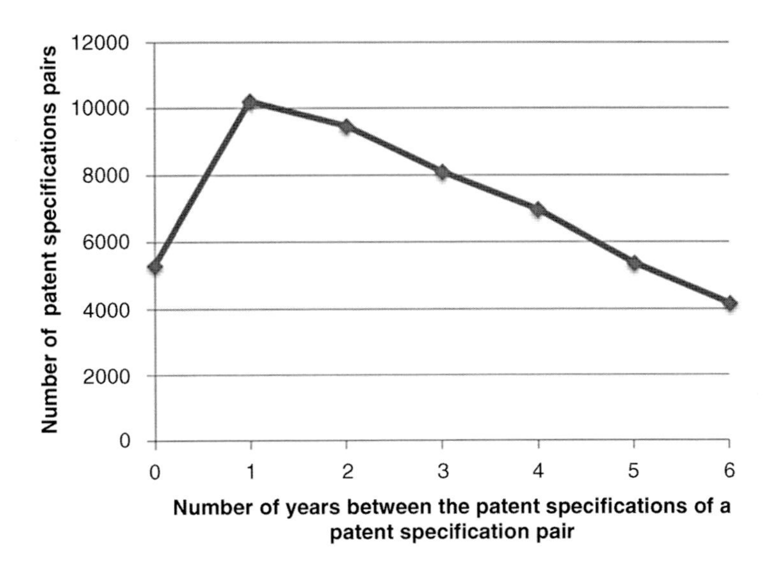

Figure 2.5 Frequency distribution of patent specification pair linked to analogue-based activities based on time between patent specification publications.

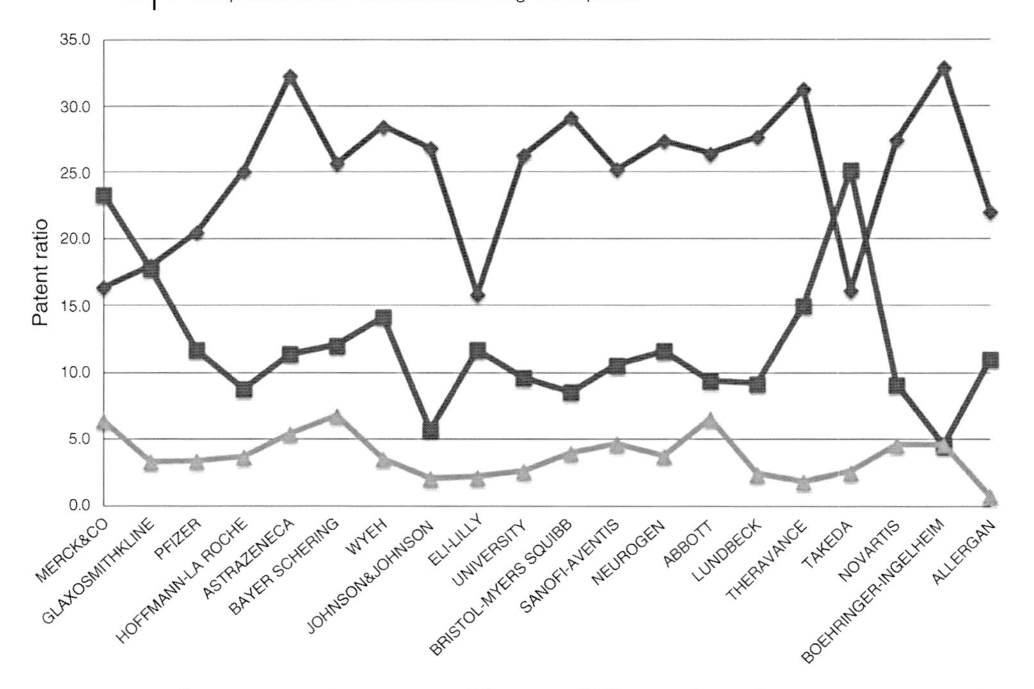

Figure 2.6 Top 20 companies and their ratio of follow-on (diamond), originator (square), and competitor (triangle) patents.

patent specifications belong to the follower class. It is of course tempting to ask the question whether there are certain organizations that are patenting more from an "originator" position than others. While Merck and Takeda display the highest number of originator patent specifications, due to the limitations of the current data set, only small, statistically nonsignificant differences between the companies can be observed (Figure 2.6).

Some originator patent specifications are more followed on than others. This might reflect the level of competitiveness in the specific area, if not the available confidence in the MoA or chemical equity. The most followed-on patent specification in the present GPCR data set is WO200046209, published in 2000 from researchers at Sanofi-Aventis (now Sanofi). In the 6 years after its original publication, it has inspired 74 follow-on patent specifications from 9 of the top 100 companies analyzed here, as shown in Table 2.1.

WO200046209 disclosed cannabinoid receptor 1 (CB1) antagonists closely related to rimonabant, as shown in Figure 2.8. Although the original patent specification covering rimonabant was published in 1993 (EP0576357A1), no follow-on patent specifications could be identified within the 6 years window considered here. As a result, WO200046209 figures as the "originator."

Analysis of the structural relationships between patent specifications from a given company is very useful. It captures the evolution of the chemical asset in terms of medicinal chemistry practices as well as patent strategy. In the Sanofi-Synthelabo

Table 2.1 Number of published patent specifications (WIPO) from the top 20 companies following on Sanofi-Synthelabo's WO200046209.

Company	2000	2001	2003	2004	2005	2006	Total
Sanofi-Synthelabo (Sanofi-Aventis)	1	1	1		2	5	11
Merck			5	2	2		9
Solvay (Abbott)			4	1	7		12
AstraZeneca			1	5	4	1	11
Roche				3	2	1	6
Pfizer				13	9	2	24
BMS					4	1	5
Janssen (J&J)					1	3	4
Bayer (Bayer-Schering)						1	1
Schering (Bayer-Schering)						1	1
Neurogen						1	1

case, after the original WO200046209 patent, two interesting applications followed in 2001 and 2003, respectively, as shown in Figure 2.7. The first one describes an interesting ring closure strategy linking the pyrazole to one of its phenyl substituents to afford new tricyclic derivatives as CB1 receptor antagonists. It is noteworthy that

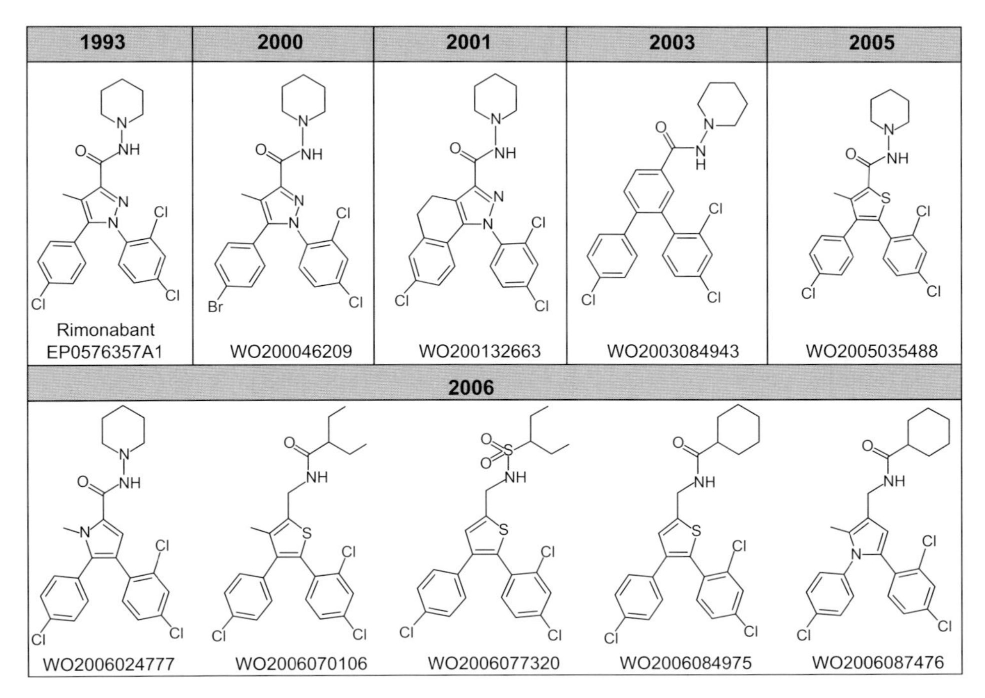

Figure 2.7 Number of published patent specifications (WIPO) targeting CB1 receptor antagonists from Sanofi-Synthelabo during the 2000–2006 period. Rimonabant is shown as a reference.

such tricyclic systems could also contain different heteroatoms in the central ring, as exemplified by compounds bearing sulfur atoms in various oxidation states. The second application, dated 2003, discloses a more conservative "scaffold hop" from the central pyrazole scaffold of rimonabant to a trisubstituted phenyl core structure, as shown in Figure 2.7.

The years 2005 and 2006 witnessed a total of six additional WIPO applications from Sanofi-Aventis covering CB1 receptor antagonists. The structural resemblance of the exemplified compounds to the original rimonabant structure is immediate, as displayed in Figure 2.7. Here, the original pyrazole framework is again swapped for similar five-membered heterocycles, notably substituted thiophenes and pyrroles. The first interpretations of amide bond bioisosteres from Sanofi-Aventis appeared as well. Sulfonamides (WO2006077320) and elongated inverse amides (WO2006070106, WO2006084975, and WO2006087476) replaced the original carboxamide derivative from EP 0576357A1. These probably represent defensive applications following the surge in CB1 receptor antagonist disclosures during 2004, as listed in Figure 2.7.

Merck was the first of the top 100 companies analyzed here to patent close analogues of the original CB1 receptor antagonist chemotype from Sanofi-Synthelabo. Their first patent specification is dated 2003 and discloses imidazole-containing CB1 receptor antagonists showing an elegant scaffold change from pyrazole to imidazole, as shown in Figure 2.8. Following the same strategy, Merck chemists also patented pyridine analogues of rimonabant (WO2003082191). Here, their initial imidazole core structure was replaced by a trisubstituted pyridine. In addition to the typical heterocycle "hop," three applications covered a very interesting ring-opening paradigm. Here, the central pyrazole ring was cut open to a 1,2-disubstituted propyl chain, and the original carboxamide was inverted to bear

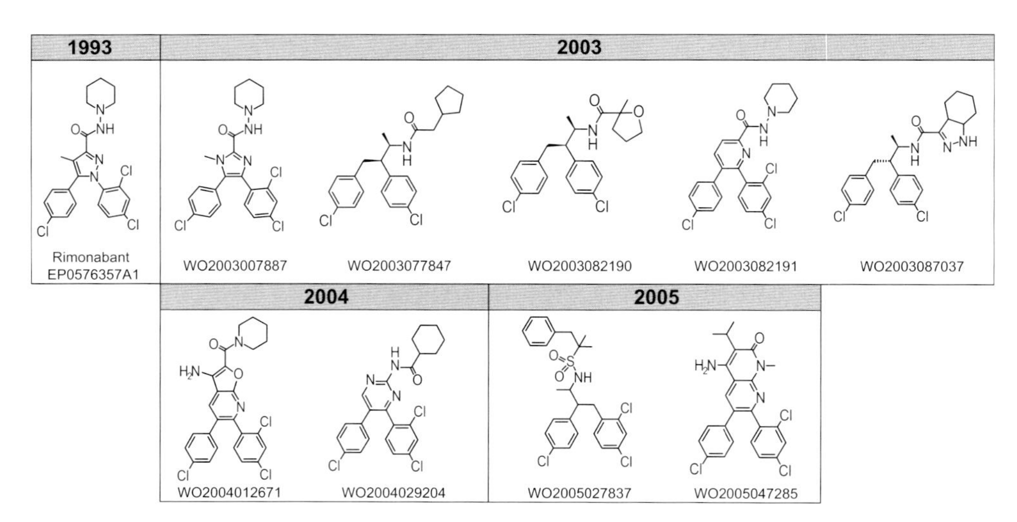

Figure 2.8 Number of published patent applications (WIPO) targeting CB1 receptor antagonists from Merck during the 2000–2006 period. Rimonabant is shown as a reference.

different types of substituents: aliphatic, spirocyclic, and aromatic (WO2003077847, WO2003082190, and WO2003087037, respectively), as displayed in Figure 2.8. In 2004, Merck followed up their core modification with an additional hop from pyridine to pyrimidine (cf. WO2003082191 and WO2004029204, Figure 2.8). They also disclosed novel derivatives bearing a central furo[2,3-*b*]pyridine scaffold (WO2004012671) as a fused heterocyclic system alternative to rimonabant's pyrazole. During 2005, the 1,2-disubstituted propyl-based chemotype was revisited by Merck, this time being decorated with a sulfonamide functionality in lieu of the previous amide (cf. WO2003087037 and WO2005027837, Figure 2.8). Analogously, the initial furo[2,3-*b*]pyridine core published in 2004 was expanded to a 1,8-naphthyridin-2-one (cf. WO2005047285 and WO2004012671).

The CB1 receptor antagonist case culminated in the discovery and launch of rimonabant, as an effective anti-obesity agent. As shown above, several other companies were inspired by the early work from Sanofi-Aventis. Unfortunately, the withdrawal of rimonabant from the market, due to the severe CNS-mediated side effects observed, prompted most of the follow-on companies to either terminate their internal programs or evaluate different compound profiles, thus reinforcing how dynamic and competitive the follow-on race actually is. A number of companies have thus actively engaged in research aiming at developing peripherally restricted CB1 receptor antagonist, as a way to mitigate the safety hazard related to CNS exposure. Aptly, researchers at 7TM Pharma disclosed compounds useful for modulating peripheral CB1 receptors that may have a reduced propensity to induce psychiatric and nervous system side effects (WO2009074782). Among these "second-generation" CB1 receptor antagonists, the amide derivative TM38328 (Figure 2.9) demonstrated weight reduction effects comparable to that of rimonabant in diet-induced obese (DIO) mice [36]. This pharmacological efficacy was achieved despite much reduced brain exposure (plasma/brain ratios: 0.42 and 10.2 for rimonabant and TM38328, respectively) [36]. Interestingly, as displayed in Figure 2.9, TM38328 is a rimonabant analogue, where the original, lipophilic 4-methylpyrazole substituent was further derivatized to a more polar acetamide as a way to reduce passive permeability. This, coupled with increased molecular weight

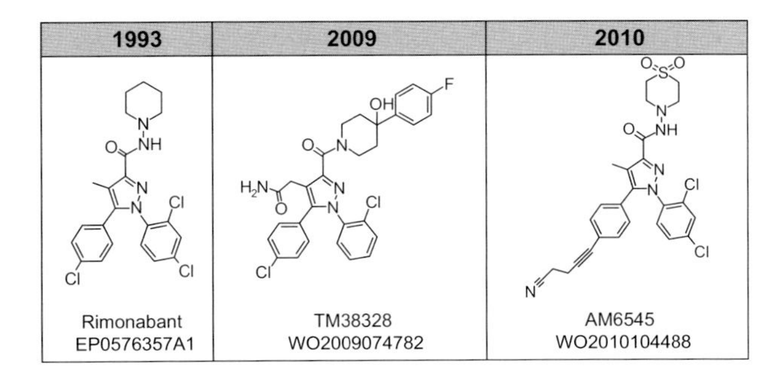

Figure 2.9 Selected "second-generation" CB1 receptor antagonists with reduced CNS distribution.

on position 3 of the pyrazole ring, provided additional gain in plasma/brain separation [36]. In 2010, scientists at the University of Connecticut published novel CB1 neutral antagonists acting preferentially on CB1 receptors located in the peripheral nervous system (WO2010104488). One of these disclosed compounds, AM6545 (Figure 2.9), was extensively profiled to assess its pharmacological, metabolic, and behavioral potential [37]. AM6545 displayed limited brain penetrance after acute administration to mice (brain/plasma ratio: 0.03 versus 0.8 for rimonabant) and was effective at reducing weight in DIO mice, but, contrarily to rimonabant, did not affect behavioral responses in mice [36]. AM6545 is also a rimonabant analogue with higher hydrophilicity (clogP: 3.3 versus 6.4 for rimonabant). As shown in Figure 2.9, replacement of a methylene by a sulfone and of a chlorine atom by a cyano-but-1-ynyl side chain are responsible for the reduced CNS exposure. It is noteworthy that these molecular changes do not alter passive diffusion but, rather, trigger active extrusion by the ABC transporter P-glycoprotein, as elegantly demonstrated by both *in vitro* and *in vivo* experiments [37].

The analysis of originator and follow-on patents can be valuable to highlight interesting chemical permutations, as summarized in Figures 2.7–2.9. Indeed, a large arsenal of medicinal chemistry tactics is on display: from ring opening to ring closure, from ring homologation and contraction to substituent walking and fine tuning, every modification could have a profound effect on key optimization parameters, as exemplified by the "second-generation" peripheral ligands. The CB1 antagonist example provides several different interpretations of the original pyrazole-3-carboxamide derivatives. While the general applicability of these variations is routinely evaluated in medicinal chemistry programs, these follow-on examples represent an important source of inspiration and medicinal chemistry experience that is now electronically available.

As patent informatics develops based on the availability of more comprehensive databases, more exhaustive enumeration techniques, and more effective structural comparison methods, direct evaluation of medicinal chemistry precedents and follow-on practices will be easier to implement. Following the PG analogues, and AI and CB1 receptor antagonist examples presented here, experimental evidence, time, and significant investments will single out the best-in-class compound from the follow-on crowd in an innovation race that does not seem to become any easier with time.

References

1 Miller, C.P. and Evans, M.J. (2010) *The Chemist's Companion Guide to Patent Law*, John Wiley & Sons, Inc., Hoboken, NJ.

2 DiMasi, J.A. and Paquette, C. (2004) The economics of follow-on drug research and development: trends in entry rates and the timing of development. *Pharmacoeconomics*, **22** (2 Suppl. 2), 1–14.

3 Schachter, A.D. and Ramoni, M.F. (2007) From the analyst's couch: clinical forecasting in drug development. *Nat. Rev. Drug Discov.*, **6**, 107–108.

4 DiMasi, J.A., Hansen, R.W., and Grabowski, H.G. (2003) The price of

innovation: new estimates of drug development costs. *J. Health Econ.*, **22**, 151–185.

5 DiMasi, J.A., Feldman, L., Seckler, A., and Wilson, A. (2010) Trends in risks associated with new drug development: success rates for investigational drugs. *Clin. Pharmacol. Ther.*, **87** (3), 272–277.

6 Kola, I. and Landis, J. (2004) Can the pharmaceutical industry reduce attrition rates? *Nat. Rev. Drug Discov.*, **3** (8), 711–715.

7 Sams-Dodd, F. (2007) Research & market strategy: how choice of drug discovery approach can affect market position. *Drug Discov. Today*, **12** (7–8), 314–318.

8 Hollis, A. (2005) Comment on "The economics of follow-on drug research and development: trends in entry rates and the timing of development". *Pharmacoeconomics*, **23** (12), 1187–1192, discussion 1193–1202.

9 Cohen, J., Cabanilla, L., and Sosnov, J. (2006) Role of follow-on drugs and indications on the WHO Essential Drug List. *J. Clin. Pharm. Ther.*, **31** (6), 585–592.

10 Dimasi, J.A. and Faden, L.B. (2011) Competitiveness in follow-on drug R&D: a race or imitation? *Nat. Rev. Drug Discov.*, **10** (1), 23–27.

11 Agarwal, R. and Gort, M. (2001) First-mover advantage and the speed of competitive entry. *J. Law Econ.*, **44**, 161–177.

12 Ueno, R., Ueno, R., and Oda, T. (1998) Preparation of prostaglandin F derivatives as vasopressors. European Patent Application EP 289349A1.

13 Stjernschantz, J. and Resul, B. (1990) Prostaglandin derivatives for the treatment of glaucoma or ocular hypertension. PCT International Application WO9002553A1.

14 Kashiwagi, K., Iizuka, Y., and Tsukuhara, S. (1999) Metabolites of isopropyl unoprostone as potential ophthalmic solutions to reduce intraocular pressure in pigmented rabbits. *Jpn. J. Pharmacol.*, **81**, 56–62.

15 Sjoquist, B., Basu, S., Byding, P., Bergh, K., and Stjernschantz, J. (1998) The pharmacokinetics of a new antiglaucoma drug, latanoprost, in the rabbit. *Drug Metab. Dispos.*, **26**, 745–754.

16 Jampel, H.D., Bacharach, J., Sheu, W., Wohl, L.G., Solish, A.M., and Christie, W. (The Latanoprost/Unoprostone Study Group) (2002) Randomized clinical trial of latanoprost and unoprostone in patients with elevated intraocular pressure. *Am. J. Ophthalmol.*, **134**, 863–871.

17 Bowman, R.M., Steele, R.E., and Browne, L.J. (1987) Preparation and testing of alpha-heterocyclyltolunitriles as aromatase inhibitors. European Patent Application EP 0236940A2.

18 Edwards, P.N. and Large, M.S. (1988) Preparation and formulation of (substituted aralkyl) heterocyclic compounds as aromatase inhibitors. European Patent Application EP 296749A1.

19 Lang, M., Batzl, C., Furet, P., Bowman, R., Hausler, A., and Bhatnagar, A.S. (1993) Structure–activity relationships and binding model of novel aromatase inhibitors. *J. Steroid Biochem. Mol. Biol.*, **44**, 421–428.

20 Browne, L.J., Gude, C., Rodriguez, H., and Steele, R.E. (1991) Fadrozole hydrochloride: a potent, selective, nonsteroidal inhibitor of aromatase for the treatment of estrogen-dependent disease. *J. Med. Chem.*, **34** (2), 725–736.

21 Browne, L.J. (1985) Substituted fused imidazole compounds as aromatase inhibitors. European Patent Application EP 165904A2.

22 Ford, N.F., Browne, L.J., Campbell, T., Gemenden, C., Goldstein, R., Gude, C., and Wasley, J.W.F. (1985) Imidazo[1,5-a] pyridines: a new class of thromboxane A2 synthetase inhibitors. *J. Med. Chem.*, **28**, 164.

23 Plourde, P.V., Dyroff, M., and Dukes, M. (1994) Arimidex: a potent and selective fourth-generation aromatase inhibitor. *Breast Cancer Res. Treat.*, **30**, 103–111.

24 Edwards, P.N. (2006) A partial view of the quest for Arimidex, a potent, selective inhibitor of aromatase, in *Smith and Williams' Introduction to the Principles of Drug Design and Action*, 4th edn, CRC Press, Boca Raton, FL, pp. 233–256.

25 Bhatnagar, A.S. (2007) The discovery and mechanism of action of letrozole. *Breast Cancer Res. Treat.*, **105**, 7–17.

26 Giordanetto, F., Boström, J., and Tyrchan, C. (2011) Follow-on drugs: how far should

chemists look? *Drug Discov. Today*, **16**, 722–732.

27 Engel, T. (2006) Basic overview of chemoinformatics. *J. Chem. Inform. Model*, **46**, 2267–2277.

28 GVKBIO (2011) http://www.gvkbio.com/informatics.html (accessed December 8, 2011).

29 Surechem (2011) http://www.surechem.org (accessed December 8, 2011).

30 IBM (2011) http://www.ibm.com/patent (accessed December 8, 2011).

31 Spangler, S., Ying, C., Kreulen, J., Boyer, S., Griffin, T., Alba, A., Kato, L., Lelescu, A., and Yan, S. (2011) Exploratory analytics on patent data sets using the SIMPLE platform. *World Patent Inform.*, **33** (4), 328–339.

32 Banville, D.L. (ed.) (2009) *Chemical Information Mining: Facilitating Literature-Based Discovery*, CRC Press, Boca Raton, FL.

33 Trippe, A.J. (2003) Patinformatics: tasks to tools. *World Patent Inform.*, **25** (3), 211–221.

34 Godden, J.W. and Bajorath, J. (2001) Differential Shannon entropy as a sensitive measure of differences in database variability of molecular descriptors. *J. Chem. Inform. Comput. Sci.*, **4**, 1060–1066.

35 Accelrys (2011) http://accelrys.com/products/scitegic (accessed December 8, 2011).

36 Receveur, J.-M., Murray, A., Linget, J.-M., Norregard, P.K., Cooper, M., Bjurling, E., Aadal Nielsen, P., and Högberg, T. (2010) Conversion of 4-cyanomethyl-pyrazole-3-carboxamides into CB1 antagonists with lowered propensity to pass the blood–brain-barrier. *Bioorg. Med. Chem. Lett.*, **20**, 453–457.

37 Tam, J., Vemuri, K., Liu, J., Batkai, S., Mukhopadhyay, B., Godlewski, G., Osei-Hyiaman, D., Ohnuma, S., Ambudkar, S.V., Pickel, J., Makriyannis, A., and Kunos, G. (2010) Peripheral CB1 cannabinoid receptor blockade improves cardiometabolic risk in mouse models of obesity. *J. Clin. Invest.*, **120**, 2953–2966.

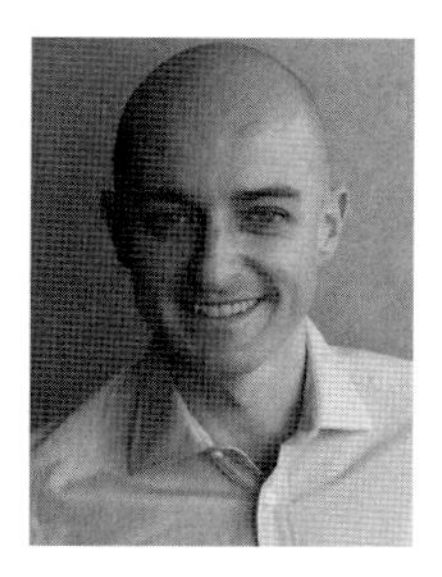

Fabrizio Giordanetto studied medicinal chemistry at the University of Genoa and obtained his Ph.D. in Computational Chemistry in 2003 from the University of London. He joined the Computational Sciences section of Pharmacia (Pfizer Group, Nerviano, Italy) in 2002, and then moved to the Medicinal Chemistry Department of AstraZeneca (Mölndal, Sweden) in 2004, where he is currently working as Principal Scientist in addition to his role as Project Leader in Drug Discovery. From hit finding to clinical candidate selection, he has a keen interest in everything that has to do with drug design, from rational chemical modifications to serendipitous realizations.

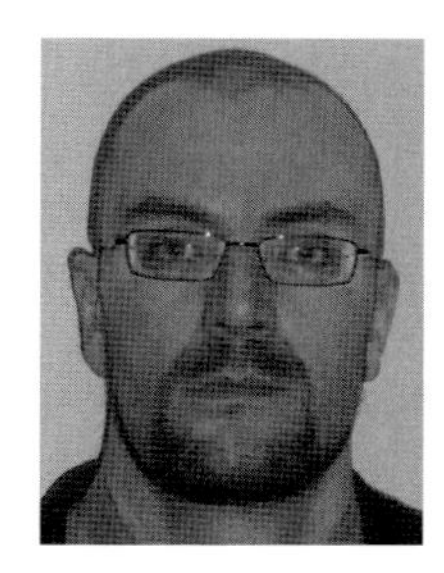

Christian Tyrchan studied chemistry with focus on pharmacology and bioinformatics, and received his Ph.D. in 2002 from the Department of Biochemistry at the University of Cologne, Germany. After holding a postdoctoral position at the Research Group for Molecular Informatics at the Cologne University BioInformatics Center (CUBIC), he joined in 2004 as a computational chemist at Euroscreen S.A. in Gosselies, Belgium, first in a postdoctoral position and then as a research scientist. In 2007, he moved to a postdoctoral position at the Chemoinformatics Group in the Discovery Enabling Capabilities and Sciences unit (DECS) of AstraZeneca in Mölndal, Sweden. Since 2008, he has been a member of the Computational Chemistry Group in the Medicinal Chemistry Department of AstraZeneca CV/GI in Mölndal, Sweden.

3
Metabolic Stability and Analogue-Based Drug Discovery

Amit S. Kalgutkar and Antonia F. Stepan

List of Abbreviations

ADME	absorption, distribution, metabolism, and excretion
AO	aldehyde oxidase
$CL_{int,app}$	apparent intrinsic clearance
CYP	cytochrome P450
DDI	drug–drug interaction
DME	drug metabolizing enzyme
GSH	reduced glutathione
HIV	human immunodeficiency virus
HLM	human liver microsomes
IADR	idiosyncratic adverse drug reaction
5-LO	5-lipoxygenase
MAO	monoamine oxidases
NADPH	nicotinamide adenine dinucleotide phosphate, reduced form
NAPQI	*N*-acetyl-*p*-benzoquinone imine
PPAR-γ	peroxisome proliferator-activated receptor-γ
QD	once a day (from Latin *quaque die*)
RM	reactive metabolite
SAR	structure–activity relationship
SULT	sulfotransferases
UGT	uridine glucuronosyl transferases

3.1
Introduction

A major focus in preclinical drug discovery involves the identification of safe and efficacious drug candidates that can be administered orally at low daily doses. During the hit-to-lead stage of drug discovery, most new chemical entities demonstrate high oxidative metabolic instability in human hepatic tissue (e.g., human liver

Analogue-based Drug Discovery III, First Edition. Edited by János Fischer, C. Robin Ganellin, and David P. Rotella.
© 2013 Wiley-VCH Verlag GmbH & Co. KGaA. Published 2013 by Wiley-VCH Verlag GmbH & Co. KGaA.

microsomes (HLMs) and human hepatocytes), principally mediated by cytochrome P450 (CYP) enzymes. The *in vivo* manifestation of high oxidative instability is suboptimal pharmacokinetics (high clearance, short elimination half-life, and poor oral bioavailability) due to extensive intestinal and first-pass metabolism by CYP enzymes [1]. Consequently, designing drug candidates with the optimal balance between efficacy and oral pharmacokinetics usually involves the introduction of metabolic resistance within the unstable lead chemical matter. For human pharmacokinetic predictions in drug discovery, much attention has been focused on the role of CYPs, since the particular enzyme system has been implicated in the metabolism of about 90% of marketed drugs. For this purpose, a high-throughput screening to facilitate structure–activity relationship (SAR) studies around these oxidative drug metabolizing enzymes (DMEs) is usually a practical starting point in most drug discovery programs. While such *in vitro* metabolic stability assays provide convenient means for "rank ordering" large numbers of compounds, information pertaining to the cause of oxidative instability cannot be discerned from such studies, and require customized mechanistic studies including the identification of metabolic "soft spots." Furthermore, it is not uncommon to find that as metabolic liability due to CYP enzymes is decreased, the molecules render themselves as substrates for other DMEs that may not be represented in the *in vitro* metabolism vector (e.g., HLM). Under such circumstances, when examined *in vivo*, an apparent *in vitro–in vivo* disconnect is revealed (i.e., greater *in vivo* metabolism is observed than would be predicted from the *in vitro* studies). The role of non-CYP enzymes in oxidative metabolism has been the subject of several recent reviews [2, 3]. Though not an exhaustive list, non-CYP DMEs that consistently reveal themselves as possible contributors to metabolism of pharmaceutical agents include (a) monoamine oxidases (MAO), (b) aldehyde oxidase (AO), and (c) uridine glucuronosyl transferases (UGTs). Unfortunately, *in vitro* tools for these enzymes that allow for high-throughput screening and prediction of human pharmacokinetics are typically not as readily available nor do they possess the fidelity for predicting human pharmacokinetics in a similar way that liver microsomes do for CYP enzymes.

In addition to manipulation of physicochemical properties (e.g., log *P*, log *D*, molecular weight, etc.), rational design of drug candidates with improved metabolic resistance also relies heavily on identification of metabolically labile sites for both phase I and phase II DMEs. Within this chapter, we will present several examples wherein SAR information from *in vitro* metabolism studies has enabled the conversion of metabolically labile lead chemical matter into "drug-like" molecules with improved absorption, distribution, metabolism, and excretion (ADME) characteristics. The value of metabolism-directed studies in the design of short-acting drug candidates (i.e., compounds with a short half-life) will also be discussed. Finally, the chapter will dwell into an analysis of rational discovery strategies/approaches for eliminating metabolism-dependent safety liabilities (e.g., reactive metabolite (RM) formation leading to genotoxicity, mechanism-based CYP inactivation, and idiosyncratic toxicity) using knowledge gathered from mechanistic drug metabolism studies.

3.2 Metabolism-Guided Drug Design

Reducing metabolic liability in the course of hit-to-lead optimization studies requires a proactive approach between medicinal chemists and drug metabolism scientists. The drug metabolism scientists identify sites of metabolism using appropriate *in vitro* metabolism vectors, information that is used by chemists to make rational structural modifications including the elimination of metabolic "soft spots" (e.g., replacement of a metabolically labile methyl group with the metabolically inert trifluoromethyl substituent), deactivating electron-rich aromatic rings prone to oxidation (e.g., substitution of phenyl with fluorophenyl or fluoropyridyl rings), and/or generally manipulating the physicochemical properties (e.g., reducing molecular weight and lipophilicity) to attenuate metabolic instability. In practice, however, this exercise is not trivial; medicinal chemistry tactics to optimize clearance could confer a detrimental effect on primary pharmacology (e.g., changes in agonist/antagonist behavior and/or subtype selectivity for target receptor or enzyme) and/or pharmacokinetic attributes. Thus, chemical intervention strategies to optimize ADME properties are often an iterative process. Of course, it will be recognized that changes in one parameter are generally not independent of others and it is likely that chemists will ultimately achieve an acceptable balance of properties rather than optimization of each aspect of the molecule. For example, excessive reduction in lipophilicity can reduce metabolism and decrease passive permeability simultaneously, which can ultimately translate into poor oral absorption via inability of the compound to permeate cellular membranes.

In the case of the major constitutively expressed human CYP isoform, that is, CYP3A4, the predominant interaction with substrates is via hydrophobic forces and overall lowering of lipophilicity can reduce metabolic lability to the enzyme. The trend for lower metabolic lability with lower lipophilicity holds regardless of structure and metabolic route [4]. An illustration of a medicinal chemistry strategy to attenuate CYP3A4 oxidative instability is evident in structure–metabolism studies on a series of *N*-arylsulfonamide-based γ-secretase inhibitors, wherein the lead compound exemplified by the lipophilic analogue **1** (Figure 3.1) suffered from extensive oxidations on the cyclohexyl motif by CYP3A4, which translated into a very high apparent intrinsic clearance ($CL_{int,app}$) in HLM [5]. Modulation of overall lipophilicity through reduction in size and introduction of polarity on the cycloalkyl region generated the corresponding tetrahydropyrans (compounds **4**–**6**) and tetrahydrofurans (compounds **7** and **8**), wherein the 3- and 4-substituted variants exhibited greater stability in HLM relative to their 2-substituted counterparts in both cases (Figure 3.1). To understand the greater metabolic resistance of 3-substituted cyclic ethers relative to the 2-substituted analogues, metabolite identification studies were performed in HLM with tetrahydropyrans **4** and **5** and tetrahydrofurans **7** and **8**. As seen in Figure 3.2, oxidative metabolism of these compounds still occurred primarily on the cycloether ring. For the tetrahydropyran and tetrahydrofuran rings, the characterization of stable hydroxycarboxylic acid metabolites was consistent with an initial CYP3A4-catalyzed oxidation(s) on the carbon α to the

		tetrahydropyrans			tetrahydrofurans		oxetanes	
IC_{50} ($A\beta_{42}$, nM)	12.3	27.9	45.2	8.58	44.5	11.2	7.99	16.9
$CL_{int,app}$ (ml/min/kg)	176	>300	136	114	210	69.8	62.1	28.6
Compound	**1**	**4**	**5**	**6**	**7**	**8**	**2**	**3**

Figure 3.1 *In vitro* γ-secretase inhibition and HLM apparent intrinsic clearance ($CL_{int,app}$) data for a representative set of *N*-arylsulfonamides.

oxygen atom, which would lead to unstable hemiacetal intermediates followed by hydrolysis to the corresponding aldehyde derivatives and further oxidation to the corresponding hydroxy acid metabolites. Based on these observations, it was speculated that the greater stability of the 3-substituted cyclic ethers (relative to the 2-substituted variants) resulted from a slower overall rate of metabolism caused by a diminished affinity for CYP binding due to a reduction in log *D* and/or unfavorable active site interactions with the 3-oxo substituent. Guided by these results, the lipophilicity of the ring system was reduced by further reducing the ring size and introducing the oxetane ring system. It was found that, relative to the other cyclic ethers, the oxetane-containing sulfonamides **2** and **3** possessed the highest degree of HLM stability and retained γ-secretase inhibitory potency in the desired nanomolar range. The relationship between oxetane ring substitution and oxidative metabolic stability followed similar trends as seen with the tetrahydropyran and tetrahydrofuran derivatives. Thus, 3-substituted oxetane **3** ($CL_{int,app}$ = 28.6 ml/min/kg) was relatively more stable in HLM than the two 2-substituted oxetane **2** ($CL_{int,app}$ = 62.1 ml/min/kg).

An example of metabolic blocking approach to minimize oxidative metabolism by CYP3A4 is evident from SAR work on human immunodeficiency virus (HIV) protease inhibitors for the treatment of HIV-1 infections. As a structural class, protease inhibitors, exemplified by indinavir, generally suffer from extensive first-pass metabolism in the small intestine and liver, which is mediated by CYP3A4. Attempts to develop agents with improved pharmacokinetics focused on blocking the sites of CYP3A4-mediated metabolism. Cheng *et al.* [6] deconstructed the metabolic liabilities of indinavir and designed in attributes that significantly enhanced

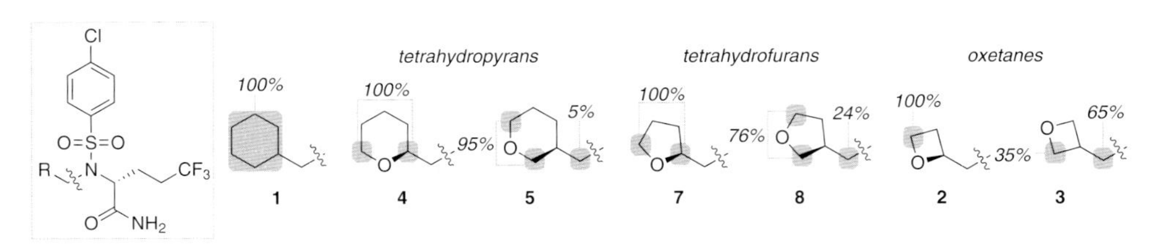

Figure 3.2 Sites of oxidative metabolism in HLM for representative *N*-arylsulfonamides.

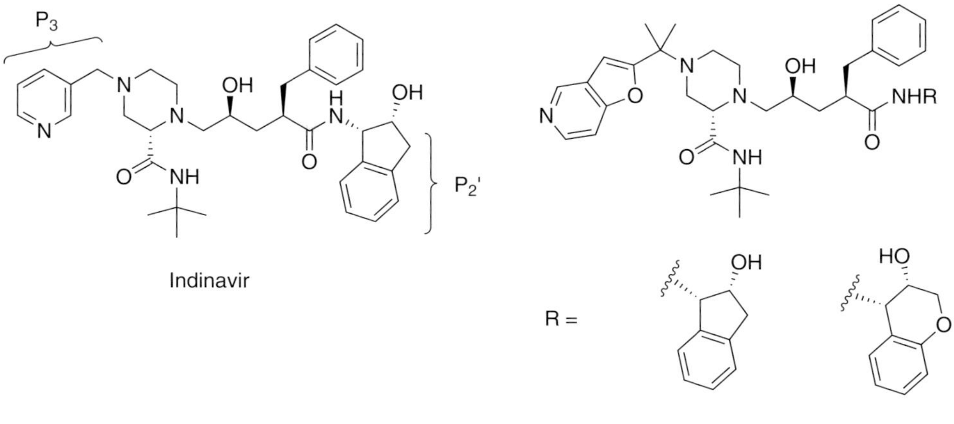

Figure 3.3 Improving oxidative metabolic liability in the HIV-1 protease inhibitor indinavir through blocking of metabolic sites.

their disposition attributes. Indinavir undergoes metabolism at two regions of the molecule designated as P_2' and P_3 (Figure 3.3). Specifically, oxidation takes place at the benzylic position of the aminoindanol moiety (P_2'), in addition to the pyridine nitrogen and the methylene linker (P_3). Incorporation of the *gem*-dimethyl and pyridylfuran functionalities in P_3 compound **9**), along with replacement of the aminoindanol with an aminochromanol moiety (compound **10**), led to analogues shown in Figure 3.3. In two markers of pharmacological activity ((i) inhibition of cleavage of a substrate by the wild-type HIV-1 protease enzyme and (ii) inhibition of the spread of viral infection in MT4 human T-lymphoid cells infected by the NL4-3 virus), both compounds showed enhanced potency compared to indinavir. When normalized for dose, compound **9** also showed twofold improvement in oral systemic exposure in dogs, while compound **10** showed a marginal improvement.

The calcium channel blocker diltiazem (Figure 3.4) is extensively metabolized via distinct pathways that include *N*-demethylation, ester hydrolysis, and *O*-demethylation. The enzyme responsible for the major route (*N*-demethylation) of clearance has been shown to be CYP3A4. Although widely used in therapy, diltiazem has a relatively short duration of action. In the search for metabolically resistant analogues, Floyd *et al.* [7] substituted the trifluoromethyl benzazepinone ring structure for the benzothiazepinone of diltiazem. Metabolism studies on this class of compound showed that the principal elimination routes were similar to that for diltiazem with *N*-demethylation, ester hydrolysis, and *O*-demethylation all occurring. Interestingly, the *N*-desmethyl metabolite was pharmacologically equipotent to the parent, and was much more resistant to metabolism. Consequently, *N*-1-pyrrolidinyl derivatives (exemplified by compound **11**) were designed to achieve metabolic stability both by a decrease in stability of the secondary amine radical (relative to tertiary amines) and by steric hindrance afforded by β-substitution (Figure 3.4).

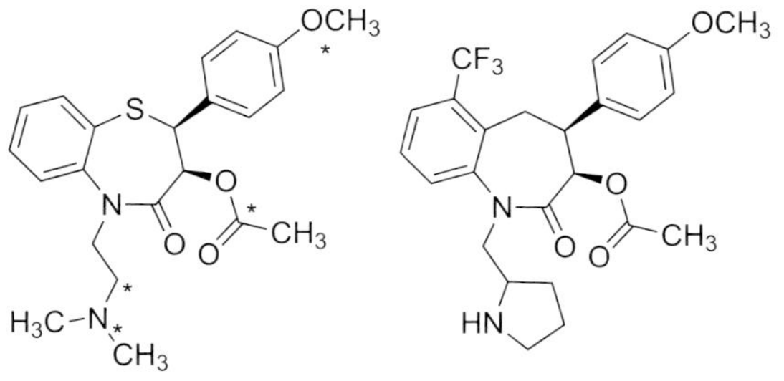

Diltiazem
* = sites of metabolism

11

Figure 3.4 Structures of diltiazem and its benzazepinone analogue **11**, which is inert to metabolism.

The success of this strategy indicates how vulnerable alkyl-substituted nitrogen functionalities can be stabilized to oxidative *N*-dealkylation.

3.3
Indirect Modulation of Metabolism by Fluorine Substitution

The effects of fluorine on ADME properties, including metabolism, have been known and exploited by medicinal chemists for some time [8]. Substituting hydrogen with fluorine at metabolically labile positions, for example, is a common approach to attenuate metabolism, although deuterium has also been considered. In the case of deuterium, the rate of metabolism via a specific pathway is attenuated, but the rate of overall substrate consumption or overall clearance is not significantly altered, due to a compensatory increase in the rate of formation of an alternate metabolite [9]. Moorjani *et al.* [10] reported on the use of fluorine substitution to enhance metabolic stability in a series of non-xanthine-selective A_{2a} antagonists for the potential treatment of Parkinson's disease. Lead compound **12** (Figure 3.5) demonstrated good antagonist activity and selectivity for the A_{2a} receptor, but was unstable in HLM. Introduction of a fluorine atom in the aromatic ring in **12** furnished **13**, which was resistant to oxidative metabolism in HLM while exhibiting single-digit nanomolar potency for the A_{2A} receptor. In this scenario, the electron-withdrawing effects of the fluorine atom most likely rendered the phenyl group resistant to CYP oxidation. A second example relates to the metabolism-directed lead optimization of *N*-(3,3-diphenylpropyl)nicotinamide (**14**), a potent inhibitor of soluble epoxide hydrolase (Figure 3.5) [11]. ADME profiling of **14** revealed a short metabolic half-life in HLM and rat liver microsomes, which was consistent with rapid clearance in rats. Metabolite identification studies indicated extensive hydroxylation on the pendant phenyl groups of the benzhydryl motif, which led to the design of the corresponding bis-(4-fluorophenyl) analogue **15** in order to block the metabolically vulnerable sites with fluorine atoms. Examination of the *in vitro* metabolic profile of **15**, however, revealed an apparent metabolic

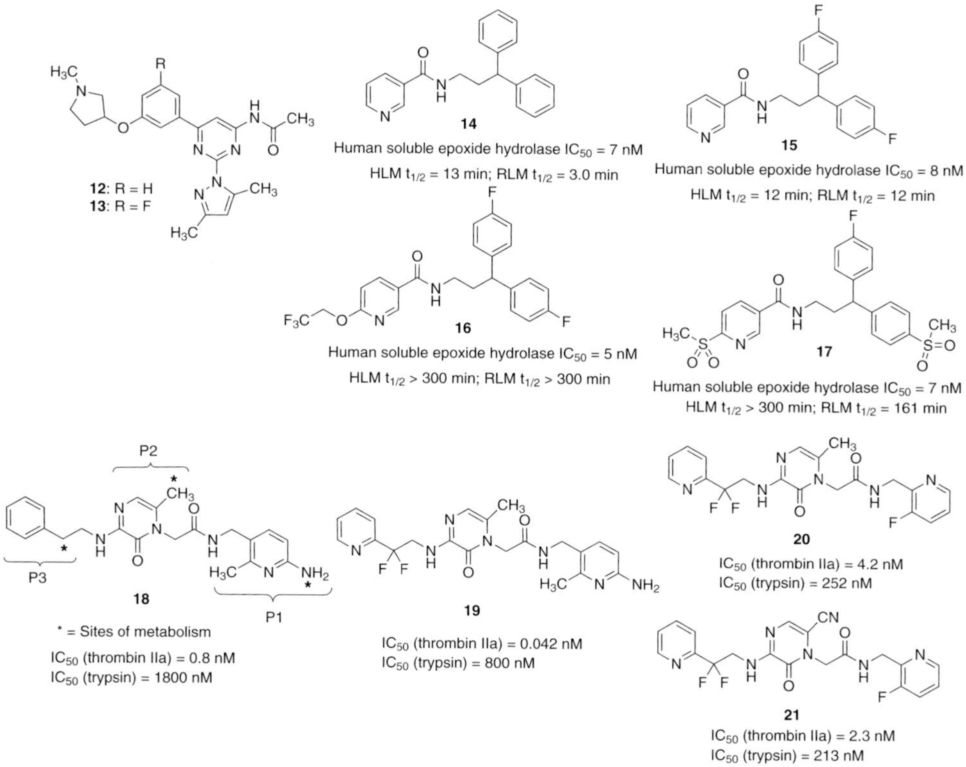

12: R = H
13: R = F

14
Human soluble epoxide hydrolase IC_{50} = 7 nM
HLM $t_{1/2}$ = 13 min; RLM $t_{1/2}$ = 3.0 min

15
Human soluble epoxide hydrolase IC_{50} = 8 nM
HLM $t_{1/2}$ = 12 min; RLM $t_{1/2}$ = 12 min

16
Human soluble epoxide hydrolase IC_{50} = 5 nM
HLM $t_{1/2}$ > 300 min; RLM $t_{1/2}$ > 300 min

17
Human soluble epoxide hydrolase IC_{50} = 7 nM
HLM $t_{1/2}$ > 300 min; RLM $t_{1/2}$ = 161 min

18
* = Sites of metabolism
IC_{50} (thrombin IIa) = 0.8 nM
IC_{50} (trypsin) = 1800 nM

19
IC_{50} (thrombin IIa) = 0.042 nM
IC_{50} (trypsin) = 800 nM

20
IC_{50} (thrombin IIa) = 4.2 nM
IC_{50} (trypsin) = 252 nM

21
IC_{50} (thrombin IIa) = 2.3 nM
IC_{50} (trypsin) = 213 nM

Figure 3.5 Modulation of oxidative metabolism by fluorine substitution.

switch in the major route of metabolism to pyridine ring hydroxylation, a feature that was consistent with lack of change in microsomal half-lives. Hypothesizing that increase in overall polarity could decrease metabolism, analogues with polar pyridine ring substituents were synthesized. From this exercise emerged **16**, which retained the soluble epoxide hydrolase inhibitory potency of **14**, and was practically inert to oxidative metabolism in microsomes. However, **16** revealed poor *in vivo* oral absorption in rats due to its poor aqueous solubility. Guided by the analysis of the costructure of **14** with soluble epoxide hydrolase, one fluorine atom in **16** was substituted for an additional polar substituent on the right-hand side benzhydryl motif with simultaneous modifications on the pyridine ring to balance physicochemical properties. These efforts culminated in the identification of potent and *in vitro* metabolically stable epoxide hydrolase inhibitors with excellent oral absorption as exemplified with compound **17**.

Burgey *et al.* also reported on the metabolism-directed optimization of a series of 3-(2-phenethylamino)-6-methylpyrazinone acetamide thrombin inhibitors (exemplified by compound **18**, Figure 3.5), which involved the use of fluorine atoms to stabilize oxidative metabolism resulting in orally bioavailable compounds [12]. Metabolic profiling of **18** revealed three principal sites of metabolism – oxidation of the P3 and P2 benzylic positions and phase II conjugation of the P1 basic amino group (Figure 3.5). A study to examine the effect of P3 benzylic substitution on thrombin inhibitory potency was initiated with the goal of sterically blocking oxidative metabolism. Incorporation of a 2-pyridyl and *gem*-difluoro modifications afforded **19**, with improved thrombin inhibitory potency and lack of obvious metabolic soft spots. Attempts to address phase II metabolism in **18** via removal of the amino group led to dramatic loss of thrombin inhibitory potency, which was regained to some degree via installation of the optimized 2,2-difluoro-2-pyridylethylamino P3 modification. Incorporation of a *meta*-substituted fluorine atom on the P1 aryl group led to **20** with inhibitory potency in the targeted range for efficacy. Compound **20** also demonstrated moderate to good oral bioavailability in rats, dogs, and monkeys. Metabolism of the P2 benzylic group was finally addressed via replacement of the problematic methyl group with a cyano functionality leading to compound **21** with excellent pharmacology and animal pharmacokinetics.

The final example involves optimization of the cholesterol absorption inhibitor (−)-SCH 48461. Metabolism studies indicated that there were four primary sites of metabolism for (−)-SCH 48461 (Figure 3.6), with metabolites resulting from *O*-demethylation, hydroxylation, and/or oxidation, and combinations thereof. The metabolism data along with the SAR studies were used as a guide in designing a metabolically more stable analogue of (−)-SCH 48461 without affecting the potency of the compound [13]. Initial attempts to prevent metabolism via substitution of the C′-3 carbon in (−)-SCH 48461 with an oxygen atom (compound **22**) were unsuccessful since this step produced an electron-rich phenoxy motif in comparison to the original phenyl group and possibly made this function more amenable to aromatic hydroxylation. Blocking aromatic oxidation with a fluorine atom introduced in the *para* position was required to produce the eventual more stable substitution ((−)-SCH 53079). Additional SAR led to the design of even more stable and

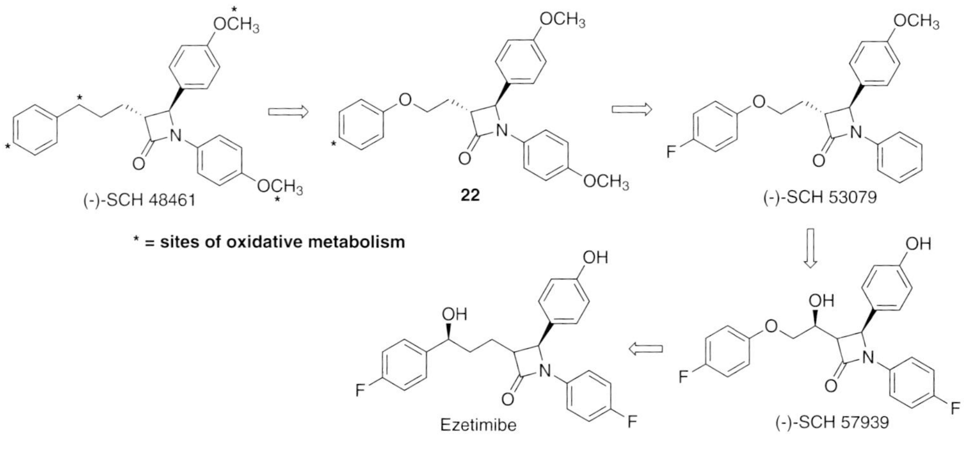

Figure 3.6 Use of fluorine to stabilize oxidative metabolism in cholesterol absorption inhibitors.

pharmacologically potent analogues exemplified by (−)-SCH 57939, and ultimately led to the discovery of ezetimibe [14, 15].

3.4 Modulation of Low Clearance/Long Half-Life via Metabolism-Guided Design

While optimization of ADME attributes usually focuses on reducing clearance and increasing half-lives, in some scenarios (e.g., mechanism-based safety concerns), engagement of the pharmacological target requires short-acting agents and/or molecules with specific clearance and half-life values. Metabolism-guided drug design has also proven very valuable in such efforts. For instance, the known lability of benzylic positions on electron-rich heteroatoms toward CYP metabolism has been exploited to decrease the unacceptably low clearance and resultant long half-life of selective cyclooxygenase-2 inhibitor lead compounds. Specifically, the anti-inflammatory agent celecoxib (Figure 3.7) exhibits a half-life of 3.5 h in rats, whereas early structural leads, represented by compounds in which celecoxib's benzylic methyl was replaced with a halogen substituent (compound **23**, Figure 3.7), possessed half-life values >220 h in rats [16]. In another illustration, short-acting calcium-sensing receptor antagonists were designed by incorporating the metabolically labile thiomethyl functionality into the metabolically stable, zwitterionic amino alcohol leads (e.g., compound **24**, Figure 3.7) to increase oxidative clearance by CYP3A4, while delivering a pharmacologically inactive sulfoxide metabolite. The efforts led to the discovery of clinical candidates **25** and **26** for the potential treatment of osteoporosis [17].

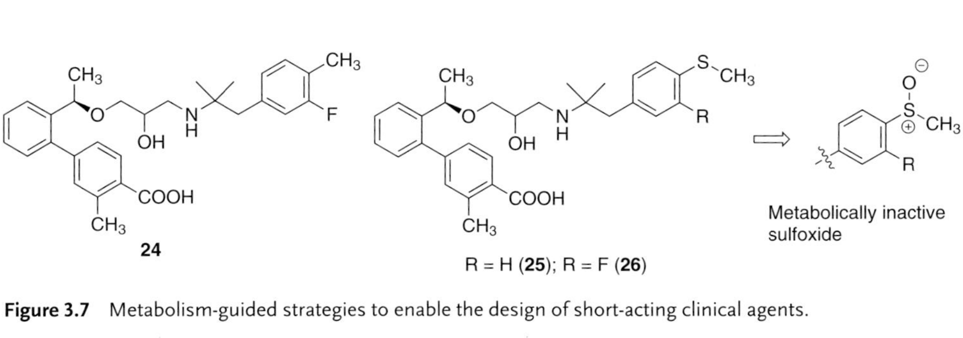

27: $R_1 = NHSO_2CH_3$; $R_2 = CF_3$
28: $R_1 = F$; $R_2 = SCH_3$
29: $R_1 = SO_2NH_2$; $R_2 = SCH_3$
30: $R_1 = SO_2NH_2$; $R_2 = S(O)CH_3$

R = H (**25**); R = F (**26**)

Metabolically inactive sulfoxide

Figure 3.7 Metabolism-guided strategies to enable the design of short-acting clinical agents.

In a slightly different approach, Middleton *et al.* report a strategy on purposely redirecting metabolism away from an undesired site on a series of serotonin reuptake inhibitors [18]. Lead compound **27** (Figure 3.7), although a promising lead, was found to undergo CYP2D6-mediated *N*-demethylation to the secondary amine metabolite, which was pharmacologically active and possessed a relatively long half-life, a phenomenon that was inconsistent with the laboratory objectives of this program. A simple thiomethyl analogue **28** was designed to explore the concept that CYP-mediated thioalkyl *S*-oxidation can be a rapid metabolic process and could potentially compete with *N*-demethylation. Further expansion of the SAR led to the sulfonamide **29**, which was potent and selective for serotonin over dopamine and norepinephrine reuptake inhibition. *In vitro*, the sulfoxide **30** was the predominant metabolite (>90%) and showed only weak pharmacological activity ($IC_{50} > 1$ μM). *In vivo*, in both rat and dog pharmacokinetic studies, the parent compound **29** retained the desired ADME properties of **27**, and indeed as predicted by the *in vitro* studies, the sulfoxide **30** was the predominant metabolite. Compound **29** possessed the desired short half-life and, furthermore, was shown to be inactive against a broad panel of other receptors, enzymes, and ion channels. Based on the cumulative knowledge, sulfonamide **29** was progressed into clinical development.

3.5 Tactics to Resolve Metabolism Liabilities Due to Non-CYP Enzymes

3.5.1 Aldehyde Oxidase

In addition to CYP isoforms, oxidative metabolic liabilities can also be encountered with AO and MAO enzymes. AO is a member of a family of enzymes referred to as molybdenum cofactor-containing enzymes, which also includes xanthine oxidase. Liver has by far the highest AO expression in all species including humans. Typical substrates of AO are compounds containing an aldehyde function, nitro/nitroso derivatives, and nitrogen-containing heterocycles. AO catalyzes the α- or γ-carbon oxidation of the imine motif ($R_1R_2C=NR_3$) in nitrogen-containing heterocycles (e.g., pyridine, pyrimidine, quinoline, quinoxaline, etc.), resulting in the formation of the corresponding lactam (α-carbon oxidation) or aminoenone (γ-carbon oxidation) metabolites, respectively [2]. Even though AO utilizes molecular oxygen as the ultimate electron acceptor, the oxygen atom that is incorporated into the product during AO-mediated hydroxylation is derived from water and not molecular oxygen. Consequently, α- and γ-carbon atoms adjacent to electron-withdrawing nitrogen atoms in nitrogen heterocycles preferentially are oxidized by AO. While the order of AO activity among animal species may vary depending on the substrate, it generally seems to be high in monkeys and humans and low in rats, whereas dogs are to a large extent deficient in activity [2].

Efforts to confer metabolic resistance into aromatic rings by virtue of introducing polar heteroatoms such as nitrogen often render the compounds susceptible to AO

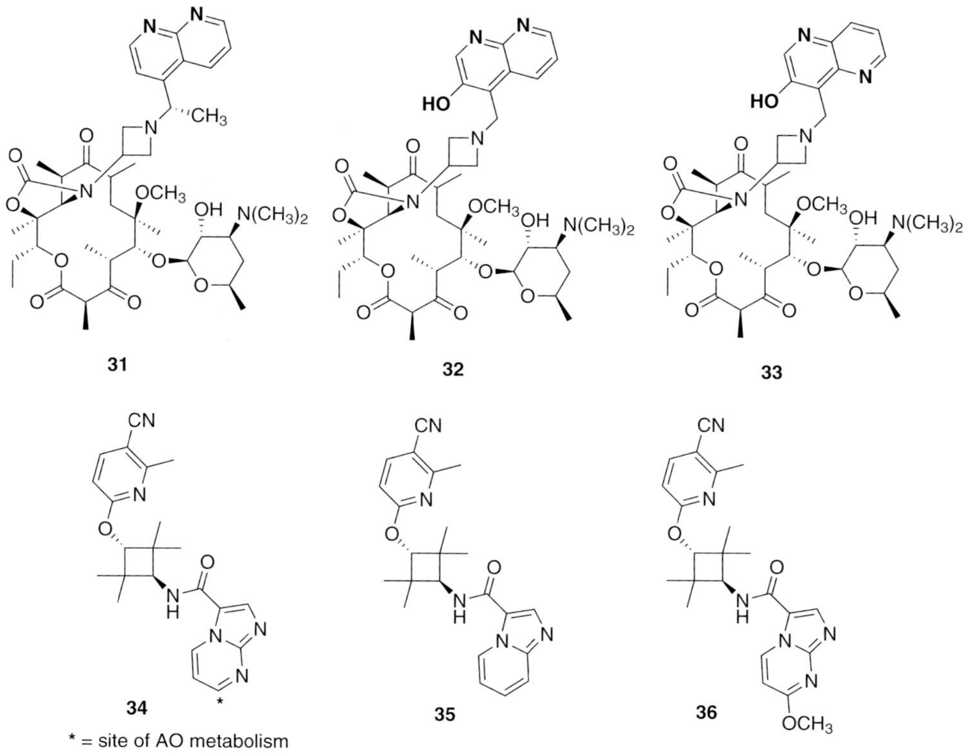

31 32 33

34 35 36

* = site of AO metabolism

Figure 3.8 SAR for AO-mediated oxidation of azetidinyl ketolide derivatives.

metabolism. In a recent account, Magee *et al.* disclosed a series of heterocycle-substituted azetidinyl ketolide derivatives as potent antibacterial agents with minimal turnover in CYPs and little to no inhibitory effects against the human CYP3A4 isoform [19]. An extensive investigation into heterocycle analogues identified a number of systems that appeared to combine favorable efficacy and metabolism properties. Compound **31** (Figure 3.8) was predicted to have low human clearance, which combined with its favorable *in vitro* profile led to pharmacokinetic studies in clinical trials. However, upon oral dosing at the predicted efficacious dose range of 300–1000 mg, the measured plasma exposures were ~20% of the predicted area under the plasma concentration–time curve values, leading to the termination of further clinical investigation with the agent. Human liver cytosolic assessment of turnover with and without raloxifene (a selective inhibitor of AO) revealed that **31** was a substrate of human AO. The 1,8-naphthyridine ring system in **31** was subsequently shown to be vulnerable to AO, although the regiochemistry of hydroxylation was not established. The AO liability was not circumvented by incorporation of polar functionalities such as hydroxyl (e.g., compound **32**), but was avoided through modification of the heteroatom arrangement. For instance, the 1,5-naphthyridine system (compound **33**) was stable in human liver cytosol and the compound was selected for clinical development [19]. In another account, AO-mediated metabolism on the imidazo[1,2-*a*]pyrimidine moiety in the androgen receptor antagonist and anticancer agent **34** was prevented by blocking the site of metabolism as well as alteration in the heterocycle as highlighted with analogues **35** and **36**, respectively (Figure 3.8) [20].

3.5.2
Monoamine Oxidases

MAO isoforms MAO-A and MAO-B are mitochondrial flavoenzymes that catalyze the oxidative deamination of structurally diverse alkyl- and arylalkyl amines [3]. Elaborate SAR studies with arylalkylamine substrates and inhibitors suggest that MAO-A and MAO-B are efficient catalysts for amines, which possess aryl group 1–3 carbons away from the amine nitrogen. Although primary and secondary amines are deaminated indiscriminately by both isozymes, tertiary amines generally display selectivity toward one form of the enzyme. From a drug metabolism perspective, MAO plays a dominant role in the clearance of the triptan class of antimigraine drugs. This class of compounds constitutes novel and highly selective serotonin receptor agonists that are used in the acute, oral treatment of migraine and cluster headaches. Members of this group of drugs include acyclic tertiary amines such as sumatriptan, almotriptan, zolmitriptan, and rizatriptan, cyclic tertiary amines such as eletriptan and naratriptan, and a secondary amine (frovatriptan). MAO-A is the principal enzyme responsible for the clearance of sumatriptan and almotriptan leading to the formation of the corresponding indoleacetic acid metabolites (Figure 3.9) [21, 22]. In the case of sumatriptan, *in vitro* studies have clearly demonstrated the involvement of MAO by using the MAO-A-specific inactivator clorgyline, which prevents sumatriptan metabolism. Rizatriptan also undergoes MAO-catalyzed oxidation leading to the indoleacetic acid derivative as the major metabolite in humans (Figure 3.9) [23]. The structurally related zolmitriptan is cleared in humans primarily via *N*-demethylation and *N*-oxidation that is mediated by CYP1A2 [24]. The *N*-demethylated metabolite undergoes selective MAO-A-catalyzed oxidation to yield the corresponding indoleacetic acid derivative (Figure 3.9) [24]. Despite their structural similarity to sumatriptan, zolmitriptan, and rizatriptan, the cyclic tertiary amines eletriptan and naratriptan and the secondary amine frovatriptan (Figure 3.9) are not substrates of MAO-A and/or MAO-B. Eletriptan is metabolized via *N*-demethylation by CYP2D6 and CYP3A4, whereas frovatriptan is metabolized by CYP1A2 [25, 26]. Naratriptan is mostly eliminated in the urine in the unchanged form (naratriptan product information). The half-lives of naratriptan, eletriptan, and, in particular, frovatriptan range from 26 to 30 h, and are longer than that of sumatriptan ($\sim$2 h) [27]. As such, most basic amine drugs do not have MAO-catalyzed metabolism as a primary clearance pathway with the exception of the triptans. The findings are probably a reflection of the low lipophilicity of the triptans and their stability to oxidative enzymes such as CYP. Overall, the findings on the MAO-A substrate properties of sumatriptan, almotriptan, rizatriptan, and the *N*-dealkylated metabolite of zolmitriptan are not surprising

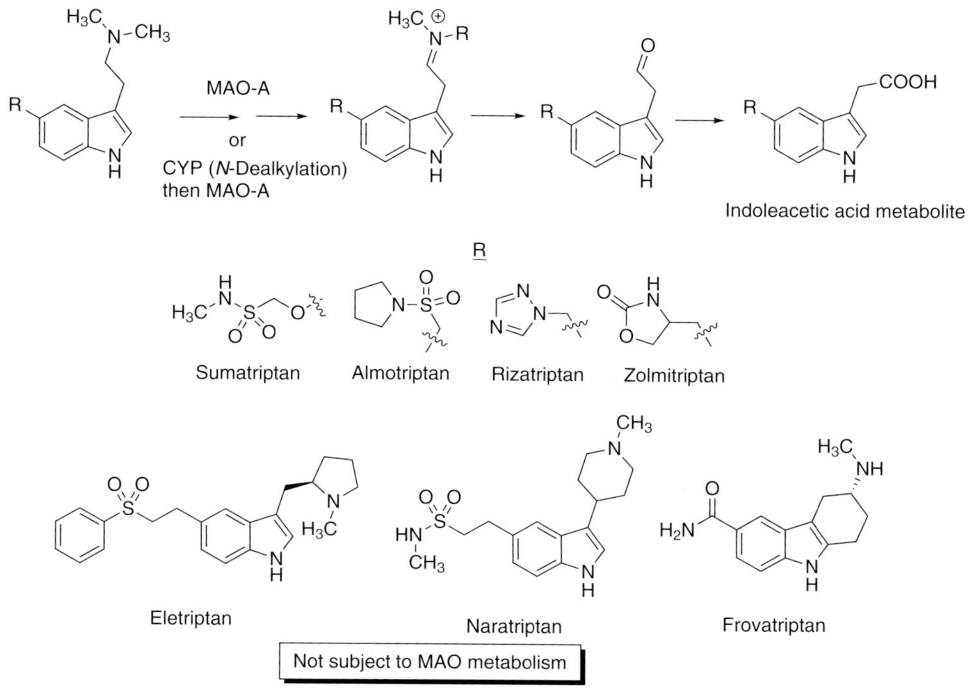

Figure 3.9 Oxidative deamination of the triptan class of antimigraine drugs by MAO-A.

considering the structural similarity with the endogenous neurotransmitter serotonin, which is a preferred MAO-A substrate [3].

3.5.3
Phase II Conjugating Enzymes (UGT and Sulfotransferases)

Conjugation with glucuronic acid or sulfate requires a nucleophilic substituent (e.g., hydroxyl, amine, etc.) present in the molecule. UGT substrates include phenol, primary, secondary, or even tertiary alcohol, or carboxylic acid derivatives, whereas substrates for sulfation catalyzed by sulfotransferases (SULTs) are usually phenolic compounds [28, 29]. In some cases, primary alcohols can also form sulfate conjugates. The most "reactive" functionality is the phenol and a simple rule of the thumb is to eliminate such a functionality unless absolutely essential for pharmacological activity. For instance, the peroxisome proliferator-activated receptor-γ (PPAR-γ) agonist troglitazone (Figure 3.10) is principally metabolized in humans via sulfation of its phenol group [30]. Related PPAR agonists pioglitazone and rosiglitazone (Figure 3.10) do not undergo this metabolic fate since they do not contain the phenol substituent. It is also noteworthy to point out that pioglitazone and rosiglitazone are significantly more potent than the PPAR-γ agonist troglitazone indicating that the phenol motif is not essential for primary pharmacology.

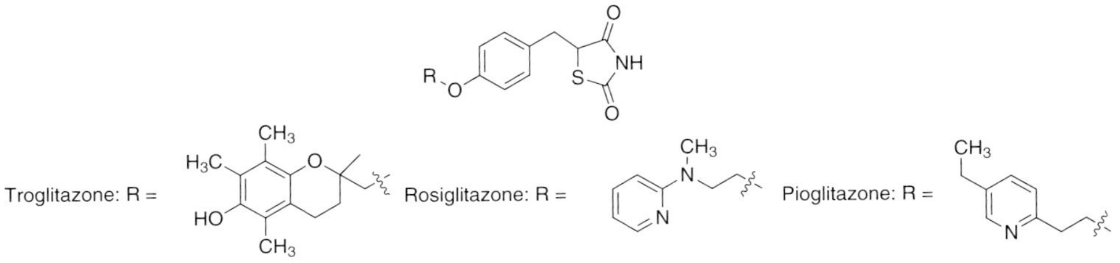

Troglitazone: R =

Rosiglitazone: R =

Pioglitazone: R =

Figure 3.10 PPAR-γ agonists troglitazone, rosiglitazone, and pioglitazone. Sulfation of the phenol group in troglitazone is the primary pathway of elimination in humans.

An example of minimizing phase II conjugation while maintaining pharmacological potency is evident with 4-(3-hydroxylphenylamino)pyrrolotriazine-based inhibitors of vascular endothelial growth factor-2 receptor [31]. The lead compounds exemplified by **37** (Figure 3.11) suffered from extensive phenol glucuronidation resulting in poor oral activity. Hence, SAR efforts were directed toward finding functionalities that would suppress glucuronidation. The solvent-exposed R_2 region of the pyrrolotriazine was considered to be the most suitable for manipulations. In the course of the SAR studies, it was observed that compounds with neutral R_2 groups (e.g., compound **37**) with basic $pK_a < 6$ exhibited high rates of glucuronidation. In contrast, introduction of a basic amino group with a calculated basic pK_a between 7 and 10 on an appendage attached to the R_2 position via different functionalities (e.g., compound **38** in Figure 3.11) led to a substantial decrease in glucuronidation rates. A second example is evident from SAR studies on a second generation of *N*-hydroxyurea-based 5-lipoxygenase (5-LO) inhibitors, wherein duration of 5-LO inhibition after oral administration in animals was optimized by

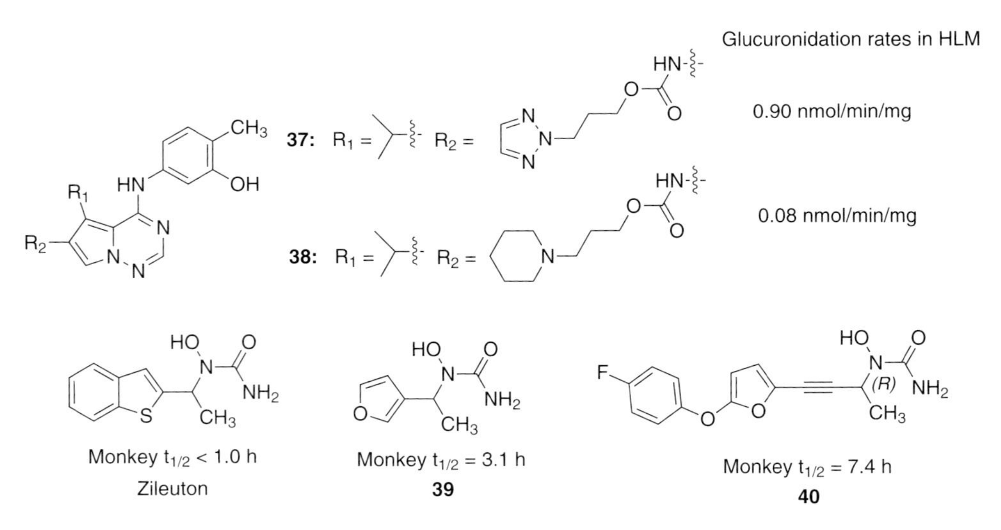

Figure 3.11 Strategies for reducing excessive glucuronidation.

reducing glucuronidation of the *N*-hydroxyurea motif [32]. The primary route of metabolism of zileuton (Figure 3.11), the first *N*-hydroxyurea-based 5-LO inhibitor, in humans involves *O*-glucuronidation of the *N*-hydroxyurea group, resulting in a relatively short plasma half-life of $\sim$3 h after oral dosing [33]. Clinical trials with zileuton in asthmatics demonstrated efficacy with oral administration of 600 mg four times daily. Validation of the therapeutic application of 5-LO inhibitors in asthma patients has provided impetus to identify an optimized compound with greater potency and longer duration of action that would in turn provide a lower and less frequent daily dose. Duration of 5-LO inhibition after oral administration in monkeys (as a model for human pharmacokinetics) was optimized by identification of structural features in the proximity of the *N*-hydroxyurea (e.g., compounds **39** and **40**), which correlated to low *in vitro* glucuronidation rates. For instance, compound **40** (phenoxyphenyl-substituted template in combination with the butynyl link) proved to be a compatible match that enhanced inhibitory potency and provided resistance to glucuronidation.

3.6 Eliminating RM Liabilities in Drug Design

Metabolic activation (also referred to as bioactivation) of innate functional groups into electrophilic RMs is considered to be an undesirable trait of drug candidates on the grounds of evidence linking this liability with genotoxicity [34], drug–drug interactions (DDIs) [35], end organ toxicity, and possibly immune-mediated idiosyncratic adverse drug reactions (IADRs) [36–39]. Most pharmaceutical companies have implemented procedures to evaluate a drug candidate's potential to form RMs with the goal of eliminating or minimizing this liability by rational structural modifications. Qualitative assessment of CYP-mediated RM formation *in vitro* usually involves "trapping" studies conducted with NADPH-supplemented HLM in the presence of reduced glutathione (GSH), amines (e.g., semicarbazide and methoxylamine), and/or cyanide ion. Microsomes can be replaced by alternate metabolism systems (e.g., liver cytosol, liver S9 fractions, hepatocytes, neutrophils, etc.), to evaluate the participation of non-CYP enzymes in RM formation. In case of RM positives, characterization of the nucleophile–RM structure provides insight into the structure of the reactive species and the mechanism leading to its formation. The information is then used, as appropriate, to modify the structure of the RM positives in order to eliminate the liability.

3.7 Eliminating Metabolism-Dependent Mutagenicity

The role of metabolism in generating RMs capable of covalently adducting with nucleic acids and leading to mutagenic lesions is well established for many endogenous and exogenous xenobiotics (including drugs). Virtually, any molecule that forms RMs possesses the propensity to modify DNA and elicit a genotoxic/carcinogenic response. Genetic toxicology testing is usually conducted in the early stages of drug development with the intent of identifying hazards associated with both the parent molecule and its metabolites. Identification of genotoxic metabolites in *in vitro* test systems is accomplished by employing metabolic activation systems (e.g., Aroclor 1254-induced rat liver S9). The *Salmonella* reverse mutation assay has become an integral part of the safety evaluation of drug candidates and is required by regulatory agencies for drug approvals worldwide. The mutagenic potential of small-molecule drug candidates is generally evaluated in genetically different strains of the *Salmonella typhimurium*, such as TA98, TA100, TA1535, and TA1537. These test strains all carry some type of defective (mutant) gene that prevents them from synthesizing the amino acid histidine in a minimal bacterial culture medium. In the presence of mutagenic chemicals, the defective gene may be mutated back to the functional state that allows the bacterium to grow in the medium. Because positive findings in the *Salmonella* reverse mutation assay have a good correlation with the outcome of rodent carcinogenicity testing, a positive result leads to the discontinuation of development, particularly for drugs intended for non-life-threatening indications.

RM trapping studies have proven useful in elucidating mutagenic mechanisms of drug candidates, and the mechanistic insights gathered have been used in the rational design of follow-on compounds that are devoid of genotoxic response. An example is evident with the anti-obesity agent and 5-hydroxytryptamine 2C agonist **41** (Figure 3.12), which was mutagenic in the bacterial *Salmonella* Ames assay in an Aroclor 1254-induced rat liver S9/NADPH-dependent fashion [40, 41]. In the *Salmonella* assay, **41** produced a significant increase of mutations only in strains TA100 and TA1537 that are known to be sensitive to mainly base-pair and frameshift mutagens, consistent with covalent adduction to DNA (rather than a simple intercalation). Studies with $[^{14}C]$-**41** revealed the irreversible and concentration-dependent incorporation of radioactivity in calf thymus DNA in an S9/NADPH-dependent fashion confirming that **41** was metabolized to a DNA-reactive metabolite. RM trapping studies in S9/NADPH incubations led to the detection of GSH and amine conjugates. Structural elucidation of these conjugates allowed an insight into the mechanism leading to the formation of DNA-reactive metabolites (Figure 3.12). The mass spectrum of the methoxylamine conjugate of **41** was consistent with condensation of amine with an electrophilic, aldehyde metabolite derived from piperazine ring scission in **41**, whereas the mass spectrum of the GSH conjugate suggested a bioactivation pathway involving initial aromatic ring hydroxylation on the 3-chlorobenzyl motif in **41** followed by β-elimination to an electrophilic quinone methide species that reacted with GSH. The observation that methoxylamine and GSH reduced mutagenicity suggested that the trapping agents competed with DNA toward reaction with the RMs. Overall, the exercise provided indirect information on the structure of DNA-reactive intermediates leading to mutagenic response with **41** and hence a rationale on which to base subsequent chemical intervention strategy for designing nonmutagenic 5-hydroxytryptamine 2C agonists such as compound **42** (Figure 3.12) [41]. In contrast with **41**, **42** cannot form the

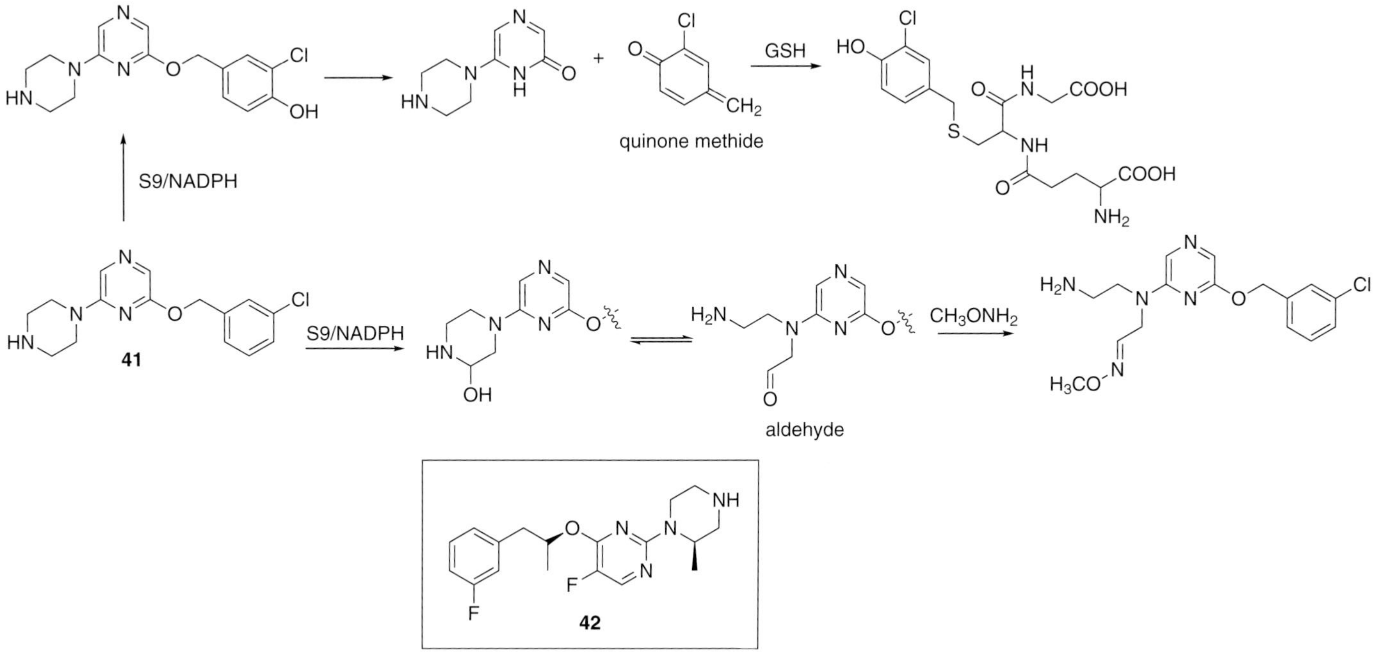

Figure 3.12 Insights into the S9/NADPH-dependent mutagenic response with the 5-hydroxytryptamine 2C agonist **41** that led to the design of nonmutagenic analogue and clinical candidate **42**.

reactive quinone methide species. Likewise, introduction of the methyl group is thought to shunt metabolism from piperazine ring opening to hydroxylation of the methyl substituent.

Another account of medicinal chemistry tactics to resolve metabolism-dependent mutagenicity is evident with the arylindenopyrimidine series of selective dual A_{2A}/A_1 adenosine receptor antagonists exemplified by 2-amino-4-phenyl-8-pyrrolidin-1-ylmethyl-indeno[1,2-*d*]pyrimidin-5-one (**43**) (Figure 3.13) [42]. Compound **43** was shown to be genotoxic in both the Ames and mouse lymphoma L5178Y assays in a rat liver S9/NADPH-dependent fashion, and also demonstrated irreversible covalent binding to calf thymus DNA in the presence of Aroclor 1254-induced rat liver S9 and NADPH. Profiling for RM formation in rat liver S9 indicated that **43** was bioactivated on its pyrrolidine ring to several electrophilic species that included endocyclic iminium ion, amino aldehyde, epoxide, and α,β-unsaturated carbonyl intermediates as judged from the detection of corresponding cyano, oxime, and GSH conjugates (Figure 3.13). The endocyclic iminium ion and amino aldehyde species appear to be the likely candidates responsible for genotoxicity based on, first, the protection afforded by both cyanide ion and methoxylamine, which reduced the potential to form covalent adducts with DNA, and, second, analogues of **43** (e.g., compounds **44** and **45**) designed with low probability to form these RMs were not genotoxic. It was concluded that **43** also had the potential to be mutagenic in humans based on the formation of the endocyclic iminium ion following incubation with a human liver S9 preparation and the commensurate detection of DNA adducts.

3.8 Eliminating Mechanism-Based Inactivation of CYP Enzymes

Modulation of CYP activity via induction or inhibition by xenobiotics including drugs can lead to clinical DDIs with consequences ranging from loss of efficacy to the introduction of adverse effects, respectively, for coadministered "victim" drugs. DDIs arising from CYP inhibition are more frequent and, in some cases, have resulted in the withdrawal of the marketed "perpetrator" drug (e.g., the antihypertensive agent mibefradil), especially those drugs associated with potent inhibition of the major constitutively expressed human CYP enzyme, CYP3A4. CYP inhibitors can be categorized as reversible (competitive or noncompetitive), quasi-irreversible, and irreversible in nature [35]. Reversible inhibition usually involves two or more agents competing for metabolism at the active site of a CYP isozyme, with one drug inhibiting the metabolism of the other agent. In contrast, drugs converted to electrophilic RMs by CYP may interact with the CYP quasi-irreversibly or irreversibly leading to enzyme destruction. Quasi-irreversible inactivation occurs when the reactive species complexes with the ferrous form of heme (product of reduction of resting state ferric enzyme by NADPH-CYP reductase) in a tight, noncovalent interaction. CYP inactivation can also arise through covalent adduction of the RM to the heme prosthetic group and/or to an active site amino acid residue in

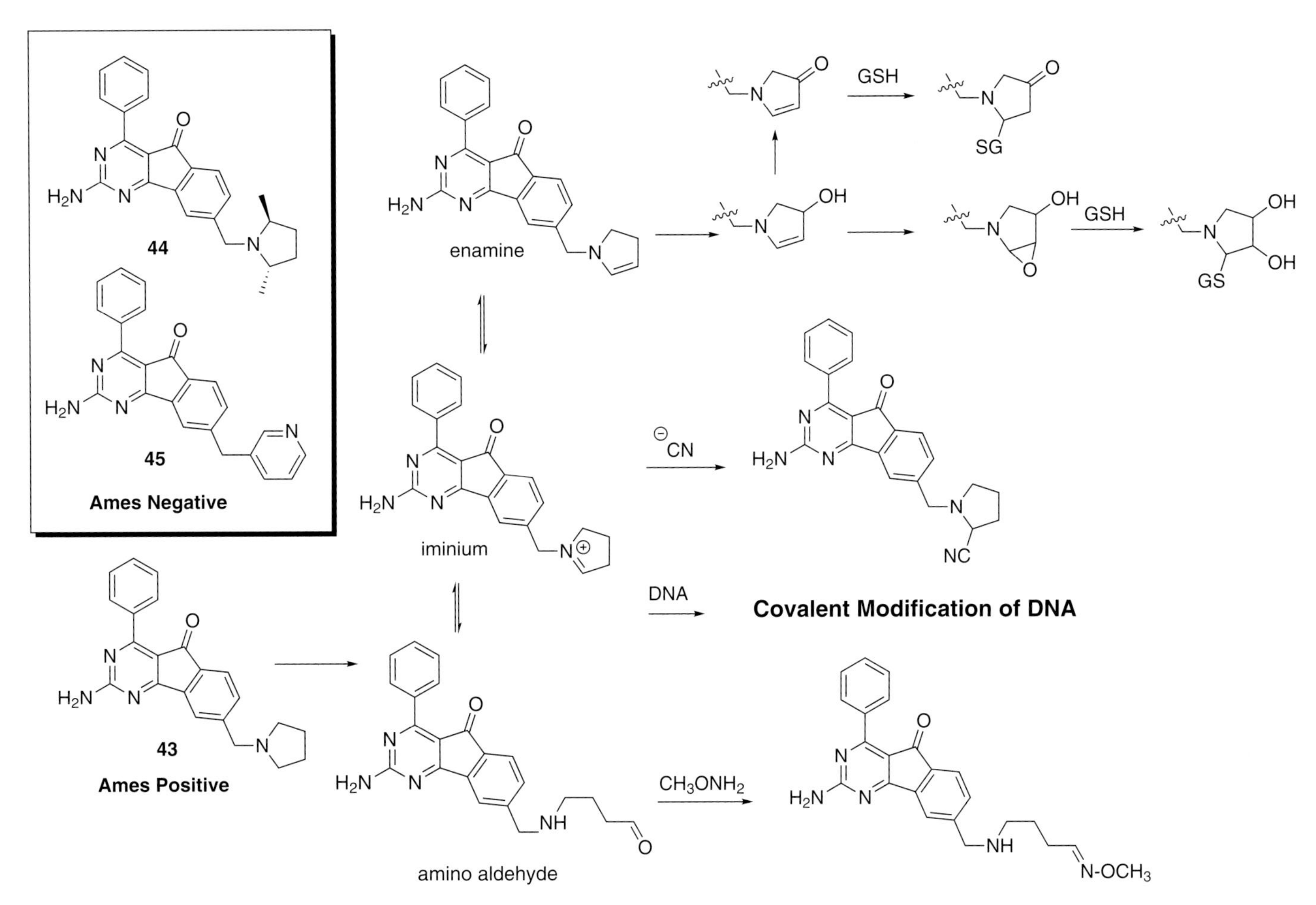

Figure 3.13 Circumventing metabolism-dependent genotoxicity of a pyrrolidine-substituted arylindenopyrimidine derivative **43**.

the apoprotein. As such, CYP isozymes inactivated via these mechanisms are rendered catalytically incompetent, and must be replenished by newly synthesized protein. The phenomenon is oftentimes referred to as time-dependent inactivation, mechanism-based inactivation, and/or suicide inactivation. Compared to reversible CYP inhibition, drug-induced time-dependent inactivation of CYPs presents a greater safety concern because of the increased propensity for pharmacokinetic interactions upon multiple dosing and the sustained duration of these interactions after discontinuation of the mechanism-based inactivator. Furthermore, depending upon the fraction of the mechanism-based inactivator that is metabolized by the inactivated CYP, an additional clinical consequence could involve supraproportional increases in systemic exposure of the inactivator itself after multiple doses. Finally, covalent modification of CYP enzymes can also lead to hapten formation and can, in some cases, trigger an autoimmune response in susceptible patients leading to idiosyncratic toxicity.

Identification of CYP inactivators with corresponding insights into the inactivation mechanism(s) is required for the rational design of compounds, devoid of the liability. Recently, several publications have demonstrated tactics to minimize and/or eliminate time-dependent inactivation of CYP enzymes without affecting primary pharmacology and/or disposition characteristics. Solutions range from modulation of lipophilicity resulting in diminished rates of metabolism (and bioactivation to RMs) to virtually eliminating the potential for RM formation via functional group manipulations. Paroxetine (Figure 3.14) is a selective serotonin reuptake inhibitor that inhibits CYP2D6 in a time- and concentration-dependent fashion consistent with mechanism-based inactivation [43]. Mechanism-based inactivation of CYP2D6 by paroxetine occurs during metabolism of the 1,3-benzdioxole ring. Thus, hydrogen atom abstraction from the methylene carbon or elimination of water from a hydroxymethylene intermediate generates a carbene intermediate, which forms a MI complex with the ferrous form of the heme iron atom in CYP2D6 resulting in a catalytically inactive enzyme (Figure 3.14) [44]. As such, 1,3-benzdioxole ring scission by CYP2D6 also represents the major metabolic pathway of paroxetine in humans, leading to the formation of a catechol intermediate, which is converted to the corresponding guaiacol isomers via the action of catechol-*O*-methyltransferase [45]. GSH conjugates resulting from Michael addition of the thiol nucleophile to electrophilic *ortho*-quinone species have also been characterized in HLM incubations of paroxetine, and may represent an additional pathway of enzyme inactivation [46]. Because CYP2D6 is responsible for paroxetine metabolism, mechanism-based inactivation of CYP2D6 activity by paroxetine is associated with nonstationary PK in CYP2D6 extensive metabolizers [47]. Likewise, DDIs with coadministered drugs whose clearance is mediated by CYP2D6 have been demonstrated [48–50]. Against this backdrop, *in vitro* metabolism studies with the doubly deuterated paroxetine analogue CTP-347 (Figure 3.14) demonstrated little to no time-dependent inactivation of CYP2D6, apparently due to a dramatic reduction in the formation of the reactive carbene intermediate [51]. CTP-347 is currently in clinical trials for the treatment of hot flashes in menopausal women. CTP-347 has been studied in a 96-patient single- and multiple-ascending dose

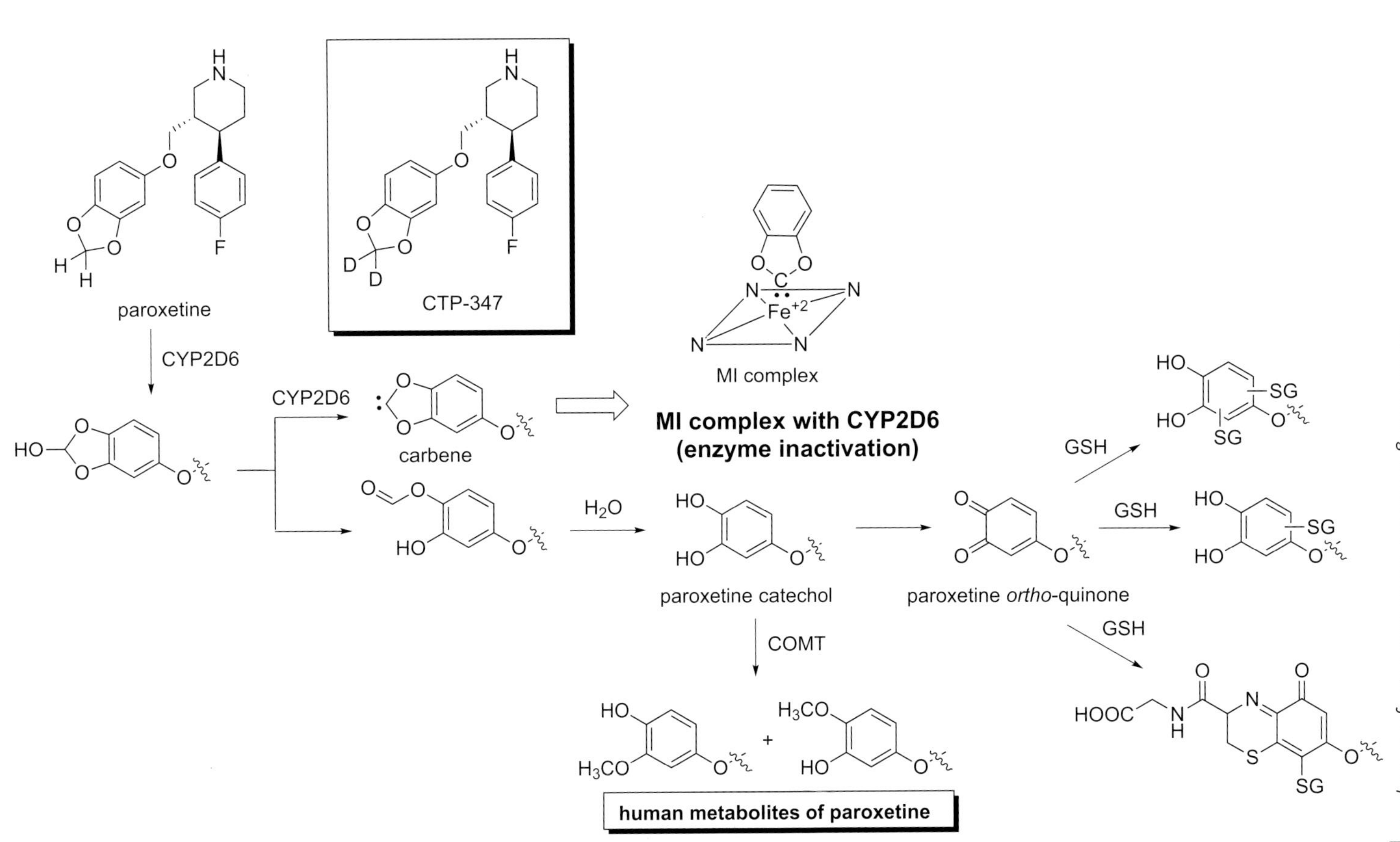

Figure 3.14 Attenuating CYP mechanism-based inactivation liability through deuterium incorporation at the metabolically labile site as illustrated with the antidepressant paroxetine.

clinical trial. The multiple-dose subjects initially received a single dose of dextromethorphan (a probe CYP2D6 substrate), followed by 14 days of treatment with CTP-347, and then another single dose of dextromethorphan. Subjects receiving CTP-347 at 20–40 mg once a day (QD) retained substantially greater ability to metabolize dextromethorphan compared to treatment with paroxetine administered at 20 mg QD (~15–20% inhibition of CYP2D6-catalyzed dextromethorphan metabolism to dextrorphan versus ~55–60% inhibition of CYP2D6 activity with paroxetine). As such, this DDI represents the first clinical demonstration that deuteration can be utilized to ameliorate DDI liabilities due to mechanism-based inactivation of CYP enzymes.

PF-562271 (Figure 3.15) is a dual inhibitor of the focal adhesion kinase and proline-rich tyrosine kinase 2 with potential utility in the treatment of ovarian cancer and osteoporosis [52]. *In vitro* metabolism studies in HLM revealed that PF-562271 is a CYP3A4 substrate and a time-dependent inactivator suggesting that the agent could inhibit its own clearance mechanism *in vivo*. The mechanism of CYP3A4 inactivation was shown to occur via a two-electron oxidation of the dianiline motif to a reactive diimine species, which was trapped with GSH (Figure 3.15) [53]. Furthermore, PF-562271 demonstrated supraproportional increases in oral systemic exposure upon repeated dosing in clinical trials, a phenomenon that was consistent with self-inactivation of its clearance mechanism. Likewise, PF-562271 also caused greater than threefold increase in the systemic exposure of the probe CYP3A4 substrate midazolam in a clinical DDI study. Insights into the mechanism of CYP3A4 inactivation allowed a rational medicinal chemistry strategy to reduce/eliminate enzyme inactivation liability [53]. Thus, simply exchanging the 5-aminooxindole nitrogen and carbonyl groups in the parent compound afforded analogues (e.g., **46**

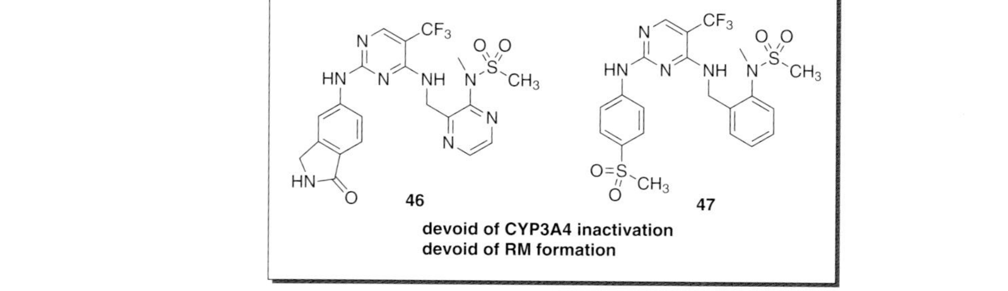

Figure 3.15 Strategies to eliminate CYP3A4 time-dependent inactivation by virtue of eliminating reactive diimine formation with oxindole-based focal adhesion kinase inhibitors.

and **47**) that were virtually devoid of CYP3A4 inactivation, while maintaining kinase potency. In general, disruption of the electron-rich dianiline structure present in PF-562271 also mitigated the formation of reactive diimine metabolites in the course of SAR studies [53].

In the course of SAR studies on a series of 1-amino-1,2,3,4-tetrahydronaphthalene-2-carboxylic acid derivatives as selective agonists for the human melanocortin-4 receptor and potential anti-obesity agents, lead compound **48** (Figure 3.16) demonstrated potent time- and concentration-dependent inactivation of CYP3A4 in a NADPH-dependent fashion, which was consistent with mechanism-based inactivation [54, 55]. Upon concomitant administration with CYP3A4 substrates in the clinic, increases in the area under the plasma concentration versus time curve for the victim drugs were expected to range from 4- to 10-fold as a result of the inactivation. The projected degree of clinical DDI was considered to be unacceptable for an anti-obesity indication and, as a result, **48** was eliminated from consideration as a development candidate. Studies were undertaken to understand the mechanism underlying **48**-mediated CYP3A4 inactivation to guide medicinal chemistry efforts. UV spectral analysis of incubations of **48** with recombinant CYP3A4 provided evidence for the formation of an MI complex between heme and

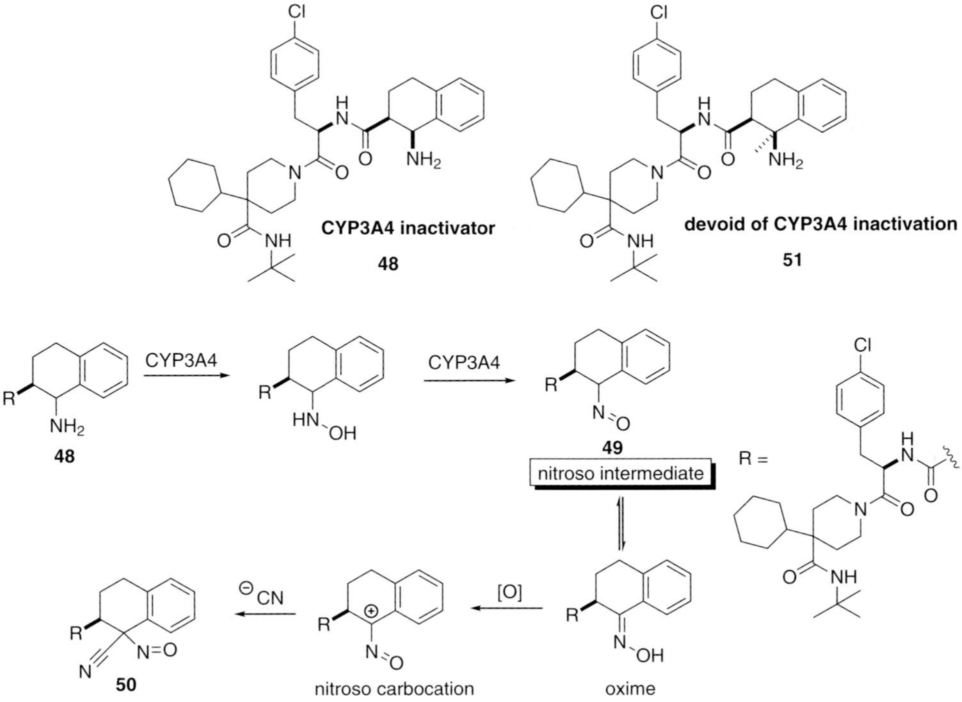

Figure 3.16 A strategy to eliminate CYP3A4 MBI liability in the selective melanocortin-4 receptor agonist **48**.

a RM of **48**. The RM was proposed to be the nitroso intermediate **49**, which is obtained from a two-electron oxidation of the initially formed hydroxylamine metabolite (Figure 3.16). Characterization of a geminal cyanonitroso adduct **50** in incubations of **48** in NADPH- and potassium cyanide-supplemented HLM was consistent with the proposed bioactivation pathway, wherein the nitroso intermediate would exist in a tautomeric equilibrium with the corresponding oxime derivative, which could be oxidized to an electrophilic nitroso carbocation and trapped by a cyanide ion [55]. Based on the insights gained from metabolism studies, it was envisioned that introducing an alkyl group α to the basic amine motif would shield this functionality from oxidation through steric hindrance, thereby reducing the probability of MI complex formation and CYP3A4 inactivation. Indeed analogue **51** (Figure 3.16) was synthesized and shown to be devoid of CYP3A4 inactivation while retaining the potent and selective melanocortin-4 receptor agonism observed with **48** [55].

3.9 Identification (and Elimination) of Electrophilic Lead Chemical Matter

Innately electrophilic compounds represent a significant liability in drug discovery because they often possess chemical reactivity similar to affinity labels (e.g., alkyl halides, Michael acceptors, and *N*-substituted maleimides); such compounds can alkylate proteins, DNA, and/or GSH, leading to toxicity. Because of the potential safety concerns, electrophilic functional groups are generally avoided in drug design. Examination of the medicinal chemistry literature, however, reveals several examples of seemingly "chemically inert" compounds, which are prone to nucleophilic displacement by GSH under nonenzymatic (pH 7.4, phosphate buffer, 37 °C) and/or enzymatic conditions. In the case of enzyme-assisted reactions, GSH conjugation to electrophilic centers is mediated by microsomal, cytosolic, and/or mitochondrial glutathione *S*-transferases. RM trapping studies have been effectively used to identify intrinsically electrophilic compounds in discovery programs. An example was recently disclosed with the oncology clinical candidate AMG458 (Figure 3.17), which covalently adducted to liver microsomal proteins in the absence of NADPH [56]. Subsequent incubations of AMG458 with GSH and *N*-acetylcysteine led to the identification of thiol conjugates derived from the nucleophilic displacement of an unanticipated electrophilic site on the molecule. Likewise, in the glucokinase activator program for treatment of type 2 diabetes, a unique metabolic liability of the 4-sulfonyl-2-pyridone ring system (e.g., compound **52**, Figure 3.17) was identified, wherein the heterocycle readily underwent conjugation with GSH under nonenzymatic as well as enzyme-catalyzed conditions [57, 58]. Identification of the electrophilic nature of 4-sulfonyl-2-pyridone motif prevented further investment in this series, and instead led to efforts centered on the optimization of a series of benzofuran derivatives, from which emerged the clinical candidate **53** (see Figure 3.17) [59].

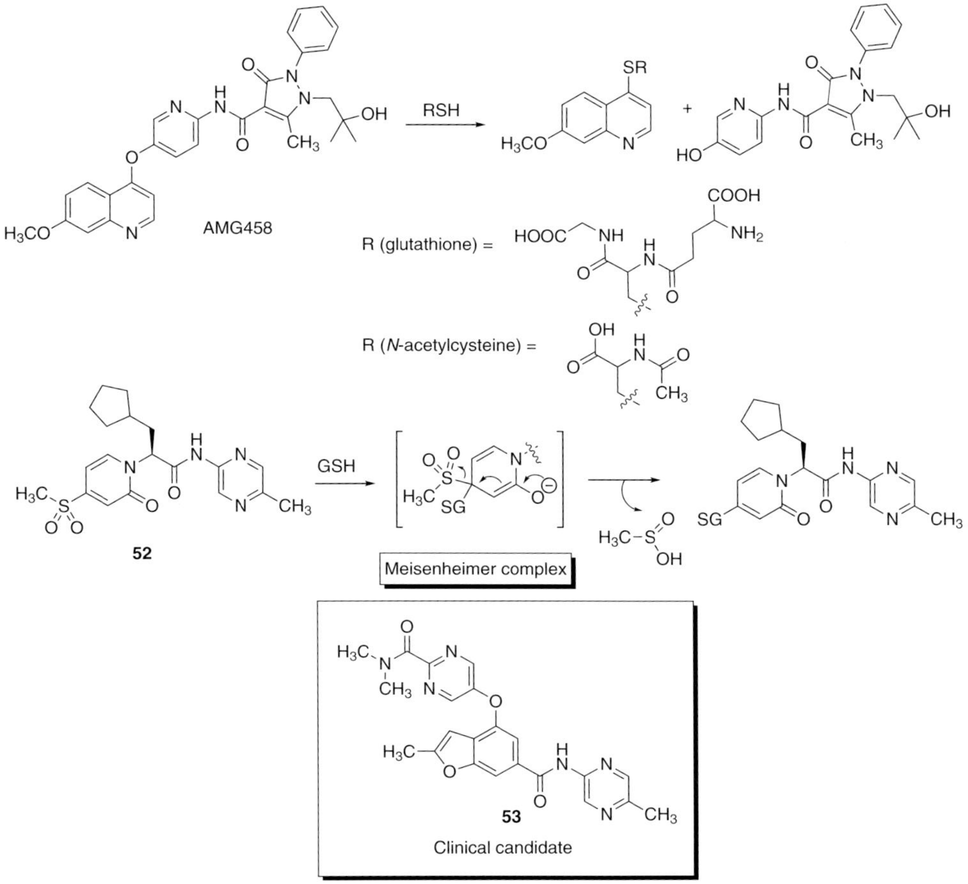

Figure 3.17 Identification of innately electrophilic lead chemical matter in drug discovery.

3.10
Mitigating Risks of Idiosyncratic Toxicity via Elimination of RM Formation

While the potential for DDI and genotoxicity can be examined directly from *in vitro* assays, the same does not often hold true for immune-mediated IADRs (e.g., hepatotoxicity, skin rashes, agranulocytosis, and aplastic anemia) in drug-treated patients. IADRs are unrelated to known drug pharmacology, and are generally dose independent (a notable exception is the dose-dependent hepatotoxicity caused by acetaminophen). Because the incidence of IADRs is very low (1 in 10 000 to 1 in 100 000), these reactions are often not detected, until the drug has gained broad exposure in a large patient population. The concept of human drug-induced hepatotoxicity via RM formation was provided from studies on the anti-inflammatory agent and hepatotoxin acetaminophen [60]. Mechanistic studies that established the CYP-mediated oxidation of acetaminophen to a reactive quinone imine intermediate NAPQI [61], capable of depleting GSH levels and/or binding covalently to liver macromolecules, have served as a paradigm for drug toxicity assessment over the decades.

An understanding of the biochemical basis for drug toxicity has aided to replace the vague perception of a chemical class effect with a sharper picture of individual molecular peculiarity. There are several instances of prototype drugs associated with IADRs that also form RM(s) and elimination of RM liability in follow-on successor agent(s) markedly improves the safety profile. Although the evidence is most often anecdotal in nature, a compelling case for chemotype-based toxicity can be inferred from such structure–toxicity analyses [62]. For instance, while clozapine use is limited by a high incidence of agranulocytosis, hepatotoxicity, and myocarditis, quetiapine and loxapine are not associated with these adverse events. Clozapine exhibits covalent binding to human neutrophil proteins *in vitro*, via myeloperoxidase-mediated oxidation of the dibenzodiazepine ring to a reactive iminium ion, which covalently binds to the target tissues and also reacts with GSH (Figure 3.18) [63]. Proteins covalently modified with clozapine have been observed in neutrophils of patients being treated with clozapine, which reaffirms the relevance of the *in vitro* studies [64]. In contrast, quetiapine and loxapine cannot form a reactive iminium [65], since the bridging nitrogen atom is replaced with a sulfur or oxygen atom, respectively (Figure 3.18). In the case of the nonsteroidal anti-inflammatory drug sudoxicam, hepatotoxicity observed in the clinic that led to its suspension in clinical trials has been attributed to thiazole ring scission yielding a reactive acylthiourea metabolite capable of oxidizing GSH and proteins (Figure 3.18) [66]. The structurally related anti-inflammatory drug meloxicam does not possess the hepatotoxic liability associated with sudoxicam. Although introduction of a methyl group at the C-5 position on the thiazole ring in meloxicam is the only structural difference, the change dramatically alters the metabolic profile such that oxidation of the C-5 methyl group to the alcohol (and carboxylic acid) metabolite(s) constitutes the principal metabolic fate of meloxicam in humans (Figure 3.18).

Because of the inability to predict and quantitate the risk of IADRs and because RMs as opposed to the parent molecules from which they are derived are thought to be responsible for the pathogenesis of many IADRs, detection of RM in the course of metabolism is considered to be an undesirable trait in preclinical drug discovery.

3.11 Case Studies on Elimination of RM Liability in Drug Discovery

Examples of medicinal chemistry tactics to eliminate RM formation are abundant in the primary literature. A recent example, which focuses on eliminating RM liability within a lead chemical series, is evident with pyrazinone-based corticotropin-releasing factor-1 receptor antagonists and potential antidepressant/anti-anxiolytic drugs [67]. A major portion of the clearance mechanism of the lead pyrazinone **54**

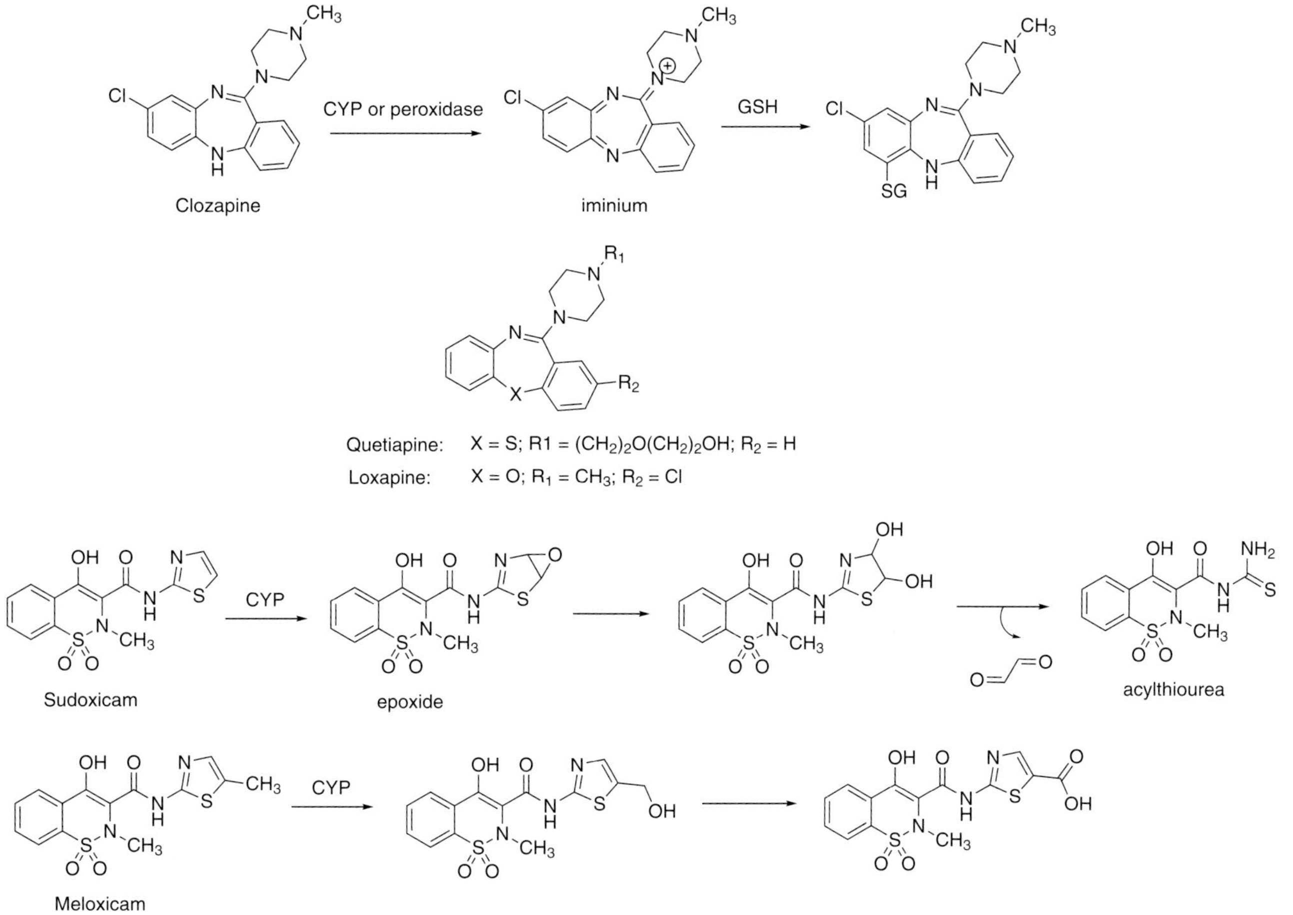

Clozapine → (CYP or peroxidase) → iminium → (GSH)

Quetiapine: X = S; R1 = $(CH_2)_2O(CH_2)_2OH$; R_2 = H

Loxapine: X = O; R_1 = CH_3; R_2 = Cl

Sudoxicam → (CYP) → epoxide → → acylthiourea

Meloxicam → (CYP) → →

Figure 3.18 Structure–toxicity relationships for idiosyncratic drug toxicity.

in rats comprised of conjugation with GSH, consistent with RM formation *in vivo* [68]. Two distinct metabolic activation pathways were deciphered (Figure 3.19): (a) oxidative metabolism on the chloropyrazinone ring to yield an electrophilic epoxide and (b) *O*-dealkylation of the difluoromethylphenoxy moiety to yield a phenol metabolite **55**, two electrons of which generated a reactive quinone imine species. To eliminate RM formation on the 2,6-dichloroaniline motif, the pyridyl group was incorporated as a bioisosteric replacement. To prevent epoxidation on the 5-chloropyrazinone ring, the chlorine atom was replaced with more strongly electron-withdrawing groups (e.g., cyano). Out of this iterative medicinal chemistry exercise emerged **56** (Figure 3.19) with sufficiently diminished RM formation in liver microsomes from rats and humans. Consistent with the *in vitro* finding, <2–4% of GSH conjugates were recovered in rat bile following *in vivo* administration of **56**. Compound **56** also retained all of the primary pharmacology and pharmacokinetic properties of **54**.

A second example is depicted with nonpeptidyl thrombopoietin receptor agonists exemplified by **57** [69]. In the course of routine metabolite identification studies, it was found that 4-(4-fluoro-3-(trifluoromethyl)phenyl)thiazol-2-amine (**58**), the product of carboxylesterase-mediated hydrolysis of **57**, formed RMs in HLM. GSH trapping studies led to the formation of two conjugates derived from the addition of the thiol nucleophile to **58** and a thiazole-*S*-oxide metabolite of **58** (i.e., compound **59**) (Figure 3.20). Mass spectral fragmentation and ^{1}H NMR analysis indicated that the site of attachment of the GSH moiety in both conjugates was the C-5 position in the thiazole ring. Based on the structures of the GSH conjugates, two metabolic activation pathways were proposed, one involving β-elimination of an initially formed hydroxylamine metabolite and the other involving direct two-electron oxidation of the electron-rich 2-aminothiazole system to RM. The mechanistic insights gained from the metabolism studies influenced subsequent medicinal chemistry strategies, which involved blocking the C-5 position with a fluorine atom (compound **60**)

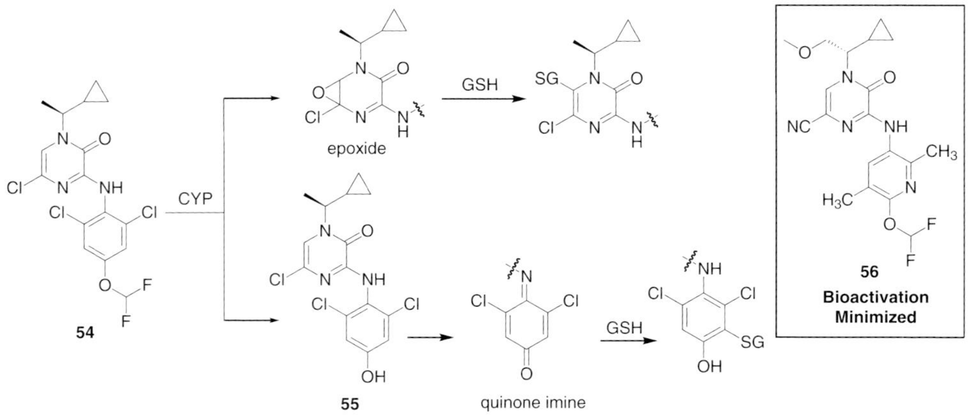

Figure 3.19 Eliminating RM liability with a series of pyrazinone-based corticotropin-releasing factor-1 receptor antagonists.

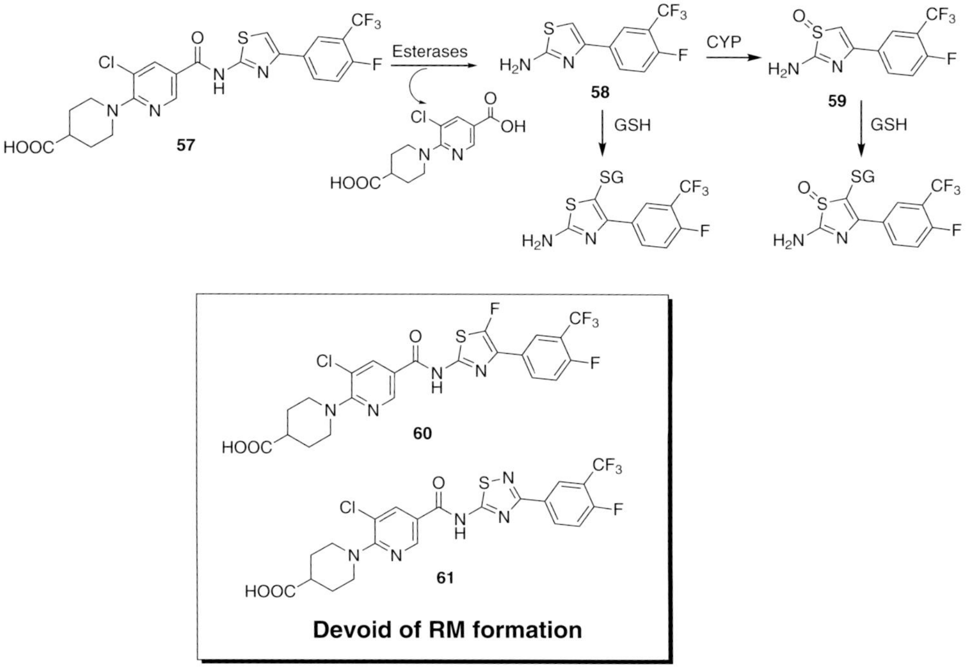

Figure 3.20 Eliminating RM liability with acetamido-thiazolyl nonpeptidyl thrombopoietin receptor agonists.

or replacing the thiazole ring with a 1,2,4-thiadiazole group (compound **61**) (Figure 3.20). These structural changes not only abrogated RM liability associated with **58** but also resulted in compounds that retained the attractive pharmacological and pharmacokinetic attributes of the prototype agent. Compound **60** was considered for further preclinical profiling as a clinical candidate [70].

Strategies toward eliminating metabolic activation of the electron-rich 4-hydroxyaniline motif have also been described by Park and coworkers with the antimalarial agent amodiaquine. The clinical use of amodiaquine is somewhat restricted by several cases of hepatotoxicity and agranulocytosis; the detection of IgG antibodies in patients exposed to the drug is consistent with an immune-mediated hypersensitivity reaction [71]. The immune-mediated toxicity is believed to arise from the metabolism of amodiaquine to a reactive quinone imine species that can covalently bind to cellular proteins or GSH (Figure 3.21) [72, 73]. Exchanging the C′-4-phenolic OH group with a fluorine atom results in compound **62** that prevents RM formation (Figure 3.21) [74]. An alternate approach to prevent RM formation involved the isomerization of the 3′- and 4′-substituents in amodiaquine; from this exercise emerged analogues **63** and **64**, which were devoid of RM formation (judged from the lack of formation of GSH conjugates) and were advanced to further profiling as the next generation of antimalarials based on their favorable pharmacokinetic and pharmacodynamic attributes (Figure 3.21) [75, 76].

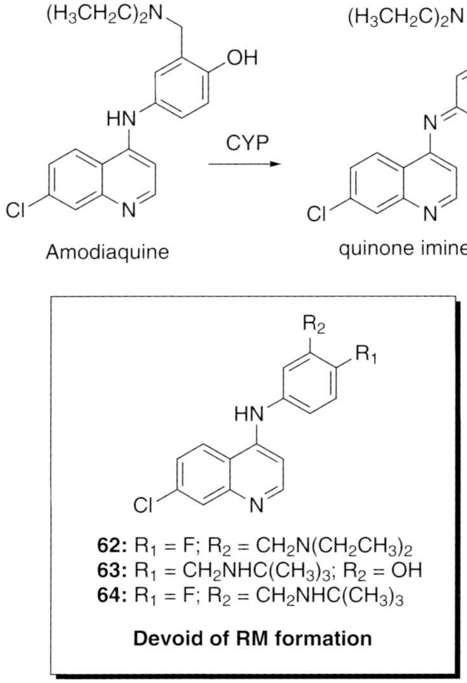

$(H_3CH_2C)_2N$ OH HN Cl N CYP $(H_3CH_2C)_2N$ O N Cl N

Amodiaquine quinone imine

R_2 R_1 HN Cl N

62: R_1 = F; R_2 = $CH_2N(CH_2CH_3)_2$
63: R_1 = $CH_2NHC(CH_3)_3$; R_2 = OH
64: R_1 = F; R_2 = $CH_2NHC(CH_3)_3$

Devoid of RM formation

Figure 3.21 Metabolism-directed efforts in the discovery of amodiaquine backup clinical candidates.

In the course of discovery efforts leading to the discovery of taranabant (Figure 3.22), a selective and potent inhibitor of the cannabinoid-1 (CB-1) receptor, and phase III clinical candidate for the treatment of obesity, lead compound **65** (Figure 3.22) revealed a high level of covalent binding to HLM in a NADPH-dependent fashion, consistent with RM formation. Elucidation of the structure of the GSH conjugate suggested that the RM was an arene oxide intermediate derived from epoxidation of the electron-rich phenoxy ring [77]. Replacement of the phenoxy ring with the trifluoromethylpyridyl ring afforded taranabant, which was devoid of RM formation, while retaining potency against the CB-1 receptor.

The final illustration concerns the antiepileptic drug felbamate, which is associated with several cases of aplastic anemia and hepatotoxicity [78]. Evidence has been presented that links felbamate-induced toxicity to its metabolism to the highly reactive α,β-unsaturated carbonyl compound atropaldehyde (2-phenylpropenal, **68**) (Figure 3.23) [79, 80]. The rate-limiting step for the formation of **68** involves amidase-mediated hydrolysis of one of the carbamate groups in felbamate to yield the corresponding primary alcohol **66**. Alcohol dehydrogenase-catalyzed oxidation of **66** yields the aldehyde intermediate **67**, which undergoes β-elimination to yield **68**, carbon dioxide, and ammonia. Compound **68**, being a α,β-unsaturated carbonyl derivative, readily reacts with GSH to afford conjugate **69**. Downstream

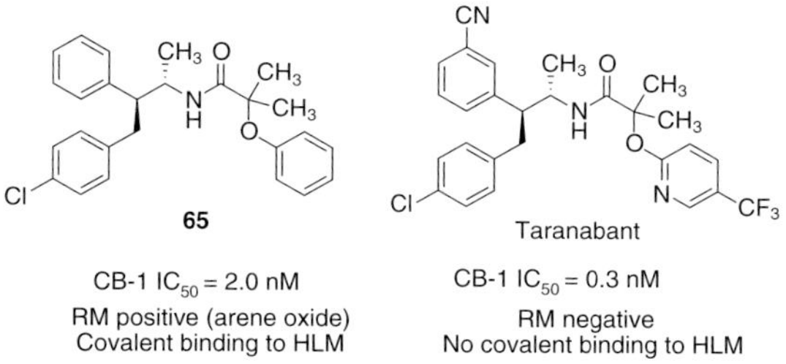

Figure 3.22 Elimination of RM liability in the discovery of taranabant, a selective and potent CB-1 receptor antagonist and anti-obesity agent.

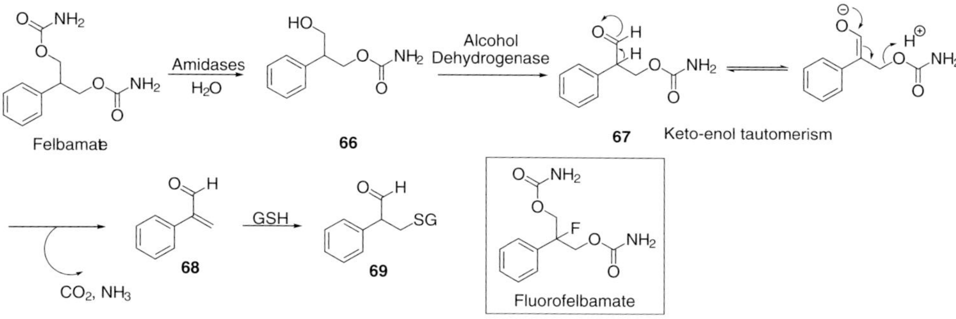

Figure 3.23 Designing a felbamate analogue that is devoid of RM formation.

mercapturic acid conjugates (breakdown products of GSH such as cysteine and *N*-acetylcysteine) of **68** have been detected in urine from patients treated with felbamate that supports the mechanistic pathway [81]. The mechanistic information on felbamate bioactivation to the electrophilic species **68** has been utilized to design fluorofelbamate, which cannot undergo the β-elimination chemistry to the reactive α,β-unsaturated carbonyl intermediate because of the replacement of the acidic benzylic hydrogen with a fluorine atom (see Figure 3.23) [82].

3.12 Concluding Remarks

It is clear from our own experience and from the general literature that the application of metabolism studies and concepts has been readily embraced by the pharmaceutical industry as an approach to mitigating attrition due to poor pharmacokinetics [83]. The real value of metabolism studies in drug discovery lies in the identification of relevant clearance mechanisms for lead chemical matter, which then dictates the choice of *in vitro* models for making projections of human pharmacokinetics prior to first-in-human testing. Similarly, the value in identifying metabolic hot spots is not the structural characterization itself, but in enabling the understanding of SAR. Recently, much effort has gone into understanding RM, and although the link between metabolism and safety is elusive, it remains prudent to continue to explore these relationships as early as possible in drug development, if for no other reason than to give chemists the option of pursuing alternate chemical series devoid of such concerns if possible.

References

1 Riley, R.J. (2001) The potential pharmacological and toxicological impact of P450 screening. *Curr. Opin. Drug Discov. Dev.*, **4** (1), 45–54.

2 Pryde, D.C., Dalvie, D., Hu, Q., Jones, P., Obach, R.S., and Tran, T.D. (2010) Aldehyde oxidase: an enzyme of emerging importance in drug discovery. *J. Med. Chem.*, **53** (24), 8441–8460.

3 Kalgutkar, A.S., Dalvie, D.K., Castagnoli, N., Jr., and Taylor, T.J. (2001) Interactions of nitrogen-containing xenobiotics with monoamine oxidase (MAO) isozymes A and B: SAR studies on MAO substrates and inhibitors. *Chem. Res. Toxicol.*, **14** (9), 1139–1162.

4 Bu, H.Z. (2006) A literature review of enzyme kinetic parameters for CYP3A4-mediated metabolic reactions of 113 drugs in human liver microsomes: structure–kinetics relationship assessment. *Curr. Drug Metab.*, **7** (3), 231–249.

5 Stepan, A.F., Karki, K., McDonald, W.S., Dorff, P.H., Dutra, J.K., Dirico, K.J., Won, A., Subramanyam, C., Efremov, I.V., O'Donnell, C.J., Nolan, C.E., Becker, S.L., Pustilnik, L.R., Sneed, B., Sun, H., Lu, Y., Robshaw, A.E., Riddell, D., O'Sullivan, T.J., Sibley, E., Capetta, S., Atchison, K., Hallgren, A.J., Miller, E., Wood, A., and Obach, R.S. (2011) Metabolism-directed design of oxetane-containing arylsulfonamide derivatives as γ-secretase inhibitors. *J. Med. Chem.*, **54** (22), 7772–7783.

6 Cheng, Y., Zhang, F., Rano, T.A., Lu, Z., Scheif, W.A., Gabryelski, L., Olsen, D.B., Stahlhut, M., Rutkowski, C.A., Lin, J.H., Jin, L., Emini, E.A., Chapman, K.T., and Tata, J.R. (2002) Indinavir analogues with blocked metabolism sites as HIV protease inhibitors with improved pharmacological profiles and high potency against PI-resistant viral strains. *Bioorg. Med. Chem. Lett.*, **12** (17), 2419–2422.

7 Floyd, D.M., Kimball, S.D., Krapcho, J., Das, J., Turk, C.F., Moquin, R.V., Lago, M. W., Duff, K.J., Lee, V.G., White, R.E., Ridgewell, R.E., Moreland, S., Brittain, R.J., Normandin, D.E., Hedberg, S.A., and Cucinotta, G.C. (1992) Benzazepinone calcium channel blockers. 2. Structure–activity and drug metabolism studies leading to potent antihypertensive agents. Comparison with benzothiazepinones. *J. Med. Chem.*, **35** (4), 756–772.

8 Park, B.K., Kitteringham, N.R., and O'Neill, P.M. (2001) Metabolism of fluorine-containing drugs. *Annu. Rev. Pharmacol. Toxicol.*, **41**, 443–470.

9 Fisher, M.B., Henne, K.R., and Boer, J. (2006) The complexities inherent in attempts to decrease drug clearance by blocking sites of CYP-mediated metabolism. *Curr. Opin. Drug Discov. Dev.*, **9** (1), 101–109.

10 Moorjani, M., Luo, Z., Lin, E., Vong, B.G., Chen, Y., Zhang, X., Rueter, J.K., Gross, R.S., Lanier, M.C., Tellew, J.E., Williams, J.P., Lechner, S.M., Malany, S., Santos, M., Crespo, M.I., Dőaz, J.-L., Saunders, J., and Slee, D.H. (2008) 2,6-Diaryl-4-acylaminopyrimidines as potent and selective adenosine A_{2A} antagonists with improved solubility and metabolic

stability. *Bioorg. Med. Chem. Lett.*, **18** (20), 5402–5405.

11 Eldrup, A.B., Soleymanzadeh, F., Taylor, S.J., Muegge, I., Farrow, N.A., Joseph, D., McKellop, K., Man, C.C., Kukulka, A., and De Lombaert, S. (2009) Structure-based optimization of arylamides as inhibitors of soluble epoxide hydrolase. *J. Med. Chem.*, **52** (19), 5880–5895.

12 Burgey, C.S., Robinson, K.A., Lyle, T.A., Sanderson, P.E.J., Lewis, S.D., Lucas, B.J., Krueger, J.A., Singh, R., Miller-Stein, C., White, R.A., Wong, B., Lyle, E.A., Williams, P.D., Coburn, C.A., Dorsey, B. D., Barrow, J.C., Stranieri, M.T., Holahan, M.A., Sitko, G.R., Cook, J.J., McMasters, D.R., McDonough, C.M., Sanders, W.M., Wallace, A.A., Clayton, F.C., Bohn, D., Leonard, Y.M., Detwiler, T.J., Jr., Lynch, J.J., Jr., Yan, Y., Chen, Z., Kuo, L., Gardell, S.J., Shafer, J.A., and Vacca, J.P. (2003) Metabolism-directed optimization of 3-aminopyrazinone acetamide thrombin inhibitors. Development of an orally bioavailable series containing P1 and P3 pyridines. *J. Med. Chem.*, **46** (4), 461–473.

13 Dugar, S., Yumibe, N., Clader, J.W., Vizziano, M., Huie, K., Van Heek, M., Compton, D.S., and Davis, H.R., Jr. (1996) Metabolism and structure activity data based drug design: discovery of (−)-SCH53079, an analog of the potent cholesterol absorption inhibitor (−)-SCH48461. *Bioorg. Med. Chem. Lett.*, **6** (11), 1271–1274.

14 Kirkup, M.P., Rizvi, R., Shanker, B.B., Dugar, S., Clader, J.W., McCombie, S.W., Lin, S.-I., Yumibe, N., Huie, K., Van Heek, M., Compton, D.S., Davis, H.R., Jr., and McPhail, A.T. (1996) (−)-SCH 57939: synthesis and pharmacological properties of a potent, metabolically stable cholesterol absorption inhibitor. *Bioorg. Med. Chem. Lett.*, **6** (17), 2069–2072.

15 Rosenblum, S.B., Huynh, T., Afonso, A., Davis, H.R., Jr., Yumibe, N., Clader, J.W., and Burnett, D.A. (1998) Discovery of 1-(4-fluorophenyl)-(3*R*)-[3-(4-fluorophenyl)-(3*S*)-hydroxypropyl]-(4*S*)-(4-hydroxyphenyl)-2-azetidinone (SCH 58235): a designed, potent, orally active inhibitor of cholesterol absorption. *J. Med. Chem.*, **41** (6), 973–980.

16 Penning, T.D., Talley, J.J., Bertenshaw, S.R., Carter, J.S., Collins, P.W., Docter, S., Graneto, M.J., Lee, L.F., Malecha, J.W., Rogers, R.S., Rogier, D.J., Yu, S.S., Anderson, G.D., Burton, E.G., Cogburn, J.N., Gregory, S.A., Koboldt, C.M., Perkins, W.E., Seibert, K., Veenhuizen, A. W., Zhang, Y.Y., and Isakson, P.C. (1997) Synthesis and biological evaluation of the 1,5-diarylpyrazole class of cyclooxygenase-2 inhibitors: identification of 4-[5-(4-methylphenyl)-3-(trifluoromethyl)-1*H*-pyrazol-1-yl]benzenesulfonamide (SC-58635, celecoxib). *J. Med. Chem.*, **40** (9), 1347–1365.

17 Southers, J.A., Bauman, J.N., Price, D.A., Humphries, P.S., Balan, G., Sagal, J.F., Maurer, T.S., Zhang, Y., Oliver, R., Herr, M., Healy, D.R., Li, M., Kapinos, B., Fate, G.D., Riccardi, K.A., Paralkar, V.M., Brown, T.A., and Kalgutkar, A.S. (2010) Metabolism-guided design of short-acting calcium-sensing receptor antagonists. *ACS Med. Chem. Lett.*, **1**, 219–223.

18 Middleton, D.S., Andrews, M., Glossop, P., Gymer, G., Hepworth, D., Jessiman, A., Johnson, P.S., MacKenny, M., Stobie, A., Tang, K., Morgan, P., and Jones, B. (2008) Designing rapid onset selective serotonin re-uptake inhibitors. Part 3. Site-directed metabolism as a strategy to avoid active circulating metabolites: structure–activity relationships of (thioalkyl)phenoxy benzylamines. *Bioorg. Med. Chem. Lett.*, **18** (19), 5303–5306.

19 Magee, T.V., Ripp, S.L., Li, B., Buzon, R.A., Chupak, L., Dougherty, T.J., Finegan, S.M., Girard, D., Hagen, A.E., Falcone, M.J., Farley, K.A., Granskog, K., Hardink, J.R., Huband, M.D., Kamicker, B.J., Kaneko, T., Knickerbocker, M.J., Liras, J.L., Marra, A., Medina, I., Nguyen, T.T., Noe, M.C., Obach, R.S., O'Donnell, J.P., Penzien, J.B., Reilly, U.D., Schafer, J.R., Shen, Y., Stone, G.G., Strelevitz, T.J., Sun, J., Tait-Kamradt, A., Vaz, A.D., Whipple, D.A., Widlicka, D.W., Wishka, D.G., Wolkowski, J.P., and Flanagan, M.E. (2009) Discovery of azetidinyl ketolides for the treatment of susceptible and multidrug resistant community-acquired respiratory tract infections. *J. Med. Chem.*, **52** (23), 7446–7457.

20 Linton, A., Kang, P., Ornelas, M., Kephart, S., Hu, Q., Pairish, M., Jiang, Y., and Guo, C. (2011) Systematic structure modifications of imidazo[1,2-*a*]pyrimidine to reduce metabolism mediated by aldehyde oxidase (AO). *J. Med. Chem.*, **54** (21), 7705–7712.

21 Dixon, C.M., Park, G.R., and Tarbit, M.H. (1994) Characterization of the enzyme responsible for the metabolism of sumatriptan in human liver. *Biochem. Pharmacol.*, **47** (7), 1253–1257.

22 McEnroe, J.D., and Fleishaker, J.C. (2005) Clinical pharmacokinetics of almotriptan, a serotonin 5-HT(1B/1D) receptor agonist for the treatment of migraine. *Clin. Pharmacokinet.*, **44** (3), 237–246.

23 Vyas, K.P., Halpin, R.A., Geer, L.A., Ellis, J.D., Liu, L., Cheng, H., Chavez-Eng, C., Matuszewski, B.K., Varga, S.L., Guiblin, A.R., and Rogers, J.D. (2000) Disposition and pharmacokinetics of the antimigraine drug, rizatriptan, in humans. *Drug Metab. Dispos.*, **28** (1), 89–95.

24 Wild, M.J., McKillop, D., and Butters, C.J. (1999) Determination of the human cytochrome P450 isoforms involved in the metabolism of zolmitriptan. *Xenobiotica*, **29** (8), 847–857.

25 Evans, D.C., O'Conner, D., Lake, B.G., Evers, R., Allen, C., and Hargreaves, R. (2003) Eletriptan metabolism by human hepatic CYP450 enzymes and transport by human P-glycoprotein. *Drug Metab. Dispos.*, **31** (7), 861–869.

26 Buchan, P., Keywood, C., Wade, A., and Ward, C. (2002) Clinical pharmacokinetics of frovatriptan. *Headache*, **42** (Suppl. 2), S54–S62.

27 Tfelt-Hansen, P., De Vries, P., and Saxena, P.R. (2000) Triptans in migraine: a comparative review of pharmacology, pharmacokinetics and efficacy. *Drugs*, **60** (6), 1259–1287.

28 Fisher, M.B., Paine, M.F., Strelevitz, T.J., and Wrighton, S.A. (2001) The role of hepatic and extrahepatic UDP-glucuronosyltransferases in human drug metabolism. *Drug Metab. Rev.*, **33** (3–4), 273–297.

29 Lindsay, J., Wang, L.L., Li, Y., and Zhou, S.F. (2008) Structure, function and polymorphism of human cytosolic sulfotransferases. *Curr. Drug Metab.*, **9** (2), 99–105.

30 Honma, W., Shimada, M., Sasano, H., Ozawa, S., Miyata, M., Nagata, K., Ikeda, T., and Yamazoe, Y. (2002) Phenol sulfotransferase, ST1A3, as the main enzyme catalyzing sulfation of troglitazone in human liver. *Drug Metab. Dispos.*, **30** (8), 944–949.

31 Borzilleri, R.M., Cai, Z.W., Ellis, C., Fargnoli, J., Fura, A., Gerhardt, T., Goyal, B., Hunt, J.T., Mortillo, S., Qian, L., Tokarski, J., Vyas, V., Wautlet, B., Zheng, X., and Bhide, R.S. (2005) Synthesis and SAR of 4-(3-hydroxyphenylamino)pyrrolo[2,1-*f*][1,2,4]triazine based VEGFR-2 kinase inhibitors. *Bioorg. Med. Chem. Lett.*, **15** (5), 1429–1433.

32 Stewart, A.O., Bhatia, P.A., Martin, J.G., Summers, J.B., Rodriques, K.E., Martin, M.B., Holms, J.H., Moore, J.L., Craig, R.A., Kolasa, T., Ratajczyk, J.D., Mazdiyasni, H., Kerdesky, F.A., DeNinno, S.L., Maki, R.G., Bouska, J.B., Young, P.R., Lanni, C., Bell, R.L., Carter, G.W., and Brooks, C.D. (1997) Structure–activity relationships of *N*-hydroxyurea 5-lipoxygenase inhibitors. *J. Med. Chem.*, **40** (13), 1955–1968.

33 Awni, W.M., Braeckman, R.A., Granneman, G.R., Witt, G., and Dube, L.M. (1995) Pharmacokinetics and pharmacodynamics of zileuton after oral administration of single and multiple dose regimens of zileuton 600 mg in healthy volunteers. *Clin. Pharmacokinet.*, **29** (Suppl. 2), 22–33.

34 Dobo, K.L., Obach, R.S., Luffer-Atlas, D., and Bercu, J.P. (2009) A strategy for the risk assessment of human genotoxic metabolites. *Chem. Res. Toxicol.*, **22** (2), 348–356.

35 Kalgutkar, A.S., Obach, R.S., and Maurer, T.S. (2007) Mechanism-based inactivation of cytochrome P450 enzymes: chemical mechanisms, structure–activity relationships and relationship to clinical drug–drug interactions and idiosyncratic adverse drug reactions. *Curr. Drug Metab.*, **8** (5), 407–447.

36 Stepan, A.F., Walker, D.P., Bauman, J., Price, D.A., Baillie, T.A., Kalgutkar, A.S., and Aleo, M.D. (2011) Structural alert/reactive metabolite concept as

applied in medicinal chemistry to mitigate the risk of idiosyncratic drug toxicity: a perspective based on the critical examination of trends in the top 200 drugs marketed in the United States. *Chem. Res. Toxicol.*, **24** (9), 1345–1410.

37 Park, B.K., Boobis, A., Clarke, S., Goldring, C.E., Jones, D., Kenna, J.G., Lambert, C., Laverty, H.G., Naisbitt, D.J., Nelson, S., Nicoll-Griffith, D.A., Obach, R. S., Routledge, P., Smith, D.A., Tweedie, D. J., Vermeulen, N., Williams, D.P., Wilson, I.D., and Baillie, T.A. (2011) Managing the challenge of chemical reactive metabolites in drug development. *Nat. Rev. Drug Discov.*, **10** (4), 292–306.

38 Kumar, S., Kassahun, K., Tschirret-Guth, R.A., Mitra, K., and Baillie, T.A. (2008) Minimizing metabolic activation during pharmaceutical lead optimization: progress, knowledge gaps and future directions. *Curr. Opin. Drug Discov. Dev.*, **11** (1), 43–52.

39 Guengerich, F.P. and MacDonald, J.S. (2007) Applying mechanisms of chemical toxicity to predict drug safety. *Chem. Res. Toxicol.*, **20** (3), 344–369.

40 Kalgutkar, A.S., Dalvie, D.K., Aubrecht, J., Smith, E.B., Coffing, S.L., Cheung, J.R., Vage, C., Lame, M.E., Chiang, P., McClure, K.F., Maurer, T.S., Coelho, R.V., Jr., Soliman, V.F., and Schildknegt, K. (2007) Genotoxicity of 2-(3-chlorobenzyloxy)-6-(piperazinyl)pyrazine, a novel 5-hydroxytryptamine 2C receptor agonist for the treatment of obesity: role of metabolic activation. *Drug Metab. Dispos.*, **35** (6), 848–858.

41 Kalgutkar, A.S., Bauman, J.N., McClure, K.F., Aubrecht, J., Cortina, S.R., and Paralkar, J. (2009) Biochemical basis for differences in metabolism-dependent genotoxicity by two diazinylpiperazine-based 5-HT2C receptor agonists. *Bioorg. Med. Chem. Lett.*, **19** (6), 1559–1563.

42 Lim, H.-K., Chen, J., Sensenhauser, C., Cook, K., Preston, R., Thomas, T., Shook, B., Jackson, P.F., Rassnick, S., Rhodes, K., Gopaul, V., Salter, R., Silva, J., and Evans, D.C. (2011) Overcoming the genotoxicity of a pyrrolidine substituted arylindenopyrimidine as a potent dual adenosine A_{2A}/A_1 antagonist by minimizing bioactivation to an iminium ion reactive intermediate. *Chem. Res. Toxicol.*, **24** (7), 1012–1030.

43 Bertelsen, K.M., Venkatakrishnan, K., Von Moltke, L.L., Obach, R.S., and Greenblatt, D.J. (2003) Apparent mechanism-based inhibition of human CYP2D6 *in vitro* by paroxetine: comparison with fluoxetine and quinidine. *Drug Metab. Dispos.*, **31** (3), 289–293.

44 Murray, M. (2000) Mechanisms of inhibitory and regulatory effects of methylenedioxyphenyl compounds on cytochrome P450-dependent drug oxidation. *Curr. Drug Metab.*, **1** (1), 67–84.

45 Haddock, R.E., Johnson, A.M., Langley, P. F., Nelson, D.R., Pope, J.A., Thomas, D. R., and Woods, F.R. (1989) Metabolic pathways of paroxetine in animals and man and the comparative pharmacological properties of its metabolites. *Acta Psychiatr. Scand. Suppl.*, **350**, 24–26.

46 Zhao, S.X., Dalvie, D.K., Kelly, J.M., Soglia, J.R., Frederick, K.S., Smith, E.B., Obach, R.S., and Kalgutkar, A.S. (2007) NADPH-dependent covalent binding of [3*H*]paroxetine to human liver microsomes and S-9 fractions: identification of an electrophilic quinone metabolite of paroxetine. *Chem. Res. Toxicol.*, **20** (11), 1649–1657.

47 Kaye, C.M., Haddock, R.E., Langley, P.F., Mellows, G., Tasker, T.C., Zussman, B.D., and Greb, W.H. (1989) A review of the metabolism and pharmacokinetics of paroxetine in man. *Acta Psychiatr. Scand. Suppl.*, **350**, 60–75.

48 Hemeryck, A., Lefebyre, R.A., De Vriendt, C., and Belpaire, F.M. (2000) Paroxetine affects metoprolol pharmacokinetics and pharmacodynamics in healthy volunteers. *Clin. Pharmacol. Ther.*, **67** (3), 283–291.

49 Spina, E., Avenoso, A., Facciola, G., Scordo, M.G., Ancione, M., and Madia, A. (2001) Plasma concentrations of risperidone and 9-hydroxyrisperidone during combined treatment with paroxetine. *Ther. Drug Monit.*, **23** (3), 223–227.

50 Belle, D.J., Ernest, C.S., Sauer, J.M., Smith, B.P., Thomasson, H.R., and Witcher, J.W. (2002) Effect of potent CYP2D6 inhibition by paroxetine on atomoxetine pharmacokinetics. *J. Clin. Pharmacol.*, **42** (11), 1219–1227.

51 Yarnell, A.T. (2009) Heavy-hydrogen drugs turn heads, again. *Chem. Eng. News*, **87** (25), 36–39.

52 Wendt, M.K., and Schiemann, W.P. (2009) Therapeutic targeting of the focal adhesion complex prevents oncogenic TGF-beta signaling and metastasis. *Breast Cancer Res.*, **11** (5), R68.

53 Walker, D.P., Bi, F.C., Kalgutkar, A.S., Bauman, J.N., Zhao, S.X., Soglia, J.R., Aspnes, G.E., Kung, D.W., Klug-McLeod, J., Zawistoski, M.P., McGlynn, M.A., Oliver, R., Dunn, M., Li, J.C., Richter, D.T., Cooper, B.A., Kath, J.C., Hulford, C.A., Autry, C.L., Luzzio, M.J., Ung, E.J., Roberts, W.G., Bonnette, P.C., Buckbinder, L., Mistry, A., Griffor, M.C., Han, S., and Guzman-Perez, A. (2008) Trifluoromethylpyrimidine-based inhibitors of proline-rich tyrosine kinase 2 (PYK2): structure–activity relationships and strategies for the elimination of reactive metabolite formation. *Bioorg. Med. Chem. Lett.*, **18** (23), 6071–6077.

54 Bakshi, R.K., Hong, Q., Olson, J.T., Ye, Z., Sebhat, I.K., Weinberg, D.H., MacNeil, T., Kalyani, R.N., Tang, R., Martin, W.J., Strack, A., McGowan, E., Tamvakopoulos, C., Miller, R.R., Stearns, R.A., Tang, W., MacIntyre, D.E., van der Ploeg, L.H.T., Patchett, A.A., and Nargund, R.P. (2005) 1-Amino-1,2,3,4-tetrahydronaphthalene-2-carboxylic acid as a Tic mimetic: application in the synthesis of potent human melanocortin-4 receptor selective agonists. *Bioorg. Med. Chem. Lett.*, **15** (14), 3430–3433.

55 Tang, W., Stearns, R.A., Wang, R.W., Miller, R.R., Chen, Q., Ngui, J., Bakshi, R. K., Nargund, R.P., Dean, D.C., and Baillie, T.A. (2008) Assessing and minimizing time-dependent inhibition of cytochrome P450 3A in drug discovery: a case study with melanocortin-4 receptor agonists. *Xenobiotica*, **38** (11), 1437–1451.

56 Teffera, Y., Colletti, A.E., Harmange, J.C., Hollis, L.S., Albrecht, B.K., Boezio, A.A., Liu, J., and Zhao, Z. (2008) Chemical reactivity of methoxy 4-*o*-aryl quinolines: identification of glutathione displacement products *in vitro* and *in vivo*. *Chem. Res. Toxicol.*, **21** (11), 2216–2222.

57 Pfefferkorn, J.A., Lou, J., Minich, M.L., Filipski, K.J., He, M., Zhou, R., Ahmed, S., Benbow, J., Perez, A.G., Tu, M., Litchfield, J., Sharma, R., Metzler, K., Bourbonais, F., Huang, C., Beebe, D.A., and Oates, P.J. (2009) Pyridones as glucokinase activators: identification of a unique metabolic liability of the 4-sulfonyl-2-pyridone heterocycle. *Bioorg. Med. Chem. Lett.*, **19** (12), 3247–3252.

58 Litchfield, J., Sharma, R., Atkinson, K., Filipski, K.J., Wright, S.W., Pfefferkorn, J. A., Tan, B., Kosa, R.E., Stevens, B., Tu, M., and Kalgutkar, A.S. (2010) Intrinsic electrophilicity of the 4-methylsulfonyl-2-pyridone scaffold in glucokinase activators: role of glutathione-*S*-transferases and *in vivo* quantitation of a glutathione conjugate in rats. *Bioorg. Med. Chem. Lett.*, **20** (21), 6262–6267.

59 Pfefferkorn, J.A., Guzman-Perez, A., Oates, P.J., Litchfield, J., Aspnes, G., Basak, A., Benbow, J., Berliner, M.A., Bian, J., Choi, C., Freeman-Cook, K., Corbett, J.W., Didiuk, M., Dunetz, J.R., Filipski, K.J., Hungerford, W.M., Jones, C.S., Karki, K., Ling, A., Li, J.-C., Patel, L., Perreault, C., Risley, H., Saenz, J., Song, W., Tu, M., Aiello, R., Atkinson, K., Barucci, N., Beebe, D., Bourassa, P., Bourbounais, F., Brodeur, A.M., Burbey, R., Chen, J., D'Aquila, T., Derksen, D.R., Haddish-Berhane, N., Huang, C., Landro, J., Lapworth, A.L., MacDougall, M., Perregaux, D., Pettersen, J., Robertson, A., Tan, B., Treadway, J.L., Liu, S., Qiu, X., Knafels, J., Ammirati, M., Song, X., DaSilva-Jardine, P., Liras, S., Sweet, L., and Rolph, T.P. (2011) Designing glucokinase activators with reduced hypoglycemia risk: discovery of *N,N*-dimethyl-5-(2-methyl-6-((5-methylpyrazin-2-yl)-carbamoyl)benzofuran-4-yloxy) pyrimidine-2-carboxamide as a clinical candidate for the treatment of type 2 diabetes mellitus. *Med. Chem. Commun.*, **2**, 828–839.

60 Liu, Z.X., and Kaplowitz, N. (2006) Role of innate immunity in acetaminophen-induced hepatotoxicity. *Expert Opin. Drug Metab. Toxicol.*, **2** (4), 493–503.

61 Dahlin, D.C., Miwa, G.T., Lu, A.Y., and Nelson, S.D. (1984) *N*-Acetyl-*p*-benzoquinone imine: a cytochrome P-450-mediated oxidation product of acetaminophen. *Proc. Natl. Acad. Sci. USA*, **81** (5), 1327–1331.

62 Kalgutkar, A.S., and Didiuk, M.T. (2009) Structural alerts, reactive metabolites, and protein covalent binding: how reliable are these attributes as predictors of drug toxicity. *Chem. Biodivers.*, **6** (11), 2115–2137.

63 Uetrecht, J.P. (1992) Metabolism of clozapine by neutrophils. Possible implications for clozapine-induced agranulocytosis. *Drug Saf.*, **7** (Suppl. 1), 51–56.

64 Gardner, I., Leeder, J.S., Chin, T., Zahid, N., and Uetrecht, J.P. (1998) A comparison of the covalent binding of clozapine and olanzapine to human neutrophils *in vitro* and *in vivo*. *Mol. Pharmacol.*, **53** (6), 999–1008.

65 Uetrecht, J., Zahid, N., Tehim, A., Fu, J.M., and Rakhit, S. (1997) Structural features associated with reactive metabolite formation with clozapine analogues. *Chem. Biol. Interact.*, **104** (2–3), 117–129.

66 Obach, R.S., Kalgutkar, A.S., Ryder, T.F., and Walker, G.S. (2008) *In vitro* metabolism and covalent binding of enol-carboxamide derivatives and anti-inflammatory agents sudoxicam and meloxicam: insights into the hepatotoxicity of sudoxicam. *Chem. Res. Toxicol.*, **21** (9), 1890–1899.

67 Hartz, R.A., Ahuja, V.T., Zhuo, X., Mattson, R.J., Denhart, D.J., Deskus, J.A., Vrudhula, V.M., Pan, S., Ditta, J.L., Shu, Y. Z., Grace, J.E., Lentz, K.A., Lelas, S., Li, Y. W., Molski, T.F., Krishnananthan, S., Wong, H., Qian-Cutrone, J., Schartman, R., Denton, R., Lodge, N.J., Zaczek, R., Macor, J.E., and Bronson, J.J. (2009) A strategy to minimize reactive metabolite formation: discovery of (*S*)-4-(1-cyclopropyl-2-methoxyethyl)-6-[6-(difluoromethoxy)-2,5-dimethylpyridin-3-ylamino]-5-oxo-4,5-dihydropyrazine-2-carbonitrile as a potent, orally bioavailable corticotropin-releasing factor-1 receptor antagonist. *J. Med. Chem.*, **52** (23), 7653–7668.

68 Zhuo, X., Hartz, R.A., Bronson, J.J., Wong, H., Ahuja, V.T., Vrudhula, V.M., Leet, J.E., Huang, S., Macor, J.E., and Shu, Y.Z. (2010) Comparative biotransformation of pyrazinone-containing corticotropin-releasing factor receptor-1 antagonists: minimizing the reactive metabolite formation. *Drug Metab. Dispos.*, **38** (1), 5–15.

69 Kalgutkar, A.S., Driscoll, J., Zhao, S.X., Walker, G.S., Shepard, R.M., Soglia, J.R., Atherton, J., Yu, Li., Mutlib, A.E., Munchhof, M.J., Reiter, L.A., Jones, C.S., Doty, J.L., Trevena, K.A., Shaffer, C.L., and Ripp, S.L. (2007) A rational chemical intervention strategy to circumvent bioactivation liabilities associated with a nonpeptidyl thrombopoietin receptor agonist containing a 2-amino-4-arylthiazole motif. *Chem. Res. Toxicol.*, **20** (12), 1954–1965.

70 Antipas, A.S., Blumberg, L.C., Brissette, W.H., Brown, M.F., Casavant, J.M., Doty, J.L., Driscoll, J., Harris, T.M., Jones, C.S., McCurdy, S.P., McElroy, E., Mitton-Fry, M., Munchhof, M.J., Reim, D.A., Reiter, L. A., Ripp, S.L., Shavnya, A., Smeets, M.I., and Trevena, K.A. (2010) Structure–activity relationships and hepatic safety risks of thiazole agonists of the thrombopoietin receptor. *Bioorg. Med. Chem. Lett.*, **20** (14), 4069–4072.

71 Tingle, M.D., Jewell, H., Maggs, J.L., O'Neill, P.M., and Park, B.K. (1995) The bioactivation of amodiaquine by human polymorphonuclear leucocytes *in vitro*: chemical mechanisms and the effects of fluorine substitution. *Biochem. Pharmacol.*, **50** (7), 1113–1119.

72 Maggs, J.L., Tingle, M.D., Kitteringham, N.R., and Park, B.K. (1988) Drug–protein conjugates. 14. Mechanisms of formation of protein-arylating intermediates from amodiaquine, a myelotoxin and hepatotoxin in man. *Biochem. Pharmacol.*, **37** (2), 303–311.

73 Tingle, M.D., Jewell, H., Maggs, J.L., O'Neill, P.M., and Park, B.K. (1995) The bioactivation of amodiaquine by human polymorphonuclear leucocytes *in vitro*: chemical mechanisms and the effects of fluorine substitution. *Biochem. Pharmacol.*, **50** (7), 1113–1119.

74 O'Neill, P.M., Harrison, A.C., Storr, R.C., Hawley, S.R., Ward, S.A., and Park, B.K. (1994) The effect of fluorine substitution on the metabolism and antimalarial activity of amodiaquine. *J. Med. Chem.*, **37** (9), 1362–1370.

75 O'Neill, P.M., Shone, A.E., Stanford, D., Nixon, G., Asadollahy, E., Park, B.K., Maggs, J.L., Roberts, P., Stocks, P.A., Biagini, G., Bray, P.G., Davies, J., Berry, N., Hall, C., Rimmer, K., Winstanley, P.A., Hindley, S., Bambal, R.B., Davis, C.B., Bates, M., Gresham, S.L., Brigandi, R.A., Gomez-de-Las-Heras, F.M., Gargallo, D. V., Parapini, S., Vivas, L., Lander, H., Taramelli, D., and Ward, S.A. (2009) Synthesis, antimalarial activity, and preclinical pharmacology of a novel series of 4′-fluoro and 4′-chloro analogues of amodiaquine. Identification of a suitable "back-up" compound for *N-tert*-butyl isoquine. *J. Med. Chem.*, **52** (7), 1828–1844.

76 O'Neill, P.M., Park, B.K., Shone, A.E., Maggs, J.L., Roberts, P., Stocks, P.A., Biagini, G.A., Bray, P.G., Gibbons, P., Berry, N., Winstanley, P.A., Mukhtar, A., Bonar-Law, R., Hindley, S., Bambal, R.B., Davis, C.B., Bates, M., Hart, T.K., Gresham, S.L., Lawrence, R.M., Brigandi, R.A., Gomez-delas-Heras, F.M., Gargallo, D.V., and Ward, S.A. (2009) Candidate selection and preclinical evaluation of *N-tert*-butyl isoquine (GSK369796), an affordable and effective 4-aminoquinoline antimalarial for the 21st century. *J. Med. Chem.*, **52** (5), 1408–1415.

77 Hagmann, W.K. (2008) The discovery of taranabant, a selective cannabinoid-1 receptor inverse agonist for the treatment of obesity. *Arch. Pharm.*, **341**, 405–411.

78 Nightingale, S.L. (1994) Recommendation to immediately withdraw patients from treatment with felbamate. *J. Am. Med. Assoc.*, **272** (13), 995.

79 Thompson, C.D., Kinter, M.T., and Macdonald, T.L. (1996) Synthesis and *in vitro* reactivity of 3-carbamoyl-2-phenylpropionaldeyde and 2-phenylpropenal: putative reactive metabolites of felbamate. *Chem. Res. Toxicol.*, **9** (8), 1225–1229.

80 Diekhaus, C.M., Thompson, C.D., Roller, S.G., and MacDonald, T.L. (2002) Mechanisms of idiosyncratic drug reactions: the case of felbamate. *Chem. Biol. Interact.*, **142** (1–2), 99–117.

81 Thompson, C.D., Barthen, M.T., Hopper, D.W., Miller, T.A., Quigg, M., Hudspeth, C., Montouris, G., Marsh, L., Perhach, J. L., Sofia, R.D., and Macdonald, T.L. (1999) Quantitation in patient urine samples of felbamate and three metabolites: acid carbamate and two mercapturic acids. *Epilepsia*, **40** (6), 769–776.

82 Roecklein, B.A., Sacks, H.J., Mortko, H., and Stables, J. (2007) Fluorofelbamate. *Neurotherapeutics*, **4** (1), 97–101.

83 Smith, D.A., Allerton, C., Kalgutkar, A., van de Waterbeemd, H., and Walker, D.K. (2012) *Pharmacokinetics and Metabolism in Drug Design*, 3rd edn, Wiley-VCH Verlag GmbH, Weinheim.

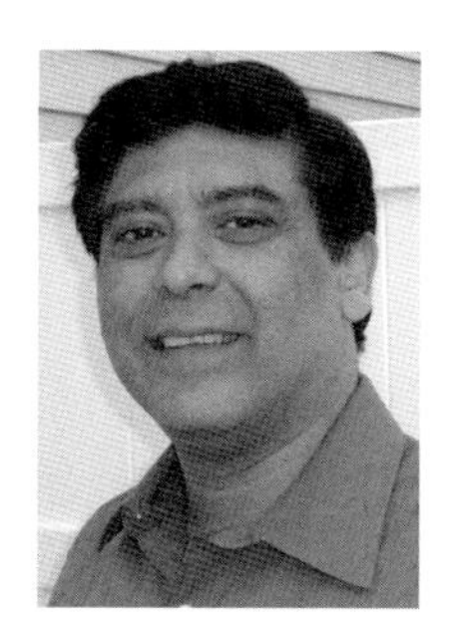

Amit S. Kalgutkar is a Research Fellow in the Drug Metabolism Group at Pfizer. He earned his Ph.D. (1993) in Organic Chemistry from Virginia Tech, and carried out postdoctoral research at the Department of Biochemistry, Vanderbilt University School of Medicine before joining Pfizer. His research interest primarily focuses on medicinal chemistry and mechanistic drug metabolism centered on biotransformation. He has been a member of the editorial board of *Chemical Research in Toxicology* (American Chemical Society) and is currently on the editorial board of Drug Metabolism and Disposition and *Xenobiotica*. Besides his current position at Pfizer, he is also an Adjunct Professor at the Department of Biomedical and Pharmaceutical Sciences, School of Pharmacy, University of Rhode Island. He has coauthored over 110 peer-reviewed papers, reviews, and book chapters and holds several patents in the area of selective COX-2 inhibition.

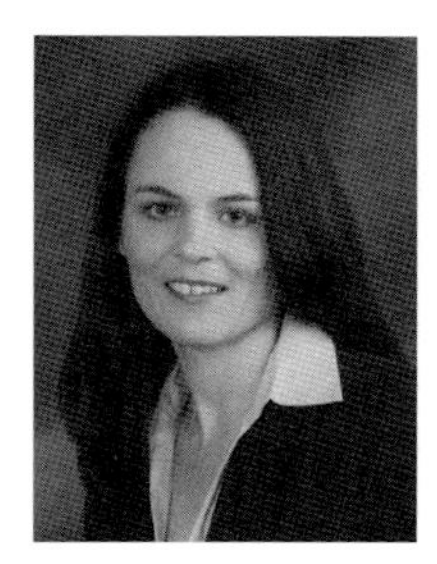

Antonia F. Stepan is a Principal Scientist in the Neuroscience Medicinal Chemistry Department at Pfizer. She earned her Ph.D. in Organic Chemistry from the University of Cambridge (UK) in 2006 and then carried out postdoctoral research at The Scripps Research Institute in La Jolla, California. In 2008, she joined the Antibacterials Medicinal Chemistry Department at Pfizer. Her research interest focuses on the discovery of novel medicines for the treatment of neurodegenerative diseases. She has coauthored 15 peer-reviewed papers, reviews, and patents.

4
Use of Macrocycles in Drug Design Exemplified with Ulimorelin, a Potential Ghrelin Agonist for Gastrointestinal Motility Disorders

Mark L. Peterson, Hamid Hoveyda, Graeme Fraser, Éric Marsault, and René Gagnon

4.1
Introduction

4.1.1
Ghrelin as a Novel Pharmacological Target for GI Motility Disorders

Ghrelin is a 28-amino acid peptide hormone isolated originally from the stomach of rats with the orthologue subsequently identified in humans, distinguished by an unusual *n*-octanoyl group modification on Ser^3 (Figure 4.1) [1]. The existence of this hormone in a wide range of species suggests a conserved and important role in normal physiological function. Indeed, since the isolation and characterization of the peptide in 1999, numerous studies have identified a range of endocrine and nonendocrine processes in which the hormone is involved [2].

The ghrelin peptide has been demonstrated to be the endogenous ligand for a previously orphan G protein-coupled receptor (GPCR), the type 1 growth hormone secretagogue receptor (GHS-R1a) [3], which, not surprisingly, was reclassified as the ghrelin receptor (GRLN) in 2005 [4]. Although ghrelin is produced primarily in the stomach [5], GRLN is found predominantly in the brain, with the highest level in the pituitary, but also is expressed throughout the gut, and a number of other tissues and organs [6]. The GHS-R1a receptor had been the focus of a significant amount of pharma industry interest in the latter part of the twentieth century due primarily, as its name suggests, to its role in stimulating growth hormone (GH) release. The goal was to develop small molecules, generically termed growth hormone secretagogues (GHS), which could activate the receptor and thereby act as oral mimics of GH, a "holy grail"-type objective that motivated drug discovery efforts by essentially all major pharmaceutical firms [7]. Despite significant success, initially with peptidomimetics, and then with traditional small molecules, in finding a number of potent, orally available GHS, the inability to generate sustained effects from these molecules eventually resulted in a waning of interest in the pharmaceutical potential of the receptor by the time ghrelin itself was identified [8, 9].

Since then, however, the myriad actions of ghrelin have led to a renaissance in exploring modulation of this receptor for therapeutic purposes [10]. Indeed,

Analogue-based Drug Discovery III, First Edition. Edited by János Fischer, C. Robin Ganellin, and David P. Rotella.
© 2013 Wiley-VCH Verlag GmbH & Co. KGaA. Published 2013 by Wiley-VCH Verlag GmbH & Co. KGaA.

Gly-Ser-Ser(Oct)-Phe-Leu-Ser-Pro-Glu-His-Gln-Arg-Val-Gln-Gln-Arg-Lys-Glu-Ser-Lys-Lys-Pro-Pro-Ala-Lys-Leu-Gln-Pro-Arg
ghrelin (human)

Figure 4.1 Primary sequence of human ghrelin.

renewed attention to many of the GHS (i.e., ghrelin agonists) developed from these previous efforts has occurred, albeit often by smaller companies that have in-licensed these compounds from the innovator firms. Interestingly, only those therapeutic indications related to the original focus on promoting GH release were being actively pursued prior to the work reported herein. For example, ghrelin and ghrelin agonists have been demonstrated to have positive effects in wasting syndromes, such as cachexia [11, 12], and as agents to counteract some effects of aging [13]. In addition, antagonism of the ghrelin receptor has been identified as a strategy for the treatment of metabolic diseases due to the intimate involvement of ghrelin in the control of energy balance and appetite [14].

In contrast, we were drawn to the effects ghrelin displayed in the gastrointestinal (GI) system [15], in large part due to the dearth of new products being developed in that therapeutic space despite GI diseases and disorders being among the most prevalent illnesses in the general population. In the United States alone, it has been estimated that there were over 104 million visits to primary care physicians with a diagnosis of a GI disorder in 2004 imposing an annual cost burden greater than $141 billion including both direct and indirect expenditures [16]. Motility disorders, which negatively impact the normal contractions and relaxation of the GI tract to ensure orderly transit of food and liquids, are among the most common of these disorders, which include gastroparesis, functional dyspepsia, constipation, and irritable bowel syndrome (IBS).

Ghrelin is intimately connected to the GI tract. It is produced mainly by oxyntic cells of the stomach [17] and has a highly potent and direct role in the stimulation of GI motility [18]. This GI prokinetic activity appears to be independent of the GH secretory action and is likely mediated by the vagal cholinergic muscarinic pathway [19]. Ghrelin acts locally in the stomach to activate and coordinate the firing of vagal afferent neurons and thereby induce gut motility. The peptide has been shown to accelerate gastric emptying in animal models [20] and successfully treat postoperative ileus (POI) in both rats and dogs [21]. These results suggested that ghrelin agonists would be able to provide a novel mechanism of action for therapeutic purposes in GI disorders characterized by dysmotility through duplicating the effects of ghrelin and accelerating the normalization of gut function [22]. This was later confirmed through studies with earlier developed GHS/ghrelin agonist compounds [23]. Also subsequent to the initiation of our work, clinical studies conclusively demonstrated the GI promotility effects of ghrelin, acting by promoting phase III of the migrating motor complex (MMC), in humans [24, 25].

Most previous efforts to develop pharmacotherapies for GI motility disorders have focused on modulation of serotonin [26] and dopamine receptors [27]. Serotonin and dopamine are major mediators of various physiological functions, both inside and outside the CNS, and exert their actions, including the stimulation of GI motility, through multiple different receptor subtypes. Unfortunately, a number of these agents have been removed from the market, or had their distribution highly restricted, due to deleterious side effects, often caused by nonselective activity at these subtypes or other receptors. For example, cisapride, a serotonin receptor modulator, originally used for nocturnal GERD, was removed from the market in 2000 due to the potential of serious cardiac arrhythmias [28]. Another serotonin receptor modulator, tegaserod, developed as a treatment for IBS with constipation, was withdrawn in 2007 due to an increased risk of ischemic events, including heart attacks and strokes [29]. Even one of the few remaining available drugs, metoclopramide, a mixed dopamine and serotonin receptor modulator with modest efficacy, had a black box warning added to its label in 2009 because of the risk of tardive dyskinesia with extended use [30]. Given this checkered history with established targets, coupled with the unmet need in the area, we felt that exploration of the potential of activation of the ghrelin receptor as a new pharmacological approach for the generation of novel GI prokinetic agents was well warranted.

4.1.2
Macrocycles in Drug Discovery

Despite the promise of combinatorial chemistry in conjunction with the many advances in genomics/proteomics, drug discovery productivity has not experienced the significant improvement originally anticipated. One of the reasons for this has been suggested to be a lack of sufficient diversity in the number of chemotypes typically investigated [31]. Hence, attention has been directed toward mining new or underexplored chemical scaffolds for interesting pharmacological activity.

One of the emerging compound classes in the underexplored category is macrocycles. Due to their presence in a wide variety of natural products that exhibit an equally broad range of bioactivity, such structures have long been recognized as a potentially fruitful pharmaceutical compound class. However, the generation of libraries of macrocycles, screening of which would be the typical starting point for the majority of current medicinal chemistry efforts, has been an impediment due to the lack of appropriate synthetic methods for their construction in a highly parallel manner. Further, concerns about the ability of these structures to possess appropriate "drug-like" properties, since typically one or more parameters fall outside the acceptable "rule of five" ranges [32], have deterred wider investigation.

Nonetheless, macrocyclic compounds possess highly attractive characteristics, including

- diverse, often complex, functionality;
- defined topological display of functionality;
- ability to interact at otherwise intractable targets.

These features often lead to stronger affinity and greater selectivity than traditional structures. Further, macrocycles usually possess enhanced metabolic stability versus the comparable linear compounds. Indeed, increasingly over the past decade, macrocyclic compounds have been reported that display biological activity against a wide range of pharmacological targets and recent reviews have summarized these efforts [33]. In many cases, such structures were accessed as a means of improving activity of linear analogues through conformational restriction, although more examples have begun to appear where macrocycles are being utilized as the core scaffold as well. With the successful discovery and development of technologies that permit larger screening libraries of macrocycles to be prepared, including that described herein, the use of macrocycles as a *de novo* source of novel chemical entities is expected to continue to expand.

4.1.3 Tranzyme Technology

Tranzyme has discovered and developed a proprietary technology for the generation of peptidomimetic macrocycles of the general structure shown in Figure 4.2 in a highly parallel fashion, thereby enabling the creation of the first library of macrocyclic structures available for screening for novel bioactivity [34].

Several features of these structures merit further comment as they have proven very advantageous for their use in drug discovery. The molecules are comprised of four building block units, three from amino acids (or their equivalents) and one a unique element, acting as a bridge between the ends of the peptidic segment, that we termed a "tether." This tether more importantly functions to constrain and define the conformation(s) of the resulting structure. In this manner, topological diversity is introduced into these compounds and can be investigated simultaneously with chemical diversity. Although initially designed in order to control and modulate the conformational population, subsequent studies have demonstrated that the tether functions as a recognition site for binding to the target as well. Further, the tether can significantly influence the physicochemical properties of the macrocycle as the current work will also illustrate.

In addition, the use of three amino acids maintains the total molecular weight within the small molecule range (400–600), yet with the capability of interacting over significant regions of three-dimensional space. Although additional amino acids can be incorporated, the screening library used for the ghrelin receptor only utilized macrocycles of the general structure of Figure 4.2. Substantial chemical diversity is provided by the standard amino acid side chains that display, as a group, a variety of polarities, hydrophobicities/hydrophilicities, sizes, and charges.

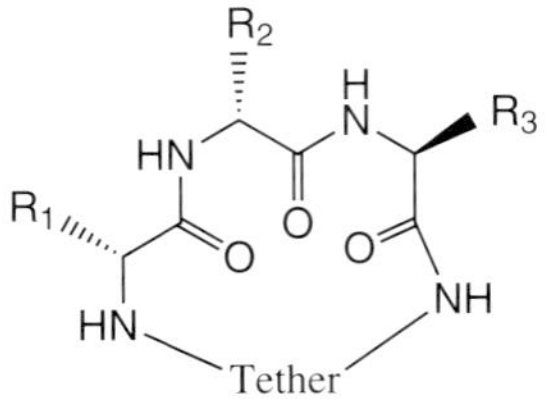

Figure 4.2 Generic structure of Tranzyme macrocyclic library (stereochemistry for illustration purposes only).

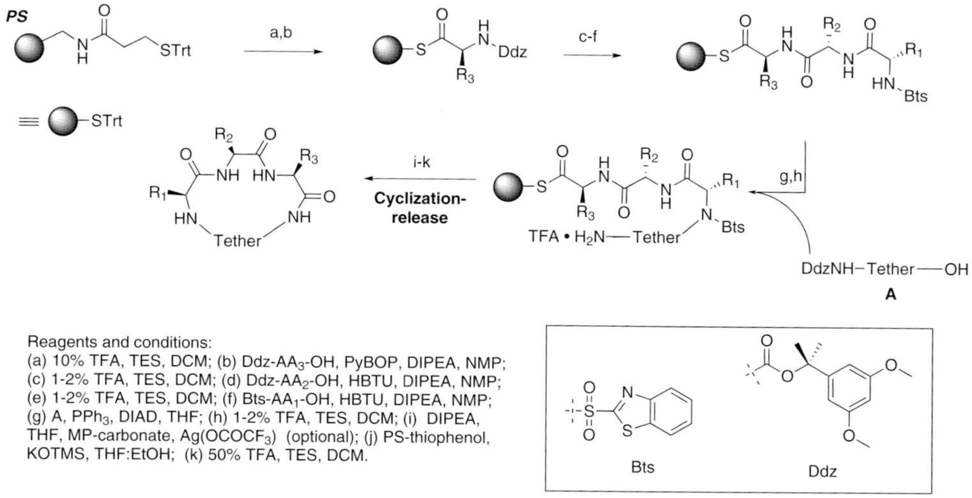
PS
STrt
a,b
Ddz
c-f
Bts
g,h
i-k
Cyclization-release
TFA • H2N—Tether
Tether
DdzNH–Tether—OH
A
Reagents and conditions:
(a) 10% TFA, TES, DCM; (b) Ddz-AA3-OH, PyBOP, DIPEA, NMP;
(c) 1-2% TFA, TES, DCM; (d) Ddz-AA2-OH, HBTU, DIPEA, NMP;
(e) 1-2% TFA, TES, DCM; (f) Bts-AA1-OH, HBTU, DIPEA, NMP;
(g) A, PPh3, DIAD, THF; (h) 1-2% TFA, TES, DCM; (i) DIPEA,
THF, MP-carbonate, Ag(OCOCF3) (optional); (j) PS-thiophenol,
KOTMS, THF:EtOH; (k) 50% TFA, TES, DCM.
Bts
Ddz

Scheme 4.1 Macrocyclic library synthetic method.

Importantly, their side chains have unquestioned biological relevance. This diversity is further enhanced through using both the natural and unnatural stereoisomers in the library construction. Our modeling efforts have shown that the amino acid configurations can have significant effects on the conformations of the resulting macrocycles, enabling the sampling of different regions of space simply by using a variety of configurations. Finally, the secondary nitrogen atom provides a handle from which further modifications can be incorporated during optimization or for salt formation to enhance solubility.

The synthetic approach utilized for these structures as shown in Scheme 4.1 has several salient features: (i) performed on solid phase to permit high numbers of compounds to be made simultaneously; (ii) utilizes a Fukuyama–Mitsunobu reaction to attach the tether; (iii) employs standard amino acid coupling chemistry for high-yielding building block assembly; (iv) incorporates a linker that permits concomitant ring closure and cleavage from the resin (i.e., cyclative release); (v) uses radiofrequency tagging methodology for compound tracking [35]; and (vi) conducts the final steps as an array in microtiter format to prepare individual, discrete compounds in each well for ease of transfer to screening. The use of cyclative release also biases the compounds toward better crude purity as only cyclized compounds are released from the resin. Difficult macrocyclizations are thus reflected in low yields rather than multiple impurities. Indeed, the primary impurity observed in most cases, as with most such cyclizations, is the macrocyclic dimer. The synthesis success rate is typically quite high, over 95%, even for a variety of amino acids and configurations.

As a final point on the general drug discovery strategy using these macrocycles, modified synthetic methods have been developed that can be used to incorporate peptide bond isosteres into these structures. Since such an approach did not produce desirable effects in the ghrelin agonist program, they will not be discussed further, but does illustrate the additional, more significant, changes that can be made to these structures during hit-to-lead optimization.

4.2 High-Throughput Screening Results and Hit Selection

As with all of our discovery efforts, the search for agonists of the ghrelin receptor (GRLN) began with high-throughput screening (HTS) of the company's HitCreate™ Library of proprietary macrocyclic small molecules (Figure 4.2). In surveying the potential platforms available for this effort, we decided on the aequorin assay, a robust system that has proven quite useful for GPCR targets [36]. In particular, the wide dynamic range and high signal-to-noise ratio, as well as low cost per assay, were attractive benefits for screening of this new compound class. Importantly, screening for agonist and antagonist activity is performed in series with the same samples, allowing a complete characterization of the functional activity to be obtained from the primary screening. As a secondary, confirmatory screen, a standard radioligand binding assay was employed.

Screening of a set of approximately 10 000 compounds led to two different series of validated hits, represented in Figure 4.3 with their most active members, **1** and **2**. The high affinity and functional activity obtained for compounds directly from the HTS efforts were quite remarkable, although a similar level was obtained in our motilin antagonist program as well [37]. The requirement for the cyclic structure was confirmed in that linear analogues of **1** and **2** were devoid of any activity. These compounds exhibited selectivity (>100-fold) versus the motilin receptor (MLNR), the most closely homologous GPCR, plus did not display cytotoxicity in HepG2 cells at concentrations up to 100 μM.

After preliminary follow-up libraries on both series, series A, despite being initially slightly weaker in bioactivity, proved to be the most fruitful for further optimization and will be the focus of the remainder of the discussion [38].

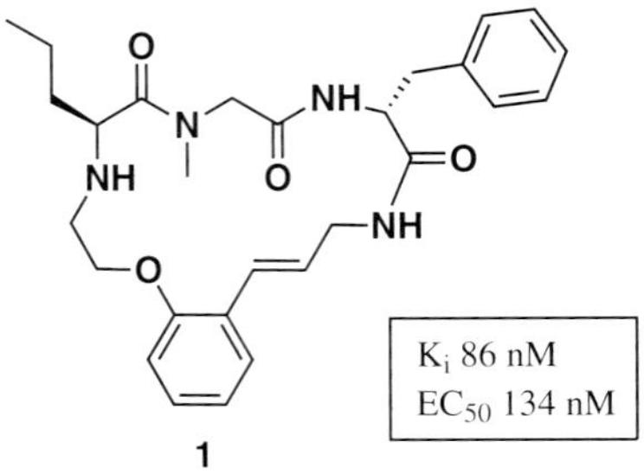

K_i 86 nM
EC_{50} 134 nM

1
(series A)

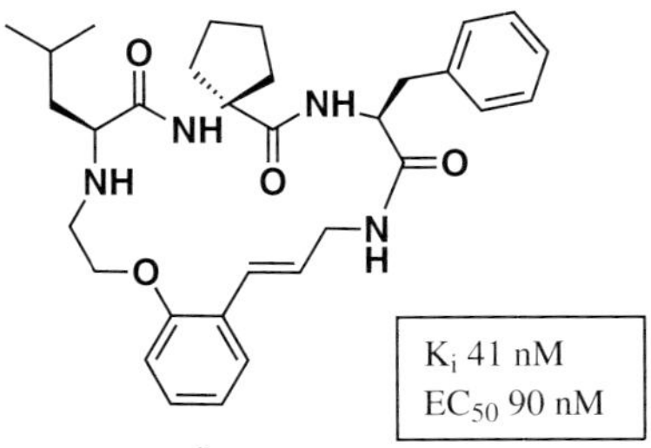

K_i 41 nM
EC_{50} 90 nM

2
(series B)

Figure 4.3 Active series obtained from HTS.

4.3 Macrocycle Structure–Activity Relationships

4.3.1 Preliminary SAR

With four individual components available for optimization and a wealth of potential diversity elements to choose from, the focus of the first phase of SAR development was to determine (1) the preferred configurations at each of the amino acid positions, (2) the steric requirements at the amino acid sites, (3) the optimal ring size, and (4) the best tether component.

In order to gain initial insight into the SAR, a library of approximately 100 compounds was prepared with each member designed to interrogate one of these questions. The same solid-phase methodology as for the synthesis of the library (Scheme 4.1) was applied to access these analogues. All compounds were purified using automated preparative HPLC to >95% purity. Selections from this library and their binding results are provided in Table 4.1.

Investigation of L- and D-stereoisomers at each of the three amino acid positions revealed strikingly different results depending on the site, although the configurations as in **1** were confirmed as preferred in all instances. For AA_1 and AA_2, a clear stereochemical preference was found, while for AA_3 the opposite stereocenter to that in **1** was much less disfavored, suggesting that this was the most promiscuous site on the structure.

From these results, the following salient characteristics of the SAR regarding the general requirements at the four diversity sites of the structure became evident (compounds that demonstrate the point shown in parentheses):

- The double bond in the tether was not necessary (**3**).
- For AA_1, the L-stereochemistry was definitely preferred (**4**) with an apparent preference for larger aliphatic side chains (**5** versus **6**).
- The D-configuration was the choice at AA_2 (**10** versus **11** and **13** versus **14**) with a limitation on the size of the side chain evident (**15** and **16**).
- The *N*-methyl group was required for AA_2 (**9**).
- AA_3 exhibited a preference for the D-stereochemistry (**18**) and it appeared that aromatic moieties were somewhat advantageous (**22** and **23**).

In particular, the benefits of Ile at AA_1 and D-NMeAla at AA_2 were considered to be significant enough to often utilize such elements as the standard reference at these positions as the optimization efforts progressed.

4.3.2 Ring Size and Tether

Turning attention next to the tether component, which allowed the exploration of different ring sizes as well, a number of alterative tether moieties to that of **1** were examined to determine if a change in the macrocyclic conformation would be

Table 4.1 Preliminary SAR selections.

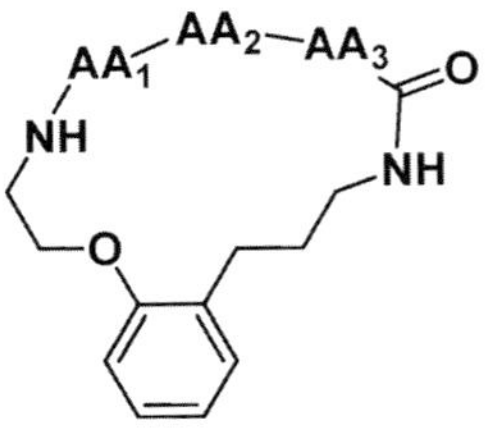

Compound	AA_1	AA_2	AA_3	K_i (nM)
1[a]	Nva	Sar	D-Phe	86
3	Nva	Sar	D-Phe	68
4	D-Nva	Sar	D-Phe	1200
5	Ala	Sar	D-Phe	4300
6	Nle	Sar	D-Phe	67
7	Phe	Sar	D-Phe	670
8	Ser	Sar	D-Phe	>10 000
9	Nva	Gly	D-Phe	820
10	Nva	Ala	D-Phe	5000
11	Nva	D-Ala	D-Phe	500
12	Ile	D-Ala	D-Phe	177
13	Nva	NMeAla	D-Phe	580
14	Nva	D-NMeAla	D-Phe	14
15	Nva	D-Leu	D-Phe	>10 000
16	Nva	D-Phe	D-Phe	8300
17	Nva	Aib	D-Phe	640
18	Nva	Sar	Phe	380
19	Nva	Sar	D-Ala	>10 000
20	Nva	Sar	Gly	>10 000
21	Nva	Sar	D-Nle	400
22	Nva	Sar	D-Tyr	120
23	Nva	Sar	D-Trp	160

a) Double bond in tether (see Figure 4.2).

beneficial. This also provided an opportunity to investigate heteroaromatic rings and modified polarities. The results of these efforts are shown in Table 4.2.

As can be seen, the majority of these alternative tether structures had dramatic detrimental effects on binding affinity to GRLN. Smaller rings also were definitely disadvantageous. Hence, the results suggest that the conformation of the macrocycle of the original hit 1 must already be at or near the optimal range. This nicely demonstrates one of the strengths of the underlying macrocyclic technology in being able to scan topological space simultaneously with chemical space to accelerate hit-to-lead-to-clinic optimization.

Therefore, more subtle modifications around the tether were tested, including shifting position of the phenyl ring, necessity of the oxygen atom, and increasing

Table 4.2 Tether SAR part 1: alternative structures.

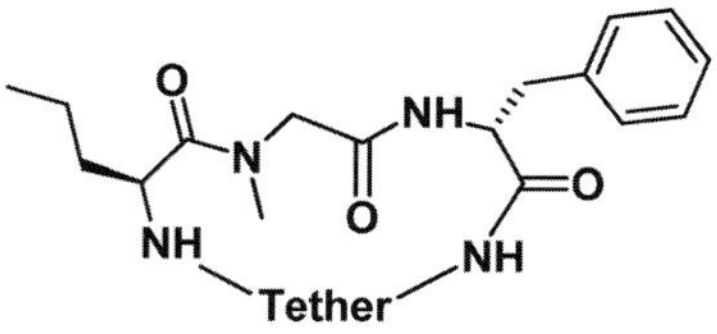

Compound	Tether	Ring size	K_i (nM)
24	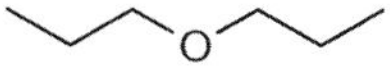	15	>10 000
25	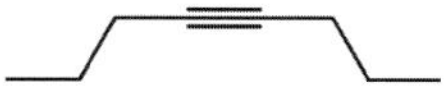	16	>10 000
26	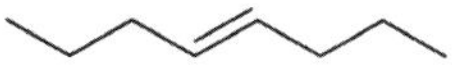	16	~ 10 000
27	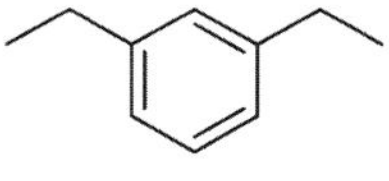	15	9200
28	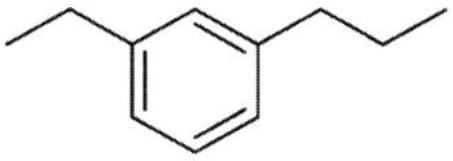	16	>10 000
29	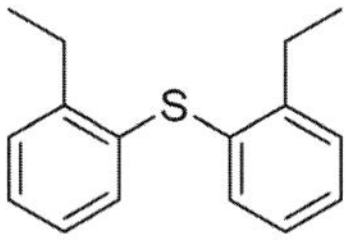	17	650
30	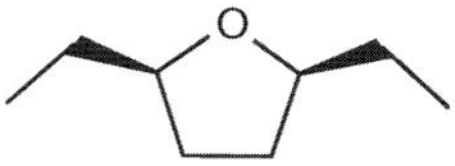	15	>10 000
31	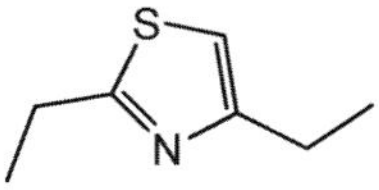	15	>10 000
32[a]	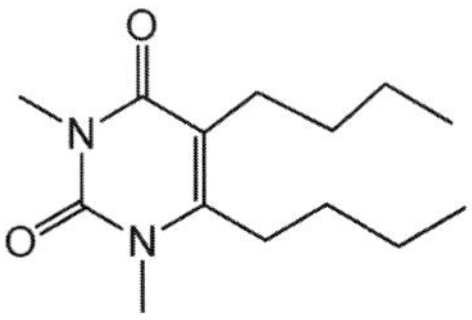	18	>10 000

a) AA_1 = Ile.

Table 4.3 Tether SAR part 2: phenyl ring presence and position.

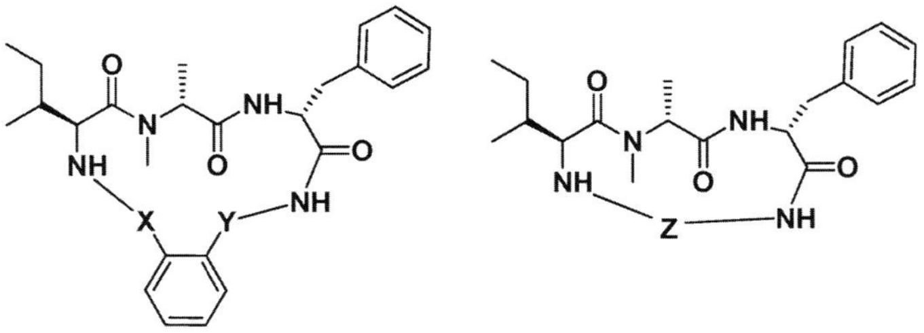

Compound	X	Y	Z	Ring size	K_i (nM)
14[a]	$(CH_2)_2O$	$(CH_2)_3$		18	14
33	$(CH_2)_3$	$(CH_2)_2$		17	400
34	$(CH_2)_2O$	$(CH_2)_2$		17	210
35	$(CH_2)_4$	$(CH_2)_2$		18	230
36	CH_2	$(CH_2)_5$		18	18
38	$(CH_2)_3$	$(CH_2)_3$		18	81
39	$(CH_2)_3$	$CH=CHCH_2$		18	10
40	$(CH_2)_3$	$(CH_2)_4$		19	78
41			$(CH_2)_7$	17	>10 000
42			$(CH_2)_8$	18	1500
43			$(CH_2)_4CH=CH(CH_2)_2$	18	160

a) AA_1 = Nva for reference.

or decreasing ring size by one atom, although the more substantial removal of the phenyl ring was also assessed (Table 4.3).

The outcome of this series was more revealing, with additional features of the SAR becoming evident:

- Removal of the phenyl was definitely unfavorable (**41** and **42**).
- Reintroduction of a conformational constraint in the form of a double bond (**43**) did restore binding, although at a level still an order of magnitude less than with the aromatic ring, confirming the importance of that moiety.
- The oxygen atom was beneficial, but not critical, as the methylene substitution only had a slightly negative effect on binding (**1** versus **38** and **33** versus **34**), which was recovered if an additional double bond was introduced (**39**). However, the oxygen-containing tether is much superior in terms of GRLN-to-MLNR selectivity (>1500 : 1) in comparison with the olefinic tether ($\leq$30 : 1).
- Smaller rings were somewhat detrimental (**33** and **34**), while larger ones (**40**) did not offer any improvement over the original 18-membered macrocycle.
- Interestingly, shifting the position of the phenyl ring with respect to the rest of the structure proved to be mixed, with positive results closer to the amine nitrogen (**36**) and negative in the opposite direction toward the amide (**35**).

Overall, these results led us to retain the tether structure of **3** and **14** as the basis for further work. Hence, it appeared that substitution on the tether, either on the phenyl ring or on the aliphatic connecting chains ("arms"), would need to be evaluated as the next stage in the optimization of this moiety.

4.3.3
Amino Acid Components

With the preferred stereochemical configuration at each amino acid position determined, although this was subjected to spot checks as analogue development continued, which confirmed the original biases, the next phase of the investigation was to conduct a thorough survey of the functionality and polarity accessible via the side chains of the proteinogenic amino acids, as well as the substantial collection of unnatural amino acids that are accessible either commercially or through synthesis. At this stage and beyond, the solid-phase procedure was often supplanted by an alternative solution-phase approach (Scheme 4.2) for the synthesis of analogues where one of the building blocks needed to be specially prepared or was available in only limited quantities.

Key results from these extensive analogue development efforts are summarized graphically in Figure 4.4. Building on the results of the preliminary SAR described

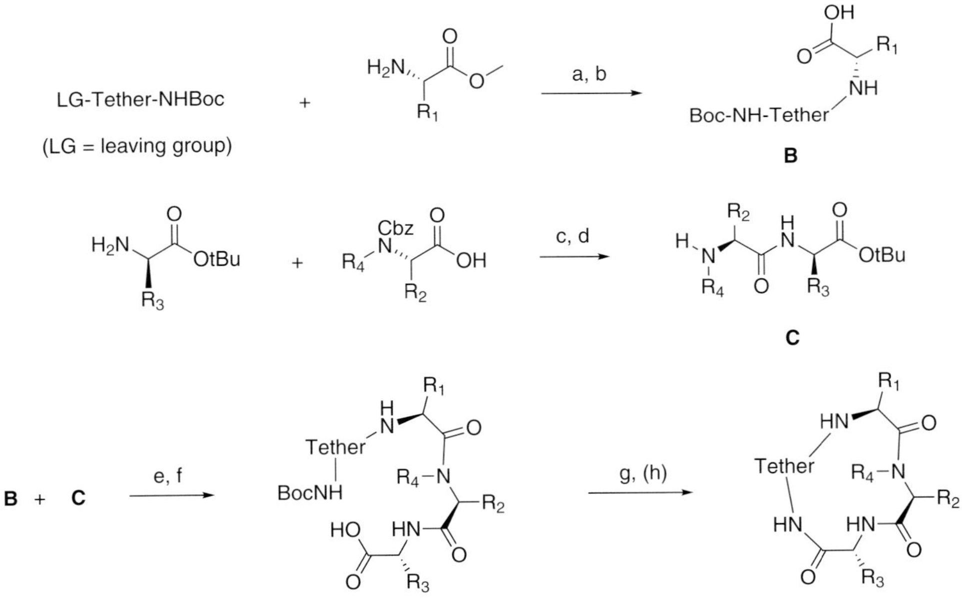

a. KI, Na_2CO_3, DMF, 105ºC; b. LiOH, THF:H_2O, :MeOH; c. HATU or EDCI/6Cl-HOBt, DIPEA, NMP; d. H_2, Pd/C, AcOEt; e. HATU, HOAt, DIPEA, NMP; f. 50% TFA/5%TES/DCM; g. DEPBT, DIPEA, THF; h. Deprotect side chains (if necessary)

Scheme 4.2 Solution-phase route to macrocycles.

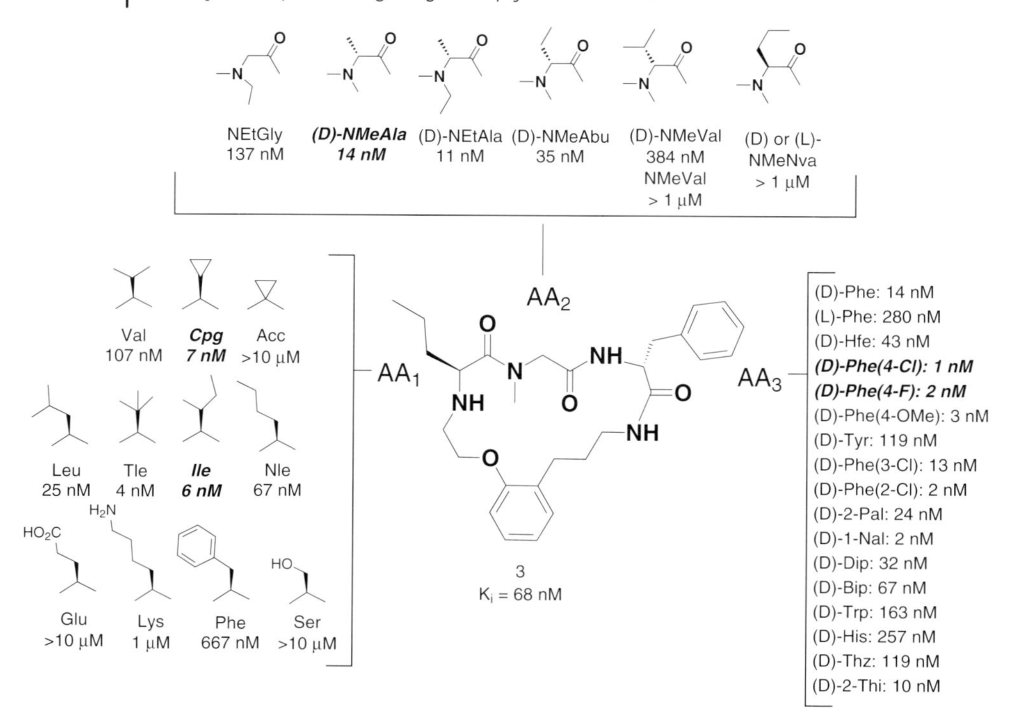

Figure 4.4 SAR amino acid components.

earlier, this study indicated greater restrictions to allowable groups at AA_1 and AA_2, with the latter very highly limited, while the other position, AA_3, was indeed more promiscuous.

For AA_1, a preference for aliphatic side chains was confirmed with the presence of basic (Lys), acidic (Glu), polar (Ser), and aromatic (Phe) groups detrimental. Slightly larger groups than methyl proved more favorable with branched alkyl moieties (Ile, Tle, and Leu) being advantageous. Of particular interest was the positive results obtained with the small cyclic amino acid cyclopropylglycine (Cpg), which had additional benefits as will be discussed later in Section 4.4.

A very tight SAR was determined for the AA_2 constituent. Charged (D-Glu and D-Lys) amino acids were essentially inactive, as were aromatic (D-Phe) side chains. Only smaller aliphatic groups, such as methyl or ethyl, were tolerated for the side chain, while the *N*-methyl group of the original hit 1 was clearly beneficial, likely due to its effect on overall molecular conformation. Since *N*-ethyl and *N*-isopropyl analogues did not result in any activity improvement and were more difficult to access synthetically, further attention at this site was deemed not to be warranted. It should be noted that *N*-methyl substitutions at the other amide nitrogens of the macrocycle proved to be unfavorable. The potential of D-Pro in this position as an alternative constrained amino acid was tested, but not found to be a fruitful avenue ($K_i = 330$ nM).

Contrastingly, a variety of different groups are permitted at the AA_3 position; however, some limitations were evident. Acidic (D-Glu), basic (D-Orn), and polar (D-Ser) derivatives, for example, failed to show GRLN binding. Small aliphatic moieties (Gly and D-Ala) were similarly ineffective; however, larger alkyl side chains (D-Nle) did exhibit binding affinity, albeit a little weaker than the worst aromatic moiety (D-His). Therefore, of all the derivatives tested at this stage, the phenyl group as originally in **1** still appeared to offer the best scaffold for additional optimization, although we were cognizant of the detrimental effects of the moiety on clogP, making this parameter higher than is typically desirable. However, as alluded to in the introduction, these macrocyclic molecules can be considered rule breakers, which do not lend themselves to standard measures of suitability for drug development.

Fortunately, many substituted phenylalanine building blocks were readily available for investigation as were alternative isosteres, such as pyridylalanine. As seen in Figure 4.4, the presence of halogen or methoxy substitution in the 4-position of the phenyl ring was particularly effective in increasing potency by an order of magnitude, with 2-halo substituents showing similar results. This provided several options to be investigated with respect to optimization of the pharmacokinetic (PK) profile (Section 4.4).

4.3.4 Further Tether Optimization

With the optimization of the three amino acid diversity elements achieved, at least with regard to the pharmacodynamic (PD) profile of the macrocycle, the tether component became the focus area. Based on the previous results (Section 4.3.2), the core tether structure of compound **3** appeared to still be the appropriate starting point for further investigation. Hence, the strategy that was taken was twofold: (1) introducing additional conformational rigidity into the arm through methyl substitutions and (2) modulation of the electronic properties of the phenyl ring through appropriate substituents. A selection of such tether variations together with their impact on the PD profile of the resulting macrocycles is presented in Table 4.4.

In considering where best to start this investigation, the all aliphatic arm connecting to the amide nitrogen did not seem to be the more fruitful avenue since removing the olefinic conformational restriction from that portion of the molecule had a minimal, actually positive, effect on activity. Hence, attention was placed on the arm joining the ether oxygen to the amine. Systematic substitution along that region led to very different results. A methyl group adjacent to the amine nitrogen (**45**) retained the binding level of the unsubstituted analogue (**44**), but hurt the functional activity[1]. In contrast, stereospecific methyl substitutions at the adjacent carbon atom resulted in both good binding affinity and functional efficacy (EC_{50}), with the (*R*)-derivative about 3.5-fold more potent than its epimer (**47**). Introducing

1) For SAR development, the focus was placed on receptor binding affinity (K_i), rather than on functional activity, since the latter is subject to potential bias due to the choice of the signal transduction pathway, as well as constitutive GRLN signaling and allosteric activation (also see Ref. [38]).

Table 4.4 Tether SAR: tether backbone substitutions.

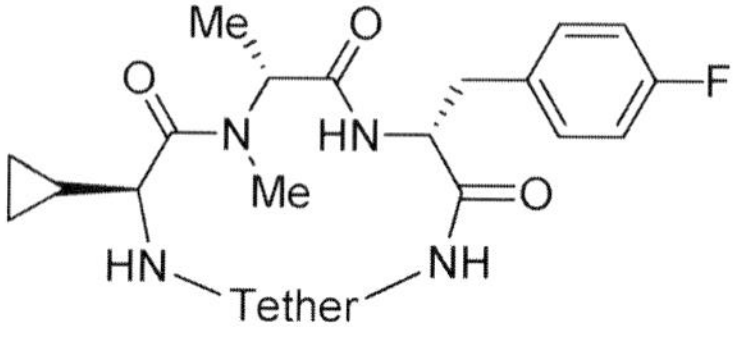

Compound	Tether	K_i (nM)	EC_{50} (nM)	Compound	Tether	K_i (nM)	EC_{50} (nM)
44	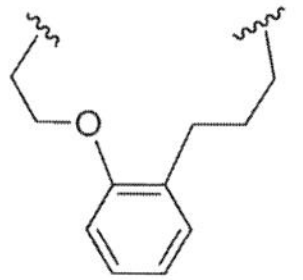	7.3	ND	**49**	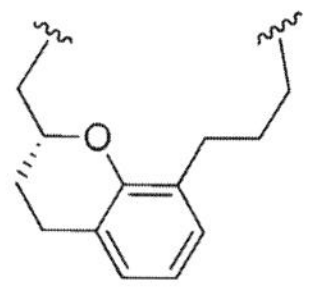	0.90	85
45	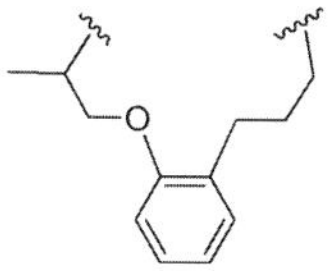	9.0	760	**50**	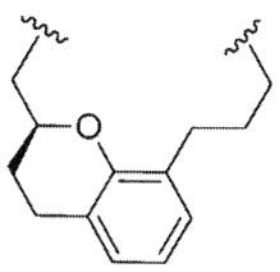	19	ND
46	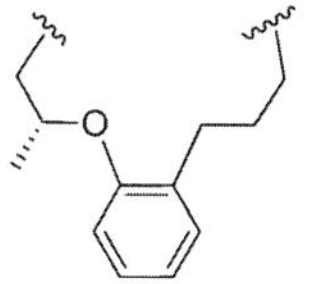	16	29	**51**	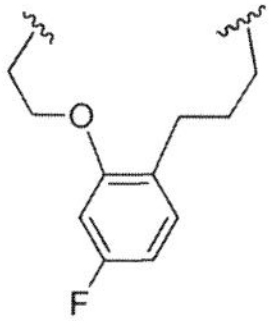	2.6	27

47		56	26	**52**		58	ND
48		12	Partial agonist[a]	**53**		61	ND

ND: not determined.

a) ~40% agonist response at 3 μM test concentration.

an additional methyl group on that atom to give the *gem*-disubstituted analogue (**48**), although displaying good binding, yielded a partial agonist, whereas all other compounds tested were full agonists. Additional restrictions on conformation by connecting the methyl to the phenyl moiety to create a dihydrobenzopyran ring provided chiral derivatives **49** and **50**. Consistent with the trends observed with the methyl derivatives, the (*R*)-analogue proved to be more potent than the (*S*)-isomer, although with a much greater effect here, exhibiting over a 20× difference in activity versus 3.5× for **46** versus **47**.

The second aspect of this investigation, substitution on the ring of the tether, displayed a clear SAR. Introduction of a fluorine substituent at the *para*-benzylic tether position (**51**) resulted in more than a twofold improvement in binding as compared with the unsubstituted compound (**44**). Shifting the fluorine substitution to the *para*-phenoxy position reduced the activity by over 20× (**52** versus **51**). Surprisingly, an analogue that combined both the tether (*R*)-methyl and phenyl fluorine beneficial substitutions (**53**) displayed worse potency than either of its singly substituted progenitors. The unexpected impact of these tether structural variants on the PK is described in the next section.

4.4 PK–ADME Considerations

Although not addressed in the discussion to this point, an assessment of the PK–ADME properties of the molecules actually was initiated at an early stage of the discovery process. Since these small molecule macrocycles represent an essentially unexplored chemical class, this work represents one of the first opportunities to extensively explore their properties. The target therapeutic indications for these ghrelin agonists were those characterized by acute GI dysmotility, such as those occurring after surgery (termed postoperative ileus), serious gastroparesis, and gastric stasis in critical care patients. For such applications, intravenous (i.v.) administration would actually be preferred since patients suffering from these conditions cannot easily take or tolerate oral medications. Hence, the primary focus was ensuring that the PK–ADME properties were optimal for i.v. administration. However, further development of a second generation of this compound class for chronic GI disorders was anticipated and these studies were expected to assist in establishing the groundwork for that effort as well. Despite the failure to meet certain traditional measurements required for oral pharmaceutical agents, such as Lipinski's rule of five referred to earlier, these macrocycles did prove amenable to optimization not only toward acceptable plasma half-life ($T_{1/2}$) and low systemic clearance rate (CL), but also toward good oral bioavailability (%F) to support their eventual development for chronic clinical applications[2)].

Shown in Table 4.5 are the PK data obtained in rats for a selection of analogues described previously. Two tether modifications in particular proved to

2) This second-generation ghrelin agonist, TZP-102, is currently being evaluated in a multinational phase 2b clinical trial as an oral treatment for diabetic gastroparesis.

Table 4.5 PK profile (i.v. administration) in rats.[a]

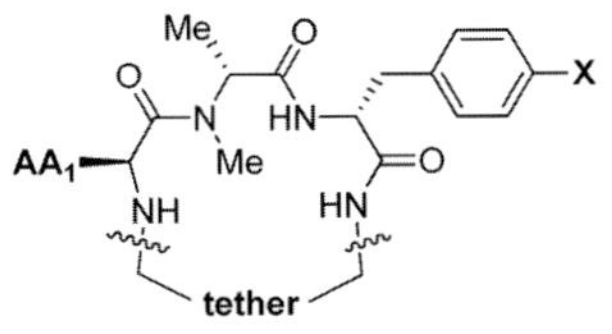

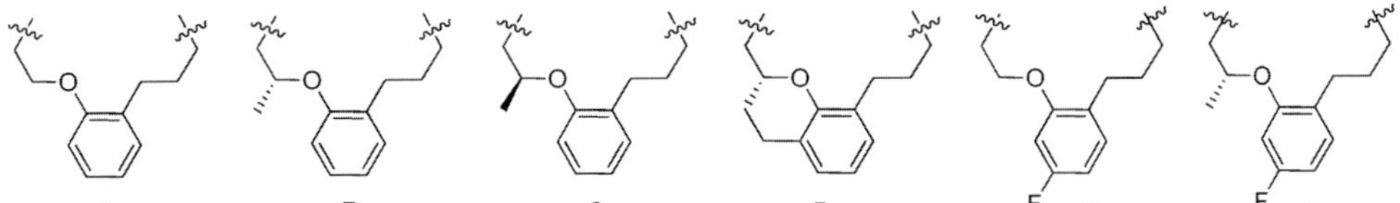

AA$_1$ Me Me O O N HN X NH HN O tether

A B C D E F

Compound	AA_1	X	Tether	K_i (nM)	EC_{50} (nM)	i.v., 2 mg/kg		
						$T_{1/2}$ (min)	V_{dss} (1/kg)	CL (ml/min/kg)
44	Cpg	F	A	7.3	ND	14	1.4	72
46	Cpg	F	B	16	29	50	1.7	24
47	Cpg	F	C	56	26	22	2.1	64
49	Cpg	F	D	0.70	85	59	1.1	13
51	Cpg	F	E	2.6	27	44	1.8	28
53	Cpg	F	F	61	ND	66	0.9	9
54	Nva	F	B	34	ND	29	1.7	41
55	Val	F	B	104	ND	34	2.0	40
56	Ile	F	B	32	ND	44	2.5	40
57	Cpg	Cl	B	15	18	41	1.4	24
58	Cpg	H	B	34	ND	32	1.3	25
59	Chg	F	B	0.38	49	74	4.7	43
60	Ile	Cl	A	0.35	20	33	3.2	67

ND: not determined.
a) Male Sprague-Dawley rats were administered compounds as an intravenous (i.v.) bolus at 2 mg/kg in physiological saline with 9% 2-hydroxypropyl-β-cyclodextrin.

have substantial impact on the PK profile: (i) stereospecific (*R*)-methyl substitution at the tether position adjacent to the oxygen atom (**46**) and (ii) substitution of the phenyl at the tether *para*-benzylic position (**51**). Indeed, a combination of these features (**53**) led to additional improvement of CL and half-life, unfortunately at the expense of potency (~4-fold reduction compared with **46**). Furthermore, an interesting difference in PK was observed for different configurations of the methyl substituent on the tether in the ether-containing arm. Analogue **46** with an (*R*)-methyl had a relatively low clearance and acceptable half-life, whereas the corresponding (*S*)-stereoisomer (**47**) was cleared at much higher rates with a much shorter $T_{1/2}$. Consistent with this trend, the benzopyran with an (*R*)-configuration at the same center (**49**) also possessed an improved PK profile with an even further reduced clearance rate, longer half-life, and a volume of distribution nearly twice that of total body water. Therefore, the additional conformational restriction introduced with the benzopyran benefited both binding affinity (18× improvement) and improved clearance. Nonetheless, analogue **46**, in comparison with **49**, possessed a threefold advantage in functional potency and, further, the synthesis of **49** was more complex than that for **46**. In contrast, compound **51** seemed to have similar functional activity and PK properties to **46**. However, after the additional *in vivo* evaluations described in Section 4.6, compound **46** (ulimorelin) proved to be a superior candidate for advancement into clinical development.

Although the tether structure had a significant impact on the PK profile of these macrocyclic compounds, there was an additional critical factor that contributed to the desirable PK profile for **46** of reduced CL and longer $T_{1/2}$. Indeed, this improved profile resulted from the (*R*)-methyl-substituted tether *together with* the cyclopropyl side chain on AA_1. Comparison of the PK results obtained with analogues **54–56**, which differ solely in the nature of the AA_1 side chain (*n*-propyl (Nva), isopropyl (Val), and isobutyl (Ile), respectively) highlights this apparent cooperative effect. Thus, **46** displayed ~2-fold improved clearance rate versus **54–56** for which significantly higher CL values were obtained. Similarly, analogue **44**, which contains only $AA_1 = Cpg$, but not the (*R*)-methyl substitution on the tether, displayed essentially flow-limited clearance along with a short $T_{1/2}$. Further, these results suggest that it is not simply metabolic blockade of that particular tether position that leads to the improved PK profile of **46**. A potential rationale for this vital cooperativity effect observed with this analogue is provided in Section 4.5.

In contrast to the crucial role of the AA_1 side chain in modulating PK, variations in the AA_3 side chain were much less impactful. For example, analogue **57** with a 4-chlorophenyl side chain at AA_3 exhibited a similar CL to **46**, containing a 4-fluorophenyl in that position. In fact, even the unsubstituted AA_3 phenyl ring (**58**) showed similar clearance rates to **46** and **57**. These results indicated that metabolism of the AA_3 phenyl ring was likely not a major elimination pathway in these macrocycles as was later confirmed from more detailed studies conducted on ulimorelin (**46**).

4.5
Structural Studies

In order to potentially gain insight into the PD and PK profiles observed with these unique macrocycles, as well as obtain confirmation of the underlying conformational control principles on which the technology was originally based, the solid-state structure of compound **46** (as its hydrochloride salt) was determined using single-crystal X-ray crystallography. In addition, solution conformation analysis of **46**·HCl was performed by a combination of NMR spectroscopy and molecular modeling[3)]. Upon analysis of bond distance and torsion angle data from the X-ray structure, the following information regarding the conformation(s) of the macrocycle could be gleaned: (i) the $C\alpha(i)$–$C\alpha(i+3)$ distances are less than 7 Å, indicative of a β-turn [39], and (ii) the torsion angles in the tripeptide segment revealed a (nonideal) closed type I′ β-turn [40]. These same features were also identified in the NMR-derived consensus solution structure where only a single conformational family was consistent with all the experimental constraints. Indeed, a very good correlation between the solid-state and solution-state structures was obtained, suggesting that the conformation was well optimized and rigidified in the final macrocycle (Figure 4.5).

Further comparison of the X-ray and NMR structures revealed another major similarity, the presence of an intramolecular hydrogen bond between the tether oxygen and the protonated secondary amine at the AA_1 position [41]. This intramolecular H-bond imparts additional conformational rigidity on the macrocyclic structure that, perhaps not surprisingly, does appear to have an impact on the activity. Recall that fluorine substitution at the *para*-phenoxy position in **52** reduced the activity by over 20× relative to the analogue with a *para*-benzylic fluoro substituent. This result is consistent with substitution of an electron-withdrawing group *para* to the oxygen lowering the basicity of that atom with concomitant weakening of this intramolecular H-bond. The possible influence that the presence of this H-bond has on the PK profile of the molecules is discussed below. Finally, in the NMR structure, the ammonium hydrogen appears associated with the carbonyl oxygen of AA_1, adding to the conformational constraints in **46**.

Additional insights into the potential role of the intramolecular H-bond between the tether oxygen and the AA_1 amine in **46** can be obtained from consideration of the somewhat unique nature of the cyclopropyl side chain. The cyclopropyl ring is almost as strong an electron-donating moiety as the cyclohexyl group[4)]. The effect of such electron donation would be to enhance the basicity of the secondary amine at AA_1, concomitantly strengthening the intramolecular H-bond[5)]. In addition, the relatively low lipophilicity of the cyclopropyl group could positively impact hepatic metabolism rates as well as the solubility. Indeed, **46** has aqueous solubility values in the 1–8 mg/ml range (at about pH 5), while related structures with

3) For a more detailed description of these studies, see Ref. [38].
4) Based upon a comparison of the Hammett σ_p and Hansch π values.
5) This is confirmed by the measured pK_a values for analogues with Cpg at AA_1, where the amine basicity is enhanced by ≥ 0.3 log units versus derivatives with an *n*-propyl side chain.

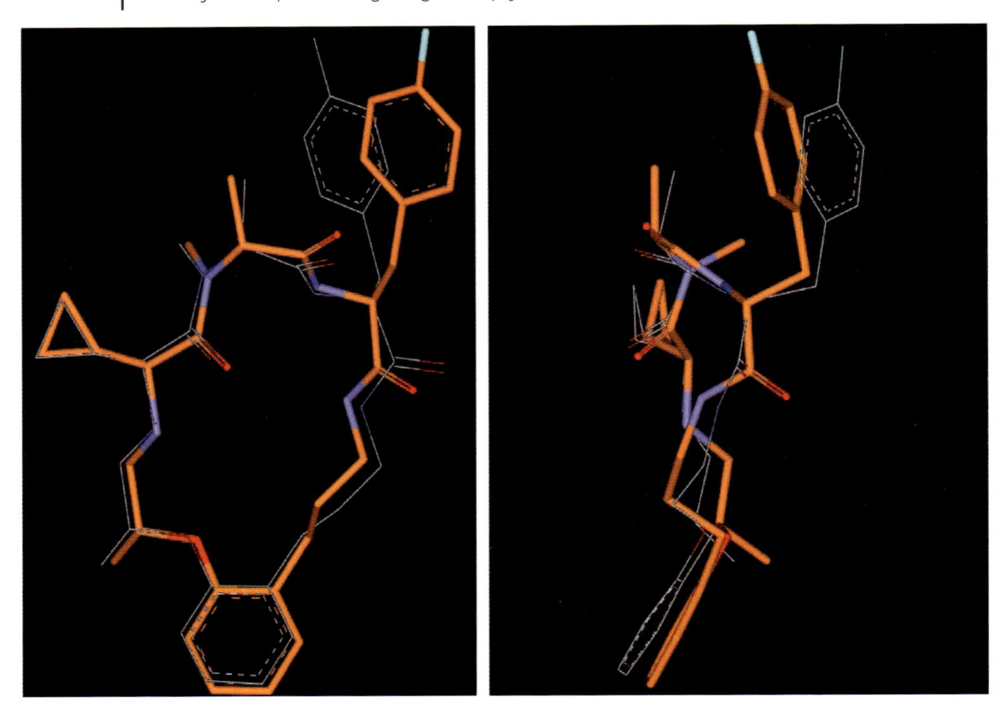

Figure 4.5 Comparison of NMR (orange) and X-ray structures for **46** (ulimorelin).

$AA_1 = Nva$ (**54**) or Ile (**56**) gave significantly lower aqueous solubility (0.1–0.5 mg/ml range) with the solubility of the Chg analogue (**59**) extremely poor ($\leq$0.01 mg/ml) under similar conditions.

Thus, the strong electron-donating ability of the cyclopropyl moiety at the AA_1 position appears to enhance the conformational rigidity in **46** by strengthening the intramolecular H-bond seen in both the X-ray and NMR structures with minimal impact on the overall lipophilicity. Further, the topological positioning of the (*R*)-Me tether substitution and the AA_1 cyclopropyl side chain on opposite faces of the core macrocyclic framework provides hydrophobic shielding of this intramolecular H-bond from both sides of the molecule, possibly protecting it from disruption by encroaching water molecules. Hence, the electronic and steric shielding effects provided by these two moieties work together to stabilize the intramolecular H-bond and further rigidify the structure, providing a potential explanation for the observed PK cooperative effect observed in **46**, which was lacking in its close analogues.

4.6 Preclinical Evaluation

A number of *in vitro* assays have become fixtures in drug discovery research in order to improve the evaluation of early stage compounds and direct attention

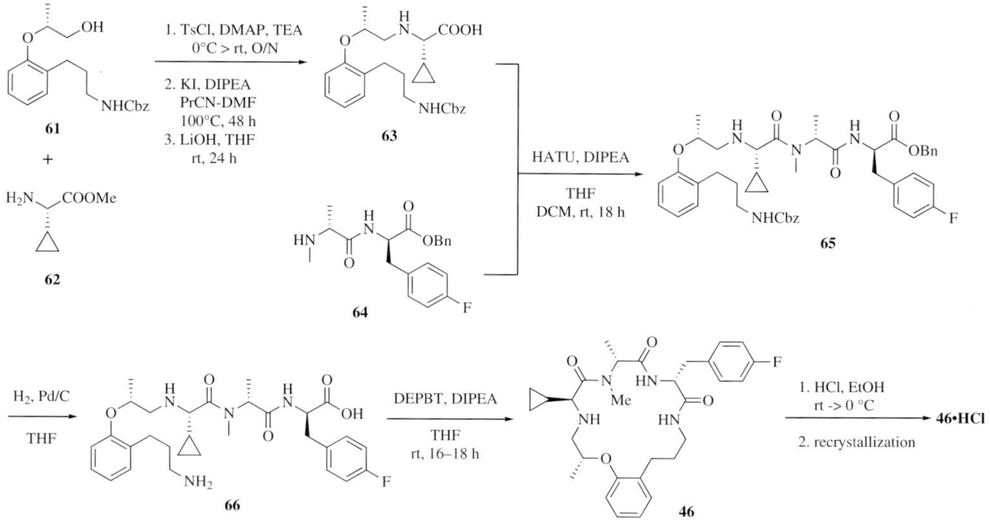

Scheme 4.3 Synthesis of ulimorelin (46).

toward compounds with favorable properties for further development [42]. In addition, the lack of an existing knowledge base regarding this particular compound class and our desire to eventually develop an oral gastroprokinetic agent prompted us to investigate applicable physicochemical parameters and oral PK of these molecules as well. To access sufficient material for more complete profiling and for *in vivo* studies, a synthetic route amenable to larger amounts of material first needed to be developed. Based upon the solution-phase procedure presented earlier, Scheme 4.3 illustrates the resulting process, which has proved viable for even clinical quantities of **46**.

4.6.1
Additional Compound Profiling

One common screen for membrane permeability, used as a predictor for oral bioavailability, is the Caco-2 assay [43]. The results in Table 4.6 demonstrate that very good membrane permeability could be obtained with the small variety of substituents tested and that the variations seen in the PK for these molecules were not duplicated in this test. Further, the near-equivalent flux rates in both directions for **46** and **60**, both of which displayed moderate permeability, indicate that neither appears to be a P-glycoprotein (Pgp) substrate. However, the results with **51** suggest that at least moderate Pgp-mediated active transport is likely occurring.

For metabolic stability, however, differences between **46** and **60** are again evident. Analogue **46** displayed greater *in vitro* stability in rat (RLM) and human hepatic liver microsomes (HLMs) as compared to **60**. This indicates that the improved CL and oral bioavailability obtained for **46** could be due to improved first-pass hepatic

Table 4.6 Physiochemical profile, permeability, and metabolic stability of advanced analogues.

					Caco-2 flux (nm/s)[b]		RLM[c]	HLM[d]
Compound	MW (g/mol)	clogP[a]	H-bond donors	H-bond acceptors	s-to-m[e]	m-to-s[e]	%cmpd[f]	$T_{1/2}$ (min)
46	538.6	5.3	3	5	140	150	68	19
51	542.6	5.1	3	5	125	198	54	41
60	557.1	6.4	3	5	150	140	86	5

a) Calculated using ChemDrawUltra v. 12.0.
b) For reference, propranolol, a high-permeability compound, displays Caco-2 flux values of ~350 nm/s.
c) RLM: rat liver microsomes.
d) As a reference, human liver microsome (HLM) $T_{1/2}$ value for propranolol was 59 min.
e) s-to-m and m-to-s represent serosal-to-mucosal and mucosal-to-serosal, respectively.
f) %cmpd refers to % of compound metabolized after 15 min.

and/or intestinal metabolism, perhaps mediated by P450 enzymes. In addition, improved RLM and HLM stability was observed for **51**, which contains a fluorophenyl tether, in comparison with **46** and **60**. Overall, these results imply that the improved rat PK profile obtained with *para*-fluorobenzylic tether moieties (**51** and **53**) may be due to both improved first-pass clearance and enhanced absorption assisted by Pgp active transport.

Following a 30 min i.v. infusion at a target dose level of 6 mg/kg in Sprague-Dawley rats, ^{14}C-labeled **46** was efficiently excreted in the feces unchanged with a recovery of 95% of the administered dose[6)]. These results are consistent with hepatobiliary elimination [44] and suggests that **46** would be subjected to liver first-pass metabolism after PO dosing. It is also noteworthy that **46** displayed a reasonably high unbound fraction in rat plasma ($f_u = 13\%$) compared to human plasma ($f_u = 1.6\%$)[7)]. Subsequent studies have determined that **46** is actually even more strongly protein bound than this in man ($\geq 99\%$), primarily to α_1-acid glycoprotein [45].

4.6.2 Additional Pharmacokinetic Data

Shown in Tables 4.7 and 4.8 are PK data in rats and monkeys, respectively, for various analogues that displayed good overall PD and PK profiles with the most advanced compounds only being examined in the latter species.

Whereas **46** displayed identical oral bioavailability in monkeys and rats, the bioavailability of compound **51** in monkeys was nearly fivefold lower than that observed in the rodent species. Parallel trends for clearance followed for these two

6) Compound was dosed in 5% dextrose in water containing sodium acetate buffer.
7) Equilibrium protein binding results were obtained using an ultracentrifugation method.

Table 4.7 PK profiles of representative analogues in rat.[a]

	PO, 8 mg/kg		i.v., 2 mg/kg			
Compound	C_{max} (μM)	$AUC_{0-\infty}$ (μM min)	$T_{1/2}$ (min)	V_{dss} (l/kg)	CL (ml/min/kg)	%F[b]
46	0.39	82.0	50	1.7	24	24
51	0.90	99.9	44	1.8	28	36
53	0.75	125	66	0.9	9	15
57	0.67	73.8	41	1.4	24	22
60	0.06	3.51	33	3.2	67	3

a) Male Sprague-Dawley rats were administered compounds either as an i.v. bolus at 2 mg/kg in physiological saline with 9% 2-hydroxypropyl-β-cyclodextrin or PO (gavage) at 8 mg/kg in physiological saline.
b) %F: absolute oral bioavailability.

compounds; thus, in monkeys, **46** was cleared 2.3 times more slowly than **51**, representing a greater disparity versus the same trends observed in rats in which both analogues cleared at similar rates.

The majority of drug–drug interactions are metabolism based and, moreover, these interactions typically involve inhibition of cytochrome P450s. Six CYP450 enzymes (CYP1A2, CYP2C8, CYP2C9, CYP2C19, CYP2D6, and CYP3A4) appear to be commonly responsible for the metabolism of most drugs and binding to these and other isoforms are often evaluated to determine potential risk from drug–drug interactions [46]. The overall cytochrome P450 profile for **46** appeared somewhat better than that of **51** (Table 4.9) even though both analogues displayed suboptimal CYP3A4 profiles that are nonetheless acceptable for the acute treatment regimen envisioned.

The data from these profiling efforts taken together with the *in vivo* efficacy results (Section 4.6.3) affirmed **46** as the clinical candidate of choice.

Table 4.8 PK profiles of advanced analogues in monkey.[a]

	PO, 8 mg/kg		IV, 2 mg/kg			
Compound	C_{max} (μM)	$AUC_{0-\infty}$ (μM min)	$T_{1/2}$ (min)	V_{dss} (l/kg)	CL (ml/min/kg)	%F[b]
46	1.4	75.4	23	0.23	8.8	24
51	0.09	10.3	29	0.66	20	7

a) Adult male cynomolgus monkeys were administered compounds either as an i.v. bolus at 0.5 mg/kg in physiological saline with 9% 2-hydroxypropyl-β-cyclodextrin or PO (gavage) at 1.5 mg/kg in physiological saline.
b) %F: absolute oral bioavailability.

Table 4.9 Human cytochrome P450 profile of advanced analogues.

Compound	CYP P450 IC_{50} (μM)				
	3A4	2D6	2C9	2C19	1A2
46	2.4	84	66	>100	>100
51	1.2	31	>100	>100	>100

Table 4.10 Gastric emptying data (i.v. administration) in rats for advanced analogues.

Compound	Gastric emptying[a] (i.v.)[b], EC_{50} (mg/kg)[c]
46	0.91
51	1.20
53	1.38
57	0.84
60	0.39

a) Conducted with overnight-fasted male Wistar rats given a 2% methylcellulose meal containing 10% phenol red administered orally at 2 ml/animal and sacrificed 15 min later. Stomach contents were measured at sacrifice by colorimetric analysis (560 nm) for determination of phenol red remaining.
b) Administered coincident with the meal in 9% 2-hydroxypropyl-β-cyclodextrin.
c) For reference, ghrelin peptide in this assay has $EC_{50} = 0.04$ mg/kg.

4.6.3
Animal Models for Preclinical Efficacy

Based upon the output from the medicinal chemistry efforts and the additional profiling just described, the most promising macrocycles were advanced into proof-of-concept testing in an animal model of gastric emptying (Table 4.10). Gratifyingly, these compounds displayed potent effects on the stimulation of GI motility as was expected from these ghrelin agonists.

As further evidence of *in vivo* prokinetic activity of ulimorelin (**46**), its effectiveness as a treatment in a rat model of POI has been reported [47]. In contrast to other classes of ghrelin agonists, ulimorelin did not appear to stimulate concurrent GH secretion in these animal models [48].

4.7
Clinical Results and Current Status

Based upon the promising preclinical data, ulimorelin (compound **46**) was advanced into the clinic in early 2006 as an intravenous treatment for restoration of GI motility following surgery. Table 4.11 summarizes the six clinical trials conducted, completed, and reported to date for ulimorelin.

Table 4.11 Clinical evaluation of ulimorelin.

Clinical phase	Design and size	Ulimorelin dose levels	Results
Phase 1a [49]	Prospective, randomized, double-blind, placebo-controlled, dose escalation trial to assess safety, tolerability, pharmacokinetics, and pharmacodynamics in 48 healthy volunteers	Single 30 min i.v. infusion, six dose ranges from 20 to 600 μg/kg or placebo	All doses were well tolerated, PK analysis revealed less than dose-proportional behavior of drug with low clearance (approximately 7 ml/h/kg), small volume of distribution (approximately 114 ml/kg), and half-life values of approximately 13 h, which were independent of dose. Pharmacodynamic analyses suggested ulimorelin, at doses as low as 40 μg/kg, expressed activity at the receptor.
Phase 1b [50]	Dose-escalating double-blind study in 12 healthy subjects, with six (6) additional at the highest dose, for evaluation of safety, tolerability, pharmacokinetics, and pharmacodynamics	30 min i.v. infusion of one of three dose levels (80, 320, and 600 μg/kg) or placebo for five consecutive days	Ulimorelin was well tolerated and safe after infusions across several dose levels with no dose-dependent drug-related events observed. PK was linear, but not dose proportional, possibly as a result of concentration-dependent protein binding. Confirmed low clearance and low volume of distribution with plasma half-life of 20 h.
Phase 1 (QTc)	Double-blind, randomized, parallel study to compare the ECG effects of ulimorelin to placebo and moxifloxacin (a positive control known to increase the QT interval) in 160 healthy men and women	Two doses daily for five consecutive days, therapeutic (160 μg/kg) and supratherapeutic dose (600 μg/kg)	No effect on cardiac parameters or morphology. Measured a multitude of electrophysiological parameters with no apparent deleterious effect on any of them.
Phase 2a [51]	Double-blind, crossover trial in 10 subjects with moderate-to-severe diabetic gastroparesis	30 min i.v. infusion of one of four doses (80, 160, 320, or 600 μg/kg) or placebo	Ulimorelin showed a statistically significant acceleration of gastric emptying ($p = 0.043$) and reduction of latency times ($p = 0.037$) of a solid radiolabeled meal relative to placebo.

(continued)

Table 4.11 *(Continued)*

Clinical phase	Design and size	Ulimorelin dose levels	Results
Phase 2b [52]	Double-blind, randomized, placebo-controlled trial in 76 diabetic patients with moderate-to-severe symptoms due to diabetic gastroparesis	Single 30 min i.v. infusion of one of six doses ranging from 20 to 600 μg/kg or placebo once daily for four consecutive days	Symptoms were evaluated daily with the Gastroparesis Cardinal Symptom Index (GCSI, consisting of nine patient-rated symptom assessments for quantifying the severity of gastroparesis. The 80 μg/kg dose was identified as the most effective dose; statistically significant improvement compared with placebo in the severity of GCSI loss of appetite and vomiting scores for that dose group ($p = 0.034$ and $p = 0.006$). In addition, the proportion of patients with at least 50% improvement in vomiting score was significantly higher with ulimorelin ($p = 0.019$) compared with placebo.
Phase 2b [53]	Multinational, multicenter, double-blind, dose-ranging, placebo-controlled trial employing an adaptive randomization design in 236 patients undergoing open partial colectomy	One of seven dose levels, 20–600 μg/kg, or placebo, single daily dose by 30 min i.v. infusion for up to seven consecutive days	Ulimorelin accelerated the time to first bowel movement in all groups, with $p = 0.056$ for the low efficacious dose (80 μg/kg) and $p = 0.03$ for the most efficacious dose (480 μg/kg). The median time to first bowel movement was reduced in all treatment groups by 10–22 h versus placebo. At the 480 μg/kg dose, the median time to readiness for hospital discharge was significantly accelerated by 20.4 h compared with placebo ($p = 0.03$). A greater number of patients who received ulimorelin achieved recovery by 72 h postsurgery compared with placebo ($p \leq 0.001$).

In summary, these studies have shown that ulimorelin

- has potent GI motility effects in humans;
- is efficacious in the treatment of two disorders characterized by GI dysmotility, POI and diabetic gastroparesis;
- possesses better PK parameters in humans than had been anticipated based upon the effects in preclinical animal models;
- gives PK profiles in both healthy subjects and patients that were less than dose proportional, most likely because of concentration-dependent protein binding;
- exhibits very good safety in humans, with no indication of the side effects that have plagued previous GI promotility agents.

Ulimorelin has just completed two multinational phase 3 studies for the treatment of restoration of GI function following partial bowel resection surgery in the United States and Europe. Each trial targeted 360 patients and was conducted at approximately 50 sites in North America and Europe. Patients in these double-blind, placebo-controlled trials were evenly randomized to one of three treatment groups: placebo, 160 μg/kg, or 480 μg/kg, doses which were selected based on data from the phase 2 trial. Topline results from these trials have been reported, which disappointingly failed to meet its primary and secondary efficacy end points [54]. While analysis of the data from these trials continues, all other NDA development activities for ulimorelin have been placed on hold.

4.8 Summary

The discovery and development of ulimorelin admirably demonstrates the tremendous utility of mining underexplored chemotypes in the search for new pharmacological activity. Drug discovery using these macrocycles proceeds with both differences and similarities to efforts with more traditional scaffolds. Although these compounds do not typically conform to certain standard measurements of druglikeness, such as the Lipinski rules, they do match better with the revised considerations advocated by Veber that emphasize polar surface area (PSA) and rotatable bond count [55].

Further, in many traditional efforts, moving from hit to clinical candidate has been seen to add molecular weight and increase lipophilicity [56]. With this macrocyclic scaffold, however, significant property modification can be achieved without such increases. Indeed, the MW of ulimorelin (**46**) was merely 9% higher than analogue **1** and clogP increased only 12%.

In conclusion, starting from a library of unique, conformationally defined macrocyclic molecules, a promising hit series was progressed through a series of approximately 500 analogues, based upon a systematic investigation of each of the four diversity components of the structures, to ultimately produce a viable clinical candidate with a novel mechanism of action, ghrelin receptor agonism, for gastrointestinal disorders. In addition, the capacity for the nature of one of these components, the tether, to have profound effects on the PK–ADME parameters suggests that there will be much new knowledge to be gained as additional investigations are conducted on this structural class.

References

1 Kojima, M., Hosoda, H., Date, Y., Nakazato, M., Matsuo, H., and Kangawa, K. (1999) Ghrelin is a growth-hormone-releasing acylated peptide from stomach. *Nature*, **402**, 656–660.

2 (a) Broglio, F., Gottero, C., Arvat, E., and Ghigo, E. (2003) Endocrine and non-endocrine actions of ghrelin. *Horm. Res.*, **59**, 109–117. (b) Hosoda, H., Kojima, M., and Kangawa, K. (2006) Biological, physiological, and pharmacological aspects of ghrelin. *J. Pharmacol. Sci.*, **100**, 398–410.

3 Howard, A.D., Feighner, S.D., Cully, D.F., Arena, J.P., Liberator, P.A., Rosenblum, C.I., Hamelin, M., Hreniuk, D.L., Palyha, O.C., Andrerson, J., Paress, P.S., Diaz, C., Chou, M., Liu, K.K., McKee, K.K., Pong, S.-S., Chaung, L.-Y., Elbrecht, A., Dashkevicz, M., Heavens, R., Rigby, M., Sirinathsighji, D.J.S., Dean, D.C., Melillo, D.G., Patchett, A.A., Nargund, R., Griffin, P.R., DeMartino, J.A., Gupta, S.K., Schaeffer, J.M., Smith, R.G., and Van der Ploeg, L.H.T. (1996) A receptor in pituitary and hypothalamus that functions in growth hormone release. *Science*, **273**, 974–977.

4 Davenport, A.P., Bonner, T.I., Foord, S.M., Harmar, A.J., Neubig, R.R., Pin, J.P., Spedding, M., Kojima, M., and Kangawa, K. (2005) International Union of Pharmacology. LVI. Ghrelin receptor nomenclature, distribution, and function. *Pharmacol. Rev.*, **57**, 541–546.

5 Ghelardoni, S., Carnicelli, V., Frascarelli, S., Ronca-Testoni, S., and Zucchi, R. (2006) Ghrelin tissue distribution: comparison between gene and protein expression. *J. Endocrinol. Invest.*, **29**, 115–121.

6 Gnanapavan, S., Kola, B., Bustin, S.A., Morris, D.G., McGee, P., Fairclough, P., Bhattacharya, S., Carpenter, R., Grossman, A.B., and Korbonits, M. (2002) The tissue distribution of the mRNA of ghrelin and subtypes of its receptor, GHS-R, in humans. *J. Clin. Endocrinol. Metab.*, **87**, 2988–2991.

7 (a) Svensson, J. (2000) Growth hormone secretagogues. *Exp. Opin. Ther. Pat.*, **10**, 1071–1080. (b) Nargund, R.P., Patchett, A.A., Bach, M.A., Murphy, M.G., and Smith, R.G. (1998) Peptidomimetic growth hormone secretagogues. Design considerations and therapeutic potential. *J. Med. Chem.*, **41**, 3103–3127. (c) Ghigo, E., Arvat, E., and Camanni, F. (1998) Orally active growth hormone secretagogues: state of the art and clinical perspective. *Ann. Med.*, **30**, 159–168. (d) Smith, R.G., Van der Ploeg, L.H.T., Howard, A.D., Feighner, S.D., Cheng, K., Hickey, G.J., Wyvratt, M.J., Jr., Fisher, M. H., Nargund, R.P., and Patchett, A.A. (1997) Peptidomimetic regulation of growth hormone secretion. *Endocr. Rev.*, **18**, 621–645.

8 (a) Smith, R.G., Sun, Y.X., Beatancourt, L., and Asnicar, M. (2004) Growth hormone secretagogues: prospects and pitfalls. *Best Pract. Res. Clin. Endocrinol. Metab.*, **18**, 333–347. (b) Fehrentz, J.-A., Martinez, J., Boeglin, D., Guerlavais, V., and Deghenghi, R. (2002) Growth hormone secretagogues: past, present and future. *IDrugs*, **5**, 804–814.

9 A peptidomimetic GHS, NN703, was also shown to cause irreversible inhibition of cytochrome P450 enzymes: Zdravkovic, M., Olse, A.K., Christiansen, T., Schulz, R., Taub, M.E., Thomsen, M.S., Rasmussen, M.H., and Ilondo, M.M. (2003) A clinical study investigating the pharmacokinetic interaction between NN703 (tabimorelin), a potential inhibitor of CYP3A4 activity, and midazolam, a CYP3A4 substrate. *Eur. J. Clin. Pharmacol.*, **58**, 683–688.

10 (a) Kojima, M. and Kangawa, K. (2006) Drug insight: the functions of ghrelin and

its potential as a multitherapeutic hormone. *Nat. Clin. Pract. Endocrinol. Metab.*, **2**, 80–88. (b) Akamizu, T. and Kangawa, K. (2006) Translational research on the clinical applications of ghrelin. *Endocr. J.*, **53**, 585–591. (c) Leite-Moreira, A.F. and Soares, J.-B. (2007) Physiological, pathological and potential therapeutic roles of ghrelin. *Drug Discov. Today*, **12**, 276–288. (d) Katergari, S.A., Milousis, A., Pagonopoulou, O., Asimakopoulos, B., and Nikolettos, N.K. (2008) Ghrelin in pathological conditions. *Endocr. J.*, **55**, 439–453.

11 (a) Kamiji, M.M. and Inui, A. (2008) The role of ghrelin and ghrelin analogues in wasting disease. *Curr. Opin. Clin. Nutr. Metab. Care*, **11**, 443–451. (b) DeBoer, M. D. (2008) Emergence of ghrelin as a treatment for cachexia syndromes. *Nutrition*, **24**, 806–814.

12 (a) Garcia, J.M. and Polvino, W.J. (2007) Effect on body weight and safety of RC-1291, a novel, orally available ghrelin mimetic and growth hormone secretagogue: results of a phase I, randomized, placebo-controlled, multiple-dose study in healthy volunteers. *Oncologist*, **12**, 594–600. (b) Strasser, F., Lutz, T.A., and Maeder, M.T. (2008) Safety, tolerability and pharmacokinetics of intravenous ghrelin for cancer-related anorexia/cachexia: a randomised, placebo-controlled, double-blind, double-crossover study. *Br. J. Cancer*, **98**, 300–308. (c) Garcia, JM. and Polvino, W.J. (2009) Pharmacodynamic hormonal effects of anamorelin, a novel oral ghrelin mimetic and growth hormone secretagogue in healthy volunteers. *Growth Horm. IGF Res.*, **19**, 267–273.

13 Smith, R.G., Sun, Y., Jiang, H., Albarran-Zeckler, R., and Timchenko, N. (2007) Ghrelin receptor (GHS-R1A) agonists show potential as interventive agents during aging. *Ann. N. Y. Acad. Sci.*, **1119**, 147–164.

14 (a) Horvath, T.L., Castañeda, T., Tang-Christensen, M., Pagotto, U., and Tschöp, M.H. (2003) Ghrelin as a potential anti-obesity target. *Curr. Pharm. Des.*, **9**, 1383–1395. (b) Cummings, D.E. (2006) Ghrelin and the short- and long-term regulation of appetite and body weight. *Physiol. Behav.*, **89**, 71–84.

15 Murray, C.D.R., Kamm, M.A., Bloom, S. R., and Emmanuel, A.V. (2003) Ghrelin for the gastroenterologist: history and potential. *Gastroenterology*, **125**, 1492–1502.

16 Everhart, J.E. (ed.) (2008) *The Burden of Digestive Diseases in the United States*, NIH Publication 09-6433, National Institute of Diabetes and Digestive and Kidney Diseases, U.S. Department of Health and Human Services, Bethesda, MD.

17 (a) Kojima, M. Hsoda, H., and Kangawa, K. (2001) Purification and distribution of ghrelin: the natural endogenous ligand for the growth hormone secretagogue receptor. *Horm. Res.*, **56** (Suppl. 1), 93–97. (b) Ariyasu, H., Takaya, K., Tagami, T., Ogawa, Y., Hosoda, K., Akamizu, T., Suda, M., Koh, T., Natsui, K., Toyooka, S., Shirakami, G., Usui, T., Shimatsu, A., Doi, K., Hosoda, H., Kojima, M., Kangawa, K., and Nakao, K. (2001) Stomach is a major source of circulating ghrelin, and feeding state determines plasma ghrelin-like immunoreactivity levels in humans. *J. Clin. Endocrinol. Metab.*, **86**, 4753–4758.

18 Inui, A., Asakawa, A., Bowers, C.Y., Mantovani, G., Laviano, A., Meguid, M. M., and Fujimiya, M. (2004) Ghrelin, appetite, and gastric motility: the emerging role of the stomach as an endocrine organ. *FASEB J.*, **18**, 439–456.

19 (a) Peeters, T.L. (2003) Central and peripheral mechanisms by which ghrelin regulates gut motility. *J. Physiol. Pharmacol.*, **54** (Suppl. 4), 95–103. (b) Edholm, T., Levin, F., Hellström, P.M., and Schmidt, P.T. (2004) Ghrelin stimulates motility in the small intestine of rats through intrinsic cholinergic neurons. *Regul. Pept.*, **121**, 25–30.

20 (a) Masuda, Y., Tanaka, T., Inomata, N., Ohnuma, N., Tanaka, S., Itoh, Z., Hosoda, H., Kojima, M., and Kangawa, K. (2000) Ghrelin stimulates gastric acid secretion and motility in rats. *Biochem. Biophys. Res. Commun.*, **276**, 905–908. (b) Fujino, K., Inui, A., Asakawa, A., Kihara, N., Fujimura, M., and Fujimiya, M. (2003) Ghrelin induces fasting motor activity of the gastrointestinal tract in conscious fed rats. *J. Physiol.*, **550**, 227–240.

21 (a) Trudel, L., Tomasetto, C., Rio, M.C., Bouin, M., Plourde, V., Eberling, P., and Poitras, P. (2002) Ghrelin/motilin-related peptide is a potent prokinetic to reverse gastric postoperative ileus in rats. *Am. J. Physiol.*, **282**, G948–G952. (b) Trudel, L., Bouin, M., Tomasetto, C., Eberling, P., St-Pierre, S., Bannon, P., L'Heureux, M. C., and Poitras, P. (2003) Two new peptides to improve post-operative gastric ileus in dog. *Peptides*, **24**, 531–534.

22 (a) This is now a well-established paradigm: Peeters, T.L. (2006) Potential of ghrelin as a therapeutic approach for gastrointestinal motility disorders. *Curr. Opin. Pharmacol.*, **6**, 553–558. (b) Sanger, G.J. (2008) Motilin, ghrelin and related neuropeptides as targets for the treatment of GI diseases. *Drug Discov. Today*, **13**, 234–239. (c) Venkova, K. and Greenwood-Van Meerveld, B. (2008) Application of ghrelin to gastrointestinal diseases. *Curr. Opin. Invest. Drugs*, **9**, 1103–1107. (d) DeSmet, B., Mitselos, A., and Depoortere, I. (2009) Motilin and ghrelin as prokinetic drug targets. *Pharmacol. Ther.*, **123**, 207–223. (e) Greenwood-Van Meerveld, B., Kriegsman, M., and Nelson, R. (2011) Ghrelin as a target for gastrointestinal motility disorders. *Peptides*, **32**, 2352–2356.

23 (a) Kitazawa, T., De Smet, B., Verbeke, K., Depoortere, I., and Peeters, T.L. (2005) Gastric motor effects of peptide and non-peptide ghrelin agonists in mice *in vivo* and *in vitro*. *Gut*, **54**, 1078–1084. (b) Poitras, P., Polvino, W.J., and Rocheleau, B. (2005) Gastrokinetic effect of ghrelin analog RC-1139 in the rat. Effect on post-operative and on morphine induced ileus. *Peptides*, **26**, 1598–1601.

24 (a) Murray, C.D.R., Martin, N.M., Patterson, M., Taylor, S., Ghatei, M.A., Kamm, M.A., Johnston, C., Bloom, S.R., and Emmanuel, A.V. (2005) Ghrelin enhances gastric emptying in diabetic gastroparesis: a double blind, placebo controlled, crossover study. *Gut*, **54**, 1693–1698. (b) Tack, J., Depoortere, I., Bisschops, R., Verbeke, K., Janssens, J., and Peeters, T. (2005) Influence of ghrelin on gastric emptying and meal-related symptoms in idiopathic gastroparesis. *Aliment. Pharmacol. Ther.*, **22**, 847–853. (c) Binn, M., Albert, C., Gougeon, A., Maerki, H., Coulie, B., Lemoyne, M., Rabasa Lhoret, R., Tomasetto, C., and Poitras, P. (2006) Ghrelin gastrokinetic action in patients with neurogenic gastroparesis. *Peptides*, **27**, 1603–1606.

25 Tack, J., Depoortere, I., Bisschops, R., Delporte, C., Coulie, B., Meulemans, A., Janssens, J., and Peeters, T. (2006) Influence of ghrelin on interdigestive gastrointestinal motility in humans. *Gut*, **55**, 327–333.

26 (a) For representative reviews, see Gershon, M.D. and Tack, J. (2007) The serotonin signaling system: from basic understanding to drug development for functional GI disorders. *Gastroenterology*, **132**, 397–414. (b) Spiller, R. (2008) Serotonin and GI clinical disorders. *Neuropharmacology*, **55**, 1072–1080.

27 Fernández, AG. and Massingham, R. (1985) Peripheral receptor populations involved in the regulation of gastrointestinal motility and the pharmacological actions of metoclopramide-like drugs. *Life Sci.*, **36**, 1–14.

28 Quigley, E.M. (2011) Cisapride: what can we learn from the rise and fall of a prokinetic? *J. Dig. Dis.*, **12**, 147–156.

29 Al-Judaibi, B., Chande, N., and Gregor, J. (2010) Safety and efficacy of tegaserod therapy in patients with irritable bowel syndrome or chronic constipation. *Can. J. Clin. Pharmacol.*, **17**, e194–200.

30 Pasricha, P.J., Pehlivanov, N., Sugumar, A., and Jankovic, J. (2006) Drug Insight: from disturbed motility to disordered movement – a review of the clinical benefits and medicolegal risks of metoclopramide. *Nat. Clin. Pract. Gastroenterol. Hepatol.*, **3**, 138–148.

31 Drewry, D.H. and Macarron, R. (2010) Enhancements of screening collections to address areas of unmet medical need: an industry perspective. *Curr. Opin. Chem. Biol.*, **14**, 289–298.

32 Lipinski, C.A., Lombardo, F., Dominy, B. W., and Feeney, P.J. (1997) Experimental and computational approaches to estimate

solubility and permeability in drug discovery and development settings. *Adv. Drug Deliv. Rev.*, **23**, 3–25.

33 (a) Driggers, E.M., Hale, S.P., Lee, J., and Terrett, N.K. (2008) The exploration of macrocycles for drug discovery – an underexploited structural class. *Nat. Rev. Drug Discov.*, **7**, 608–624. (b) Terrett, N.K. (2010) Methods for the synthesis of macrocycle libraries for drug discovery. *Drug Discov. Today*, **7** (2), e97–e104. (c) Marsault, E.M. and Peterson, M.L. (2011) Macrocycles are great cycles: applications, opportunities, and challenges of synthetic macrocycles in drug discovery. *J. Med. Chem.*, **54**, 1961–2004.

34 Marsault, E., Hoveyda, H.R., Gagnon, R., Peterson, M.L., Vézina, M., Saint-Louis, C., Landry, A., Pinault, J.-F., Ouellet, L., Beauchemin, S., Beaubien, S., Mathieu, A., Benakli, K., Wang, Z., Brassard, M., Lonergan, D., Bilodeau, F., Ramaseshan, M., Fortin, N., Lan, R., Li, S., Galaud, F., Plourde, V., Champagne, M., Doucet, A., Bhérer, P., Gauthier, M., Olsen, G., Villeneuve, G., Bhat, S., Foucher, L., Fortin, D., Peng, X., Bernard, S., Drouin, A., Déziel, R., Berthiaume, G., Dory, Y.L., Fraser, G.L., and Deslongchamps, P. (2008) Efficient parallel synthesis of macrocyclic peptidomimetics. *Bioorg. Med. Chem. Lett.*, **18**, 4731–4735.

35 Xiao, X.Y., Li, R., Zhuang, H., Ewing, B., Karunaratne, K., Lillig, J., Brown, R., and Nicolaou, K.C. (2000) Solid-phase combinatorial synthesis using MicroKan reactors, Rf tagging, and directed sorting. *Biotechnol. Bioeng.*, **71**, 44–50.

36 Le Poul, E., Hisada, S., Mizuguchi, Y., Dupriez, V.J., Burgeon, E., and Detheux, M. (2002) Adaptation of aequorin functional assay to high throughput screening. *J. Biomol. Screen.*, **7**, 57–65.

37 Marsault, E., Hoveyda, H.R., Peterson, M. L., Saint-Louis, C., Landry, A., Vézina, M., Ouellet, L., Wang, Z., Ramaseshan, M., Beaubien, S., Benakli, K., Beauchemin, S., Déziel, R., Peeters, T., and Fraser, G.L. (2006) Discovery of new class of macrocyclic antagonists to the human motilin receptor. *J. Med. Chem.*, **49**, 7190–7197.

38 For additional discussions on the development of ulimorelin, see Hoveyda, H.R., Marsault, E., Gagnon, R., Mathieu, A.P., Vézina, M., Landry, A., Wang, Z., Benakli, K., Beaubien, S., Saint-Louis, C., Brassard, M., Pinault, J.F., Ouellet, L., Bhat, S., Ramaseshan, M., Peng, X., Foucher, L., Beauchemin, S., Bhérer, P., Veber, D.F., Peterson, M.L., and Fraser, G. L. (2011) Optimization of the potency and pharmacokinetic properties of a macrocyclic ghrelin receptor agonist. Part I. Development of ulimorelin (TZP-101) from hit to clinic. *J. Med. Chem.*, **54**, 8305–8320.

39 Rose, G.D., Gierasch, L.M., and Smith, J.A. (1985) Turns in peptides and proteins. *Adv. Protein Chem.*, **37**, 1–109.

40 Tyndall, J.D.A., Pfeiffer, B., Abbenante, G., and Fairlie, D.P. (2005) Over one hundred peptide-activated G protein coupled receptors recognize ligands with turn structure. *Chem. Rev.*, **105**, 793–826.

41 Since distances are significantly shorter than the sum of the van der Waals radii: Bondi, A. (1964) van der Waals volumes and radii. *J. Phys. Chem.*, **68**, 441–451.

42 (a) Di, L. and Kerns, E.H. (2003) Profiling drug-like properties in discovery research. *Curr. Opin. Chem. Biol.*, **7**, 402–408. (b) Li, A.P. (2005) Preclinical *in vitro* screening assays for drug-like properties. *Drug Discov. Today Technol.*, **2**, 179–185.

43 van Breemen, R.B. and Li, Y. (2005) Caco-2 cell permeability assays to measure drug absorption. *Expert Opin. Drug Metab. Toxicol.*, **1**, 175–185.

44 (a) Biliary excretion is commonly observed in cyclic peptides or peptidomimetics; see, for example, Veber, D.F., Saperstein, R., Nutt, R.F., Freidinger, R.M., Brady, S.F., Curley, P., Perlow, D.S., Paleveda, W.J., Colton, C.D., Zacchei, A.G., Tocco, D.J., Hoff, D.A., Vandlen, R.L., Gerich, J.E., Hall, L., Mandarino, L., Cordes, E.H., Anderson, P.S., and Hirschmann, R. (1984) A super active cyclic hexapeptide analog of somatostatin. *Life Sci.*, **34**, 1371–1378. (b) Llinàs-Burnet, M., Bailey, M.D., Bolger, G., Brochu, C., Faucher, A.-M., Ferland, J.M., Garneau, M., Ghiro, E., Gorys, V., Grand-Maôtre, C., Halmos, T., Lapeyre-Paquette, N., Liard, F., Poirier,

M., Rhéaume, M., Tsantrizos, Y.S., and Lamarre, D. (2004) Structure–activity study on a novel series of macrocyclic inhibitors of the hepatitis C virus NS3 protease leading to the discovery of BILN 2061. *J. Med. Chem.*, **47**, 1605–1608.

45 Wargin, W., Thomas, H., Clohs, L., St-Louis, C., Ejskjaer, N., Gutierrez, M., Shaughnessy, L., and Kosutic, G. (2009) Contribution of protein binding to the pharmacokinetics of the ghrelin receptor agonist TZP-101 in healthy volunteers and adults with symptomatic gastroparesis: two randomized, double-blind studies and a binding profile study. *Clin. Drug Invest.*, **29**, 409–418.

46 White, R.E. (2000) High-throughput screening in drug metabolism and pharmacokinetic support of drug discovery. *Annu. Rev. Pharmacol. Toxicol.*, **40**, 133–157.

47 (a) Venkova, K., Fraser, G., Hoveyda, H.R., and Greenwood-Van Meerveld, B. (2007) Prokinetic effects of a new ghrelin receptor agonist TZP-101 in a rat model of postoperative ileus. *Dig. Dis. Sci.*, **52**, 2241–2248. (b) Fraser, G.L., Venkova, K., Hoveyda, H.R., Thomas, H., and Greenwood-Van Meerveld, B. (2009) Effect of the ghrelin receptor agonist TZP-101 on colonic transit in a rat model of postoperative ileus. *Eur. J. Pharmacol.*, **604**, 132–137.

48 Fraser, G.L., Hoveyda, H.R., and Tannenbaum, G.S. (2008) Pharmacological demarcation of the growth hormone, gut motility and feeding effects of ghrelin using a novel ghrelin receptor agonist. *Endocrinology*, **149**, 6280–6288.

49 Lasseter, K.C., Shaughnessy, L., Cummings, D., Pezzullo, J.C., Wargin, W., Gagnon, R., Oliva, J., and Kosutic, G. (2008) Ghrelin agonist (TZP-101): safety, pharmacokinetics and pharmacodynamic evaluation in healthy volunteers: a phase I, first-in-human study. *J. Clin. Pharmacol.*, **48**, 193–202.

50 Gutierrez, M., Shaughnessy, L., Cummings, D., Pezzullo, J., Reeve, R., Reilly, R., and Kosutic, G. (2007) Ghrelin agonist (TZP-101): pharmacokinetics and pharmacodynamics: a multi-dose evaluation in healthy volunteers. *Neurogastrol. Motil.*, **19**, 428–429.

51 Ejskjaer, N., Vestergaard, E.T., Hellström, P.M., Gormsen, L.C., Madsbad, S., Madsen, J.L., Jensen, T.A., Pezzullo, J.C., Christiansen, J.S., Shaughnessy, L., and Kosutic, G. (2009) Ghrelin receptor agonist (TZP-101) accelerates gastric emptying in adults with diabetes and symptomatic gastroparesis. *Aliment. Pharmacol. Ther.*, **29**, 1179–1187.

52 (a) Ejskjaer, N., Dimcevski, G., Wo, J., Hellström, P.M., Gormsen, L.C., Sarosiek, I., Sùfteland, E., Nowak, T., Pezzullo, J.C., Shaughnessy;, L., Kosutic, G., and McCallum, R. (2010) Safety and efficacy of ghrelin agonist TZP-101 in relieving symptoms in patients with diabetic gastroparesis: a randomized, placebo-controlled study. *Neurogastroenterol. Motil.*, **22**, 1069–1078. (b) Wo, J.M., Ejskjaer, N., Hellström, P.M., Malik, R.A., Pezzullo, J. C., Shaughnessy, L., Charlton, P., Kosutic, G., and McCallum, R.W. (2011) Randomised clinical trial: ghrelin agonist TZP-101 relieves gastroparesis associated with severe nausea and vomiting – randomised clinical study subset data. *Aliment. Pharmacol. Ther.*, **33**, 679–688.

53 Popescu, I., Fleshner, P.R., Pezzullo, J.C., Charlton, P.A., Kosutic, G., and Senagore, A.J. (2010) The ghrelin agonist TZP-101 for management of postoperative ileus after partial colectomy: a randomized, dose-ranging, placebo-controlled clinical trial. *Dis. Colon Rectum*, **53**, 126–134.

54 Tranzyme (2012) *Corporate Press Release.* Available at http://ir.tranzyme.com/releasedetail.cfm?ReleaseID=656438 (last accessed March 12, 2012).

55 Veber, D.F., Johnson, S.R., Cheng, H.Y., Smith, B.R., Ward, K.W., and Kopple, K.D. (2002) Molecular properties that influence the oral bioavailability of drug candidates. *J. Med. Chem.*, **45**, 2615–2623.

56 Keserü, G.M. and Makara, G.M. (2009) The influence of lead discovery strategies on the properties of drug candidates. *Nat. Rev. Drug Discov.*, **8**, 203–212.

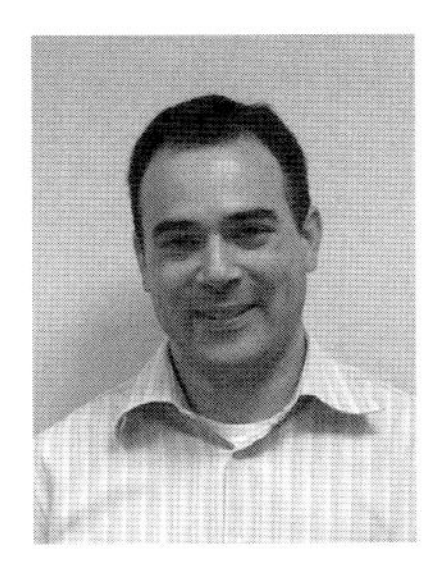

Graeme Fraser has more than 17 years of industry experience in both management and technical roles. Prior to his current position as Director, Drug Discovery at Euroscreen SA, Dr. Fraser was Vice President, Drug Discovery at Tranzyme Pharma, where he led the discovery and preclinical development activities for a pipeline of GPCR small-molecule programs. Earlier, he managed preclinical development activities at Viron Therapeutics (London, Ontario) and led specific GPCR target validation activities at Astra Pain Control AB (Södertälje, Sweden and Montreal, Quebec). In total, he has directed research activities for three products currently in clinical development. Dr. Fraser received a Ph.D. from McGill University and is an author of over 50 publications and research abstracts, including nine patents and two IND filings.

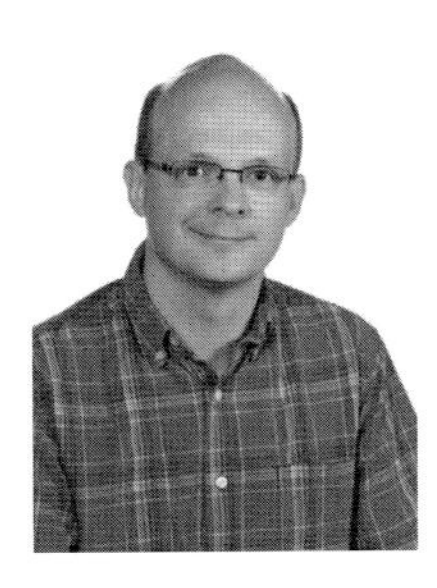

René Gagnon earned his Ph.D. in Organic Chemistry from the University of Laval. He conducted postdoctoral studies with Stanley Roberts at the University of Exeter (UK). After research positions with the Armand-Frappier Institute and the University of Sherbrooke (UdeS), he joined NéoKimia (now Tranzyme Pharma), where he eventually became Manager, Analytical Chemistry & QC. He has expertise in the use of enzymes in organic synthesis, total synthesis, small-molecule library characterization, drug substance and drug product analysis, pharmacokinetic and stability studies, and purification and formulation of new chemical entities. After leaving Tranzyme, he worked as an Associate Professor at the Biomedical Genetics Department (UdeS) and is presently Manager of the Mass Spectrometry Facility at the UdeS Chemistry Department.

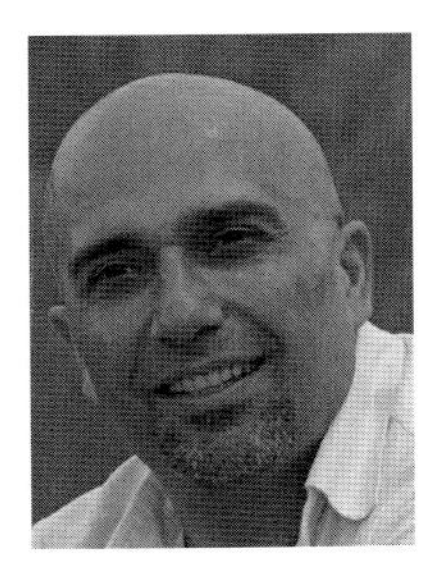

Hamid Hoveyda is currently the Director of Medicinal Chemistry & Development at Euroscreen SA, Belgium. He received his Ph.D. from the University of British Columbia (UBC) and conducted postdoctoral research at Harvard. His first contribution to clinical candidate discovery was an insulin mimetic agent discovered during his doctoral studies at UBC. He began his industrial career in 1997 at Affymax Research Institute, where he worked on applications of diversity-oriented synthesis in drug discovery. Later, at Tranzyme Pharma, he contributed to improvements in the proprietary macrocyclic chemistry platform technology and then led several medicinal chemistry projects that culminated in the discovery of ulimorelin and the follow-up oral candidate TZP-102. Dr. Hoveyda is an author/inventor on 25 peer-reviewed papers and over 50 patent applications.

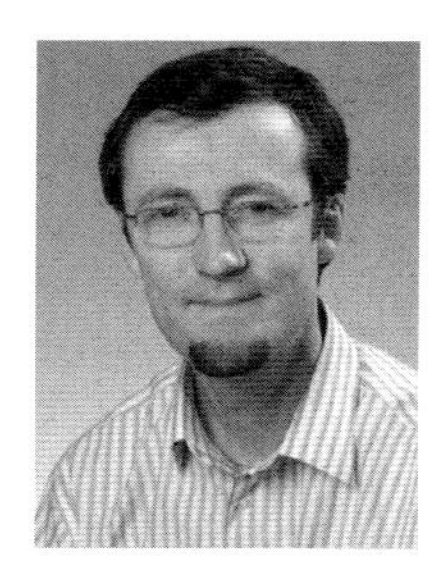

Éric Marsault is an Associate Professor at the Institut de Pharmacologie de Sherbrooke (IPS). He earned his Ph.D. in Organic Chemistry from McGill University. After working for Sanofi (Milan, Italy) as a Visiting Scientist and performing postdoctoral studies at the University of Sherbrooke (UdeS), he became a Research Scientist at NéoKimia (now Tranzyme Pharma), where he rose through the ranks, culminating as Director of Medicinal Chemistry. In 2009, he joined the faculty at UdeS in the Pharmacology Department. His research focuses on validating emerging pharmacological targets and emerging approaches to existing targets, with the goal to provide new avenues for drug discovery. Particular research interests include macrocycles, peptidomimetics, GPCR signaling in metabolic disorders, infectious diseases, and pain, as well as emerging antibacterial targets.

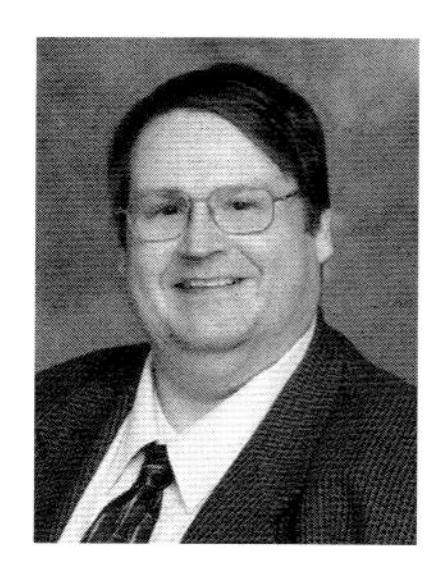

Mark L. Peterson is currently Vice President, IP and Operations at Tranzyme Pharma. He was previously with Monsanto and Advanced ChemTech, where he worked in a variety of research areas including structure-based design, solid-phase organic chemistry, combinatorial libraries, synthetic automation, heterocycles, unnatural amino acids, peptides, and peptidomimetics. With Tranzyme Pharma since 1999, Dr. Peterson led the chemistry R&D efforts during the technology development stage of the company and the initiation of its drug discovery programs. He received his Ph.D. in Organic Chemistry from Washington State University and conducted postdoctoral research at the University of Minnesota. He is author or coauthor of over 80 publications and abstracted presentations plus two book chapters, as well as co-inventor on over 20 patents.

Part II
Drug Classes

Analogue-based Drug Discovery III, First Edition. Edited by János Fischer, C. Robin Ganellin, and David P. Rotella.
© 2013 Wiley-VCH Verlag GmbH & Co. KGaA. Published 2013 by Wiley-VCH Verlag GmbH & Co. KGaA.

5
The Discovery of Anticancer Drugs Targeting Epigenetic Enzymes

A. Ganesan

List of Abbreviations

5-azaC	5-azacytidine
5-aza-dC	5-aza-2′-deoxycytidine
AML	acute myelogenous leukemia
CpG	cytosine phosphate guanine dinucleotide
CTCL	cutaneous T-cell lymphoma
DMSO	dimethyl sulfoxide
DNMT	DNA methyltransferase
EGFR	epidermal growth factor receptor
FDA	Food and Drug Administration
HATU	(2-(7-aza-1*H*-benzotriazole-1-yl)-1,1,3,3-tetramethyluronium hexafluorophosphate
HDAC	histone deacetylase
HER2	human epidermal growth factor receptor
IL	interleukin
IND	investigational new drug
MBD	methyl binding domain
MDS	myelodysplastic syndromes
NAD	nicotinamide adenine dinucleotide
NCI	National Cancer Institute
QT	Q and T waves
SAHA	suberoylanilide hydroxamic acid
SAM	*S*-adenosylmethionine
ST	S and T waves
STAT	signal transducer and activator of transcription

Analogue-based Drug Discovery III, First Edition. Edited by János Fischer, C. Robin Ganellin, and David P. Rotella.
© 2013 Wiley-VCH Verlag GmbH & Co. KGaA. Published 2013 by Wiley-VCH Verlag GmbH & Co. KGaA.

5.1
Epigenetics

Sixty years ago, Conrad Waddington first defined epigenetics as "the branch of biology which studies the causal interactions between genes and their products" in his article titled "The epigenotype" [1]. Subsequently, our understanding of gene structure and function has led to the currently accepted definition of epigenetics as the study of heritable changes in an organism's phenotype without underlying changes in genotype. For example, there are dramatic differences between humans although we share 99% identity at the genome level. Within a single individual, there are dramatic differences between tissues and organs in the body although the genome is 100% identical. These phenotypic variations are due to gene regulation as not all genes are equally expressed in different cells or different individuals. The physical basis for gene regulation in eukaryotes is the science of epigenetics and at the molecular level it takes place by a complex pattern of chemical alterations of DNA and their associated histone proteins at specific regions of a chromosome. Unlike the genome of DNA sequences, the epigenome of DNA/histone modifications is dynamically changing in response to signals and the environment and it can be partially transmitted to future generations. From the drug discovery perspective, there is one major difference between genetics and epigenetics: once a gene mutation has occurred, it is permanent and cannot be reversed. Epigenetic modifications, on the other hand, are catalyzed by enzymes. In principle, they are reversible by a small molecule enzyme inhibitor that can then reverse a disease state back to the normal phenotype.

In eukaryotic cell nuclei, the genetic material is tightly packaged with histone proteins. The basic repeating unit is the nucleosome composed of 146 base pairs of DNA wound around four pairs of histone proteins H2A, H2B, H3, and H4 stapled with the linker histone H1A. Together with linker DNA, the nucleosomes form "beads on a string" that leads to the higher order structures of chromatin and chromosomes. Chromatin exists in two forms: heterochromatin is formed when nucleosomes are tightly condensed and genes are transcriptionally silent, whereas euchromatin is a relaxed state that allows access to the transcription machinery and gene expression. Recently, it has become evident that the transition between different states of chromatin is due to extensive and reversible structural modifications of the DNA and histone proteins. In DNA, the major alteration is the conversion of cytosine to 5-methylcytosine that has a gene silencing effect (Figure 5.1).

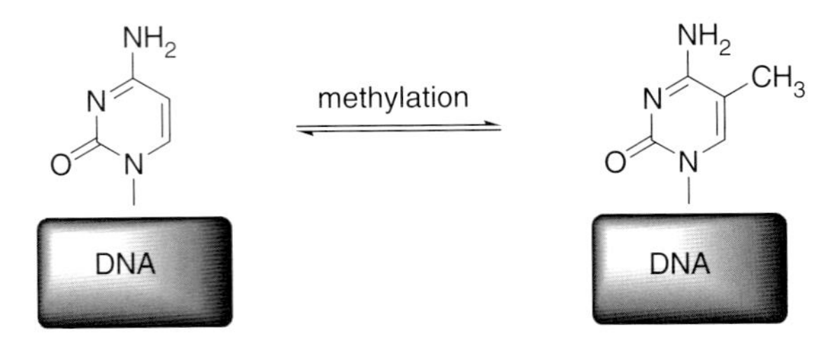

Figure 5.1 The methylation of cytosine residues in DNA to 5-methylcytosine.

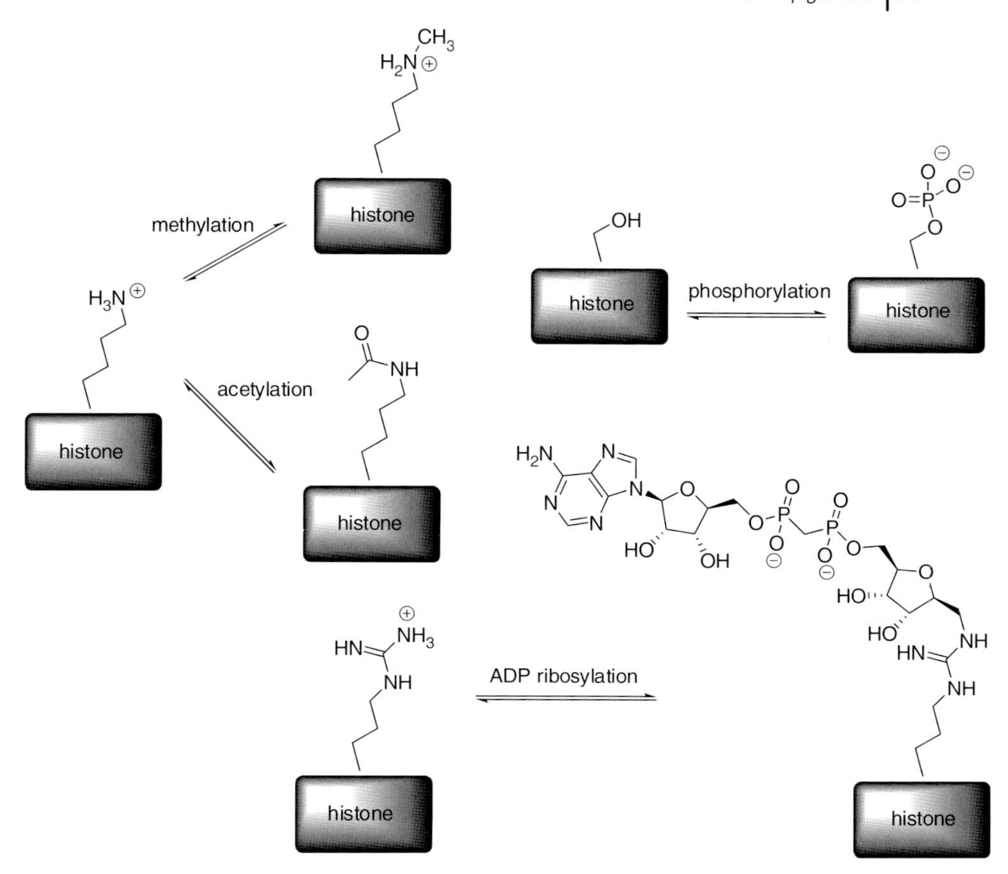

Figure 5.2 Examples of histone post-translational modification.

In histone proteins, the basic N-terminal regions are subject to a plethora of post-translational modifications including methylation, acetylation, malonylation, crotonylation, biotinylation, polyADP-ribosylation, ubiquitinylation, and sumoylation of lysine; methylation and polyADP-ribosylation of arginine; phosphorylation of serine and threonine; and *cis–trans* isomerization of proline (Figure 5.2).

Together, this complex pattern of DNA and histone modification regulates gene expression in two ways. First, the modifications can alter the intrinsic affinity between DNA and histones leading to unwinding of the nucleic acid off the nucleosome into a transcriptionally active state. Second, the modifications serve as chemical signals that are recognized by specific binding partners that act as activators or repressors of transcription. The pattern of DNA/histone modification is often referred to as the "epigenetic code" [2]. The code, if it exists, is highly complex as there are multiple sites for DNA and histone modification and their consequences for gene regulation can be context dependent. Nevertheless, it is already clear that the epigenome is at least partially heritable in addition to the genetic sequence and that aberrant changes in the epigenome contribute to many human diseases.

There are three major sets of proteins involved in epigenetics:

1) **Writers:** enzymes that chemically modify DNA or histone proteins, for example, DNA methyltransferases and histone acetyltransferases.
2) **Erasers:** enzymes that remove the modifications introduced by writers, for example, histone deacetylases and lysine demethylases.
3) **Readers:** protein domains that recognize and bind to modified DNA or histones, for example, methyl-binding proteins that recognize 5-methylcytosine and bromodomains that recognize acetyl-lysine residues.

All three classes of epigenetic modulators are of great interest as drug discovery targets. Attention has been primarily focused on epigenetic modulation for anticancer therapy as there is genetic and clinical evidence that readers, writers, and erasers are overexpressed in a variety of human cancers. *In vitro* proof-of-concept studies with small molecules have confirmed the anticancer effects of epigenetic modulators and in some cases this has progressed to *in vivo* models and proof of efficacy in humans. At the present time, two inhibitors of DNA methyltransferase and two inhibitors of Zn-dependent histone deacetylases have received FDA approval as anticancer drugs [3].

5.2 DNA Methyltransferases

The DNMTs catalyze the C-5 methylation of cytosine by the cofactor *S*-adenosylmethionine (SAM). The reaction primarily occurs within CpG dinucleotides present in highly repeated transposable elements in DNA. The methylated cytosine residues protrude into the DNA major groove and interfere with binding of the transcription machinery and gene transcription. Furthermore, methylated cytosine is specifically recognized by methyl CpG binding domains (MBDs) that function as adaptors between DNA and other chromatin modifying enzymes. Together, these effects lead to gene silencing. Programmed changes in DNA methylation are essential during normal embryological development and play a crucial role in chromatin remodeling, X chromosome inactivation, and genomic imprinting. Cancer cells are globally hypomethylated compared to normal cells, but hypermethylated upstream of CpG islands of silenced genes [4]. These silenced genes often encode for tumor suppressors and a DNMT inhibitor would activate their transcription leading to re-establishment of pathways of cell repair, apoptosis, and suppression of proliferation.

In mammals, three DNA methyltransferases have been identified: DNMT1 and DNMT3A/B. Among these enzymes, DNMT1 is ubiquitous and the most abundant and primarily methylates hemimethylated DNA. Thus, it is referred to as a maintenance methyltransferase responsible for maintaining the pattern of methylation during DNA replication. DNMT3A/B methylate both nonmethylated and hemimethylated DNA and are hence *de novo* methyltransferases that establish methylation patterns during embryogenesis. In addition, there are nonfunctional DNMTs:

DNMT2 is a tRNA methyltransferase while DNMT3L has a mutated active site that is catalytically inactive and is involved in recruiting other binding partners to chromatin.

In double-stranded DNA, Watson–Crick base pairing and stacking with adjacent base pairs place the purine and pyrimidine heterocycles in the interior and unexposed toward enzymatic reaction. X-ray crystallographic studies with DNMTs show that the enzyme flips the cytosine substrate out of the double helix in order for catalysis to take place. The DNMT mechanism (Figure 5.3) is composed of three steps: (i) Transient protonation of cytosine N-3 by a glutamic acid residue increases the pyrimidine electrophilicity and promotes Michael addition of an active site cysteine residue to generate the imino form of the heterocycle. (ii) Nucleophilic attack of the SAM cofactor by the imine methylates C-5. (iii) Deprotonation of the C-5

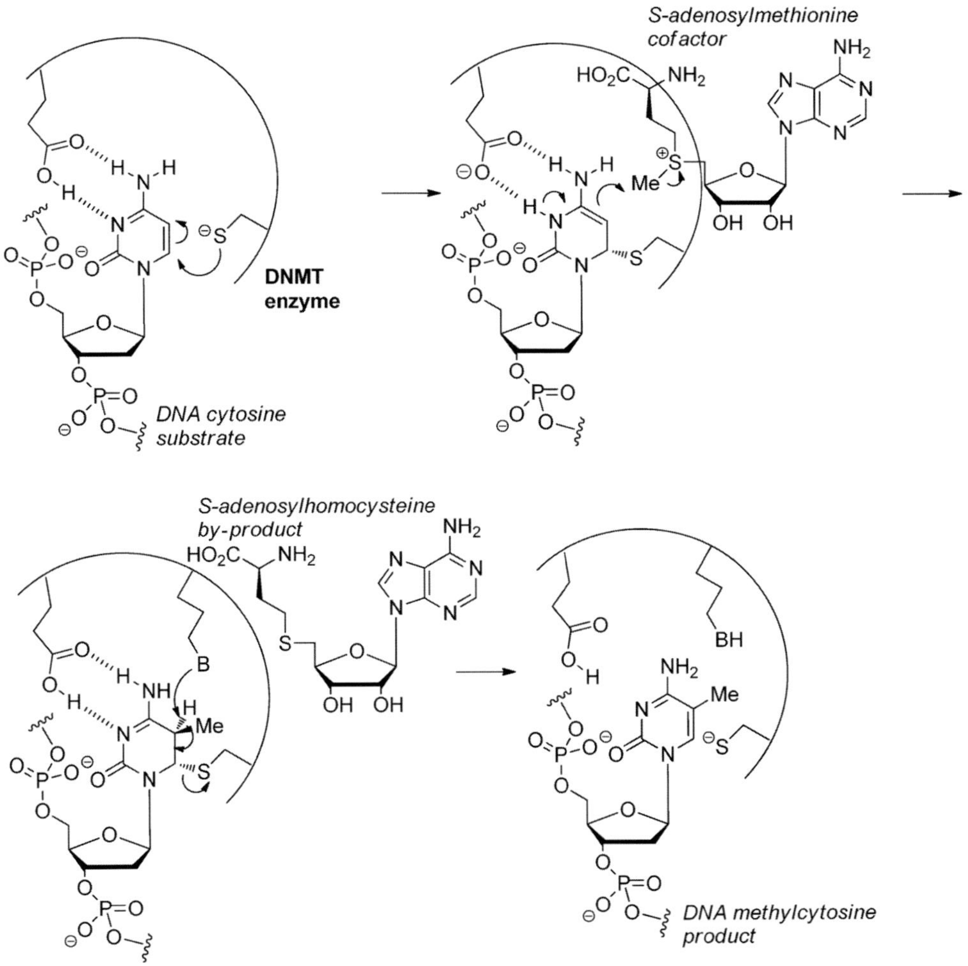

Figure 5.3 The catalytic reaction mechanism of DNA methyltransferases.

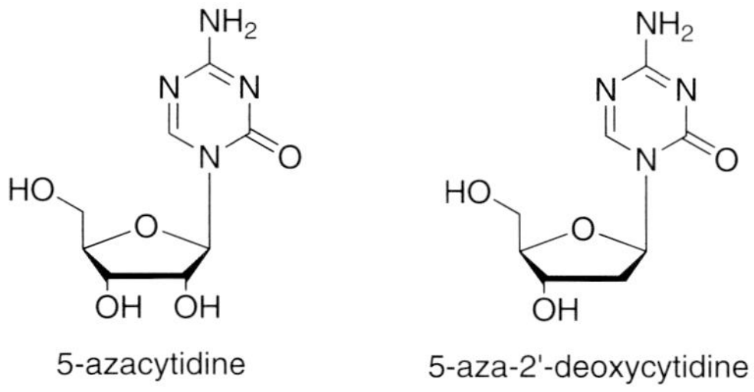

Figure 5.4 Structures of 5-azacytidine and 5-aza-2′-deoxycytidine.

proton by a basic enzyme residue or the DNA backbone causes β-elimination of the cysteine to release the 5-methylcytosine product and regenerate the enzyme. Overall, the mechanism of DNMTs is similar to that of RNA methyltransferases and thymidylate synthase [5].

One strategy for enzyme inhibition would be to compete with SAM for the cofactor binding pocket. Indeed, the cofactor by-product *S*-adenosylhomocysteine is a competitive inhibitor of DNMTs. However, it lacks specificity and would affect other SAM-dependent enzymes. Another approach is the design of substrate analogues that are recognized by the enzyme but do not result in catalytic turnover. Although not rationally designed to work in this manner, the two clinically approved DNMT inhibitors 5-azacytidine and 5-aza-2′-deoxycytidine (Figure 5.4) serendipitously follow this principle.

5.3 5-Azacytidine (Azacitidine, Vidaza) and 5-Aza-2′-deoxycytidine (Decitabine, Dacogen)

The structural elucidation of DNA led to the hypothesis that compounds interfering with nucleic acid biosynthesis would have a damaging effect on cell division and inhibit the proliferation of tumor cells. There was a substantial interest by medicinal chemists in the synthesis of such purine and pyrimidine antimetabolites and a number of these are widely used anticancer drugs including 5-fluorouracil and mercaptopurine (Figure 5.5).

With a similar goal in mind of preparing cytostatic antimetabolites, Alois Piskala and Frantisek Sorm at the Czech Academy of Sciences reported the synthesis of

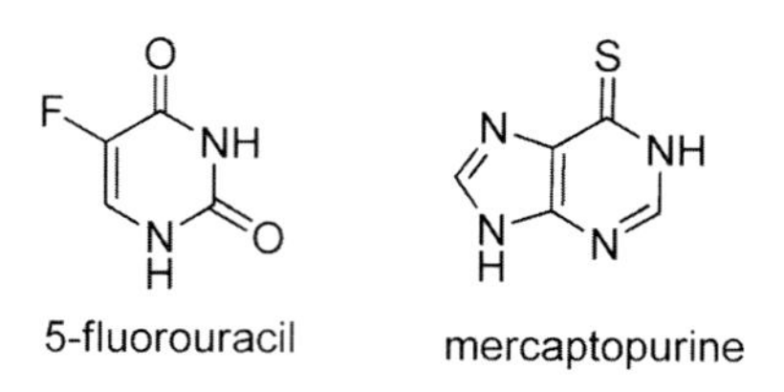

Figure 5.5 Examples of antimetabolite drugs.

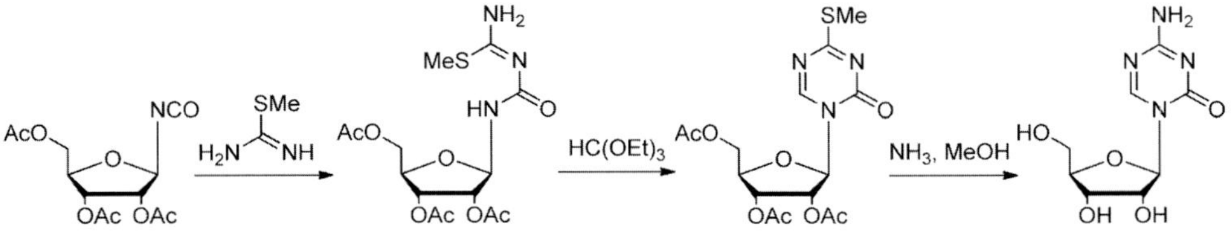

Figure 5.6 The Piskala and Sorm synthesis of 5-azacytidine.

5-azaC and 5-aza-dC in 1964 [6]. The azapyrimidine heterocycle was constructed starting from a ribosyl isocyanate (Figure 5.6). Later, 5-azaC was identified as a natural product from an extract of *Streptoverticillium ladakanus* [7].

5-AzaC demonstrated the ability to induce chromosomal breakage and had high activity against lymphatic leukemia in cell lines and mouse *in vivo* cancer models. Clinical trials of 5-azaC were initiated in Europe in 1967 and in the United States in 1970. In 1971, the US National Cancer Institute (NCI) filed an FDA application for IND status for the use of 5-azaC in the treatment of multiple cancers. The clinical trial data were promising for acute myelogenous leukemia (AML), especially in patients who did not respond to conventional chemotherapy. However, responses were low or absent in other cancer types and drug treatment was accompanied by toxicity with 73% of 745 patients suffering from nausea and vomiting within 3 h of administration. Consequently, the IND application was rejected.

Interest in 5-azaC was rekindled in 1980 by Peter Jones and Shirley Taylor at the University of California, Los Angeles (UCLA), who reported that the drug inhibits DNA methylation [8]. *In vivo*, 5-azaC acts as a prodrug converted by a series of phosphorylations to 5-azacytidine triphosphate that can then be incorporated into RNA. Partially, 2′-reduction of the sugar by ribonucleotide reductase produces 5-aza-2′-deoxycytidine diphosphate that is further phosphorylated to 5-aza-2′-deoxycytidine triphosphate. The deoxycytidine triphosphate is then incorporated into DNA and this is the fate of approximately 10% of administered 5-azaC. DNA containing 5-azaC is recognized as a substrate by DNMTs. While the Michael addition by the enzyme and methyl transfer from SAM can take place, the final elimination step is impossible and the drug remains as an irreversible covalent adduct leading to depletion of cellular DNMT and loss of genomic methylation (Figure 5.7).

The growing evidence highlighting the importance of methylation in cancer cells and the elucidation of DNMT as the molecular target of 5-azaC led to a second IND application submitted by Pharmion (later acquired by Celgene) for the treatment of myelodysplastic syndromes (MDS). MDS are a collection of hematopoietic stem cell disorders characterized by bone marrow dysplasia and peripheral blood cytopenia with a propensity for transformation into AML. As the standard treatment consists of supportive measures such as blood transfusions, and administration of hematopoetic factors and antibiotics to treat opportunistic infections, there is a pressing need for new therapeutic agents that specifically target MDS. In this predominantly elderly population, a positive response was observed with low doses of 5-azaC leading to a significant decrease in onset of leukemia and an increase in

in vivo phosphorylation and deoxygenation

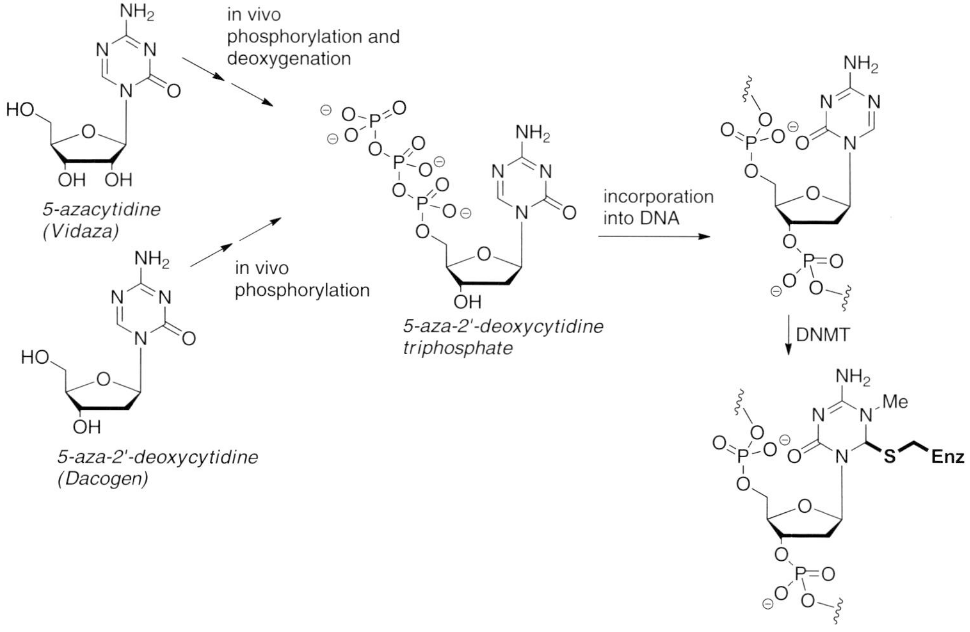

5-azacytidine (Vidaza)

in vivo phosphorylation

5-aza-2'-deoxycytidine (Dacogen)

5-aza-2'-deoxycytidine triphosphate

incorporation into DNA

DNMT

Enz

Figure 5.7 The mechanism of DNMT inhibition by 5-azacytidine and 5-aza-2′-deoxycytidine.

quality of life [9]. Based on the Pharmion clinical trial data, in 2004 the FDA approved 5-azaC (azacitidine, trade name Vidaza) as the first drug for the treatment of all five subtypes of MDS. Thus, the journey from Piskala and Sorm's initial synthesis culminated in clinical approval four decades later. Pharmion has patented a more efficient route to 5-azaC compared to the original synthesis using Vorbruggen coupling that can be performed as a one-pot process (Figure 5.8). Clinically, Vidaza is administered subcutaneously or intravenously at a dose of 100 mg for 7 days per month and has a half-life of ~41 min.

Alongside 5-azaC, Piskala and Sorm had reported 5-aza-2′-deoxycytidine in 1964. As described above, 5-azaC is a prodrug of 5-aza-dC triphosphate that is the actual

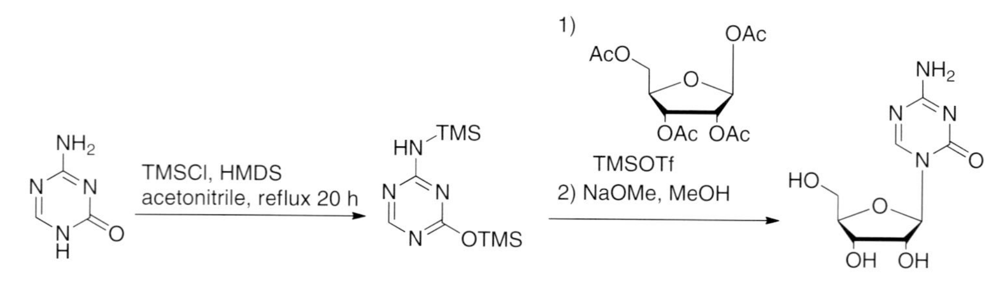

Figure 5.8 The Pharmion route to 5-azacytidine.

molecule incorporated into DNA. However, this requires 2′-reduction of the ribose sugar and the major metabolic pathway is phosphorylation without deoxygenation to give 5-azaC triphosphate. 5-AzaC triphosphate is incorporated into RNA and hence the drug has a number of effects independent of DNA methylation including disruption of ribosome and tRNA biosynthesis. The RNA pathway may be responsible for some of the side effects as well as some of the clinical benefits of 5-azaC. Meanwhile, 5-aza-dC offers an opportunity to bypass the formation of 5-azaC triphosphate as the 2′-deoxysugar can only be incorporated into DNA. Both *in vitro* and *in vivo* evidence indicate that 5-aza-dC shows 10-fold or higher activity compared to 5-azaC [10]. In 2004, MGI Pharma (later acquired by Eisai) submitted a new drug application (NDA) to the FDA and in 2006 5-aza-dC (decitabine, trade name Dacogen) received approval as the only drug for 5-day dosing in previously treated and untreated, intermediate, and intermediate and high-risk MDS [11]. Dacogen is administered by intravenous infusion for either 3 days in a 6-week cycle or 5 days in a 4 week cycle.

The success of 5-azaC and 5-aza-dC stems from their novel mechanism of action as DNMT inhibitors and their clinical value of reactivating silenced tumor suppressors in the treatment of MDS. These drugs are highly cytotoxic with dose-limiting myelosuppression and work best when administered at low doses over long periods. MDS primarily affects elderly patients and there is a dearth of chemotherapy options available – a situation that favors the prolonged low dosing suitable for the two drugs. It is likely that DNMTs do not play a special role in the progression of MDS but rather the high cytotoxicity of azacytosines complicates the more aggressive dosing needed in other cancers [12].

Besides the high cytotoxicity, another drawback of 5-azaC and 5-aza-dC is their susceptibility to base hydrolysis and removal of the 5-azapyrimidine. This occurs at neutral or basic pH and the drug solution has to be freshly prepared for prolonged infusion [13]. Both the 5′-elaidic acid ester [14] of 5-azaC and the 5-azaCpG dinucleotide [15] (Figure 5.9) are undergoing evaluation as more stable and bioavailable derivatives of 5azaC.

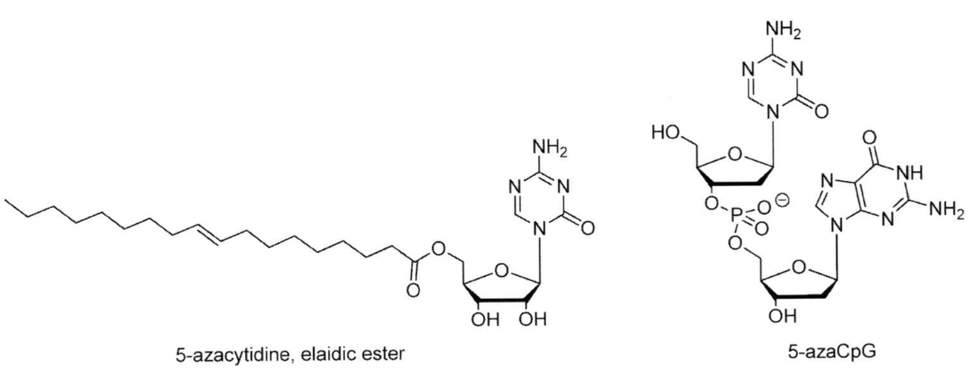

5-azacytidine, elaidic ester

5-azaCpG

Figure 5.9 5-AzaC derivatives with improved bioavailability.

5.4
Other Nucleoside DNMT Inhibitors

The poor stability, lack of oral bioavailability, and high cytotoxicity are shortcomings of 5-azaC and 5-aza-dC. Several other nucleoside DNMT inhibitors that work by a similar mechanism were investigated and have reached clinical trials (Figure 5.10). In 1979, Beisler *et al.* reported the synthesis of fazarabine, the 5-azaC analogue with arabinose instead of ribose as the sugar moiety [16]. In parallel, Beisler *et al.* had synthesized dihydro-5-azacytidine whereby the 5,6-imino bond of the pyrimidine is reduced [17]. This leads to improved aqueous stability over 5-azaC and the opportunity to dose the drug by slow infusion to avoid acute toxicity. Like 5-azaC, fazarabine and dihydro-5-azacytidine are prodrugs that are partially metabolized *in vivo* to the 2′-deoxysugar triphosphate that is incorporated into DNA and inhibits DNMT. Both compounds are active against cancer cell lines and tumor xenograft animal models. However, a lack of activity was observed in phase II trials and further clinical development of these agents has been discontinued [18].

Zebularine is a cytidine analogue lacking the exocyclic C-4 amine and was first synthesized in 1961 by Funakoshi *et al.* [19]. Initial investigations focused on its bacteriostatic properties and later on inhibition of cytidine deaminase [20] before its potential as a DNMT inhibitor was realized [21]. Zebularine is stable and orally bioavailable unlike 5-azaC and 5-aza-dC. Following conversion to 2′-deoxyzebularine triphosphate, it is incorporated into DNA. The absence of the pyrimidine amino group results in loss of one hydrogen bond in Watson–Crick base pairing to the adjacent DNA strand. Consequently, there is less of an energy penalty for the base to be flipped out and bind to DNMTs. Compared to cytosine, the absence of the C-4 amine increases the reactivity toward Michael addition of the DNMT active site cysteine while inhibiting the β-elimination release of the methylated DNA. 2′-Deoxyzebularine itself is not phosphorylated *in vivo* and is inactive. To bypass this metabolic block and the inefficient 2′-reduction needed to reach zebularine, the 3′- and 3′,5′-phosphoramidite analogues of 2′-deoxyzebularine have been prepared [22].

Based on the antitumor properties of 5-fluorouracil, the analogous 5-fluoro-2′-deoxycytidine was expected to have similar activity and its synthesis was reported in 1961 [23]. 5-Fluoro-2′-deoxycytidine is incorporated into DNA, whereupon it acts

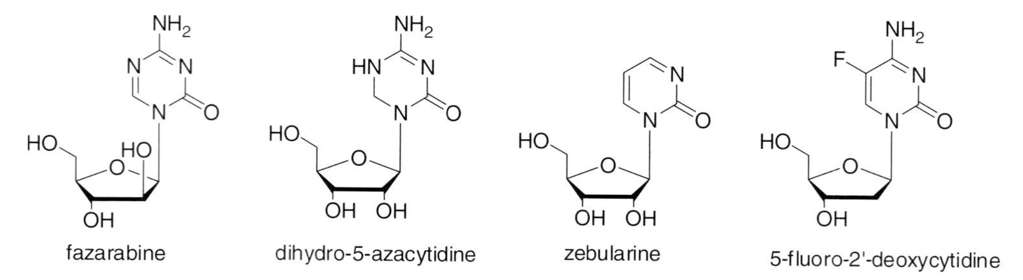

Figure 5.10 Nucleoside DNMT inhibitors that have reached clinical trials.

as a DNMT inhibitor [24]. The Michael addition of cysteine occurs, but the absence of the C-5 proton makes the final elimination step impossible and the drug forms a covalent adduct. The mechanism is identical to the inhibition of thymidylate synthase by 5-fluorouracil. As the drug is already a 2′-deoxysugar, its metabolism is not complicated by incorporation into RNA. Clinical trials with zebularine and 5-fluoro-2′-deoxycytidine are ongoing. Like the other nucleoside prodrugs, the active triphosphate is only formed after a series of metabolic conversions.

5.5 Preclinical DNMT Inhibitors

A diverse range of natural products and some known drugs have been reported as DNMT inhibitors (Figure 5.11) [25]. Although these leads are at the early stages of drug discovery, it is possible that further optimization may result in a clinical candidate. Unlike the nucleoside DNMT inhibitors, they bind directly to DNMT without being incorporated into nucleic acids. The known antihypertensive drug hydralazine and the anesthetic procainamide are DNMT inhibitors. Molecular modeling suggests that hydralazine binds to the active site by a set of hydrogen bonds similarly to the cytosine substrate [26]. Among the natural products reported to be DNMT inhibitors are epigallocatechin gallate, a component of green tea, and nanaomycin A that is selective for inhibition of DNMT3b [27]. Molecular modeling and virtual screening of compound libraries have led to DNMT inhibitors such as the tryptophan derivative RG108 designed to bind to the active site of DNMT1 [28]. The quinoline SGI-1027 is a micromolar inhibitor of DNMTs and competes with the SAM cofactor [29].

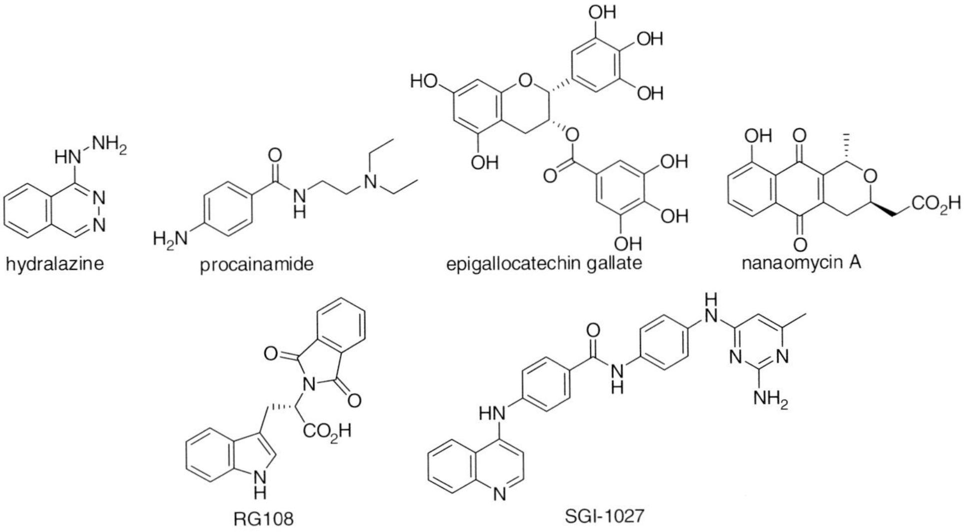

Figure 5.11 Examples of preclinical non-nucleoside DNMT inhibitors.

5.6
Zinc-Dependent Histone Deacetylases

Acetylation of lysine residues is an important epigenetic mark. It converts the positively charged lysine to a neutral acetamide, thus reducing its affinity for the negatively charged DNA backbone. In addition, protein bromodomains specifically recognize acetyllysine and help recruit binding partners involved in gene transcription. The chemical reversal of acetyllysine to lysine is catalyzed by histone deacetylases. There are 18 HDACs in the human genome and these are subdivided according to their catalytic mechanism, sequence homology, and localization [30]. HDACs 1–11 are metallohydrolases that employ zinc as the active site catalyst while the sirtuins SIRTs 1–7 use the cofactor NAD^+ for catalysis. Both activators and inhibitors of sirtuins are of interest as therapeutic agents. As these are at the preclinical stage, they will not be discussed further [31]. The zinc-dependent HDACs are further classified as class I (HDACs 1, 2, 3, and 8), class II (HDACs 4, 5, 6, 7, 9, and 10), and class IV (HDAC 11). Class I HDACs are localized in the cell nucleus whereas the larger class II HDACs shuttle between the nucleus and cytoplasm. HDAC 11, the sole member of class IV, has similarities to both class I and class II HDACs and is primarily nuclear. The primary effect of a HDAC inhibitor on cancer cells is to reactivate repair pathways that are suppressed leading to cell differentiation and apoptosis [32]. In this respect, the phenotypic outcome is similar to that of DNMT inhibitors. It is important to appreciate that the HDACs do not exclusively deacetylate histones but have a large number of other substrates in the nucleus and cytoplasm. While the nuclear class I HDACs that act on histones appear to be the most important in cancer, some of the therapeutic benefits and side effects of HDAC inhibitors may be due to effects on nonhistone proteins [33].

The X-ray structures of several zinc-dependent HDACs have been solved and indicate a catalytic mechanism similar to other metallohydrolases such as matrix metalloproteinases and angiotensin-converting enzyme [34]. The acetyllysine substrate is accommodated in a narrow tunnel approximately 12 Å in length with the active site zinc atom at the end coordinated to two aspartic acid residues and one histidine. The carbonyl group of the acetyllysine then binds to the zinc and a conserved tyrosine or histidine residue and this serves to activate the amide bond toward hydrolysis (Figure 5.12). The attacking water molecule is made more nucleophilic by interactions with the zinc and charge relay with the active site residues and addition to the carbonyl gives a tetrahedral intermediate that collapses to the hydrolysis products.

The inhibition of metallohydrolases in drug discovery is usually accomplished by designing molecules that reversibly bind to the active site metal cation [35]. Achieving selectivity between metalloenzymes needs to take advantage of differences in active site geometry. In the case of zinc-dependent HDACs, inhibitors can be described by a simple dumbbell-shaped pharmacophore consisting of a warhead, a spacer, and a cap. At one end of the molecule is a reversible zinc binding warhead and at the other is a "cap". In between is a linear spacer that fits into the narrow hydrophobic substrate binding channel. The critical interaction between a HDAC

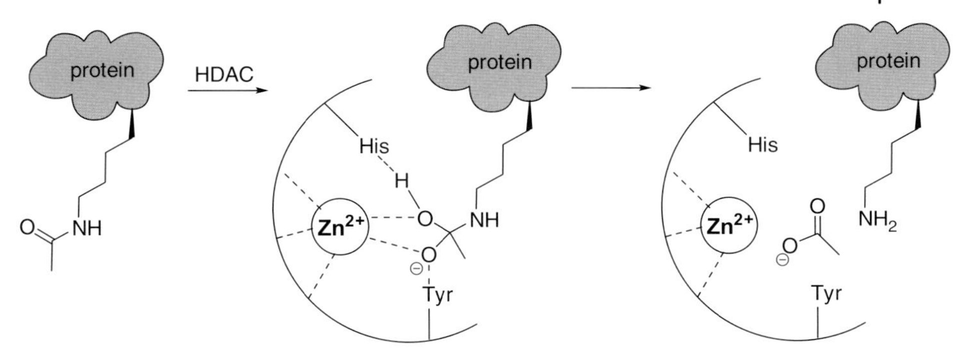

Figure 5.12 The catalytic reaction mechanism of zinc-dependent HDACs.

inhibitor and its enzyme target is binding to the active site zinc. Discrimination between HDACs and other metalloenzymes is promoted by the long linear spacer that is typically not accommodated by unrelated enzymes. Discrimination within the HDAC family is through the "cap" that interacts with a region of the enzyme referred to as the "rim" at the top of the narrow channel. The channel and active site are relatively conserved among HDACs, whereas the isoforms diverge from one another in the rim. Differential binding to the rim can thus give rise to a selective HDAC inhibitor. Although the understanding of enzyme structure has aided the structure-based design of inhibitors, the early compounds were developed without the hindsight of this information. Indeed, the two currently approved HDAC inhibitors were discovered on the basis of phenotypic activity before the human HDACs were even identified.

5.7 Suberoylanilide Hydroxamic Acid (SAHA, Vorinostat, Zolinza)

Remarkably, the lead for the first approved HDAC inhibitor SAHA was the simple molecule DMSO. Charlotte Friend had observed that DMSO caused differentiation of murine leukemia cells and this sparked collaboration between Paul Marks and Ronald Breslow at Columbia University to understand the mechanism. It was discovered that other polar small molecules could induce differentiation although none were particularly potent. *N*-Methylacetamide had an optimal effect at 30 mM and Breslow then synthesized a series of bisacetamides with a linker of 2–8 methylene units. The compound with a spacer of six methylenes, hexamethylene bisacetamide (Figure 5.13), induced differentiation of 95% of the cells at 5 mM [36]. The bisamides with seven and eight methylenes were slightly more potent but more cytotoxic. On the basis of promising *in vitro* and *in vivo* results, an IND was filed for hexamethylene bisacetamide and the compound reached phase II clinical trials [37]. While some remissions were observed in MDS and AML, these were reversed upon cessation of treatment and higher doses were not tolerated by patients. Additional bis-, tri-, and tetraamides were investigated although further

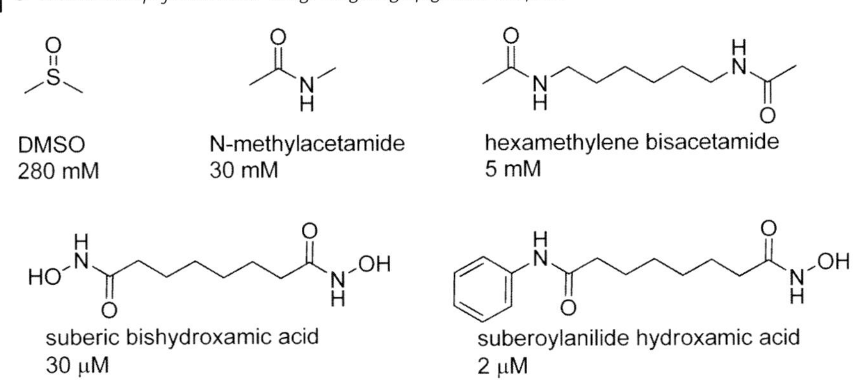

Figure 5.13 The evolution of SAHA from DMSO with potencies in cell differentiation indicated.

gains of potency were not achieved. It was then postulated that the amides might act by hydrogen bonding or metal binding at the receptor. This led to studies with a hydroxamic acid series as an amide isostere with a linker of 2–10 methylene units. The compound with six methylene units, suberic bishydroxamic acid, was significantly more potent than the bisacetamide with an optimum concentration of 30 μM in cell differentiation [38]. Further optimization involved the synthesis of more than 600 compounds. One design consideration was that the distance between the two hydroxamic acids was too large for simultaneous binding to a metal ion and one should be sufficient. Compounds with a hydroxamic acid at one end and a hydrophobic amide at the other were prepared and SAHA emerged as the candidate, inducing differentiation at 2 μM [39].

Up to this point, the molecular targets of the bisamides and hydroxamic acids were unknown. Meanwhile, Minoru Yoshida in Japan had characterized the natural product trichostatin A as a HDAC inhibitor [40]. The structural resemblance between trichostatin A and SAHA (Figure 5.14) suggested that the latter too was a HDAC inhibitor and this was quickly verified by *in vitro* studies. Interestingly, the lead precursor hexamethylene bisacetamide is not a HDAC inhibitor and its target remains unidentified. An X-ray structure of SAHA bound to a HDAC-like bacterial protein confirmed that the hydroxamic acid is chelated to the active site zinc while the phenyl ring extends into the enzyme rim [41]. Thus, SAHA fits the HDAC pharmacophore of warhead, spacer, and cap and its potency is driven primarily by zinc binding and occupancy of the enzyme channel. The small phenyl cap does not

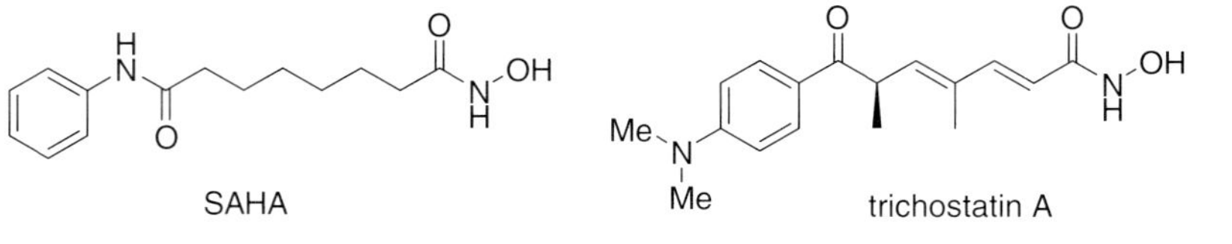

Figure 5.14 Comparison between SAHA and trichostatin A.

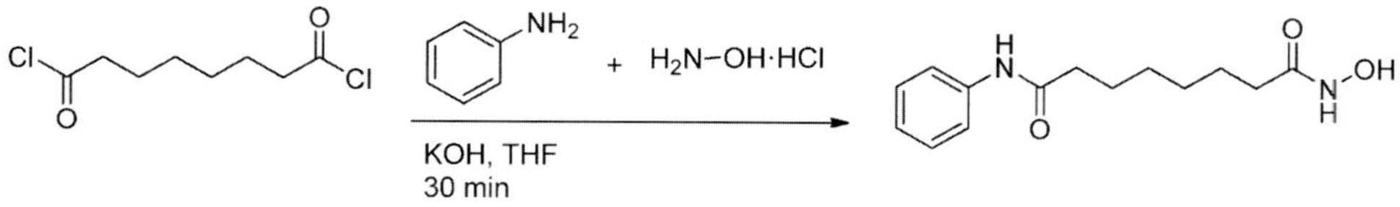

KOH, THF
30 min

+ $H_2N-OH \cdot HCl$

Figure 5.15 One-pot synthesis of Zolinza.

discriminate between isoforms and SAHA is a pan-HDAC inhibitor with IC_{50} values ~50 nM against individual HDACs.

SAHA analogues with higher potency were discovered in the course of Breslow's optimization. However, they also had higher toxicity and SAHA was deliberately chosen as the clinical candidate with medium potency and efficacy without an unacceptable level of side effects. SAHA progressed to phase I clinical trials in 2000 and the compound was licensed to the spinout company Aton Pharmaceuticals (acquired by Merck in 2004). SAHA (vorinostat, trade name Zolinza) received FDA approval for the treatment of cutaneous T-cell lymphoma (CTCL) in 2006 [42]. While the initial trials used intravenous infusion, Zolinza is now administered orally with a maximum dose of 400 mg once daily with food. The drug is 71% bound to plasma proteins and has a half-life of ~2 h with two major metabolic pathways: O-glucuronidation and hydrolysis of the hydroxamic acid followed by β-oxidation. Synthetically, Zolinza can be prepared in one step from the bis-acid chloride of suberic acid by reaction with aniline and hydroxylamine (Figure 5.15) [43].

The identification of trichostatin A and Zolinza as HDAC inhibitors and the availability of X-ray crystallographic data spurred many medicinal chemistry programs directed at this target. More than 10 hydroxamic acid HDAC inhibitors have reached clinical trials (Figure 5.16) [44]. They range from pyroxamide, a closely related Zolinza analogue with a pyridine replacing the aniline, to more complex structures such as CHR-3996. Besides the aliphatic hydroxamic acid motif present in Zolinza, these compounds feature more rigid variants such as cinnamoyl, benzoyl, and hetaryl hydroxamic acids while the presence of a larger cap provides gains in potency and Class I isoform stability for JNJ-26481585 and CHR-3996. The second-generation hydroxamic acids usually have increased oral bioavailability compared to Zolinza. The Curis compound CUDC-101 is unique in being rationally designed as a dual-acting HDAC and tyrosine kinase inhibitor combining erlotinib and vorinostat with nanomolar IC_{50} values against HDACs, HER2 and EGFR. Numerous other hydroxamic acid HDAC inhibitors at the preclinical stage have been reported with varying degrees of isoform selectivity.

5.8 FK228 (Depsipeptide, Romidepsin, Istodax)

A high-throughput screening campaign at Fujisawa Pharmaceutical Co., Ltd. investigated natural product extracts for the ability to revert a *ras*-transformed phenotype to normal cells. They reported the isolation of the cyclic depsipeptide FR901228

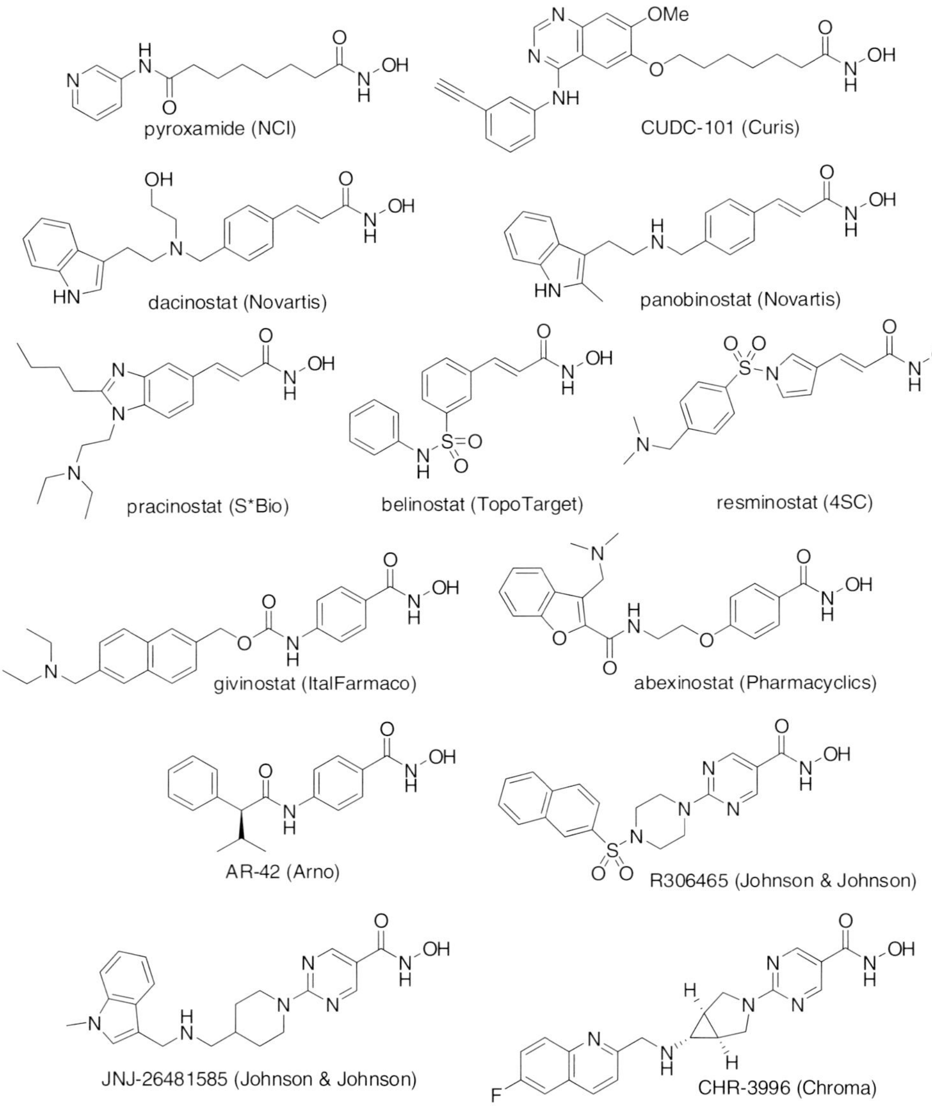

pyroxamide (NCI)
CUDC-101 (Curis)
dacinostat (Novartis)
panobinostat (Novartis)
pracinostat (S*Bio)
belinostat (TopoTarget)
resminostat (4SC)
givinostat (ItalFarmaco)
abexinostat (Pharmacyclics)
AR-42 (Arno)
R306465 (Johnson & Johnson)
JNJ-26481585 (Johnson & Johnson)
CHR-3996 (Chroma)

Figure 5.16 Hydroxamic acid HDAC inhibitors that have reached clinical trials.

(later named FK228) based on this assay from a culture of *Chromobacterium violaceum* No. 968 in 1994 [45]. The compound displayed potent antitumor activity *in vitro* and in murine xenograft models while its structure (Figure 5.17) was unrelated to known natural products. Mechanistic studies by Yoshida *et al.* later confirmed that FK228, like trichostatin A, was a HDAC inhibitor [46]. At first sight, the structure does not fit the HDAC pharmacophore of warhead, spacer, and cap. The natural product is in fact a prodrug that undergoes intracellular reductive

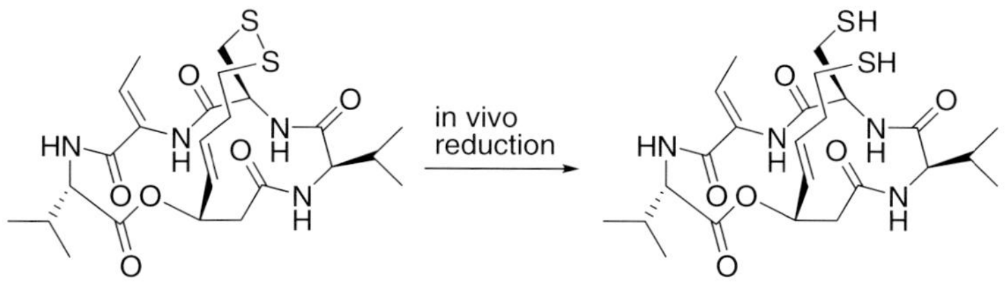

Figure 5.17 Structure of FK228 and the active drug formed by metabolism.

cleavage of the disulfide bridge. This releases a free thiol-bearing side chain and it is the thiol that binds to the active site zinc. Recently, support for this mechanism has been obtained from the X-ray structure of HDAC8 bound to largazole, a depsipeptide natural product with the same thiol zinc binding warhead as FK228 [47].

Compared to the synthetic HDAC inhibitor SAHA, FK228 has a number of unique features. The zinc binding warhead is a thiol rather than the higher affinity bidentate chelating hydroxamic acid. Nevertheless, FK228 is a more potent inhibitor of HDACs and cancer cells *in vitro* with an $IC_{50} \sim 1\,nM$. This is because FK228 has a large macrocyclic scaffold as the cap and this extends out into the HDAC rim to provide additional binding interactions with the enzyme. Furthermore, as the rim is divergent between HDACs, FK228 is isoform selective and is particularly potent in the inhibition of class I HDACs – fortuitously the ones that are linked to cancer.

FK228 was licensed by Fujisawa to Gloucester Pharmaceuticals (later acquired by Celgene) and phase I clinical trials for CTCL were initiated in 2004. As asymptomatic T-wave flattening and ST segment depression were observed in the phase I trials, cardiac evaluation was incorporated into the phase II study. While there was no evidence of acute or cumulative cardiac toxicity, one sudden death occurred and the protocol excluded patients with heart disease. FK228 (romidepsin, trade name Istodax) received FDA approval for the treatment of CTCL in 2009, becoming the second HDAC inhibitor to reach the market [48]. A dose of 10 mg is administered intravenously over 4 h on days 1, 8, and 15 of a 28-day cycle. Due to the potential risk of cardiac side effects, potassium and magnesium electrolyte levels should be within the normal range before administration and cardiac monitoring is recommended for patients at risk of QT prolongation. Some cardiac effects have been observed in clinical trials of other HDAC inhibitors of unrelated structure, suggesting that this is a common on-target side effect of the mechanism of action. Romidepsin is 92–94% bound to plasma proteins and has a half-life of ~3 h. *In vivo* metabolism is complex with over a dozen metabolites identified [49]. Romidepsin is a substrate of P-glycoprotein and transporter-mediated efflux appears to be the major mechanism of drug resistance [50].

Industrially, romidepsin is produced by bacterial fermentation. Several total syntheses have been reported that involve Mitsunobu esterification to assemble the cyclic depsipeptide. However, the reaction needs careful optimization and an alternative route (Figure 5.18) uses macrolactamization instead [51]. The synthesis involves building up a D-Val-D-Cys-Dha tripeptide that is combined with a fragment

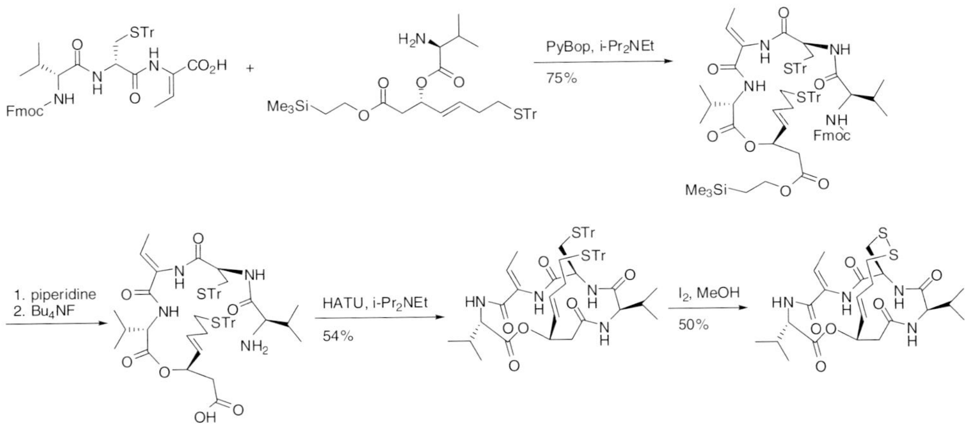

Figure 5.18 A macrolactamization-based total synthesis of FK228.

containing the zinc binding warhead in protected form. The linear *seco*-amino acid undergoes HATU mediated intramolecular coupling to give the macrocycle. In the final step, oxidation forms the disulfide bridge.

Although total synthesis of the depsipeptides is unlikely to compete with the fermentation process in efficiency, it provides access to unnatural analogues. These have shed valuable light on the structure–activity relationship (SAR) of the natural product (Figure 5.19) [52]. The macrocyclic ester is essential as linear uncyclized compounds are inactive. The stereochemistry of the ester is essential as the epimer is virtually inactive. The amino acids present in the peptide macrocycle can be substituted by others without loss in activity. The dehydroalanine Michael acceptor is not needed and it is speculated that its function is to tie up the thiol from the Cys residue upon disulfide ring opening. The zinc-binding thiol warhead needs to be protected to ensure efficient cell uptake, whether as a disulfide as in FK228 or as a thioester in synthetic analogues and the related natural product largazole.

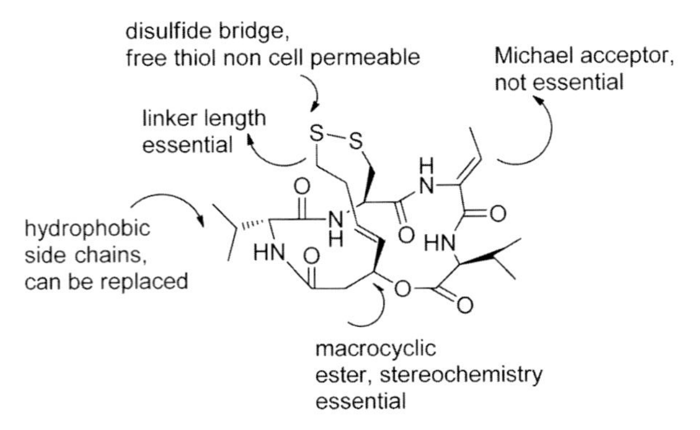

Figure 5.19 Key structural features of FK228.

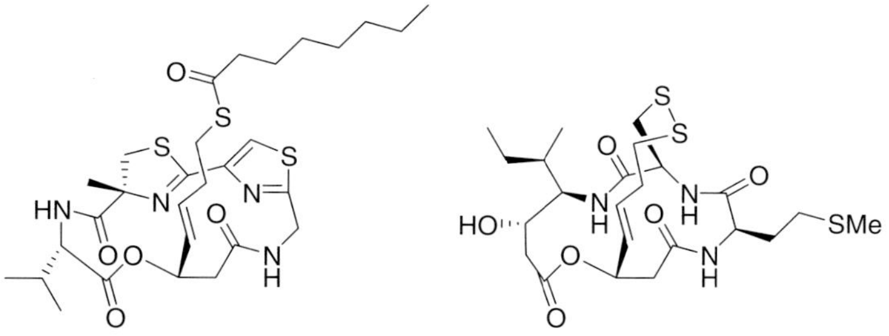

largazole

burkholdac B

Figure 5.20 Structure of largazole and burkholdac B.

Subsequent to the discovery of FK228, other natural product HDAC inhibitors containing the same zinc binding warhead have been isolated. Two noteworthy examples are largazole from the marine cyanobacterium *Symploca* sp. and burkholdac B from *Burkholderia thailandensis* (Figure 5.20). Largazole features extensive modification of the peptide backbone to form a thiazole and thiazoline ring. Unlike FK228, the zinc binding warhead is protected as a thioester prodrug rather than a disulfide. Largazole is exceptionally potent in HDAC enzyme assays with a picomolar IC_{50} and many academic groups have worked on its total synthesis as well as analogue preparation [53]. Despite its potent HDAC inhibition, largazole suffers from two shortcomings. First, there is no gain in potency of antiproliferative effects compared to FK228 and other depsipeptides indicating a loss of activity in cells relative to HDAC inhibition. Second, the thioester prodrug is highly labile in liver microsomes and undergoes hydrolysis in less than 2 min [54]. The disulfide in FK228 appears to be a more stable prodrug and a better approach for protection of the zinc binding thiol. Burkholdac B (= thailandepsin A) is the most recent member of the depsipeptide HDAC inhibitors to be isolated. In cell proliferation assays, it outperforms FK228 with a picomolar IC_{50} and is the most potent compound within this class [55]. The initial report did not assign the stereochemistry of the chiral centers and this was later unambiguously determined by the total synthesis of multiple diastereomers [56].

5.9 Carboxylic Acid and Benzamide HDAC Inhibitors

Besides the hydroxamic acid present in Zolinza and the thiol in FK228, a variety of other zinc binding warheads have been employed in HDAC inhibitors. In an example of drug repositioning, three short-chain carboxylic acids – butyric, valproic, and phenylbutyric acid – as well as a butyrate prodrug have progressed to clinical trials (Figure 5.21). These compounds are already used for other indications and their pharmacokinetics is well understood. Nevertheless, the short-chain carboxylic acids are modest micromolar HDAC inhibitors at best and have short half-lives. This is to be expected from a consideration of the HDAC pharmacophore as they contain a

butyric acid phenylbutyric acid valproic acid AN-9 azumamide E

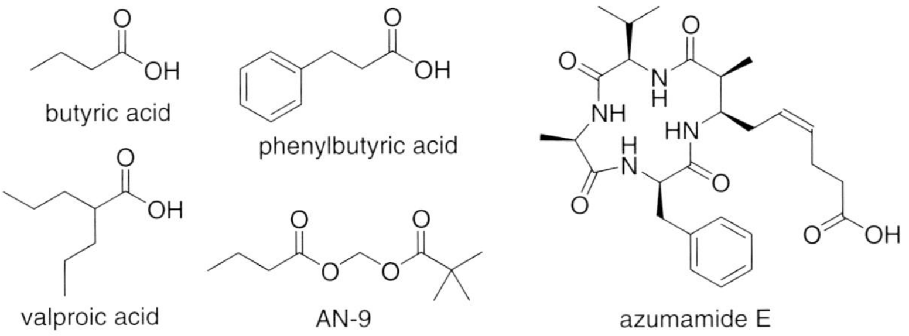

Figure 5.21 Examples of carboxylic acid HDAC inhibitors.

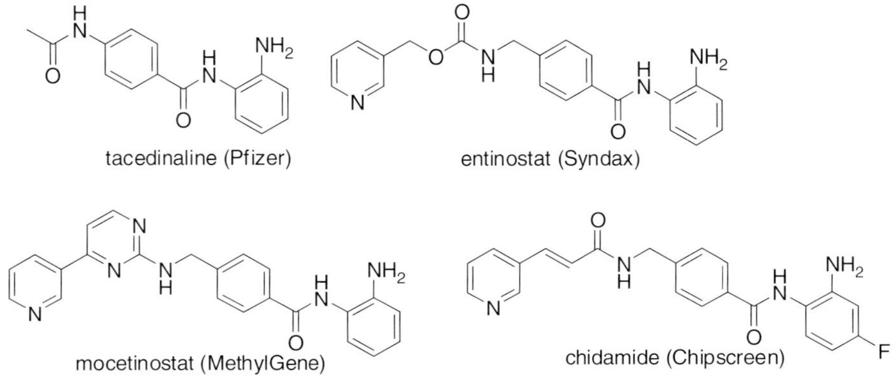

tacedinaline (Pfizer) entinostat (Syndax) mocetinostat (MethylGene) chidamide (Chipscreen)

Figure 5.22 Examples of benzamide HDAC inhibitors.

relatively weak monodentate zinc binding warhead and lack a cap. The only carboxylic acid HDAC inhibitor with a submicromolar IC_{50} is the marine natural product azumamide E [57]. In this case, the macrocyclic cap provides additional binding to the enzyme rim. Synthetic replacement of the carboxylic acid by the superior hydroxamic acid warhead provided an azumamide E derivative with enhanced HDAC inhibition [58].

Benzamides are the most recent family of HDAC inhibitors to reach clinical trials. The two nitrogens coordinate to the active site zinc in a bidentate manner similar to hydroxamic acids. *In vitro* and *in vivo*, benzamides are low micromolar to nanomolar in efficacy. Development of the early example tacedinaline is now discontinued due to toxicity while second-generation compounds (Figure 5.22) are currently in clinical trials.

5.10 Prospects for HDAC Inhibitors

Like DNMT inhibitors, the clinical trial data for HDAC inhibitors have been disappointing for solid and hematological tumors. Zolinza and Istodax are approved only for the treatment of CTCL and even in this indication only a minority of patients show complete response. The underlying biology that enables HDAC inhibitors to succeed against this particular cancer is unclear. *In vitro* studies show that HDAC inhibitors strongly downregulate cytokine signaling in CTCL, particularly IL-10, IL-2, IL-4, and STAT3 and this may be the reason for their antiproliferative effect [59]. For the future, two major developments can be foreseen. First, the true potential of HDAC inhibitors may lie in combination therapy rather than use as single agents. Multiple clinical trials are currently underway to test this hypothesis and early results are promising [60]. Second, there is growing evidence from *in vitro* and *in vivo* models for the use of HDAC inhibitors in other therapeutic indications besides cancer [61]. Such applications will benefit from the ongoing development of isoform-selective HDAC inhibitors.

5.11 Epigenetic Drugs – A Slow Start but a Bright Future

The importance of epigenetics and the identification of epigenetic targets for drug discovery is a recent phenomenon. In spite of the short timeline, four epigenetic drugs are already approved. These DNMT and HDAC inhibitors were earmarked for development based solely on their promising phenotypic effects in inhibition of cell proliferation without knowledge of the mechanism of action. Three of the drugs originated from academic laboratories and all reached the clinic championed by small biotech firms rather than big pharma. Interestingly, all these biotech firms were later acquired by larger organizations. The clinical development owed a lot to the NCI running pivotal clinical trials and working out appropriate dosing schedules.

Today, the situation has changed dramatically. Many of the molecular players in epigenetics have been identified and it is now possible to run high-throughput screening campaigns against such targets. This approach is being pursued by a number of biotech firms that focus exclusively on epigenetics as well as big pharma. At the time of writing, GlaxoSmithKline's bromodomain inhibitor [62] is about to enter clinical trials while there are promising preclinical compounds targeting lysine methyltransferase [63] and lysine demethylase [64], among others. Epigenetics has become an accepted strategy in drug discovery and is now as competitive a field as any other. One can expect many more epigenetic drugs to reach the clinic and to receive approval for multiple therapeutic indications. In addition to targeted drugs, nutraceuticals can play a role as many nutrients and food components have been shown to inhibit specific epigenetic enzymes [65].

Acknowledgments

I am grateful to Professors Manfred Jung (University of Freiburg, Germany) and Andrew MacMillan (University of Alberta, Canada) for helpful comments on the chapter and to the COST Action TD0905 "Epigenetics: From Bench to Bedside" for financial assistance.

References

1 Waddington, C.H. (1942) The epigenotype. *Endeavour*, **1**, 18–20.

2 (a) Szyf, M. (2009) Epigenetics, DNA methylation, and chromatin modifying drugs. *Annu. Rev. Pharmacol. Toxicol.*, **49**, 243–263. (b) Chi, P., Allis, C.D., and Wang, G.G. (2010) Covalent histone modifications – miswritten, misinterpreted and mis-erased in human cancers. *Nat. Rev. Cancer*, **10**, 457–469. (c)Portela, A. and Esteller, M. (2010) Epigenetic modifications and human disease. *Nat. Biotechnol.*, **28**, 1057–1068. (d) Henikoff, S. and Shilatifard, A. (2011) Histone modification: cause or cog? *Trends Genet.*, **10**, 389–396.

3 (a) Mai, A. and Altucci, L. (2009) Epi-drugs to fight cancer: from chemistry to cancer treatment, the road ahead. *Int. J. Biochem. Cell Biol.*, **41**, 199–213. (b) Ganesan, A., Nolan, L., Crabb, S.J., and Packham, G. (2009) Epigenetic therapy: histone acetylation, DNA methylation and anti-cancer drug discovery. *Curr. Cancer Drug Targets*, **2**, 963–981. (c) Jüngel, A., Ospelt, C., and Gay, S. (2010) What can we learn from epigenetics in the year 2009? *Curr. Opin. Rheumatol.*, **22**, 284–292.

4 Esteller, M. (2008) Cancer epigenomics: DNA methylomes and histone-modification maps. *Nat. Rev. Genet.*, **8**, 286–298.

5 (a) Christman, J.K. (2002) 5-Azacytidine and 5-aza-2′-deoxycytidine as inhibitors of DNA methylation: mechanistic studies and their implications for cancer therapy. *Oncogene*, **21**, 5483–5495. (b) Gowher, H. and Jeltsch, A. (2004) Mechanism of inhibition of DNA methyltransferases by cytidine analogs in cancer therapy. *Cancer Biol. Ther.*, **3**, 1062–1068.

6 (a) Piskala, A. and Sorm, F. (1964) Nucleic acids components and their analogues. LI. Synthesis of 1-glycosyl derivatives of 5-azauracil and 5-azacytosine. *Collect. Czech. Chem. Commun.*, **29**, 2060–2076. (b) Pliml, J. and Sorm, F. (1964) Synthesis of 2′-deoxy-D-ribofuranosyl-5-azacytosine. *Collect. Czech. Chem. Commun.*, **29**, 2576–2577. (c) Sorm, F., Piskala, A., Cihak, A., and Vesely, J. (1964) 5-Azacytidine, a new, highly effective cancerostatic. *Experientia*, **20**, 202–203.

7 Hanka, L.J., Evans, J.S., Mason, D.J., and Dietz, A. (1966) Microbiological production of 5-azacytidine. I. Production and biological activity. *Antimicrob. Agents Chemother.*, **6**, 619–624.

8 Jones, P.A. and Taylor, S.M. (1980) Cellular differentiation, cytidine analogs and DNA methylation. *Cell*, **20**, 85–93.

9 (a) Oki, Y. and Issa, J.P.J. (2007) Treatment options in advanced myelodysplastic syndrome, with emphasis on epigenetic therapy. *Int. J. Hematol.*, **86**, 306–314. (b) Howell, P.M., Jr., Liu, Z., and Khong, H.T. (2010) Demethylating agents in the treatment of cancer. *Pharmaceuticals*, **3**, 2022–2044.

10 Lyko, F. and Brown, R. (2005) DNA methyltransferase inhibitors and the development of epigenetic cancer therapies. *J. Natl. Cancer Inst.*, **97**, 1498–1506.

11 Gore, S.D., Jones, C., and Kirkpatrick, P. (2006) Decitabine. *Nat. Rev. Drug Discov.*, **5**, 891–892.

12 Issa, J.-P.J., Kantarjian, H.M., and Kirkpatrick, P. (2005) Azacitidine. *Nat. Rev. Drug Discov.*, **4**, 275–276.

13 Stresemann, C. and Lyko, F. (2008) Modes of action of the DNA methyltransferase inhibitors azacytidine and decitabine. *Int. J. Cancer*, **123**, 8–13.

14 Brueckner, B., Rius, M., Markelova, M.R., Fichtner, I., Hals, P.-A., Sandvold, M.L., and Lyko, F. (2010) Delivery of 5-azacytidine to human cancer cells by elaidic acid esterification increases therapeutic drug efficacy. *Mol. Cancer Ther.*, **9**, 1256–1264.

15 Yoo, C.B., Jeong, S., Egger, G., Liang, G., Phiasivongsva, P., Tang, C., Redkar, S., and Jones, P.A. (2007) Delivery of 5-aza-2′-deoxycytidine to cells using oligodeoxynucleotides. *Cancer Res.*, **67**, 6400–6408.
16 Beisler, J.A., Abbasi, M.M., and Driscoll, J. S. (1979) Synthesis and antitumor activity of 5-azacytosine arabinoside. *J. Med. Chem.*, **22**, 1230–1234.
17 Beisler, J.A., Abbasi, M.M., Kelley, J.A., and Driscoll, J.S. (1977) Synthesis and antitumor activity of dihydro-5-azacytidine, a hydrolytically stable analogue of 5-azacytidine. *J. Med. Chem.*, **20**, 806–812.
18 Goffin, J. and Eisenhauer, E. (2002) DNA methyltransferase inhibitors – state of the art. *Ann. Oncol.*, **13**, 1699–1716.
19 Funakoshi, R., Irie, M., and Ukita, T. (1961) Synthesis of unnatural pyrimidine nucleosides. *Chem. Pharm. Bull.*, **9**, 406–409.
20 Kim, C.H., Marquez, V.E., Mao, D.T., Haines, D.R., and McCormack, J.J. (1986) Synthesis of pyrimidin-2-one nucleosides as acid-stable inhibitors of cytidine deaminase. *J. Med. Chem.*, **29**, 1374–1380.
21 (a) Hurd, P.J., Whitmarsh, A.J., Baldwin, G.S., Kelly, S.M., Waltho, J.P., Price, N.C., Connolly, B.A., and Hornby, D.P. (1999) Mechanism-based inhibition of C5-cytosine DNA methyltransferases by 2-*H* pyrimidinone. *J. Mol. Biol.*, **286**, 389–401. (b) Zhou, L., Cheng, X., Connolly, B. A., Dickman, M.J., Hurd, P.J., and Hornby, D.P. (2002) Zebularine: a novel DNA methylation inhibitor that forms a covalent complex with DNA methyltransferases. *J. Mol. Biol.*, **321**, 591–599.
22 Yoo, C.B., Valente, R., Congiatu, C., Gavazza, F., Angel, A., Siddiqui, M.A., Jones, P.A., McGuigan, C., and Marquez, V.E. (2008) Activation of p16 gene silenced by DNA methylation in cancer cells by phosphoramidate derivatives of 2′-deoxyzebularine. *J. Med. Chem.*, **51**, 7593–7601.
23 Wempen, I., Duschinsky, R., Kaplan, L., and Fox, J.J. (1961) Thiation of nucleosides. IV. The synthesis of 5-fluoro-2′-deoxycytidine and related compounds. *J. Am. Chem. Soc.*, **83**, 4755–4766.
24 Osterman, D.G., DePillis, G.D., Wu, J.C., Matsuda, A., and Santi, D.V. (1988) 5-Fluorocytosine in DNA is a mechanism-based inhibitor of HhaI methylase. *Biochemistry*, **27**, 5204–5210.
25 Martinet, N., Michel, B.Y., Bertrand, P., and Benhida, R. (2012) Small molecules DNA methyltransferases inhibitors. *Med. Chem. Commun.*, **3**, 263–273.
26 Singh, N., Duenas-Gonzalez, A., Lyko, F., and Medina-Franc, J.L. (2009) Molecular modeling and molecular dynamics studies of hydralazine with human DNA methyltransferase 1. *ChemMedChem*, **4**, 792–799.
27 Kuck, D., Caulfield, T., Lyko, F., and Medina-Franco, J.L. (2010) Nanaomycin A selectively inhibits DNMT3B and reactivates silenced tumor suppressor genes in human cancer cells. *Mol. Cancer Ther.*, **9**, 3015–3023.
28 Brueckner, B., Garcia, B.R., Siedlecki, P., Musch, T., Kliem, H.C., Zielenkiewicz, P., Suhai, S., Wiessler, M., and Lyko, F. (2005) Epigenetic reactivation of tumor suppressor genes by a novel small-molecule inhibitor of human DNA methyltransferases. *Cancer Res.*, **65**, 6305–6311.
29 Datta, J., Ghoshal, K., Denny, W.A., Gamage, S.A., Brooke, D.G., Phiasivongsa, P., Redkar, S., and Jacob, S. (2009) A new class of quinoline-based DNA hypomethylating agents reactivates tumor suppressor genes by blocking DNA methyltransferase 1 activity and inducing its degradation. *Cancer Res.*, **69**, 4277–4285.
30 (a) Yang, X.J. and Seto, E. (2008) The Rpd3/Hda1 family of lysine deacetylases: from bacteria and yeast to mice and men. *Nat. Rev. Mol. Cell Biol.*, **9**, 206–218. (b) Imai, S.I. and Guarente, L. (2010) Ten years of NAD-dependent SIR2 family deacetylases: implications for metabolic diseases. *Trends Pharmacol. Sci.*, **31**, 212–220.
31 Carafa, V., Nebbioso, A., and Altucci, L. (2012) Sirtuins and disease: the road ahead. *Front. Pharmacol.*, **3**, 4.
32 Witt, O., Deubzer, H.E., Milde, T., and Oehme, I. (2009) HDAC family: what are

the cancer relevant targets? *Cancer Lett.*, **277**, 8–21.

33 (a) Choudary, C., Kumar, C., Gnad, F., Nielsen, M.L., Rehman, M., Walther, T.C., Olsen, J.V., and Mann., M. (2009) Lysine acetylation targets protein complexes and co-regulates major cellular functions. *Science*, **325**, 834–840. (b) Singh, B.N., Zhang, G.H., Hwa, Y.L., Li, J.P., Dowdy, S. C., and Jiang, S.W. (2010) Nonhistone protein acetylation as cancer therapy targets. *Expert Rev. Anticancer Ther.*, **10**, 935–954.

34 Paris, M., Porcelloni, M., Binaschi, M., and Fattori, D. (2008) Histone deacetylase inhibitors: from bench to clinic. *J. Med. Chem.*, **51**, 1505–1529.

35 (a) Jacobsen, F.E., Lewis, J.A., and Cohen, S.M. (2007) The design of inhibitors for medicinally relevant metalloproteins. *ChemMedChem*, **2**, 152–171. (b) Rouffet, M. and Cohen, S.M. (2011) Emerging trends in metalloprotein inhibition. *Dalton Trans.*, **40**, 3445–3454.

36 Reuben, R.C., Wife, R.L., Breslow, R., Rifkind, R.A., and Marks, P.A. (1976) A new group of potent inducers of differentiation in murine erythroleukemia cells. *Proc. Natl. Acad. Sci. USA*, **73**, 862–866.

37 Andreeff, M., Stone, R., Michaeli, J., Young, C.W., Tong, W.P., Sogoloff, H., Ervin, T., Kufe, D., Rifkind, R.A., and Marks, P.A. (1992) Hexamethylene bisacetamide in myelodysplastic syndrome and acute myelogenous leukemia: a phase II clinical trial with a differentiation-inducing agent. *Blood*, **80**, 2604–2609.

38 Breslow, R., Jursic, B., Yan, Z.F., Friedman, E., Leng, L., Ngo, L., Rifkind, R.A., and Marks, P.A. (1991) Potent cytodifferentiating agents related to hexamethylenebisacetamide. *Proc. Natl. Acad. Sci. USA*, **88**, 5542–5546.

39 Richon, V.M., Webb, Y., Merger, R., Sheppard, T., Jursic, B., Ngo, L., Civoli, F., Breslow, R., Rifkind, R.A., and Marks, P.A. (1996) Second generation hybrid polar compounds are potent inducers of transformed cell differentiation. *Proc. Natl. Acad. Sci. USA*, **93**, 5705–5708.

40 Yoshida, M., Kijima, M., Akita, M., and Beppu, T. (1990) Potent and specific inhibition of mammalian histone deacetylase both *in vivo* and *in vitro* by trichostatin A. *J. Biol. Chem.*, **265**, 17174–17179.

41 Finnin, M.S., Donigian, J.R., Cohen, A., Richon, V.M., Rifkind, R.A., Marks, P.A., Breslow, R., and Pavletich, N.P. (1999) Structures of a histone deacetylase homologue bound to the TSA and SAHA inhibitors. *Nature*, **401**, 188–193.

42 (a) Grant, S., Easley, C., and Kirkpatrick, P. (2007) Vorinostat. *Nat. Rev. Drug Discov.*, **6**, 21–22. (b) Marks, P.A. and Breslow, R. (2007) Dimethyl sulfoxide to vorinostat: development of this histone deacetylase inhibitor as an anticancer drug. *Nat. Biotechnol.*, **25**, 84–90.

43 Breslow, R., Marks, P.A., Rifkind, R.A., and Jursic, B. (1991) Potent inducers of terminal differentiation and methods of use thereof. US Patent 5,369,108.

44 Jones, P. (2012) Development of second generation epigenetic agents. *Med. Chem. Commun.*, **3**, 135–161.

45 (a) Ueda, H., Nakajima, H., Hori, Y., Fujita, T., Nishimura, M., Goto, T., and Okuhara, M. (1994) FR901228, a novel antitumor bicyclic depsipeptide produced by *Chromobacterium violaceum* No. 968. I. Taxonomy, fermentation, isolation, physico-chemical and biological properties, and antitumor activity. *J. Antibiot.*, **47**, 301–310. (b) Shigematsu, N., Ueda, H., Takase, S., Tanaka, H., Yamamoto, K., and Tada, T. (1994) FR901228, a novel antitumor bicyclic depsipeptide produced by *Chromobacterium violaceum* No. 968. II. Structure determination. *J. Antibiot.*, **47**, 311–314. (c) Ueda, H., Manda, T., Matsumoto, S., Mukumoto, S., Nishigaki, F., Kawamura, I., and Shimomura, K. (1994) FR901228, a novel antitumor bicyclic depsipeptide produced by *Chromobacterium violaceum* No. 968. III. Antitumor activities on experimental tumors in mice. *J. Antibiot.*, **47**, 315–323.

46 (a) Nakajima, H., Kim, Y.B., Terano, H., Yoshida, M., and Horinouchi, S. (1998) FR901228, a potent antitumor antibiotic, is a novel histone deacetylase inhibitor.

Exp. Cell Res., **241**, 126–133. (b) Furumai, R., Matsuyama, A., Kobashi, N., Lee, K.-H., Nishiyama, N., Nakajima, H., Tanaka, A., Komatsu, Y., Nishino, N., Yoshida, M., and Horinouchi, S. (2002) FK228 (depsipeptide) as a natural prodrug that inhibits class I histone deacetylases. *Cancer Res.*, **62**, 4916–4921.

47 Cole, K.E., Dowling, D.P., Boone, M.A., Phillips, A.J., and Christianson, D.W. (2011) Structural basis of the antiproliferative activity of largazole, a depsipeptide inhibitor of the histone deacetylases. *J. Am. Chem. Soc.*, **133**, 12474–12477.

48 VanderMolen, K.M., McCulloch, W., Pearce, C.J., and Oberlies, N.H. (2011) Romidepsin (Istodax, NSC 630176, FR901228, FK228, depsipeptide): a natural product recently approved for cutaneous T-cell lymphoma. *J. Antibiot.*, **64**, 525–531.

49 (a) Xiao, J.J., Byrd, J., Marcucci, G., Grever, M., and Chan, K.K. (2003) Identification of thiols and glutathione conjugates of depsipeptide FK228 (FR901228), a novel histone protein deacetylase inhibitor, in the blood. *Rapid Commun. Mass Spectrom.*, **17**, 757–766. (b) Tozuka, Z., Strupat, W.M., Shiraga, T., Ishimura, R., Hashimoto, T., Kawamura, A., and Kagayama, A. (2005) LTQ FT MS accurate mass and SRM data dependent exclusion MS_n measurements for structure determination of FK228 and its metabolites. *J. Mass Spectrom. Jpn.*, **53**, 89–99.

50 Robey, R.W., Chakraborty, A.R., Basseville, A., Luchenko, V., Bahr, J., Zhan, Z., and Bates, S.E. (2011) Histone deacetylase inhibitors: emerging mechanisms of resistance. *Mol. Pharm.*, **8**, 2021–2031.

51 Wen, S., Packham, G., and Ganesan, A. (2008) Macrolactamization versus macrolactonization: total synthesis of FK228, the depsipeptide histone deacetylase inhibitor. *J. Org. Chem.*, **73**, 9353–9361.

52 Yurek-George, A., Cecil, A., Mo, A.H.K., Wen, S., Rogers, H., Habens, F., Maeda, S., Yoshida, M., Packham, G., and Ganesan, A. (2007) The first biologically active synthetic analogues of FK228, the depsipeptide histone deacetylase inhibitor. *J. Med. Chem.*, **50**, 5720–5726.

53 Hong, J. and Luesch, H. (2012) Largazole: from discovery to broad-spectrum therapy. *Nat. Prod. Rep.*, **29**, 449–456.

54 Benelkebir, H., Marie, S., Hayden, A.L., Lyle, J., Loadman, P.M., Crabb, S.J., Packham, G., and Ganesan, A. (2011) Total synthesis of largazole and analogues: HDAC inhibition, antiproliferative activity and metabolic stability. *Bioorg. Med. Chem.*, **19**, 3650–3658.

55 (a) Biggins, J.B., Gleber, C.D., and Brady, S.F. (2011) Acyldepsipeptide HDAC inhibitor production induced in *Burkholderia thailandensis*. *Org. Lett.*, **13**, 1536–1539. (b) Wang, C., Henkes, L.M., Doughty, L.B., He, M., Wang, D., Meyer-Almes, F.J., and Cheng, Y.Q. (2011) Thailandepsins: bacterial products with potent histone deacetylase inhibitory activities and broad-spectrum antiproliferative activities. *J. Nat. Prod.*, **74**, 2031–2038.

56 Benelkebir, H., Donlevy, A.M., Packham, G., and Ganesan, A. (2011) Total synthesis and stereochemical assignment of burkholdac B, a depsipeptide HDAC inhibitor. *Org. Lett.*, **13**, 6334–6337.

57 Nakao, Y., Yoshida, S., Matsunaga, S., Shindoh, N., Terada, Y., Nagai, K., Yamashita, J.K., Ganesan, A., van Soest, R.W.M., and Fusetani, N. (2006) Azumamides A-E: histone deacetylase inhibitory cyclic tetrapeptides from the marine sponge *Mycale izuensis*. *Angew. Chem., Int. Ed.*, **45**, 7553–7557.

58 Wen, S., Carey, K.L., Nakao, Y., Fusetani, N., Packham, G., and Ganesan, A. (2007) Total synthesis of azumamide A and azumamide E, evaluation as histone deacetylase inhibitors, and design of a more potent analogue. *Org. Lett.*, **9**, 1105–1108.

59 Tiffon, C.E., Adams, J.E., van der Fits, L., Wen, S., Townsend, P.A., Ganesan, A., Hodges, E., Vermeer, M.H., and Packham, G. (2011) The histone deacetylase inhibitors vorinostat and romidepsin downmodulate IL-10 expression in cutaneous T-cell lymphoma cells. *Br. J. Pharmacol.*, **162**, 1590–1602.

60 (a) Ellis, L. and Pili, R. (2010) Histone deacetylase inhibitors: advancing therapeutic strategies in hematological and solid malignancies. *Pharmaceuticals*, **3**, 2441–2469. (b) Kim, H.J. and Bae, S.C. (2011) Histone deacetylase inhibitors: molecular mechanisms of action and clinical trials as anti-cancer drugs. *Am. J. Transl. Res.*, **3**, 166–179.

61 (a) Dinarello, C.A., Fossati, G., and Mascagni, P. (2011) Histone deacetylase inhibitors for treating a spectrum of diseases not related to cancer. *Mol. Med.*, **17**, 333–352. (b) Ververis, K. and Karagiannis, T.C. (2011) Potential non-oncological applications of histone deacetylase inhibitors. *Am. J. Transl. Res.*, **3**, 454–467.

62 Prinjha, R.K., Witherington, J., and Lee, K. (2012) Place your BETs: the therapeutic potential of bromodomains. *Trends Pharmacol. Sci.*, **33**, 146–153.

63 Yost, J.M., Korboukh, I., Liu, F., Gao, C., and Jin, J. (2011) Targets in epigenetics: inhibiting the methyl writers of the histone code. *Curr. Chem. Genomics*, **5**, 72–84.

64 Suzuki, T. and Miyata, N. (2011) Lysine demethylases inhibitors. *J. Med. Chem.*, **54**, 8236–8250.

65 Huang, J., Plass, C., and Gerhauser, C. (2011) Cancer chemoprevention by targeting the epigenome. *Curr. Drug Targets*, **12**, 1925–1956.

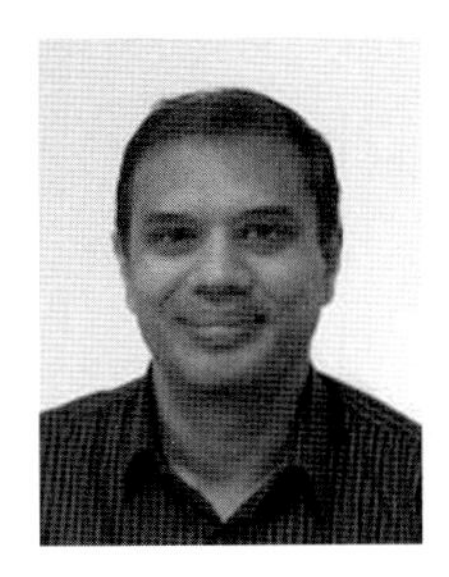

A. Ganesan received his B.Sc. degree from the National University of Singapore (1986), followed by a Ph.D. from the University of California-Berkeley (1992), and postdoctoral studies at Harvard University. Between 1993 and 1999, he worked at the Institute of Molecular and Cell Biology in Singapore, heading the Medicinal and Combinatorial Chemistry Group. In 1999, he joined the University of Southampton's Combinatorial Centre of Excellence as a Reader. Since 2011, he is Professor of Chemical Biology in the School of Pharmacy at the University of East Anglia in Norwich (UK). He is a co-founder of Karus Therapeutics, a drug discovery spinout company.

6
Thienopyridyl and Direct-Acting P2Y$_{12}$ Receptor Antagonist Antiplatelet Drugs

Joseph A. Jakubowski and Atsuhiro Sugidachi

List of Abbreviations

AA	arachidonic acid
ACS	acute coronary syndrome
ADP	adenosine 5′-diphosphate
AMP	adenosine 5′-monophosphate
ASA	acetyl salicylic acid (aspirin)
AUC	area under time–concentration curve
BRIDGE	maintenance of platelet inhibition with cangrelor after discontinuation of thienopyridines in patients undergoing surgery
CABG	coronary artery bypass graft
CAD	coronary artery disease
CAPRIE	clopidogrel versus aspirin in patients at risk of ischemic events
CD	cluster of differentiation
CHAMPION	cangrelor versus standard therapy to achieve optimal management of platelet inhibition
C_{max}	maximum observed concentration
CURE	clopidogrel in unstable angina to prevent recurrent events
CYP	cytochrome P450
ECLIPSE	elinogrel to clarify the optimal inhibition of platelets in secondary prevention
ED_{50}	effective dose that reduces response by 50%
FDA	Food and Drug Administration
hCE	human carboxyl esterase
INNOVATE-PCI	randomized, double-blind, active-controlled trial to evaluate intravenous and oral PRT060128, a selective and reversible P2Y$_{12}$ inhibitor, versus clopidogrel, as a novel antiplatelet therapy in patients undergoing non-urgent PCI
MI	myocardial infarction
PCI	percutaneous coronary intervention
PD	pharmacodynamic

Analogue-based Drug Discovery III, First Edition. Edited by János Fischer, C. Robin Ganellin, and David P. Rotella.
© 2013 Wiley-VCH Verlag GmbH & Co. KGaA. Published 2013 by Wiley-VCH Verlag GmbH & Co. KGaA.

PK	pharmacokinetic
PLATO	the study of platelet inhibition and patient outcomes
SH	sulfhydryl (reactive thiol)
TIMI	thrombolysis in myocardial infarction
T_{max}	observed time of C_{max}
TRITON	trial to assess improvement in therapeutic outcomes by optimizing platelet inhibition with prasugrel
TXA_2	thromboxane A_2
wt	wild type

6.1 Introduction

6.1.1 Platelet Involvement in Atherothrombosis

Atherothrombosis is a term coined to describe the formation of a partially or fully occlusive arterial thrombus at sites of atherosclerotic plaque. Multiple lines of evidence support the involvement of platelets both in the formation and progression of atherosclerotic plaques and in thrombus formation subsequent to plaque disruption. Platelets initially adhere to exposed subendothelial collagen, von Willebrand factor, and other adhesive proteins at sites of vascular injury or atherosclerotic plaque erosion/rupture (Figure 6.1) [1–3]. Platelet activation following these initial adhesive interactions results in the secretion from the activated platelets of adenosine 5′-diphosphate (ADP), thromboxane A_2 (TXA_2), and other mediators. Released ADP promotes platelet activation via the G-protein-coupled P2Y$_1$ and P2Y$_{12}$ purinergic receptors leading to further platelet activation, aggregation, and other platelet functions such as platelet shape change and granular secretion [4–6]. Thromboxane A_2, generated *de novo* upon platelet activation, similarly amplifies platelet activation, aggregation, and other platelet functions, albeit via a separate set of receptors and signaling pathways. These pathways just described are largely responsible for recruiting additional platelets to sites of coronary plaque rupture forming aggregates that may lead to platelet-rich thrombi, vascular occlusion, tissue ischemia, and myocardial necrosis in what is collectively known as acute coronary syndrome (ACS). Accordingly, agents that inhibit platelet activation and aggregation (antiplatelet agents) are widely used in patients with atherothrombotic disease [7–9]. Understanding the above roles of ADP and TXA_2 in platelet recruitment and aggregation, it is not surprising that the most commonly used antiplatelet agents target the ADP and TXA_2 pathways, namely, P2Y$_{12}$ antagonists and aspirin, respectively. P2Y$_{12}$ antagonists will be discussed in detail below. Aspirin interrupts the TXA_2 pathway by irreversible inhibition of platelet cyclooxygenase, the enzyme responsible for the initial step of TXA_2 formation. Aspirin and P2Y$_{12}$ antagonists individually have shown efficacy in the treatment of ischemic cardiovascular disease; however, their distinct modes of action also allow for combination

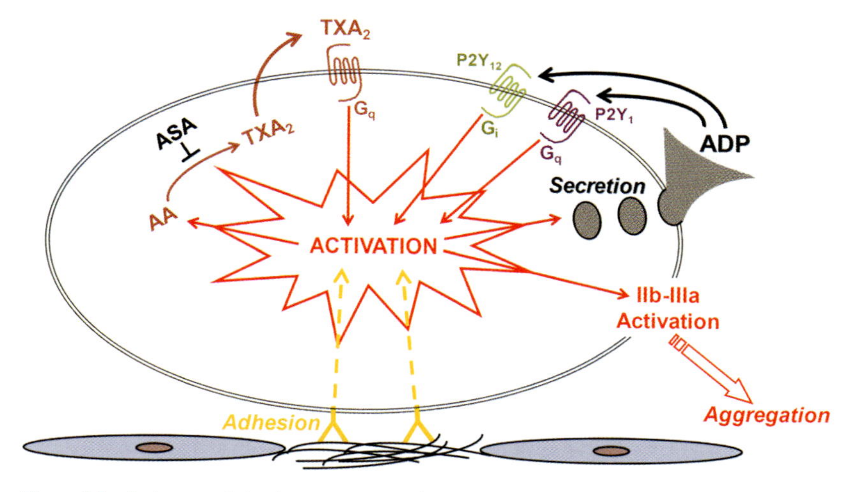

Figure 6.1 Pathways of platelet activation and aggregation. (Modified from Ref. [10].)

therapy (dual antiplatelet therapy), typically resulting in efficacy that is greater than that provided by either agent alone. Given the platelets' physiological role in the promotion of hemostasis, antiplatelet therapy is associated with a bleeding liability.

6.2 Thienopyridines

The thienopyridines are the best-known family of $P2Y_{12}$ targeted oral antiplatelet agents. They are all prodrugs and require *in vivo* metabolism to an active metabolite. Each active metabolite contains a reactive thiol (SH) group that binds specifically to the platelet $P2Y_{12}$ ADP receptor. Platelets also contain a second G-protein-coupled purinergic (ADP) receptor, $P2Y_1$, but this is unaffected by the thienopyridines. Much of our more detailed mechanistic information about the mechanism of action of the thienopyridines has been obtained from studies of clopidogrel and prasugrel. It is of interest to note that less specific information is available for ticlopidine since at the time of its development, clinical evaluation, and regulatory approval neither the structure of the active receptor antagonist nor the target receptor itself had been described.

The thienopyridine prodrugs, by definition, are all inactive *in vitro* as platelet aggregation inhibitors. While several publications describe *in vitro* activities of the parent molecules, these observations are mostly at very high concentrations that would not be sustained following administration at approved doses. Thus, it is generally accepted that single active metabolite for each thienopyridine provides the established pharmacological effects of the thienopyridines. The labile reactive thiol-containing active metabolites bind irreversibly to $P2Y_{12}$ via cysteines 97 and 175 that are close to the ligand binding site in the transmembrane region of

$P2Y_{12}$ [11, 12]. Thus, when administered at doses that singly result in submaximal inhibition, the magnitude of inhibition increases on a daily basis up to the target level of inhibition that ultimately reflects the daily dose given [13]. Steady-state platelet inhibition is typically reached in 3–7 days. This "cumulative inhibition" reflects the irreversible nature of active metabolite binding to the platelet and the circulating platelet's inability to generate and express new $P2Y_{12}$. Recovery of platelet function after cessation of thienopyridine administration also reflects the irreversibility of AM binding to $P2Y_{12}$ and the requisite entry of new platelets into the circulation. Accordingly, recovery of platelet function may take up to 7 days following the last administered dose of thienopyridine. Full restoration of platelet function, which is not necessarily required to provide hemostasis, reflects the level of inhibition present at the time of discontinuation [14].

6.2.1 Ticlopidine: 5-[(2-Chlorophenyl)methyl)-4,5,6,7-tetrahydrothieno[3,2-*c*]pyridine

The discovery of ticlopidine, which has been addressed elsewhere by Savi and Herbert [15], resulted from an *in vivo*/*ex vivo* screening process in which rodents were orally administered the test agents and *ex vivo* platelet aggregation response was used as the bioassay. Screened agents with antiplatelet activity would have shown an attenuated aggregation response compared to control values. Interestingly, while the bioassay was inhibition of platelet aggregation, this was used as a surrogate to identify molecules with potential anti-inflammatory utility. A detailed structure–activity relationship has not been reported. However, ticlopidine was ultimately developed and approved as an antiplatelet agent. Following evaluation of ticlopidine in animal models of *ex vivo* platelet inhibition and *in vivo* thrombus formation, it moved into the clinical arena and first reports of its phase 1 studies confirmed its antiplatelet activity in man [16, 17]. Following a series of phase 2 and phase 3 efficacy trials, ticlopidine was approved for clinical use with indications for use in the primary and secondary prevention of stroke. As would be expected with administration of a platelet inhibitory agent, ticlopidine use was associated with increased bleeding. However, more troublesome side effects included neutropenia, which occurred at an overall rate of 2.4% of which 0.8% were considered severe, and thrombotic thrombocytopenic purpura[1]. While not approved for such cases, ticlopidine was widely used as adjunctive therapy in percutaneous coronary intervention (PCI) and stent placement. This use emerged from several studies indicating that ticlopidine was more effective at reducing recurrent ischemia and with fewer hemorrhagic events compared with standard therapy at the time [18–21].

The approved daily dose of ticlopidine is 500 mg given as 250 mg twice per day. After several daily doses, steady-state platelet inhibition is achieved and maintained thereafter at approximately 40% inhibition of ADP-induced platelet

1) Ticlid (US package insert). Available at http://www.accessdata.fda.gov/drugsatfda_docs/nda/2001/19-979S018_Ticlid_prntlbl.pdf (accessed May 11, 2012).

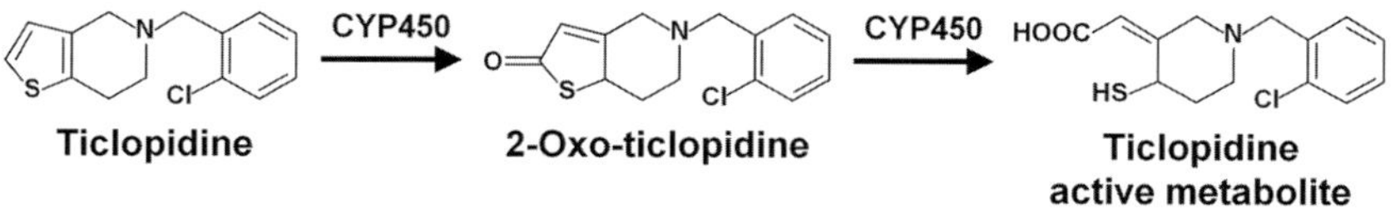

Figure 6.2 Structure and activation of ticlopidine.

aggregation [22]. Relatively little information is available on the pharmacokinetic profile of ticlopidine and its active metabolite. This in part reflects the lack of knowledge of ticlopidine's active metabolite at the time of its initial development and clinical evaluation. While initial FDA approval for ticlopidine was obtained in October of 1991, it was not until 2000 that its active metabolite structure was deduced following identification of clopidogrel's and prasugrel's active metabolite structures [23, 24] and later more definitively disclosed [25]. The pathway from ticlopidine to its active metabolite is shown in Figure 6.2. The initial step from ticlopidine to its 2-oxo intermediate is mediated by cytochrome P450 (CYP) 2C19 and CYP2B6 [26, 27]; this metabolite is not active at $P2Y_{12}$ and presumably requires further oxidation by members of the CYP enzyme family to the SH-containing active metabolite.

Despite the limitations of ticlopidine (lack of understanding of its mode of action and target receptor, bid dosing, and serious hematological side effects), ticlopidine played an early, pivotal role in enabling the widespread adoption of coronary artery stenting. However, a "next-generation" molecule that would provide the clinical benefit of ticlopidine's antiplatelet effects but with a more acceptable safety and "convenience" profile resulted in the development of clopidogrel. It is considered one of the "blockbuster" cardiovascular drugs of the twenty-first century with annual sales in 2011 of approximately 8 billion dollars.

6.2.2 Clopidogrel: (+)-(*S*)-α-(2-Chlorophenyl)-6,7-dihydrothieno[3,2-*c*]pyridine-5(4*H*) acetate

As may be seen from the chemical structures (Figure 6.3), clopidogrel has a different substitution pattern at the benzylic carbon, namely, a methoxycarbonyl (methyl ester) group. This molecule was originally described (as PCR 4099) together with its increased potency over ticlopidine by Maffrand *et al.* [28] and subsequently Defreyn *et al.* [29] and has been extensively reviewed (e.g., see Ref. [15]). Like ticlopidine, clopidogrel itself is inactive *in vitro* and was identified based on its platelet inhibition profile following administration to rodents and assessment of *ex vivo* platelet aggregation. Introduction of the methyl ester at the benzylic center introduces a chiral center into the molecule that was not present in its predecessor ticlopidine. However, preclinical studies indicated that the *R*-enantiomer lacked *in vivo* activity; accordingly, the *S*-enantiomer advanced for clinical evaluation. Preclinical studies in rodents indicated that following oral dosing clopidogrel was substantially more potent than ticlopidine in terms of *ex vivo* inhibition of platelet aggregation

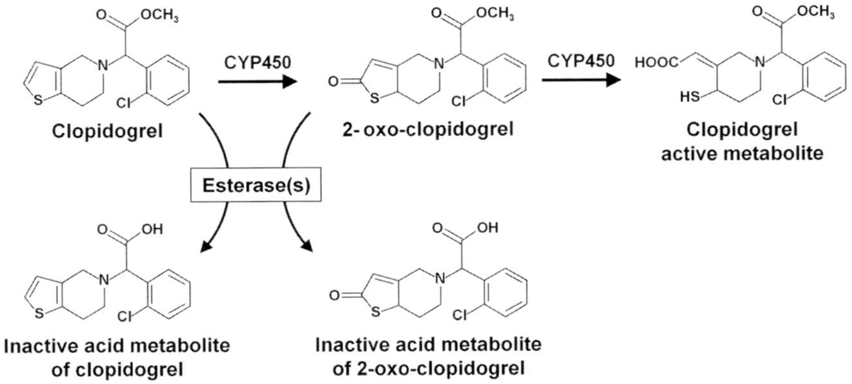

Figure 6.3 Structure and metabolism of clopidogrel.

and inhibition of thrombus formation [23]. Early clinical pharmacology trials in humans confirmed the increased activity of clopidogrel compared to ticlopidine and, at steady-state platelet inhibition, the levels of inhibition associated with ticlopidine's approved dosing regimen of 500 mg/day were achieved with clopidogrel at daily doses of just 50–75 mg [22]. Based on further clinical evaluation, 75 mg of clopidogrel was chosen as the daily dose to explore in pivotal phase 3 trials. This dose was in part chosen on the basis of it providing similar levels of inhibition as ticlopidine at its approved doses with the anticipation that similar clinical efficacy would be achieved but in the absence of the blood dyscrasias associated with ticlopidine. In addition, once a day dosing would be preferable to the bid dosing required for ticlopidine. Ultimately several phase 3 studies of clopidogrel demonstrated that clopidogrel did have a superior side effect profile than ticlopidine [30]. While 75 mg is the approved daily (maintenance) dose of clopidogrel, providing approximately 40% inhibition of ADP-induced platelet aggregation, achieving this steady-state level of inhibition takes several days of dosing. Accordingly in those situations where higher levels of inhibition are required more rapidly, loading doses of 300–600 mg are used. Clopidogrel has a wide range of indications in patients with ischemic cardiovascular disease either as monotherapy or, in combination with aspirin, as dual antiplatelet therapy. Based on the results of the CAPRIE clinical trial, clopidogrel gained its first regulatory approval as monotherapy for the secondary prevention of atherothrombotic disease [31]. Its indications were broadened as a result of the CURE trial [32] and associated CURE-PCI [33], the collective results of which documented the superiority of clopidogrel plus aspirin over aspirin alone. Further details of the clinical trials supporting these and other indications can be found elsewhere [15, 34]. Despite the similarity in structure of clopidogrel to ticlopidine, clopidogrel therapy is associated with much lower rates of neutropenia than those found with ticlopidine (see above). Given that there is no generally accepted mechanistic basis for the neutropenia associated with ticlopidine, it is not possible to explain the different rates found among the thienopyridine family of compounds.

Like ticlopidine, clopidogrel is converted to its active metabolite by metabolism of the thiophene ring at the position adjacent to the sulfur (Figure 6.3). Initial oxidation to the 2-oxo derivative is mediated by CYP enzymes with CYP2C19, CYP1A2, and CYP2B6 playing major roles [35]. As with ticlopidine's 2-oxo intermediate, 2-oxo-clopidogrel is devoid of platelet inhibitory activity and requires further oxidation to open the thiophene ring generating the SH ("reactive thiol")-containing active metabolite. The CYP enzymes involved in this second step include CYP3A, CYP2B6, CYP2C9, and CYP2C19 [35]. The structure of the active metabolite as shown in Figure 6.3 was first definitively described in 2000 [24] with follow-on studies on its stereochemistry appearing subsequently [36].

While introduction of the methyl ester group increased the *in vivo* antiplatelet activity, this substitution also renders clopidogrel susceptible to hydrolysis by human carboxyl esterases (hCEs). Carboxyl esterases are ubiquitous in humans and other species and are acknowledged to act on a wide range of ester- and amide-containing xenobiotics [37]. Thus, approximately 80% of the administered dose of clopidogrel is hydrolyzed to an inactive carboxylic acid metabolite[2)] [38] (Figure 6.3). Recent evidence indicates that 2-oxo-clopidogrel, the intermediate *en route* to the active metabolite, also appears susceptible to hydrolysis [38]. Overall, the consequence of hCE activities would appear to be a reduction in the efficiency of conversion of the administered dose clopidogrel to its active metabolite with perhaps as little as 10% of the administered dose ending up as the active metabolite. It was only recently that reliable assays for the active metabolite of clopidogrel were developed [39].

As with many other pharmaceutical agents, genetic polymorphisms resulting in reduced function alleles encoding for the CYP enzyme lead to altered pharmacokinetics of clopidogrel. Notably, Brandt *et al.* initially demonstrated that polymorphisms in CYP2C19, which is involved in both oxidative steps of clopidogrel's transformation to its active metabolite, and to a lesser extent CYP2C9, resulted in reduced exposure to clopidogrel's active metabolite and reduced platelet inhibition [40]. Consistent with these observations on impaired activation of clopidogrel and reduced platelet inhibition was the finding that patients treated with clopidogrel who had at least one loss of function allele in CYP2C19 had an approximately 1.55-fold increase in the rate of death, heart attack, and stroke compared to non-carriers [41, 42]. The above association of loss of function alleles for CYP2C19 and reduced clinical effectiveness are currently reflected in the prescribing information for clopidogrel[2)].

6.2.3
Prasugrel: 5-[(1*RS*)-2-Cyclopropyl-1-(2-fluorophenyl)-2-oxoethyl]-4,5,6,7-tetrahydrothieno[3,2-*c*]pyridin-2-yl acetate

Prasugrel (originally known as CS-747 and LY640315), which is inactive *in vitro*, was identified by an *in vivo*/*ex vivo* screening approach and first described by

2) Plavix (US package insert). Available at http://www.accessdata.fda.gov/drugsatfda_docs/label/2011/020839s055lbl.pdf (accessed May 11, 2012).

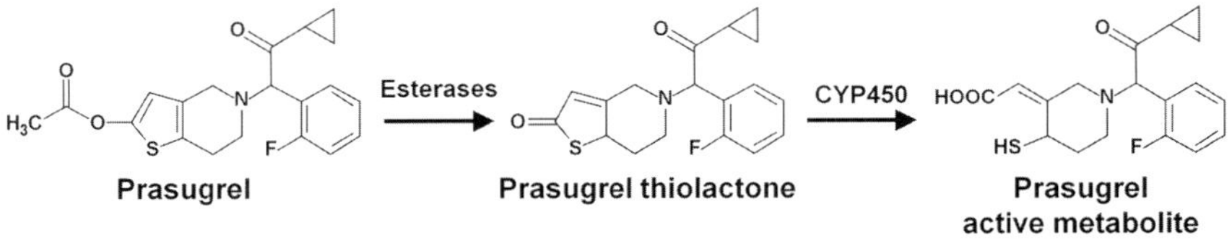

Esterases
CYP450
Prasugrel
Prasugrel thiolactone
Prasugrel active metabolite

Figure 6.4 Structure and activation of prasugrel.

Sugidachi *et al.* [23]. Prasugrel's structure is shown in Figure 6.4; in contrast to clopidogrel, the benzylic carbon is substituted with a cyclopropyl carbonyl group. In addition, the individual *R* and *S* enantiomers at this position in prasugrel undergo spontaneous racemization in solution. Accordingly, prasugrel was developed as the racemate rather than as one of the individual enantiomers. Further differences in prasugrel compared to clopidogrel are found in the substitution pattern in the thiophene ring in which prasugrel contains an acetoxy group at position 2 and in the halide moiety in the phenyl ring (fluoro- versus chloro-).

Early rodent studies demonstrated that following oral dosing, prasugrel produced dose-related inhibition of ADP-induced platelet aggregation that was approximately 10- and 100-fold more potent than clopidogrel and ticlopidine, with ED_{50} doses of 1.2, 16, and >300 mg/kg, respectively [23]. The antithrombotic effects of prasugrel were also investigated and compared to clopidogrel and ticlopidine in a rat arteriovenous shunt thrombosis model. Consistent with the relative platelet inhibitory profile, prasugrel, on a mg/kg basis, had approximately 10 and 100 times more antithrombotic activity compared with clopidogrel and ticlopidine, exhibiting ED_{50} values of 0.68, 6.2, and >300 mg/kg, respectively (Figure 6.5). Further preclinical evaluation of prasugrel indicated that combined administration of prasugrel and

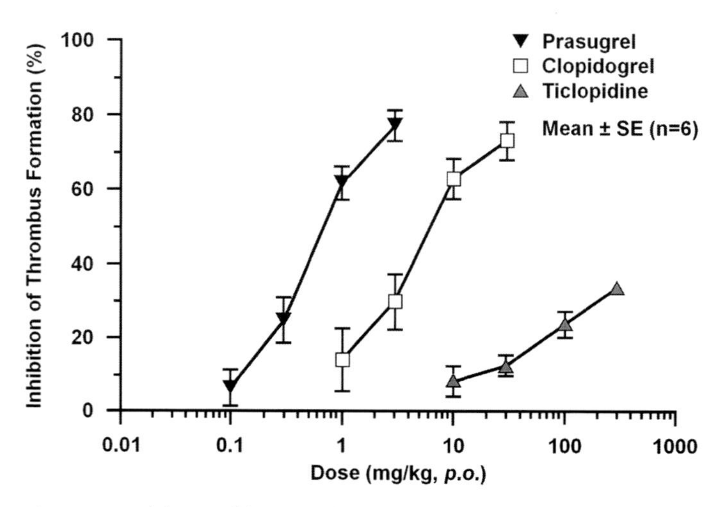

Figure 6.5 Inhibition of thrombus formation in the rat arteriovenous shunt model following oral dosing with thienopyridines. (Derived from Ref. [23].)

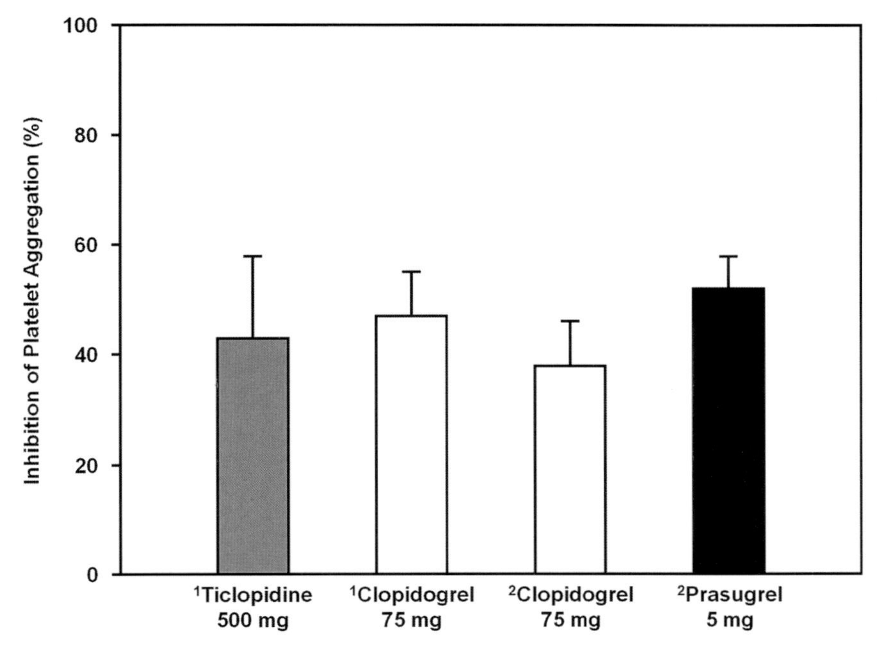

Figure 6.6 Levels of inhibition of human platelet aggregation achieved with clinically relevant doses of thienopyridines. (Derived from (1) Ref. [22] and (2) Ref. [13].)

aspirin produced greater inhibition of both platelet aggregation and thrombus formation compared to either drug alone in rats [43]. These data are consistent with the alternate pathways that these agents inhibit.

A series of phase 1 and phase 2 clinical studies that assessed the safety, pharmacokinetics, and pharmacodynamics of both loading and maintenance doses of prasugrel, the majority of which included clopidogrel as the comparator, have been completed [10]. In summary, these studies indicated that prasugrel was well tolerated and exhibited an acceptable side effect profile. The most common observed side effect being the impaired hemostasis that would be expected with effective platelet inhibition. Consistent with the rodent studies, following oral administration in humans prasugrel was found to be approximately 10- and 100-fold more potent than clopidogrel [10, 13] and ticlopidine, respectively, at inhibiting ADP-induced platelet aggregation. Figure 6.6 illustrates data collected from two studies that collectively illustrate the relative platelet inhibitory activities of the three thienopyridines. As described earlier, the approved maintenance dose of clopidogrel (75 mg) provides approximately the same level of ADP-induced platelet aggregation as the approved maintenance dose of ticlopidine (500 mg), while prasugrel provides similar levels of inhibition at a dose of 5 mg/day.

Based on the results of phase 1 and 2 studies, a loading dose of 60 mg and maintenance doses of 10 mg/day were chosen to take forward into the pivotal phase 3 study of prasugrel. This study, Trial to Assess Improvement in Therapeutic Outcomes by Optimizing Platelet Inhibition with Prasugrel Thrombolysis in

Myocardial Infarction (TRITON-TIMI 38), was a randomized, double-blind, parallel group, multinational clinical trial that randomized a total of 13 608 ACS patients undergoing PCI to prasugrel or standard dose clopidogrel. The primary objective was to test the hypothesis that prasugrel is superior to clopidogrel on a background of aspirin in the treatment of patients with ACS who are to undergo PCI measured by the composite end point of cardiovascular death, nonfatal MI, or nonfatal stroke. The results showed that the primary efficacy end point occurred in 12.1% of patients receiving clopidogrel and 9.9% of patients receiving prasugrel, a statistically significantly reduction of 19% [44]. However, prasugrel-treated patients experienced significantly more major bleeding than the clopidogrel-treated patients (2.8% versus 1.4%, respectively).

Detailed metabolic, pharmacokinetic, pharmacodynamic, and pharmacogenomic studies have provided great insight into the relative disposition of prasugrel and clopidogrel. These studies were in part enabled by the development of reliable assays for the determination of plasma concentrations of both clopidogrel's and prasugrel's active metabolites [39, 45]. Of note, these assays were not available during the clinical development of ticlopidine and clopidogrel. Figure 6.7 shows the notable difference in exposure to the aforementioned active metabolites following loading dose administration in humans. It can be seen that despite being administered at one-fifth the dose of clopidogrel (i.e., 60 mg versus 300 mg), prasugrel resulted in substantially greater active metabolite exposure than did clopidogrel. This was reflected in the C_{max} and AUC for prasugrel's active metabolite that were approximately 14- and 12-fold greater than those for clopidogrel's active metabolite, and greater and more consistent platelet inhibition [46, 47]. On a dose-adjusted basis, this represents an approximately 60-fold greater active metabolite exposure following prasugrel.

Numerous factors contribute to the greater exposure to prasugrel's active metabolite [48, 49]. In contrast to the methyl ester found at the benzylic carbon of clopidogrel that is susceptible to esterase activity, the cyclopropyl carbonyl group at the corresponding position in prasugrel cannot be hydrolyzed by hCE activity. Conversely, the acetoxy group at position 2 in prasugrel is susceptible to hydrolysis, albeit by different carboxyl esterases (hCE-2, present in the intestinal wall) resulting in rapid generation of prasugrel's intermediate metabolite (prasugrel thiolactone). Thus, following absorption/hydrolysis, only a single CYP-mediated oxidative step is required to generate prasugrel's active metabolite. This oxidative step is mediated by CYP3A4 and CYP2B6, and to a lesser extent by CYP2C9 and CYP2C19 [50]. In contrast to CYP2C19, genetic variation in CYP3A4 does not result in a meaningful loss of function phenotype. The lack of impact of CYP2C19 loss of function alleles on prasugrel's pharmacokinetics/pharmacodynamics is illustrated in Figure 6.8. It can be seen that for clopidogrel, compared to fully functional CYP2C19 (wt/wt), the presence of one loss of function allele (wt/*2) results in decreased active metabolite exposure (a) and resulting loss of platelet inhibition (c), and with the presence of two loss of function alleles (*2/*2) the effect is further increased. In contrast, neither hetero- nor homozygous loss of function results in altered active metabolite

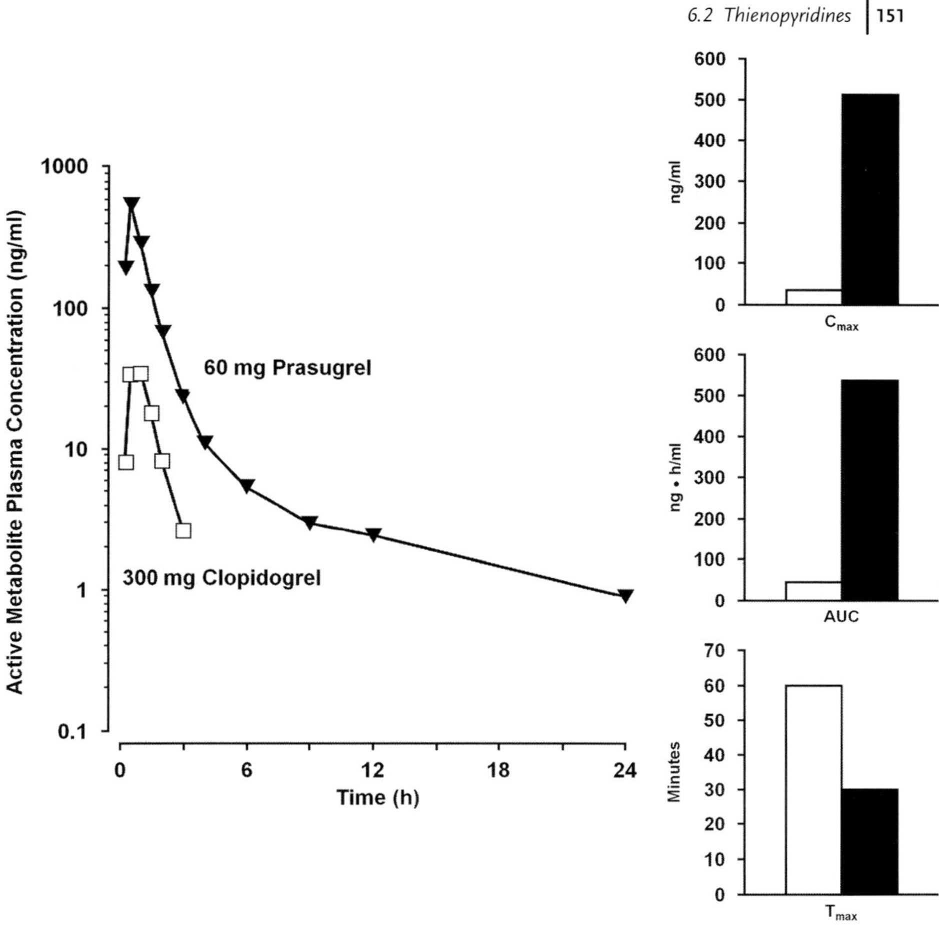

Figure 6.7 Exposure to clopidogrel's and prasugrel's active metabolites following oral dosing: C_{max}, maximum concentration; AUC, area under the concentration–time curve; T_{max}, time of C_{max}. (Modified from Ref. [10].)

exposure or platelet inhibition in prasugrel-treated subjects (Figure 6.8b and c). Taken together, the above factors explain in large part the more efficient conversion of prasugrel to its active metabolite compared to the fate of clopidogrel following administration to humans. It should be noted that loss of function alleles are found in approximately 30% of the Caucasian population and at a higher frequency in certain Asian populations. As described above, the negative impact of CYP2C19 loss of function on exposure to clopidogrel's active metabolite and inhibition of platelet aggregation were consistent with poor outcome in patients treated with clopidogrel [41]. Similar analysis for prasugrel likewise demonstrated that the PK/PD data were consistent with the clinical course in that CYP2C19 loss of function did not lead to a poorer outcome in ACS patients undergoing intervention and stent placement [42].

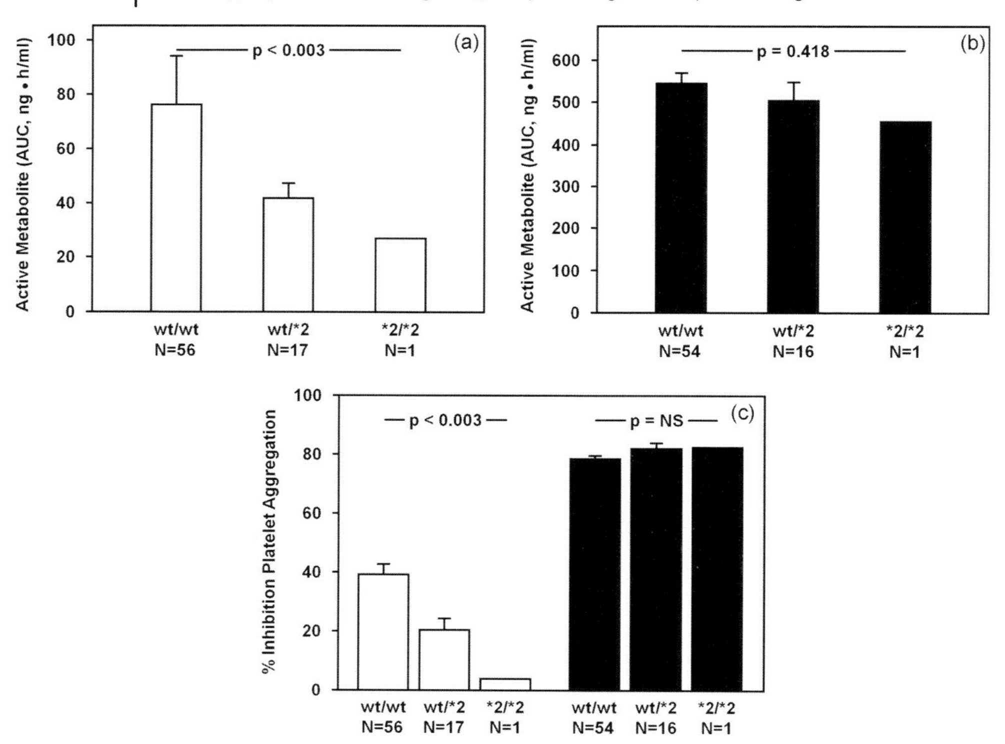

Figure 6.8 Influence of loss of function allele (*2) in CYP2C19 on the pharmacokinetics of clopidogrel's (a) and prasugrel's (b) active metabolites, and on inhibition of ADP-induced platelet aggregation (c) (clopidogrel, white bars; prasugrel, black bars). Integrated data from crossover studies in which all subjects received loading doses of both thienopyridines. (Derived from Ref. [40].)

More detailed reviews of prasugrel's early and later stage development program can be found elsewhere [10, 51].

6.3 Direct-Acting $P2Y_{12}$ Antagonists

6.3.1 Nucleoside-Containing Antagonists

The early observation that ATP was an antagonist of ADP-induced platelet aggregation [52] led to the original quest for more rationally designed antagonists of the platelet ADP receptor. While ATP is an antagonist, it would be in its own right unsuitable as a clinically useful antagonist given its interaction with many different purinergic receptors and its rapid degradation by the ecto-ADPase CD39 to metabolites such as ADP, AMP, and adenosine that themselves possess diverse pharmacological activities.

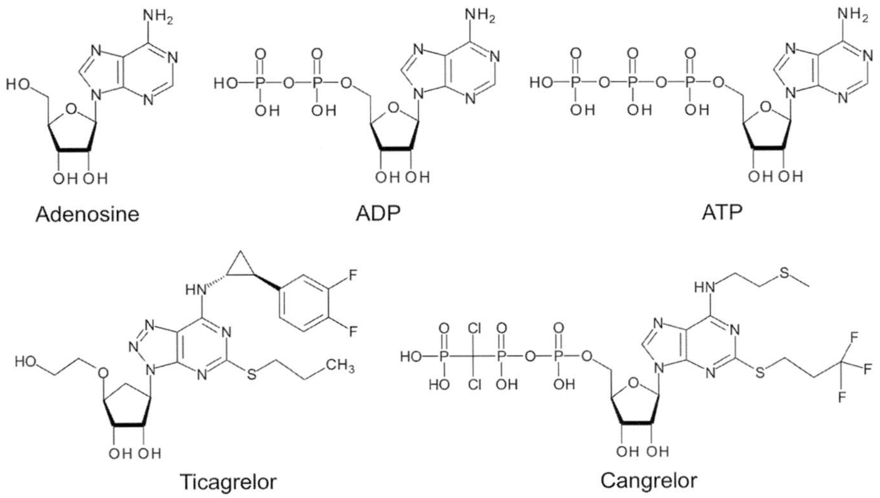

Adenosine ADP ATP

Ticagrelor Cangrelor

Figure 6.9 Structures of adenosine, the adenine nucleotides ADP and ATP, and the $P2Y_{12}$ antagonist analogues thereof.

6.3.1.1 Cangrelor: [Dichloro-[[[(2*R*,3*S*,4*R*,5*R*)-3,4-dihydroxy-5-[6-(2-methylsulfanylethylamino)-2-(3,3,3-trifluoropropylsulfanyl)purin-9-yl]oxolan-2-yl]methoxy-hydroxyphosphoryl]oxy-hydroxyphosphoryl]methyl]phosphonic acid

Cangrelor (formerly AR-C69931MX) is a direct-acting and competitive antagonist of ADP-induced platelet aggregation. Its similarity to the naturally occurring purinergic ligand ATP is readily apparent in Figure 6.9. Modifications to ATP were aimed to improve potency, specificity, and stability and resulted in a molecule with nM affinity for the $P2Y_{12}$ (originally known as P_{2T}) ADP receptor [53]. In contrast to the thienopyridines that are inactive *in vitro*, several *in vitro* studies have shown that cangrelor is a direct-acting inhibitor of ADP-induced platelet aggregation that does not require activation *in vivo* [54]. The rapid recovery of platelet function after termination of cangrelor administration made it suitable as an acute intravenous agent. Pharmacologically, cangrelor infusions in ACS patients resulted in time- and dose-dependent inhibition of ADP-induced platelet aggregation with doses of 2 μg/kg/min and above resulting in near maximal inhibition of platelet aggregation [55]. Following termination of infusion, recovery of reactivity to ADP was both dose and time dependent with full recovery being approached at 1 h at doses up to 2 μg/kg/min; however, at doses of 4 μg/kg/min 40% platelet inhibition was still present 1 h after termination of infusion [55]. Plasma concentrations dropped rapidly after ending infusions and appeared to somewhat outpace recovery of platelet inhibition. Further studies with cangrelor in patients with acute myocardial infarction suggested utility of cangrelor for this indication [56]. Two phase 3 efficacy trials of cangrelor in ACS patients undergoing PCI were recently completed. The trials were designed to assess whether cangrelor, when administered acutely at the time of PCI, improved short-term outcomes.

The clinical efficacy of cangrelor was assessed in the CHAMPION trials. CHAMPION PCI randomized patients either to a bolus and short-term infusion of cangrelor or to a 600 mg loading dose of clopidogrel. At the end of the cangrelor infusion, a 600 mg loading dose of clopidogrel was administered to the cangrelor patients. The primary composite end point of major adverse cardiovascular events in the cangrelor group was not significantly different from the clopidogrel arm [57]. A similar lack of differentiation between clopidogrel loading dose and cangrelor infusion was found in a parallel phase 3 PCI study in ACS [58]. As will be discussed later, it would appear that dyspnea is a common side effect noted with the administration of direct-acting $P2Y_{12}$ antagonists, and this was also observed in the CHAMPION studies.

It has been proposed that a possible reason for the failure of cangrelor to show efficacy over clopidogrel in the CHAMPION trials resulted from the presence of residual cangrelor on the platelet at the time of subsequent clopidogrel loading. As has previously been demonstrated, cangrelor prevents the binding of clopidogrel's active metabolite to platelet $P2Y_{12}$ [59]. This hindrance, combined with a relatively short exposure to clopidogrel's active metabolite, raises the possibility that by the time cangrelor is fully cleared from the platelet there is insufficient active metabolite of clopidogrel present to effectively inhibit the platelet $P2Y_{12}$ receptor. Support for this competitive interaction has indeed been provided in *ex vivo* studies of clopidogrel administration at the time of cangrelor termination [60]. Such an interaction does not occur when switching among the thienopyridines [61].

Cangrelor's relatively short half-life is consistent with its utility in weaning patients off of oral $P2Y_{12}$ antagonists in preparation for major surgery where dual antiplatelet therapy may pose a serious bleeding risk. However, extended periods of time while "washing out" the oral agent, resulting in less effective platelet inhibition in patients with recent ACS events, may result in the recurrence of ischemic events, thus the concept of maintaining patients on a cangrelor infusion during the washout phase and termination of the cangrelor infusion just proximal to surgery. The feasibility of such a study was recently tested in the BRIDGE study [62].

6.3.1.2 Ticagrelor: (1*S*,2*S*,3*R*,5*S*)-3-[7-[(1*R*,2*S*)-2-(3,4-Difluorophenyl)cyclopropylamino]-5-(propylthio)-3*H*-[1,2,3]triazolo[4,5-*d*]pyrimidin-3-yl]-5-(2-hydroxyethoxy)cyclopentane-1,2-diol

Ticagrelor (formerly AZD6140) is a direct-acting nucleoside analogue-containing $P2Y_{12}$ antagonist. As described previously, the identification of cangrelor resulted from modifications to the natural ligand ATP. In turn, the discovery of ticagrelor reflects further chemical modifications to cangrelor aimed at identifying an orally available agent while maintaining potency and selectivity. In brief, the route from ATP to ticagrelor has been described by Springthorpe *et al.* [63] as follows: (a) introduction of affinity-enhancing 5,7-hydrophobic substituents; (b) replacement of the labile triphosphate group; (c) changing the core purine to a triazolopyrimidine, increasing affinity >100-fold; (d) finding the first non-acidic reversible antagonists; (e) introduction of a *trans*-2-phenylcyclopropylamino substituent, increasing affinity >10-fold; and (f) identifying metabolically stable neutral compounds by modifying the hydrophobic phenylcyclopropyl group and the hydroxylic side chain substituent.

As can be seen in Figure 6.9, ticagrelor retains elements of the naturally occurring adenine nucleotides and the intravenous $P2Y_{12}$ antagonist cangrelor and is similarly classified as a reversible antagonist. However, in contrast to cangrelor, ticagrelor is available by the oral route; it also differs from cangrelor in that its interaction with $P2Y_{12}$ is noncompetitive whereas cangrelor under certain assay conditions would appear to be competitive [64]. While ticagrelor has inherent $P2Y_{12}$ receptor antagonistic activity, following oral administration a major active metabolite is formed by *O*-dealkylation mediated by CYP3A4/5 isoforms [65]. This metabolite (AR-C124910XX) has $P2Y_{12}$ antagonist activity approximately equal to the parent and approximates 40% of the exposure to ticagrelor (Figure 6.10). The half-lives of ticagrelor and AR-C124910XX are 8.4 and 11.5 h, respectively.

Detailed pharmacokinetic and pharmacodynamic studies of ticagrelor have been reported [66, 67] and indicate that reduction in ADP-induced platelet aggregation occurs within 2 h after oral dosing consistent with peak plasma concentrations being achieved at 2 h after dosing. More consistent inhibition of platelet aggregation was achieved with twice daily dosing (bid) and at doses >50 mg bid inhibition was greater than that achieved by standard clopidogrel dosing. Additional studies in aspirin-treated CAD patients indicated that doses of ≥90 mg bid dosing provided platelet inhibition that was consistently greater than that achieved by clopidogrel [68].

Phase 3 evaluation of ticagrelor in aspirin-treated patients with ACS managed both invasively and noninvasively was performed in the PLATO study. The results indicated that ticagrelor (180 mg loading dose and 90 mg bid maintenance dose)

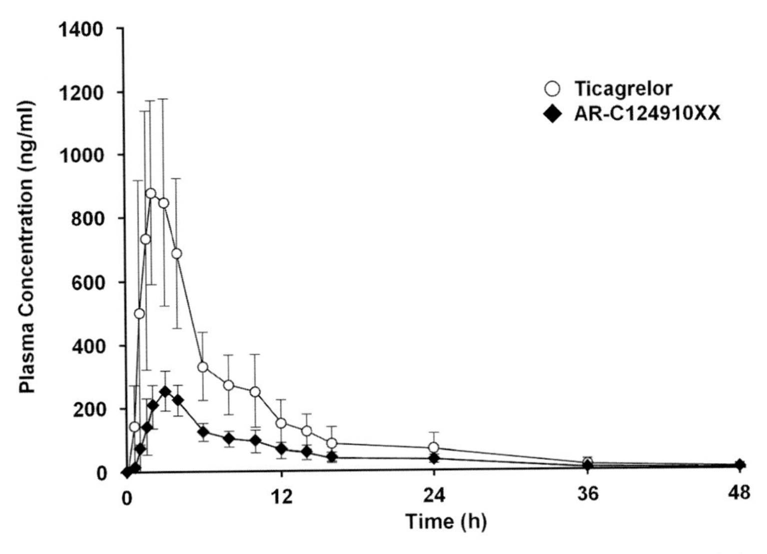

Figure 6.10 Pharmacokinetics of ticagrelor and its major circulating active metabolite (AR-C124910XX), following ticagrelor administration to healthy subjects. (Modified from Ref. [65].)

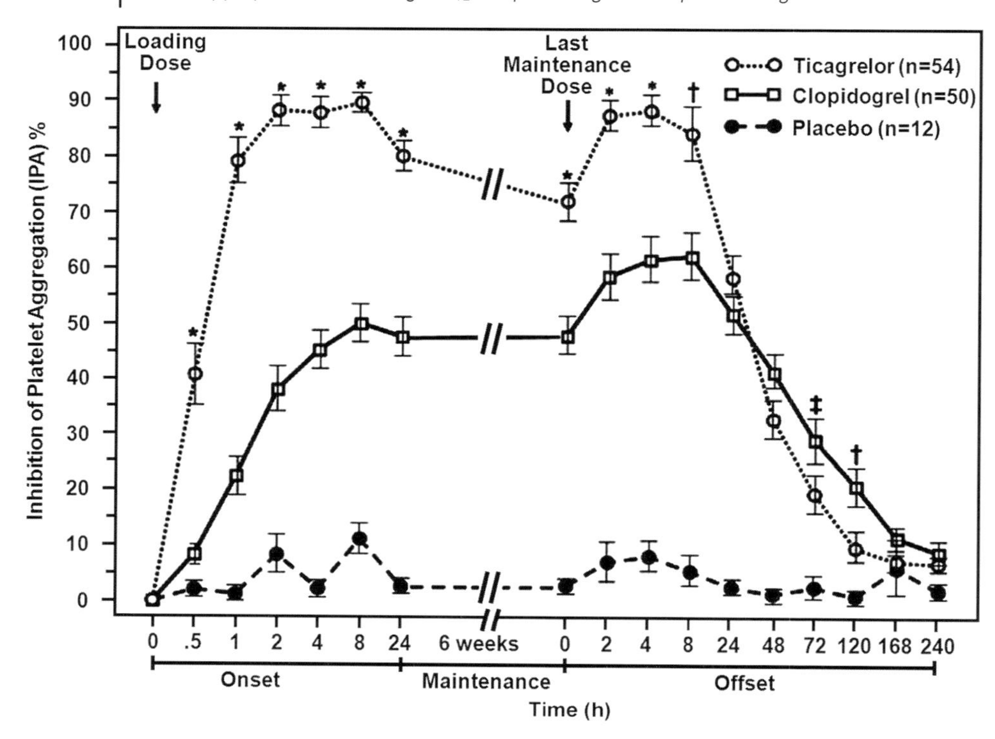

Figure 6.11 Time course of induction of and recovery from platelet inhibition following ticagrelor administration. (Used with permission from Ref. [71].)

plus aspirin resulted in a 16% relative risk reduction in the composite of vascular death, MI, or stroke compared to clopidogrel plus aspirin, including a statistically significant reduction in all-cause mortality. Ticagrelor was associated with an increase in major bleeding and compared to clopidogrel TIMI non-CABG major bleeding was increased by 25% [69]. As with prasugrel, genetic polymorphisms associated with CYP loss of function did not compromise the benefit of ticagrelor over clopidogrel [70]. In detailed parallel pharmacodynamic studies in CAD patients at doses of ticagrelor and clopidogrel utilized in PLATO, Gurbel *et al.* [71] have demonstrated rapid induction of platelet inhibition following the 180 mg loading dose with high levels being maintained with 90 mg bid (Figure 6.11). Interestingly, following cessation of ticagrelor, recovery of platelet function was delayed requiring approximately 5 days to be fully restored to baseline levels. This is in apparent contrast to the pharmacokinetic profile of ticagrelor and its active metabolite that are undetectable at 48 h postdosing (Figure 6.10) and suggests that other factors are at play at the platelet and/or $P2Y_{12}$ level.

There has been much speculation over the possibility that ticagrelor may be metabolized to adenosine *in vivo* and that adenosine mediates off-target side effects [72]. Chemically, this is unlikely; however, the discussion has been driven by the observation of increased rates of dyspnea, ventricular pauses, and hyperuricemia in clinical trials of ticagrelor [69, 73, 74]. While these may indeed be side effects of adenosine, there is, to date, no evidence that increased plasma adenosine levels explain the manifestation of these side effects in ticagrelor-treated patients (see also discussion of elinogrel below). An alternative mechanism for adenosine-like side effects is the possibility that local concentrations of adenosine may increase as a result of ticagrelor inhibiting adenosine reuptake by the erythrocyte [75]. However, the potency of this effect may be too low and has recently been questioned and alternative mechanisms proposed [76].

6.3.2 Non-Nucleoside $P2Y_{12}$ Antagonists

6.3.2.1 Elinogrel: *N*-[(5-Chlorothiophen-2-yl)sulfonyl]-*N*′-{4-[6-fluoro-7-(methylamino)-2,4-dioxo-1,4-dihydroquinazolin-3(2*H*)-yl]phenyl}urea

Elinogrel (formerly PRT060128 or PRT128), as may be appreciated from the structure below (Figure 6.12), is neither a thienopyridine nor a nucleoside-containing antagonist. Elinogrel thus constitutes a third chemical class, and is a substituted quinazolinedione phenyl thiophenyl sulfonylurea $P2Y_{12}$ antagonist [77].

Elinogrel differs from the other direct-acting agents in that it is a competitive inhibitor of $P2Y_{12}$ and may be administered either via the intravenous or via oral route, with the latter route requiring twice daily dosing. The requirement for twice daily dosing is consistent with the pharmacokinetic profile of orally administered elinogrel that, in response to a 60 mg dose, shows peak plasma concentrations being achieved approximately 4 h after dosing and returning to negligible levels by 24 h [78]. In contrast to other direct-acting $P2Y_{12}$ antagonists, there would appear to be a consistent relationship between exposure and pharmacodynamic effect with inhibition of platelet reactivity to ADP reaching a peak at 4 h and fully recovering by 24 h. Intravenous bolus doses of 10–60 mg were well tolerated in ACS patients undergoing primary PCI [79].

Phase 2 studies of elinogrel (INNOVATE-PCI) indicated that high levels of platelet inhibition could be achieved in 30–120 min following combined administration of an intravenous bolus and concomitant oral formulation of elinogrel and that inhibition could be maintained with oral twice daily dosing of 100–150 mg/day [80].

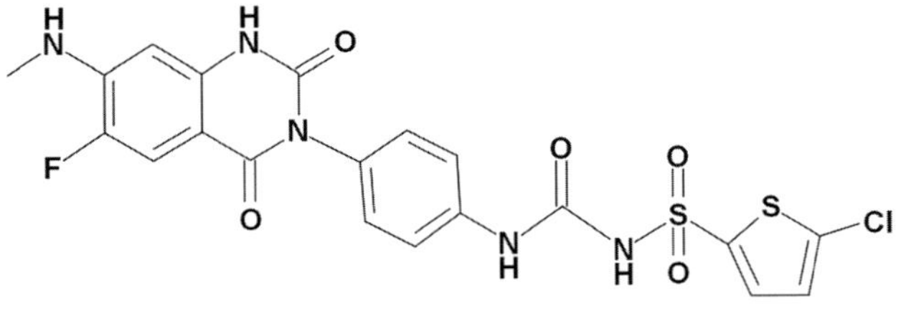

Figure 6.12 Structure of elinogrel.

Consistent with the reversible nature of the antagonist, partial recovery of platelet function to those levels associated with clopidogrel administration was evident between doses. Interestingly, in this phase 2 study elinogrel was associated with an increased rate of dyspnea, which while being reported as mild and transient was three times more common in patients treated with elinogrel compared to those treated with clopidogrel. Since elinogrel is a non-nucleoside $P2Y_{12}$ antagonist, induction of dyspnea would appear to not be the result of adenosine, as has been speculated for ticagrelor, but rather an off (platelet) target effect(s) of the direct-acting, non-thienopyridine, $P2Y_{12}$ antagonists. An additional concern raised by the INNOVATE-PCI trial was an approximately four- to fivefold increase in liver enzyme levels [80].

At present, the future development program for elinogrel is unclear following the recent company announcement that it would not proceed with its planned phase 3 study of elinogrel in patients with prior history of MI, the ECLIPSE study.

6.4 Summary

Following the serendipity of the initial development of ticlopidine, newer generations of $P2Y_{12}$ antagonists with improved pharmacodynamic profiles have been developed. This progress has in part been achieved with the development and use of a variety of technologies applied in an integrated fashion [81]. As a result, today's cardiologist has a broader armamentarium of agents that can be used in patients with coronary artery diseases.

References

1 Roth, G.J. and Majerus, P.W. (1975) The mechanism of the effect of aspirin on human platelets. I. Acetylation of a particulate fraction protein. *J. Clin. Invest.*, **56**, 624–632.

2 de Gaetano, G. (2001) Historical overview of the role of platelets in hemostasis and thrombosis. *Haematologica*, **86**, 349–356.

3 McNicol, A. and Israels, S.J. (2003) Platelets and antiplatelet therapy. *J. Pharmacol. Sci.*, **93**, 381–396.

4 Hollopeter, G., Jantzen, H.M., Vincent, D., Li, G., England, L., Ramakrishnan, V., Yang, R.B., Nurden, P., Nurden, A., Julius, D. *et al.* (2001) Identification of the platelet ADP receptor targeted by antithrombotic drugs. *Nature*, **409**, 202–207.

5 Dorsam, R.T. and Kunapuli, S.P. (2004) Central role of the P2Y12 receptor in platelet activation. *J. Clin. Invest.*, **113**, 340–345.

6 Gachet, C. and Hechler, B. (2005) The platelet P2 receptors in thrombosis. *Semin. Thromb. Hemost.*, **31**, 162–167.

7 Braunwald, E., Antman, E.M., Beasley, J.W., Califf, R.M., Cheitlin, M.D., Hochman, J.S., Jones, R.H., Kereiakes, D., Kupersmith, J., Levin, T.N. *et al.* (2002) ACC/AHA Guidelines for the Management of Patients with Unstable Angina Non-ST Segment Elevation Myocardial Infarction. Available at http://www.acc.org/qualityandscience/clinical/guidelines/unstable/incorporated/UA˙incorporated.pdf (accessed May 2, 2007).

8 Massberg, S., Schulz, C., and Gawaz, M. (2003) Role of platelets in the

pathophysiology of acute coronary syndrome. *Semin. Vasc. Med.*, **3**, 147–162.

9 Antman, E.M., Anbe, D.T., Armstrong, P. W., Bates, E.R., Green, L.A., Hand, M., Hochman, J.S., Krumholz, H.M., Kushner, F.G., Lamas, G.A. *et al.* (2004) ACC/AHA Guidelines for the Management of Patients with ST-Elevation Myocardial Infarction. Available at http://www.acc.org/qualityandscience/clinical/guidelines/stemi/Guideline1/index.pdf (accessed May 1, 2007).

10 Jakubowski, J.A., Winters, K.J., Naganuma, H., and Walletin, L. (2007) Prasugrel: a novel thienopyridine antiplatelet agent. A review of preclinical and clinical studies and the mechanistic basis for its distinct antiplatelet profile. *Cardiovasc. Drug Rev.*, **25**, 358–374.

11 Algaier, I., Jakubowski, J.A., Asai, F., and von Kügelgen, I. (2008) Interaction of the active metabolite of prasugrel, R-138727, with cysteine 97 and cysteine 175 of the human P2Y12 receptor. *J. Thromb. Haemost.*, **11**, 1908–1914.

12 Ding, Z., Bynagari, Y.S., Mada, S.R., Jakubowski, J.A., and Kunapuli, S.P. (2009) Studies on the role of the extracellular cysteines and oligomeric structures of the P2Y12 receptor when interacting with antagonists. *J. Thromb. Haemost.*, **7**, 232–234.

13 Jakubowski, J.A., Matsushima, N., Asai, F., Brandt, J.T., Hirota, T., Freestone, S., and Winters, K.J. (2007) A multiple dose study of prasugrel (CS-747), a novel thienopyridine $P2Y_{12}$ inhibitor, compared with clopidogrel in healthy humans. *Br. J. Clin. Pharmacol.*, **63**, 421–430.

14 Price, M.J. and Teirstein, P.S. (2008) Dynamics of platelet functional recovery following a clopidogrel loading dose in healthy volunteers. *Am. J. Cardiol.*, **102**, 790–795.

15 Savi, P. and Herbert, J.-M. (2005) Clopidogrel and ticlopidine. *Semin. Thromb. Haemost.*, **31**, 174–183.

16 Thebault, J.J., Blatrix, C.E., Blanchard, J.F., and Panak, E.A. (1975) Effects of ticlopidine, a new platelet aggregation inhibitor in man. *Clin. Pharmacol. Ther.*, **18**, 485–490.

17 Thebault, J.J., Blatrix, C.E., Blanchard, J.F., and Panak, E.A. (1977) The interactions of ticlopidine and aspirin in normal subjects. *J. Int. Med. Res.*, **5**, 405–411.

18 Schömig, A. *et al.* (1996) A randomized comparison of antiplatelet and anticoagulant therapy after the placement of coronary-artery stents. *N. Engl. J. Med.*, **334**, 1084–1089.

19 Leon, M.B. *et al.* (1998) A clinical trial comparing three antithrombotic-drug regimens after coronary-artery stenting. Stent Anticoagulation Restenosis Study Investigators. *N. Engl. J. Med.*, **339**, 1665–1671.

20 Bertrand, M.E. *et al.* (1998) Anticoagulation versus aspirin and ticlopidine (FANTASTIC) study. Antiplatelet therapy in unplanned and elective coronary stenting. *Circulation*, **98**, 1597–1603.

21 Urban, P. *et al.* (1998) Randomized evaluation of anticoagulation versus antiplatelet therapy after coronary stent implantation in high-risk patients: the multicenter aspirin and ticlopidine trial after intracoronary stenting (MATTIS). *Circulation*, **98**, 2126–2132.

22 Thebault, J.J., Kieffer, G., Lowe, W.S., and Cariou, R. (1999) Repeated dose pharmacodynamics of clopidogrel in healthy subjects. *Semin. Thromb. Hemost.*, **25** (Suppl. 2), 9–14.

23 Sugidachi, A., Asai, F., Ogawa, T., Inoue, T., and Koike, H. (2000) The *in vivo* pharmacological profile of CS-747, a novel antiplatelet agent with platelet ADP receptor antagonist properties. *Br. J. Pharmacol.*, **129**, 1439–1446.

24 Savi, P., Pereillo, J.M., Uzabiaga, M.F. *et al.* (2000) Identification and biological activity of the active metabolite of clopidogrel. *Thromb. Haemost.*, **84**, 891–896.

25 Yoneda, K., Iwamura, R., Kishi, H. *et al.* (2004) Identification of the active metabolite of ticlopidine from rat *in vitro* metabolites. *Br. J. Pharmacol.*, **142**, 551–557.

26 Ha-Duong, N.T., Dijols, S., Macherey, A.C. *et al.* (2001) Ticlopidine as a selective mechanism-based inhibitor of human

cytochrome P450 2C19. *Biochemistry*, **40**, 12112–12122.

27 Richter, T., Mürdter, T.E., Heinkele, G. *et al.* (2004) Potent mechanism based inhibition of human CYP2B6 by clopidogrel and ticlopidine. *J. Pharmacol. Exp. Ther.*, **308**, 189–197.

28 Maffrand, J.P., Vallee, E., Bernat, A. *et al.* (1985) Animal pharmacology of PCR 4099. A new thienopyridine compound. *Thromb. Haemost.*, **54**, 133.

29 Defreyn, G., Bernat, A., Delebassee, D., and Maffrand, J.-P. (1989) Pharmacology of ticlopidine: a review. *Semin. Thromb. Hemost.*, **15**, 159–166.

30 Bhatt, D.L. *et al.* (2002) Meta-analysis of randomized and registry comparisons of ticlopidine with clopidogrel after stenting. *J. Am. Coll. Cardiol.*, **39**, 9–14.

31 CAPRIE Steering Committee (1996) A randomised, blinded, trial of clopidogrel versus aspirin in patients at risk of ischaemic events (CAPRIE). *Lancet*, **348**, 1329–1339.

32 Yusuf, S. *et al.* (2001) Effects of clopidogrel in addition to aspirin in patients with acute coronary syndromes without ST-segment elevation. *N. Engl. J. Med.*, **345**, 494–502.

33 Mehta, S.R. *et al.* (2001) Effects of pretreatment with clopidogrel and aspirin followed by long-term therapy in patients undergoing percutaneous coronary intervention: the PCI-CURE study. *Lancet*, **358**, 527–533.

34 Yousuf, O. and Bhatt, D.L. (2001) The evolution of antiplatelet therapy in cardiovascular disease. *Nat. Rev. Cardiol.*, **8**, 547–559.

35 Kazui, M. *et al.* (2010) Identification of the human cytochrome P450 enzymes involved in the two oxidative steps in the bioactivation of clopidogrel to its pharmacologically active metabolite. *Drug Metab. Dispos.*, **38**, 92–99.

36 Pereillo, J.M., Maftouh, M., Andrieu, A. *et al.* (2002) Structure and stereochemistry of the active metabolite of clopidogrel. *Drug Metab. Dispos.*, **30**, 1288–1295.

37 Satoh, T. and Hosokawa, M. (1998) The mammalian carboxylesterases, from molecules to functions. *Annu. Rev. Pharmacol. Toxicol.*, **38**, 257–288.

38 Hagihara, K., Kazui, M., Yoshiike, M. *et al.* (2008) A possible mechanism of poorer and more variable response to clopidogrel than prasugrel. *Circulation*, **118** (Suppl. 2), S820.

39 Takahashi, M., Pang, H., Kawabata, K. *et al.* (2008) Quantitative determination of clopidogrel active metabolite in human plasma by LC–MS/MS. *J. Pharm. Biomed. Anal.*, **48**, 1219–1224.

40 Brandt, J.T., Close, S.L., Iturria, S.J. *et al.* (2007) Common polymorphisms of CYP2C19 and CYP2C9 affect the pharmacokinetic and pharmacodynamic response to clopidogrel but not prasugrel. *J. Thromb. Haemost.*, **5**, 2429–2436.

41 Mega, J.L. *et al.* (2009) Cytochrome P-450 polymorphisms and response to clopidogrel. *N. Engl. J. Med.*, **360**, 354–362.

42 Mega, J.L., Close, S.L., Wiviott, S.D. *et al.* (2009) Cytochrome P450 genetic polymorphisms and the response to prasugrel: relationship to pharmacokinetic, pharmacodynamic, and clinical outcomes. *Circulation*, **119**, 2553–2560.

43 Niitsu, Y., Jakubowski, J.A., Sugidachi, A., and Asai, A. (2005) Pharmacology of CS-747 (prasugrel, LY640315), a novel, potent antiplatelet agent with *in vivo* $P2Y_{12}$ receptor antagonist activity. *Semin. Thromb. Hemost.*, **31**, 184–194.

44 Wiviott, S.D. *et al.* (2007) Prasugrel versus clopidogrel in patients with acute coronary syndromes. *N. Engl. J. Med.*, **357**, 2001–2015.

45 Farid, N.A., McIntosh, M., Garofolo, F. *et al.* (2007) Determination of the active and inactive metabolites of prasugrel in human plasma by liquid chromatography/tandem mass spectrometry. *Rapid Commun. Mass Spectrom.*, **21**, 169–179.

46 Payne, C.D., Brandt, J.T., Weerakkody, G.J., Farid, N.A., Small, D.S., Ernest, C.S., Jansen, M., Jakubowski, J.A., Naganuma, H., Wiviott, S.D. *et al.* (2005) Superior inhibition of platelet aggregation following a loading dose CS-747 (prasugrel, LY640315) versus clopidogrel: correlation with pharmacokinetics of active metabolite generation. *J. Thromb. Haemost.*, **3** (Suppl. 1), P0952.

47 Brandt, J.T., Payne, C.D., Wiviott, S.D., Weerakkody, G., Farid, N.A., Small, D.S., Jakubowski, J.A., Naganuma, H., and Winters, K.J. (2007) A comparison of prasugrel and clopidogrel loading doses on platelet function: magnitude of platelet inhibition is related to active metabolite formation. *Am. Heart J.*, **153**, 66.e9–66.e16.

48 Farid, N.A., Kurihara, A., and Wrighton, S.A. (2010) Metabolism and disposition of the thienopyridine antiplatelet drugs ticlopidine, clopidogrel, and prasugrel in humans. *J. Clin. Pharmacol.*, **50**, 126–142.

49 Small, D.S., Farid, N.A., Payne, C.D., Konkoy, C.S., Jakubowski, J.A., Winters, K.J., and Salazar, D.E. (2010) Effect of intrinsic and extrinsic factors on the clinical pharmacokinetics and pharmacodynamics of prasugrel. *Clin. Pharmacokinet.*, **49**, 777–798.

50 Rehmel, J.L., Eckstein, J.A., Farid, N.A. *et al.* (2006) Interactions of two major metabolites of prasugrel, a thienopyridine antiplatelet agent, with the cytochromes P450. *Drug Metab. Dispos.*, **34**, 600–607.

51 Jakubowski, J.A., Riesmeyer, J.R., Close, S.L., Leishman, A.G., and Erlinge, D. (2011) TRITON and beyond: new insights into the profile of prasugrel. *Cardiovasc. Ther.*, **30** (4), e174–e182.

52 McFarlane, D. and Mills, D. (1975) The effect of ATP on platelets: evidence against the central role of released ADP in primary aggregation. *Blood*, **46**, 309–320.

53 Ingall, A.H., Dixon, J., Bailey, A., Coombs, M.E., Cox, D., McInally, J.I., Hunt, S.F., Kindon, N.D., Teobald, B.J., Willis, P.A., Humphries, R.G., Leff, P., Clegg, J.A., Smith, J.A., and Tomlinson, W. (1999) Antagonists of the platelet P2T receptor: a novel approach to antithrombotic therapy. *J. Med. Chem.*, **42**, 213–220.

54 Storey, R.F., Wilcox, R.G., and Heptinstall, S. (2002) Comparison of the pharmacodynamic effects of the platelet ADP receptor antagonists clopidogrel and AR-C69931MX in patients with ischaemic heart disease. *Platelets*, **13**, 407–412.

55 Storey, R.F., Oldroyd, K.G., and Wilcox, R.G. (2001) Open multicentre study of the P2T receptor antagonist AR-C69931MX assessing safety, tolerability and activity in patients with acute coronary syndromes. *Thromb. Haemost.*, **85**, 401–407.

56 Greenbaum, A.B., Grines, C.L., Bittl, J.A. *et al.* (2006) Initial experience with an intravenous P2Y12 platelet receptor antagonist in patients undergoing percutaneous coronary intervention: results from a 2-part, phase II, multicenter, randomized, placebo and active-controlled trial. *Am. Heart J.*, **151**, 689.e1–689.e10.

57 Harrington, R.A., Stone, G.W., McNulty, S. *et al.*(CHAMPION PCI Investigators) (2009) Platelet inhibition with cangrelor in patients undergoing PCI. *N. Engl. J. Med.*, **361**, 2318–2329.

58 Bhatt, D.L., Lincoff, A.M., Gibson, C.M. *et al.*(CHAMPION PLATFORM Investigators) (2009) Intravenous platelet blockade with cangrelor during PCI. *N. Engl. J. Med.*, **361**, 2330–2334.

59 Dovlatova, N., Jakubowski, J., Sugidachi, A. *et al.* (2008) The reversible P2Y12 antagonist cangrelor influences the ability of the active metabolites of clopidogrel and prasugrel to produce irreversible inhibition of platelet function. *J. Thromb. Haemost.*, **6**, 1153–1159.

60 Steinhubl, S.R., Oh, J.J., Oestreich, J.H. *et al.* (2008) Transitioning patients from cangrelor to clopidogrel: pharmacodynamic evidence of a competitive effect. *Thromb. Res.*, **121**, 527–534.

61 Jakubowski, J.A., Payne, C.D., Li, Y.G., Farid, N.A., Brandt, J.T., Small, D.S., Salazar, D.E., and Winters, K.J. (2008) The use of the VerifyNow P2Y12 point-of-care device to monitor platelet function across a range of P2Y12 inhibition levels following prasugrel and clopidogrel administration. *Thromb. Haemost.*, **99**, 409–415.

62 Angiolillo, D.J., Firstenberg, M.S., Price, M.J., Tummala, P.E., Hutyra, M., Welsby, I.J., Voeltz, M.D., Chandna, H., Ramaiah, C., Brtko, M., Cannon, L., Dyke, C., Liu, T., Montalescot, G., Manoukian, S.V., Prats, J., and Topol, E.J. (BRIDGE Investigators) (2012) Bridging antiplatelet therapy with cangrelor in patients undergoing cardiac surgery: a randomized controlled trial. *J. Am. Med. Assoc.*, **18**, 307, 265–274.

63 Springthorpe, B., Bailey, A., Barton, P., Birkinshaw, T.N., Bonnert, R.V., Brown, R.C., Chapman, D., Dixon, J., Guile, S.D., Humphries, R.G., Hunt, S.F., Ince, F., Ingall, A.H., Kirk, I.P., Leeson, P.D., Leff, P., Lewis, R.J., Martin, B.P., McGinnity, D. F., Mortimore, M.P., Paine, S.W., Pairaudeau, G., Patel, A., Rigby, A.J., Riley, R.J., Teobald, B.J., Tomlinson, W., Webborn, P.J., and Willis, P.A. (2007) From ATP to AZD6140: the discovery of an orally active reversible P2Y12 receptor antagonist for the prevention of thrombosis. *Bioorg. Med. Chem. Lett.*, **17**, 6013–6018.

64 van Giezen, J.J.J. and Humphries, R.G. (2005) Preclinical and clinical studies with selective reversible direct P2Y12 antagonists. *Semin. Thromb. Haemost.*, **31**, 195–204.

65 Teng, R., Oliver, S., Hayes, M.A., and Butler, K. (2010) Absorption, distribution, metabolism, and excretion of ticagrelor in healthy subjects. *Drug Metab. Dispos.*, **38**, 1514–1521.

66 Husted, S., Emanuelsson, H., Heptinstall, S., Sandset, P.M., Wickens, M., and Peters, G. (2006) Pharmacodynamics, pharmacokinetics, and safety of the oral reversible P2Y12 antagonist AZD6140 with aspirin in patients with atherosclerosis: a double-blind comparison to clopidogrel with aspirin. *Eur. Heart J.*, **27**, 1038–1047.

67 Butler, K. and Teng, R. (2010) Pharmacokinetics, pharmacodynamics, safety and tolerability of multiple ascending doses of ticagrelor in healthy volunteers. *Br. J. Clin. Pharmacol.*, **70**, 65–77.

68 Storey, R.F., Husted, S., Harrington, R.A., Heptinstall, S., Wilcox, R.G., Peters, G., Wickens, M., Emanuelsson, H., Gurbel, P., Grande, P., and Cannon, C.P. (2007) Inhibition of platelet aggregation by AZD6140, a reversible oral P2Y12 receptor antagonist, compared with clopidogrel in patients with acute coronary syndromes. *J. Am. Coll. Cardiol.*, **50**, 1852–1856.

69 Wallentin, L., Becker, R.C., Budaj, A. *et al.* (2009) Ticagrelor versus clopidogrel in patients with acute coronary syndromes. *N. Engl. J. Med.*, **361**, 1045–1057.

70 Wallentin, L., James, S., Storey, R.F. *et al.* (2010) Effect of CYP2C19 and ABCB1 single nucleotide polymorphisms on outcomes of treatment with ticagrelor versus clopidogrel for acute coronary syndromes: a genetic substudy of the PLATO trial. *Lancet*, **376**, 1320–1328.

71 Gurbel, P.A., Bliden, K.P., Butler, K. *et al.* (2009) Randomized double-blind assessment of the onset and offset of the antiplatelet effects of ticagrelor versus clopidogrel in patients with stable coronary artery disease: the ONSET/OFFSET study. *Circulation*, **120**, 2577–2585.

72 Serebruany, V. (2011) Adenosine release: a potential explanation for the benefits of ticagrelor in the PLATelet Inhibition and Clinical Outcomes trial? *Am. Heart J.*, **161**, 1–4.

73 Cannon, C.P., Husted, S., Harrington, R.A. *et al.* (2007) Safety, tolerability, and initial efficacy of AZD6140, the first reversible oral adenosine diphosphate receptor antagonist, compared with clopidogrel, in patients with non-ST-segment elevation acute coronary syndrome: primary results of the DISPERSE-2 trial. *J. Am. Coll. Cardiol.*, **50**, 1844–1851.

74 Storey, R.F., Bliden, K., Patil, S.B. *et al.* (2010) Incidence of dyspnea and assessment of cardiac and pulmonary function in patients with stable coronary artery disease receiving ticagrelor, clopidogrel or placebo in the ONSET/OFFSET study. *J. Am. Coll. Cardiol.*, **56**, 185–193.

75 van Giezen, J.J.J., Sidaway, J., Glaves, P., Kirk, I., and Bjorkman, J.A. (2012) Ticagrelor inhibits adenosine uptake *in vitro* and enhances adenosine-mediated hyperemia responses in a canine model. *J. Cardiovasc. Pharmacol. Ther.*, **17** (2), 164–172.

76 Ohman, J., Kudira, R., Albinsson, S., Olde, B., and Erlinge, D. (2012) Ticagrelor induces adenosine triphosphate release from human red blood cells. *Biochem. Biophys. Res. Commun.*, **418**, 754–758.

77 Ueno, M., Rao, S.V., and Angiolillo, D.J. (2010) Elinogrel: pharmacological principles, preclinical and early phase

clinical testing. *Future Cardiol.*, **6**, 445–453.

78 Gurbel, P., Bliden, K., Antonino, M. *et al.* (2009) The effect of elinogrel on high platelet reactivity during dual antiplatelet therapy and the relation to CYP 2C19*2 genotype: first experience in patients. *J. Thromb. Haemost.*, **8**, 43–53.

79 Berger, J.S., Roe, M.T., Gibson, C.M., Kilaru, R., Green, C.L., Melton, L., Blankenship, J.D., Metzger, D.C., Granger, C.B., Gretler, D.D., Grines, C.L., Huber, K., Zeymer, U., Buszman, P., Harrington, R.A., and Armstrong, P.W. (2009) Safety and feasibility of adjunctive antiplatelet therapy with intravenous elinogrel, a direct-acting and reversible P2Y12 ADP-receptor antagonist, before primary percutaneous intervention in patients with ST-elevation myocardial infarction: the Early Rapid ReversAl of platelet thromboSis with intravenous Elinogrel before PCI to optimize reperfusion in acute Myocardial Infarction (ERASE MI) pilot trial. *Am. Heart J.*, **158**, 998.e1–1004.e1.

80 Rao, S. (2010) A randomized, double-blind, active controlled trial to evaluate intravenous and oral PRT060128 (elinogrel), a selective and reversible P2Y12 receptor inhibitor, vs. clopidogrel, as a novel antiplatelet therapy in patients undergoing non-urgent percutaneous coronary interventions (INNOVATE-PCI). Presented at the 2010 ESC Congress, August 28–September 1, 2010, Stockholm, Sweden.

81 Jakubowski, J.A. (2011) Platelet functional testing: value in the aggregate. *Biomarkers Med.*, **5**, 5–8.

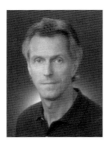

Joseph A. Jakubowski received an M.Sc. degree in Nutrition from the University of London (UK) and Ph.D. in Clinical Science from the Australian National University, Canberra, Australia, studying human platelet reactivity. He continued his platelet studies at Boston University School of Medicine where he was Assistant Professor of Medicine. Dr. Jakubowski joined Lilly Research Laboratories in 1988 and established a Platelet Research Group that was responsible for the identification and clinical evaluation of several antiplatelet agents. He has published extensively on the pharmacological control of platelet reactivity by antiplatelet agents and holds several issued patents. He is an Adjunct Assistant Professor at Indiana University School of Medicine and is an elected member of the European Society of Cardiology (ESC) Working Group on Thrombosis.

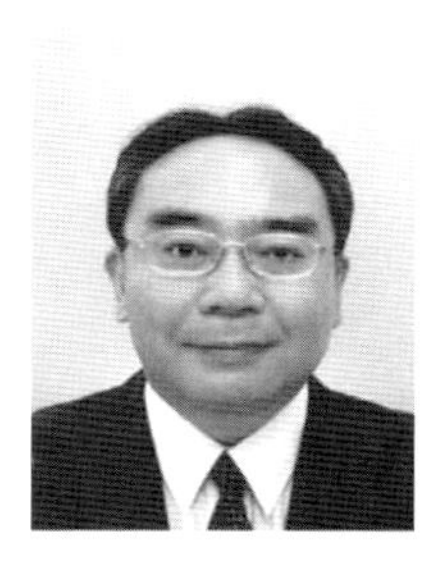

Atsuhiro Sugidachi studied biochemistry at the Faculty of Pharmaceutical Sciences, Tohoku University, Japan. In 1989, he joined the Thrombosis Research Group, Biological Research Laboratories, Sankyo Co., Ltd., participating in the $P2Y_{12}$ antagonist project. In 1996, he received his Ph.D. in Pharmaceutical Sciences from Tohoku University, Japan. Between 2000 and 2002, he was a Visiting Scientist in the laboratory of Dr. Lawrence F. Brass at The University of Pennsylvania School of Medicine. In 2005, he became Group Director of The Pharmacology and Molecular Biology Research Laboratories of Sankyo Co., Ltd., overseeing projects on cardiovascular and metabolic diseases. Since 2007, he has been a Senior Director of The Biological Research Laboratories of Daiichi Sankyo Co., Ltd., where his group has been working on several drug targets for cardiovascular diseases.

7
Selective Estrogen Receptor Modulators

Amarjit Luniwal, Rachael Jetson, and Paul Erhardt

List of Abbreviations

ABDD	analogue-based drug discovery
CoAc	coactivators
CoRe	corepressors
CYP	cytochrome P450
DES	diethylstilbestrol
ER	estrogen receptor
ERE	estrogen responsive elements
FDA	Food and Drug Administration
FMO	flavin-containing monooxygenase
GnRH	gonadotropin releasing hormone
HERS	Heart Estrogen/Progesterone Replacement Study
HRT	hormone replacement therapy
HSP	heat shock proteins
ICI	Imperial Chemical Industries
MORE	Multiple Outcomes of Raloxifene Evaluation
NDA	New Drug Application
PCOS	polycystic ovarian syndrome
RUTH	Raloxifene's Use for The Heart
SAR	structure–activity relationship
SERD	selective estrogen receptor downregulator
SERM	selective estrogen receptor modulator
STAR	Study of Tamoxifen and Raloxifene
WHI	The Women's Health Initiative

Analogue-based Drug Discovery III, First Edition. Edited by János Fischer, C. Robin Ganellin, and David P. Rotella.
© 2013 Wiley-VCH Verlag GmbH & Co. KGaA. Published 2013 by Wiley-VCH Verlag GmbH & Co. KGaA.

7.1
Introduction

7.1.1
Working Definition

Coined by workers at Eli Lilly during the 1990s [1], the acronym "SERM" (selective estrogen receptor modulator) has come to serve as the common classification for molecules that can display a multiplicity of effects due to differential modulation of the estrogen receptor (ER) pathways at different sites [2]. Scheme 7.1 conveys how the interaction of various SERM ligands with ERs can lead to different responses at numerous points along the cascade normally triggered by estrogens like 17β-estradiol (**1** in Figure 7.1) so as to eventually lead to DNA transcription. Unlike estrogens that are uniformly agonists, and antiestrogens that are uniformly antagonists, the SERMs exert selective agonist or antagonist effects on various estrogen target tissues [3]. Thus, a drug like fulvestrant, **2**, which is sometimes referred to as a "selective antagonist" or a "selective estrogen receptor downregulator" (SERD), is not a true SERM because it demonstrates only a pure antiestrogenic profile on all genes and in all tissues [2]. Following this definition in its strictest sense,

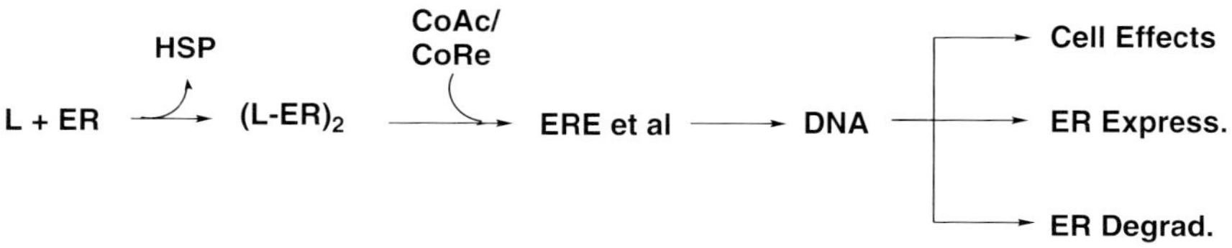

L + ER —(HSP)→ $(L\text{-}ER)_2$ —(CoAc/CoRe)→ ERE et al → DNA → Cell Effects / ER Express. / ER Degrad.

Scheme 7.1 Simplified cartoon of how SERM ligands (L) can interact with estrogen receptors (ER) to cause a multiplicity of effects. This depiction represents a composite of information conveyed in several reviews and additional references cited therein [1–6]. Points that can lead to variable effects include the following: (1) there are two types of ER (namely ERα and ERβ) differentially populated in time across normal tissues, as well as in various pathologies. (2) Relative to the estrogens, L can begin to bind with ER as agonists, partial agonists, or antagonists of varying competitive or noncompetitive potency. (3) Binding may sometimes accommodate more than one L and in all cases continues to proceed through distinct mutual molding processes wherein there are unique conformational subtleties for each SERM that represent a continuum of graded possibilities ranging between the initial agonist and antagonist modes of interaction. (4) Binding releases heat shock proteins (HSP) from their association with ER and causes the ER to dimerize ($(L\text{-}ER)_2$) in either a homo- or hetero-fashion. The type of dimer varies according to the expression levels and degradation rates of the two ER. (5) Depending upon the nature of the still maturing complex, different coactivators (CoAc) or corepressors (CoRe) can be additionally recruited. Types and concentrations of CoAc and CoRe vary in time across normal cells, as well as in various pathologies. Differences in the latter are especially important to recruitment and the eventual responses that become generated. (6) Interaction of the final complex with DNA primarily engages estrogen responsive elements (ERE) but can also involve other responsive elements. (7) DNA signaling can be either enhanced or attenuated relative to various transcriptional pathways. (8) Likewise, expression of ER can be either induced or inhibited, as can expression of factors associated with the pathway that degrades ER.

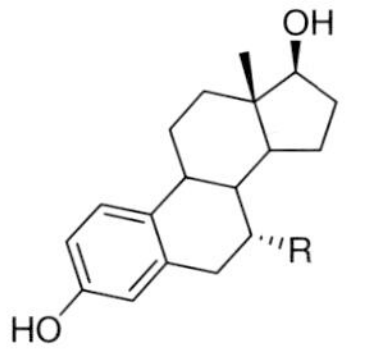

17β-Estradiol (**1**): R = H
Fulvestrant (**2**):
R = $(CH_2)_9SO(CH_2)_3CF_2CF_3$

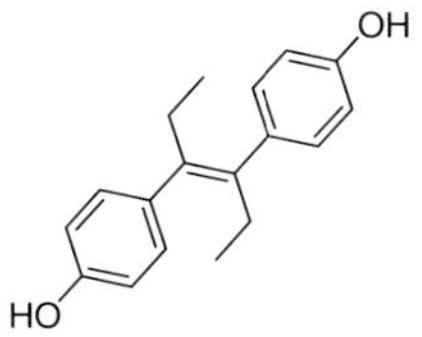

Diethylstilbestrol (DES) (**3**)

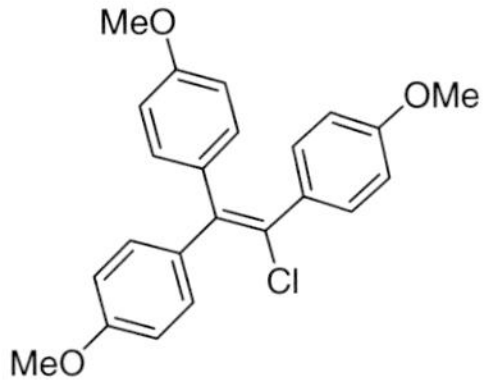

Chlorotrianisene (TACE) (**4**)

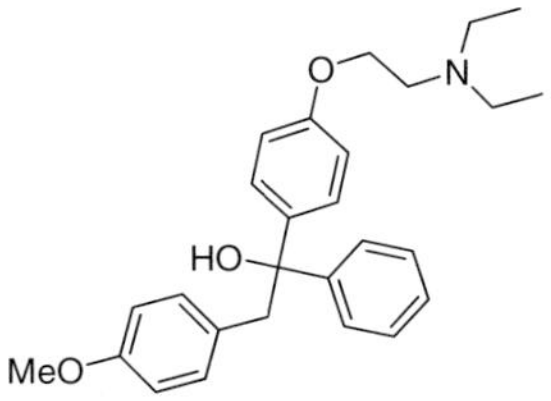

Ethamoxytriphetol (MER-25) (**5**)

Figure 7.1 One of the endogenous estrogens (**1**), a synthetic steroid analogue (**2**), and three of the early nonsteroidal analogues (**3–5**). See the text for details.

compounds that are purely estrogenic or purely antiestrogenic will only be mentioned in passing as the SERMs become further elaborated within this chapter.

7.1.2
Early ABDD Leading to a Pioneer SERM

Analogue-based drug discovery (ABDD) leading to SERM molecules can be traced back to a period well before the 1990s. For example, the work of Dodds *et al.* during the late 1930s [7, 8] established fundamental structure–activity relationships (SAR) that demonstrated that estrogenic activity could be produced by compounds lacking the steroid ring characteristic of the estrogens (e.g., **1**), those efforts culminating in diethylstilbestrol (DES, **3**) that eventually became marketed as a nonsteroidal estrogen. Chlorotrianisene (TACE, **4**) was discovered shortly thereafter and it represents the first triphenylethylene-containing synthetic estrogen to eventually reach the market in the early 1950s [4]. Alternatively, work by Lerner *et al.* during this period [9] demonstrated that the same type of scaffold could be substituted so as to produce an antiestrogenic compound, namely, ethamoxytriphetol (MER-25, **5**). Although MER-25 never became a commercially available pharmaceutical product, it underwent preliminary clinical investigation during the late 1950s and early 1960s as an estrogen antagonist [4]. Essentially devoid of estrogenic activity, an exciting property of MER-25 was its antifertility actions in laboratory animals, an observation that prompted a search for more potent agents by numerous pharmaceutical companies [1]. Subsequent research in the field of nonsteroidal antiestrogens tended to retain a focus upon the triphenylethylene nucleus, its cyclized counterparts, and their reduced versions [10]. Clomiphene (**6** in Scheme 7.2),

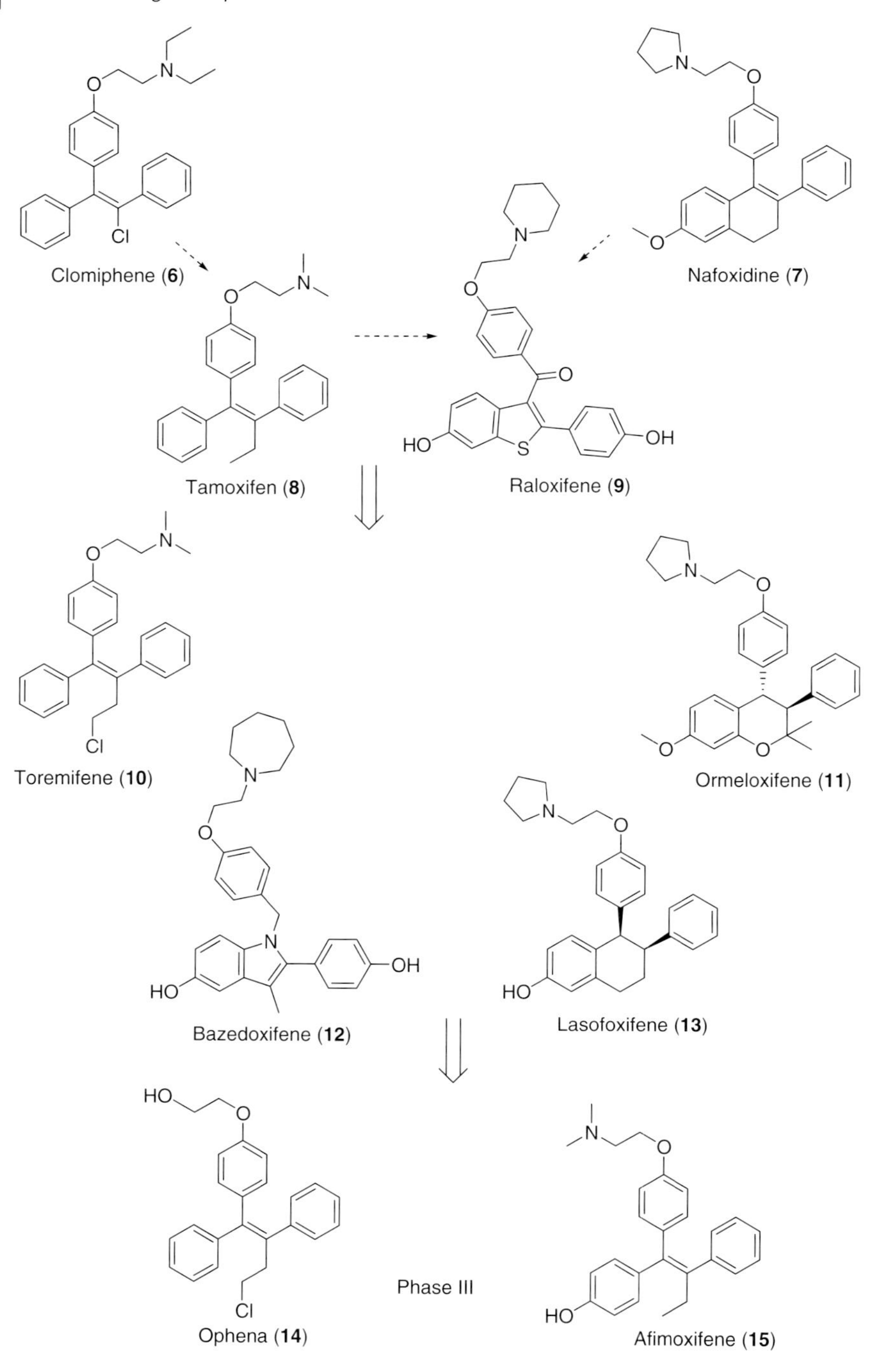

Scheme 7.2 Evolution of marketed SERMs suggested by ABDD analyses (see the text for details). Compounds **14** and **15** are progressing favorably through phase III clinical studies such that they may become marketed in the near future.

nafoxidine (7), and tamoxifen (8) were all the result of that search, but clinical application as postcoital contraceptives was found to be inappropriate [1]. Instead, because they induced ovulation in subfertile women, **6** and initially **8** were eventually approved as profertility drugs for the induction of ovulation [1]. While several compounds from the composite of drugs arising during this period might be regarded as the "pioneer SERM," our attempt to trace the lineage of these agents by tracking their initial syntheses, patents, and introductions to the marketplace moved clomiphene to the forefront. Thus, a brief description of its specific discovery and pharmacological properties follows.

7.1.3
Discovery and Development of Clomiphene

Palopoli *et al.* first synthesized **6** in the mid-1950s as its citrate salt [4], the latter still being deployed effectively in today's formulations. Coupled with preliminary biological data, a patent pertaining to this immediate family of analogues was issued in 1959 [11]. Based upon clinical studies associated with TACE and MER-25, criteria to select a lead compound from among various development stage analogues became (i) less estrogenic than TACE; (ii) more pituitary gonadotropin inhibiting activity than MER-25; (iii) some estrogen antagonizing action; and (iv) a dosage approaching that of TACE and hopefully about one-tenth of that necessary with MER-25 that was still undergoing clinical trials at that time [4]. Clomiphene was selected because it displayed the best overall profile across these criteria. Among its potential clinical indications that included oral contraception, use in certain types of estrogen-dependent tumors, and induction of ovulation, the last one was pursued at the highest priority [4]. Initial clinical results were reported in 1961 [12]: although the mechanism of action was not clear, **6** held exceptional promise of inducing ovulatory type menses with considerable regularity in anovulatory women. A New Drug Application (NDA) was filed in 1965 and within 2 years **6** was approved for marketing by prescription in the United States [4].

Clomiphene is marketed as a mixture of its *E* and *Z* stereoisomers in about a 6 : 4 ratio. Initially given the wrong designations as isomers "A" and "B" [12], this situation was corrected in 1976 by Ernst *et al.* [13] and the names "enclomiphene" and "zuclomiphene" were instead adopted [14, 15]. Enclomiphene is essentially antiestrogenic while zuclomiphene is mildly estrogenic but also capable of serving as an antiestrogen in certain settings. Importantly, zuclomiphene is about five times more potent in inducing ovulation. Metabolism is subject to considerable individual variation based, in part, on body weight [16]. As a result, dosage is sometimes required to be adjusted for body weight. In order to optimize penetration into the brain so as to occupy central and pituitary receptor sites, the total daily dose of **6** must be taken at one time. The drug is excreted primarily through the intestines, 51% being accounted for within 5 days after oral administration. However, excretion then continues for at least another 6 weeks [17]. Thus, repeated administration at 28-day intervals is cumulative with base levels increasing by nearly 50% per month [17] and **6** becomes more effective during the second and later cycles of treatment [4]. The beneficial mechanisms are thought to involve competitive antagonism of estradiol (**1**) at the level of the cytoplasmic nuclear receptor in the hypothalamic arcuate nucleus that, in turn, leads to an increase in gonadotropin releasing hormone (GnRH) [18]. In a complimentary fashion, **6** also increases the pituitary sensitivity to GnRH in a manner similar to **1** [19] such that follicle stimulating hormone and luteinizing hormone secretions are increased [20]. Finally, **6** may have a direct effect on the ovary, rendering granulose cells more sensitive to pituitary gonadotropin [4].

The introduction of **6** revolutionized the treatment of infertility in general and of polycystic ovarian syndrome (PCOS) in particular [4]. While early drawbacks included failed conception despite apparent ovulation and a supposed increase in natural abortions, additional clinical studies have been able to resolve these issues by using vaginal ultrasound to select for potentially problematic individuals. Clomiphene remains an effective drug for women suffering from anovulation and ovulating women with inadequate follicular or luteal development. Large studies have subsequently shown that **6** is effective through at least six cycles of treatment, and that there is no evidence for significant increases in spontaneous abortion, ectopic pregnancy rates, or decreases in the number of male births [4].

7.1.4 SERM-Directed ABDD: General Considerations

From this backdrop of early activities within the field of estrogen-related medicinal chemistry and our description of **6** to represent the pioneer SERM among several allied agents that additionally arose during that period, the remainder of this chapter can now specifically consider its intended subject matter, namely, *SERM-directed ABDD*. Toward this end, Table 7.1 lists several SERMs that either became marketed or are nearing market launch as a result of pursuing new agents for this class. Scheme 7.2 provides the structures for these compounds while also suggesting how they can be related to one another according to ABDD principles. Our ABDD analyses rely upon a combination of structural similarity and apparent evolution of the latter through logical advances in medicinal chemistry-derived SAR, coupled with lineage determinations derived from first-synthesized, first-patented, and first-marketed dates whenever possible. It must be emphasized, however, that unexplained gaps in the progression of a given agent at any point in the overall drug discovery and development process cannot always be identified and accounted for. Such gaps, in turn, can sometimes lead to misalignment of the associated structures within these types of ABDD schema. Alternatively and without potential shortcomings about the perfect evolutionary history of any given agent, Scheme 7.2 does provide a clear view of the overall structural landscape presently occupied by the marketed SERMs from across the globe. Two additional compounds that appear to be favorably traversing phase III clinical testing are included as well. Besides clomiphene (**6**) and nafoxidine (**7**), a quick count indicates that there are eight structures residing in this landscape. Given constraints in chapter length, just two of these agents have been chosen for a thorough description of their

Table 7.1 Marketed SERMs.

Generic name	Company	Launch	Country	Use
Clomiphene	Merrell	1961	USA	Anovulation (infertility)
Tamoxifen citrate	ICI	1977	USA	Breast cancer
Toremifene citrate	Orion	1988	EU	Breast cancer
Ormeloxifene	3M	1991	India	Contraceptive
Raloxifene	Eli Lilly	1997	USA	Osteoporosis
Fulvestrant[a]	AstraZeneca	2002	USA	Breast cancer
Bazedoxifene	Wyeth	2009	EU	Postmenopausal osteoporosis
Lasofoxifene	Pfizer	2009	EU	Osteoporosis and vaginal atrophy
Ospemifene[b]	Orion	Phase III		
Afimoxifene[b]	ASCEND	Phase III		

a) Not a SERM by strict definition, but rather a pure “antiestrogen.”
b) These compounds are progressing favorably through phase III clinical studies.

SERM-directed ABDD, namely, tamoxifen (**8**) and raloxifene (**9**). Both of these agents are taken from the first ABDD tier after clomiphene and both have interesting medicinal chemistry histories to convey. Readers interested in any of the newer agents can utilize the associated information listed within Table 7.1 as convenient starting points for further study. We likewise encourage readers to purview any of the numerous books and reviews that also cover the earlier period leading to the discovery of **6**, as well as those available for some of clomiphene’s subsequent relatives [1–6, 21–35]. Although not emphasizing ABDD themes as distinctly intended herein, many of these reports are extremely comprehensive and provide excellent discussions about the medicinal chemistry, pharmacology, and clinical data associated with specific SERMs and the field in general.

7.2 Tamoxifen

7.2.1 Early Development

Tamoxifen (Nolvadex®; ICI 46474; **8**) was discovered nearly 50 years ago by Imperial Chemical Industries (ICI; now AstraZeneca) who like many other companies at that time were pursuing the development of nonsteroidal antiestrogens as oral contraceptives [36]. Studies in laboratory animals with triphenylchloroethylene and triphenylmethylethylene against breast cancer showed that the latter had higher estrogenic activity than the chloro analogue. These results, along with the basic amine found on clomiphene (**6**; discussed above), led to the synthesis of **16** (Figure 7.2a) that later was found to possess antifertility effects in mice at a lower dose than needed for estrogenic activity. This led to the further design of a series of related structures to be developed as nonsteroidal

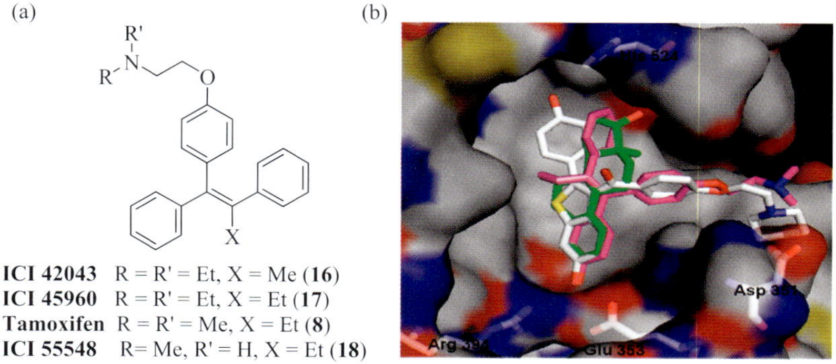

(a)

ICI 42043 R = R' = Et, X = Me (**16**)
ICI 45960 R = R' = Et, X = Et (**17**)
Tamoxifen R = R' = Me, X = Et (**8**)
ICI 55548 R= Me, R' = H, X = Et (**18**)

(b)

Figure 7.2 (a) Tamoxifen and its immediate family of analogues. (b) ERα active site surface depiction with estradiol (**1**), 4-hydroxytamoxifen (**15**), and raloxifene (**9**). Nitrogens and oxygens are shown in red and blue, respectively, the carbon atoms of protein and **9** are in silver, while carbon atoms for **1** and **15** are in green and purple, respectively. Raloxifene bound ERα structural data [45] were used for receptor surface generation. ERα bound conformations of **1** [45], **15** [46], and **9** were used for superimposition. Several amino acid residues covering the top of the ligand surface were removed to provide for better visualization of the receptor binding pocket. Likewise, not shown in the case of **1** is the helix 12 that moves across the northeast quadrant of the pocket.

contraceptives. Figure 7.2a shows some of the key representatives from this series [36]. Eventually, it was found that only the "*Z*" rather than "*E*" isomers possessed antiestrogenic activity [37, 38]. For example, after the initial synthesis of **8** (first reported in 1962 [37]), the structures of its two isomers were resolved by X-ray crystallography in 1970 so as to make the proper connection with biological activity [39]. Numerous secondary amines such as **18**, "desoxy" analogues where the ether oxygen is removed, and the saturated alkane derivatives were prepared as part of the overall series. None of these derivatives offered any benefit over **8** [36]. During this period, structural modifications to the triphenylethylene derivative chlorotrianisene (**4**), a nonsteroidal estrogen, had led to the discovery of compounds with antiestrogenic activity such as MER-25 (**5**) [9] and clomiphene (**6**), a gonadotropin inhibitor [40]. Moreover, the understanding that hormone-dependent breast cancer could be intervened by oophorectomy [41], adrenalectomy [42], or hormonal treatment led to a quest for drugs that antagonize the actions of estrogen with minimal side effects [43, 44]. This led to testing of tamoxifen against hormone-dependent breast cancer. Based on the latter's success, the US Food and Drug Administration (FDA) approved the use of tamoxifen for treatment of breast cancer in 1977 [43].

7.2.2
Clinical Indications and Molecular Action

Tamoxifen has been used clinically against breast cancer for almost four decades and is regarded as a standard therapy. It is currently used (i) to treat

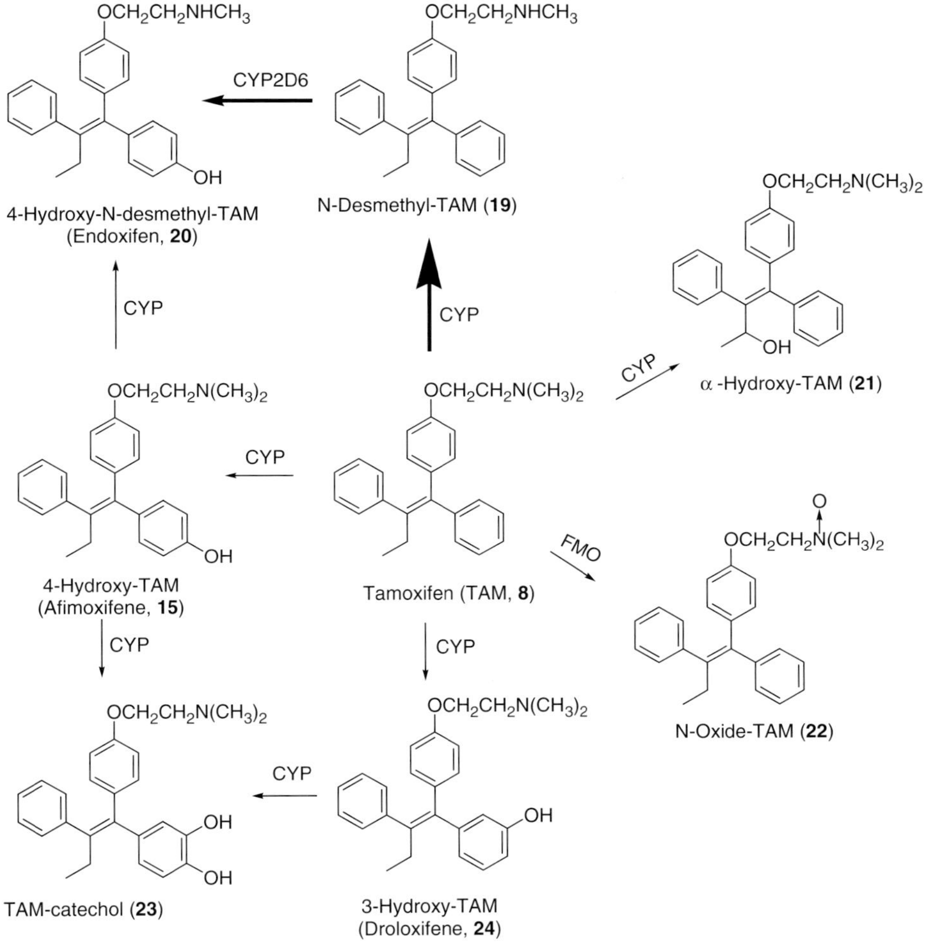

Scheme 7.3 Key metabolic pathways of tamoxifen.

metastatic breast cancer; (ii) as an adjuvant for treating node-positive and node-negative breast cancer; (iii) to lower the risk of invasive breast cancer; and (iv) as a preventative agent to decrease breast cancer occurrence in high-risk women [47]. Tamoxifen is an antiestrogenic prodrug. Scheme 7.3 shows the key metabolic pathways for **8**. The active metabolites, 4-hydroxytamoxifen (4-OHT; **15**) and 4-hydroxy-*N*-desmethyltamoxifen (endoxifen; **20**) bind with estrogen receptors and block ER-mediated transcriptional activation in breast tissues. Figure 7.2b depicts comparative binding orientations for **1**, **15**, and **9** within the ERα binding pocket. 4-OHT has key interactions with Arg394 and Glu353 through its phenolic hydroxyl group. The basic side chain on **15** extends out of the active site cavity and establishes weak ionic interactions with Asp351 [31]. This could distort the receptor conformation in a manner similar to other partial ER antagonists [45] such that the helix 12 cannot move to a position that is suitable for coactivator binding with the ER–ligand complex. Although structural data are unavailable at this point in time, it is believed that **15** interacts with ERβ in a similar fashion. Until recent reports [48, 49], **15** was considered to be the main metabolite that competitively blocked ERs. However, owing to its higher plasma concentration and equipotency to **15**, endoxifen is now believed to be the key active metabolite. This is further supported by the observation that the efficacy of **8** shows a dependency upon the CYP2D6 enzyme, which is thought to mediate the biotransformation depicted in Scheme 7.3. It is likely that endoxifen binds with ERα in a manner that is similar to what is depicted in Figure 7.2 for **15**. Finally, preliminary data suggest that **8** may enhance the degradation of the ERα receptor, rather than simply serving as a competitive receptor antagonist in breast cancer cells [50, 51]. This is based upon Western blot analyses, which indicate that **20**'s action in breast tissues appears to be different from that of **15** because it causes degradation of the ERα [51].

7.2.3
Pharmacokinetics and Major Metabolic Pathways

Tamoxifen is administered orally as its citrate salt. Steady-state plasma concentrations for **8** and its major metabolite *N*-desmethyltamoxifen (**19**) are achieved in about 4 and 8 weeks, respectively. Tamoxifen is extensively metabolized by microsomal enzymes into several active metabolites that are primarily eliminated via the intestinal route as polar conjugates. The terminal half-lives of **8** and **19** are 5–7 and 9–14 days, respectively [52].

Several studies show that the cytochrome P450 (CYP) system is primarily responsible for the biotransformation of **8** into various oxidation metabolites (Scheme 7.3) [53–55]. In addition, hepatic flavin-containing monooxygenase (FMO) converts **8** into its *N*-oxide metabolite (**22**) that can be reduced back to **8**. Thus, **22** could act as a reservoir for the drug in various body tissues [56, 57].

Tamoxifen undergoes extensive biotransformation after oral administration, mainly into **19** as the major primary metabolite with retention of similar low potency. 4-Hydroxytamoxifen (**15**) and α-hydroxytamoxifen (**21**) are the other primary metabolites. Alternatively, **20** is the major secondary active metabolite [53]. Although both **20** and **15** show similarly high potency compared to the parent drug, **20** is more abundant than **15** in the plasma. The significant increase in 8's activity after first-pass metabolism is the reason why it is classified as a prodrug. In this regard, **20** is now considered to be primarily responsible for the clinical efficacy of **8** [48] even though several reports previously attributed **8**'s activity to **15** [1]. Endoxifen (**20**) is mainly formed via oxidative biotransformation of **19** by CYP2D6 (Scheme 7.3). Consequently, the widespread interpatient variation in the clinical effectiveness and side effects of **8** can now be attributed to interindividual variation in CYP2D6 activity due to genetic polymorphism in the CYP2D6 genotype [48, 49, 53, 58].

7.2.4
Clinical Toxicity and New Tamoxifen Analogues

A major side effect of **8** is that it can increase endometrial cancer in women during adjuvant therapy [59]. Other serious toxicity includes pulmonary embolism and stroke [52]. Some reports have implicated **8**'s propensity toward carcinogenicity to result from the ability of its metabolites, such as α-hydroxytamoxifen (**21**) and the *N*-desmethyl derivatives, to form DNA adducts within normal cells [31, 60].

Several derivatives of **8** have been evaluated to potentially provide drugs that are less toxic and more efficacious. Other than toremifene, many have been discontinued because they were found to be either less efficacious than tamoxifen or still have serious side effects [31, 47]. For instance, both 3-hydroxytamoxifen (**24**) and idoxifene (metabolically stable since it has an iodo substitution at the 4 position) [31] were found to increase the incidence of uterine prolapses [61] and had no significant improvement in therapeutic efficacy; thus, their development was terminated [47]. Toremifene (Fareston or chlorotamoxifen, **10**) as the citrate salt is currently used in the clinic against estrogen receptor positive or unknown ER status metastatic breast cancer. Comparative clinical analyses with **8** showed that both drugs exhibit similar efficacy and side effect profiles [31, 47]. Alternatively, **10** shows a better lipid profile and lower carcinogenicity in rats than **8**. It has been suggested that the presence of the chloro group sterically hinders α-hydroxylation and thus forms less DNA adducts in comparison to **8** [62]. Afimoxifene (**15**) is being developed as a transdermal gel formulation to treat cyclical mastalgia, and as a SERM by ASCEND Pharmaceuticals [63]. Finally, ospemifene (Ophena™, **14**) is under investigation as a SERM to treat postmenopausal vulvovaginal atrophy [64]. It is being developed by QuatRx Pharmaceuticals.

7.3
Raloxifene

Raloxifene hydrochloride (Evista®) is a distinct SERM molecule first developed by Eli Lilly in the early 1980s [65]. Raloxifene (**9**, Scheme 7.2) was the first SERM for the prevention and the treatment of osteoporosis and has since been approved for the prevention of breast cancer in postmenopausal women [66]. This drug is of great interest in that it acts as an antagonist at ERα in the breast and uterus and works as an agonist at ERβ in the bone [67]. These effects are accompanied by fewer side effects and different potencies than tamoxifen [68–70]. Raloxifene is still being studied extensively for additional uses and it continues to be used as a scaffold for new SERM development.

This section will first describe the motivation for the design and development of **9**. Information on different raloxifene trials including their relevance and the key results will be covered next. It will conclude by outlining the strengths and weaknesses of **9** while assessing its potential as a scaffold for future SERM development.

7.3.1
Need for New Antiestrogens

As mentioned in the prior section, the early 1980s saw a heightened search for new multifunctional antiestrogens. These agents were designed to be nonsteroidal and have greater antagonism accompanied by lower intrinsic estrogenicity than previous drug molecules. At that time, **8** had already been developed and information on its side effects and drug resistance was increasing. It was also known that **8** existed in two different isomers, namely, the *E* and *Z* forms as described in the previous section. The *Z* metabolite isomer is the active form, yet when administered, a mixture of *E* and *Z* metabolites is formed making dosing difficult. Overall, it was hoped that new SERM molecules could be developed that would be equally or more effective against breast cancer, while existing as only one isomeric form and having fewer side effects [65].

7.3.2
Design and Initial Biological Data on Raloxifene

When designing **9**, Eli Lilly wanted an antiestrogen having a structure similar to **8**, but with less potential for isomerization. To do this they made an ABDD series with added rigidity, which according to previous research could be accomplished by using a variety of different atoms to form a heterocycle on the scaffold backbone [65]. In the end, they selected a benzothiophene scaffold, which had shown to give antiestrogenic effects in past research [71]. Other research had also shown for **8** that retention of the basic side chain (amine-containing side chain) contributed to the antiestrogenic effects of the drug, so Eli Lilly's overall structural motif retained the basic side chain portion of the molecule, yet the groups attached to the amine were varied [65]. There was also precedent to attach the side chain by adding a ketone linker to the phenyl ether as found in **8** [72].

Synthesis was conducted to form a series of benzothiophene analogues and biological data were obtained for all of the analogues. These studies looked for estrogenic and nonestrogenic properties of the compounds using an immature rat uterotrophic assay and the results were compared to that of a control, estradiol (**1**, Figure 7.1), as well as to that of **8**. One of the analogues, LY139481, showed impressive biological properties. It had an uterotrophic effect at a low dose that did not increase with concentration. It was also able to inhibit the effects of **1** at similar and higher concentrations [65].

With the exciting results pointing to LY139481 as an antiestrogen lead compound, the need for an improved synthesis at the multigram level was investigated. This route needed to be more efficient and provide better yields than what had been deployed during the front-line screening. This goal was accomplished by Eli Lilly soon after the original synthesis and was done using a one-pot synthesis that increased the yield to 75%. The new route allowed for multigram syntheses of the lead [65].

With a process-scale synthesis available, further tests were conducted on the hydrochloride form of the analogue of interest to determine its efficacy in uterotrophic and antitumor assays. The hydrochloride salt was referred to as analogue LY156758 and later became known as "keoxifene." Studies were continued on cell cultures and followed with animal studies using immature rats [73] as well as rats having *N*-nitrosomethylurea-induced mammary carcinoma [74]. In these trials, it was determined that keoxifene was not as effective as **8** in the uterotrophic and antitumor models and due to these biological results, further studies on the analogue were almost abandoned [75, 76]. In the late 1980s, it was determined that antiestrogens have estrogenic effects in the bone and new trials began on keoxifene, yet this time it was referred to as raloxifene (**9**) [76]. Raloxifene was studied for its use in the treatment and prevention of osteoporosis where it was then determined that it was able to increase spinal bone density in postmenopausal women. Following these studies, Eli Lilly submitted to the FDA for raloxifene's approval for the prevention and treatment of osteoporosis in postmenopausal women. In 1997, Evista® was approved by the FDA for the prevention of osteoporosis in postmenopausal women. In 1999, Evista® was then approved for the treatment of osteoporosis in postmenopausal women with osteoporosis [77]. Following the new excitement of Evista®'s use for osteoporosis, further studies followed to determine **9**'s potential in combating other diseases, especially for treatment and prevention of breast cancer and cardiovascular diseases.

7.3.3 RUTH Study

The "Raloxifene's Use for The Heart" (RUTH) trial began in 1998; this trial was a double-blind, international study. The trial's objectives were to determine the effects of **9** on coronary events as well invasive breast cancer in postmenopausal women. Over 10 000 women participated and each was given either a 60 mg tablet of Evista® or a placebo every day for a period of 1 year. The results of this study showed that **9** had no effect on coronary heart disease or any other coronary effect, in that these parameters did not increase or decrease from the amount found in the placebo. It was found that **9** did significantly reduce the amount of breast cancer and spinal fractures in comparison to placebo [69]. These data were evaluated initially by two groups referred to as "Heart Estrogen/Progesterone Replacement Study" (HERS) and "The Women's Health Initiative" (WHI). A secondary evaluation was then performed by "Multiple Outcomes of Raloxifene Evaluation" (MORE). All studies ended with the same conclusions that **9** showed benefits as a potential breast cancer treatment [3].

7.3.4 STAR Study

The "Study of Tamoxifen and Raloxifene" (STAR) was a double-blind phase III clinical trial sponsored by the National Cancer Institute in 1999. The trial was conducted to compare the effectiveness of **9** in comparison to **8** in the prevention of invasive breast cancer in postmenopausal women. This study was one of the largest cancer prevention clinical trials, enrolling close to 20 000 postmenopausal women that were at high risk for breast cancer. All participants were given either 60 mg of **9** or 20 mg of **8** daily over a period of 5 years.

Results of this study proved that both **9** and **8** were effective in the prevention of breast cancer in postmenopausal women with 50% effectiveness for **8** and 35% for **9**. Raloxifene had a lower instance of thromboembolic events, cataracts, and a lower instance of gynecological, bladder, and vasomotor problems as well as less leg cramping. Tamoxifen had a lower incident of musculoskeletal problems, dyspareunia, and weight gain. There was no notable change in physical or mental health for **8** or **9**, and both had the same instance of fractures, other cancers, heart disease, and stroke. At the end of this study, it was determined that **9** was as effective as **8** in the prevention of invasive breast cancer in postmenopausal women with fewer major side effects. Following a variety of additional trials that studied the effectiveness of **9** as a preventative medication for breast cancer, applications for this new use were submitted [68, 70]. On September 14, 2007 the FDA announced that they had determined that the benefits of **9** outweighed the risks and then approved **9** for the prevention of breast cancer in postmenopausal women that are at high risk for invasive forms of the disease. This was only the second drug allowed by the FDA for this use at the time [77].

7.3.5 Binding to the Estrogen Receptor

With expansion of the clinical studies being conducted on raloxifene, data about its mechanism of action and efficacy grew in importance. The belief is that the mechanism of action for estrogens was due to binding of **1** at ERα and ERβ causing dissociation from heat shock proteins followed by dimerization and recruitment of coactivators, resulting in transcription complex [76]. For SERMs, the same overall mechanism of action would be true, yet they are believed to cause coactivator recruitment in some tissue and corepressor recruitment in others [78] (Scheme 7.1).

To further justify the mechanism of action while equating binding interactions at ERs to the necessity of the specific structural features (given in the design portion of this section), comparisons of binding motifs were done for **9**, **1**, and **15** (a metabolite of **8** discussed in Section 7.1) within the ERα pocket. These comparisons are shown in Figure 7.2b. Binding for **1**, **15**, and **9** occurs through hydrogen bonding at amino acids Arg394 and Glu353. Further hydrogen bonding can be formed in the case of **1** and **9** with His524 residue. The antiestrogenic effects found in **9** and **8** are attributed to the amine side chain that has an ionic interaction with Asp351 [79]. The interaction with aspartic acid prevents helix 12 from reorienting like it does when **1** binds, and this, in turn, leads to a conformation that does not allow coactivator recruitment. In the case of **9**, there is also an ionic interaction in ERβ between the amine and Asp303 giving it a similar type of effect as seen in ERα [31, 45, 75].

7.3.6 ADME

The absorption, distribution, metabolism, and excretion of **9** are other important factors to consider when determining other uses for the drug, as well as when designing new drug analogues. Raloxifene is administered as a 60 mg tablet taken daily [69]. After oral administration, **9** is absorbed through the gastrointestinal tract and distributed throughout the body [80]. It is metabolized rapidly through first-pass phase II metabolism in the intestine, forming primarily glucuronide conjugates [81]. The drug has a very low bioavailability of 2%, yet the half-life is 27.7 h after a single dose and is 32.5 h following multiple doses [80, 82]. Elimination proceeds through the liver with more than 90% of the metabolites found in the feces [80].

7.3.7 Further Research

Raloxifene continues to serve as one of the SERM classical prototypes. While it was the first SERM for the treatment of osteoporosis, it was also found to have further antiestrogenic effects that are useful in breast cancer prevention in postmenopausal women. Raloxifene has a unique potency that is effective at low concentrations and its efficacy is not concentration dependent. Raloxifene is also of importance in that its use is still common today, making it an excellent prototype to help lead new SERM ABDD.

New developments in the area of **9** itself are also needed in that the drug is not devoid of its own problems. With the known side effects of the drug, a success rate lower than that of **8** in the breast, and its very low bioavailability, **9** has specific areas that need significant improvement. For example, the next tier of ABDD-derived SERMs, as depicted by the four compounds **10–13** in Scheme 7.2, exhibit differences in their overall profiles and offer some clinical improvements. Uterine data for bazedoxifene suggest that it is a more selective SERM than raloxifene such that it may not stimulate the uterus and breast [83] during postmenopausal, hormone replacement therapy (HRT) [84]. Nevertheless, raloxifene is a SERM of significant importance because it remains successful as a therapeutic agent for osteoporosis and has fewer side effects than most other marketed SERMs.

7.4 Summary

Research and clinical development of nonsteroidal ER ligands over the past 60 years has gradually evolved from estrogenic compounds intended as hormone replacement therapies to antiestrogenic compounds initially intended for birth control and later as treatments for hormone-dependent cancers, and finally to the SERMs from which their differing selective actions can be redirected toward the above uses as well as toward a variety of other clinical indications, all with less concomitant general ER-related side effects. Exemplifying the latter, clomiphene remains effective for the induction of ovulation in subfertile women, tamoxifen for the treatment and prevention of postmenopausal ER-positive breast cancer, and raloxifene for the treatment and prevention of postmenopausal osteoporosis while affording greater breast and uterine safety. Several newer agents expand the potential uses even further. Among the longer standing clinically available SERMs that can be considered for hormone replacement therapy, two major limitations have arisen, namely, that they are only weak estrogen agonists and they (can) aggravate hot flashes [3]. The latter represent a particularly confounding situation in that they are also one of the frequent symptoms for the prescription of HRT.

Marked by the discovery of ERβ as a second estrogenic system, the gradually increasing knowledge about the complexity of the ER pathways contributed significantly to the evolution of the SERMs across this period, as well as to our today's understanding about how SERMs work. Nevertheless, there still remains no unifying theory that has explained the target site-specific actions of SERMs [1]. Likewise, advances in estrogen-related medicinal chemistry and its SAR have served to drive the evolution of the SERMs to its present structural landscape. However and in sharp contrast to the variety of biological profiles that have been achieved to date, structural motifs proceeding to the marketplace have yet to depart significantly from the original triphenylethylene scaffold arrangement and the latter's cyclized possibilities with or without reduction and the use of heteroatoms. While ABDD, in turn, can certainly be ascribed to contributing toward the present lack of structural diversity, its "plus" side in this same regard has resulted in the variety of biological profiles and distinct clinical indications that have been able to be delivered to the marketplace. Furthermore, the status of SAR and X-ray-derived ER structural details have now evolved to the point where together they can allow ABDD to also adopt scaffold hopping explorations in a rational manner. Thus, novel structural types should soon be on the horizon for the SERMs.

As the clinical performances of the latest agents become elaborated and the nuances of the ER pathways continue to unfold in parallel with our expanding knowledge about their associated medicinal chemistry, pursuit of new SERMs by ABDD geared toward producing novel chemical structures should pave the way toward the development of "ideal" SERMs for clinical practice [2]. These "next-generation" SERMs will be distinctly tailored for their specific indications. Ultimately providing dramatic new paradigms for maintaining the health of women [2], indications will continue to include induction of ovulation, reduction of menopausal symptoms, and bone preservation. Toward improving the health of both men and women, indications will include cholesterol reduction and chemotherapy of hormone-related cancers.

References

1 Jordan, V.C. (2003) Antiestrogens and selective estrogen receptor modulators as multifunctional medicines. 1. Receptor interactions. *J. Med. Chem.*, **46**, 883–908.

2 Osborne, C.K., Zhao, H., and Fuqua, S.A. (2000) Selective estrogen receptor modulators: structure, function, and clinical use. *J. Clin. Oncol.*, **18**, 3172–3186.
3 Riggs, B.L. and Hartmann, L.C. (2003) Selective estrogen-receptor modulators – mechanisms of action and application to clinical practice. *N. Engl. J. Med.*, **348**, 618–629.
4 Dickey, R.P. and Holtkamp, D.E. (1996) Development, pharmacology and clinical experience with clomiphene citrate. *Hum. Reprod. Update*, **2**, 483–506.
5 Clarke, B.L. and Khosla, S. (2009) New selective estrogen and androgen receptor modulators. *Curr. Opin. Rheumatol.*, **21**, 374–379.
6 Minutolo, F., Macchia, M., Katzenellenbogen, B.S., and Katzenellenbogen, J.A. (2011) Estrogen receptor beta ligands: recent advances and biomedical applications. *Med. Res. Rev.*, **31**, 364–442.
7 Dodds, E.C., Goldberg, L., Lawson, W., and Robinson, R. (1938) Estrogenic activity of alkylated stilboestrols. *Nature*, **142**, 34.
8 Dodds, E.C. and Lawson, W. (1938) Molecular structure in relation to estrogenic activity: compounds without a phenanthrene nucleus. *Proc. R. Soc. Lond. Ser. B*, **125**, 222–232.
9 Lerner, L.J., Holthaus, F.J., Jr., and Thompson, C.R. (1958) A non-steroidal estrogen antiagonist 1-(*p*-2-diethylaminoethoxyphenyl)-1-phenyl-2-*p*-methoxyphenyl ethanol. *Endocrinology*, **63**, 295–318.
10 Jones, C.D., Jevnikar, M.G., Pike, A.J., Peters, M.K. *et al.* (1984) Antiestrogens. 2. Structure–activity studies in a series of 3-aroyl-2-arylbenzo[*b*]thiophene derivatives leading to [6-hydroxy-2-(4-hydroxyphenyl) benzo[*b*]thien-3-yl]-[4-[2-(1-piperidinyl) ethoxy]-phenyl]methanone hydrochloride (LY156758), a remarkably effective estrogen antagonist with only minimal intrinsic estrogenicity. *J. Med. Chem.*, **27**, 1057–1066.
11 Allen, R.E., Palopoli, F.P., Schumann, E.L., and Van Campen, M.G., Jr. (1959) Amine Derivatives of Triphenylethanol US Patent 2,914,562 (to the Wm. S. Merrell Co.).
12 Palopoli, F.P., Feil, V.J., Allen, R.E., Holtkamp, D.E., and Richardson, A., Jr., (1967) Substituted aminoalkoxytriarylhaloethylenes. *J. Med. Chem.*, **10**, 84–86.
13 Ernst, S., Hite, G., Cantrell, J.S., Richardson, A., Jr., and Benson, H.D. (1976) Stereochemistry of geometric isomers of clomiphene: a correction of the literature and a reexamination of structure–activity relationships. *J. Pharm. Sci.*, **65**, 148–150.
14 Clark, J.H. and Guthrie, S.C. (1981) Agonistic and antagonistic effects of clomiphene citrate and its isomers. *Biol. Reprod.*, **25**, 667–672.
15 Jordan, V.C., Haldemann, B., and Allen, K.E. (1981) Geometric isomers of substituted triphenylethylenes and antiestrogen action. *Endocrinology*, **108**, 1353–1361.
16 Shepard, M.K., Balmaceda, J.P., and Leija, C.G. (1979) Relationship of weight to successful induction of ovulation with clomiphene citrate. *Fertil. Steril.*, **32**, 641–645.
17 Mikkelson, T.J., Kroboth, P.D., Cameron, W.J., Dittert, L.W. *et al.* (1986) Single-dose pharmacokinetics of clomiphene citrate in normal volunteers. *Fertil. Steril.*, **46**, 392–396.
18 Clark, J.H. and Markaverich, B.M. (1988) *The Physiology of Reproduction* (eds E. Knobil and J. Neill), Raven Press, New York, pp. 675–723.
19 Hsueh, A.J., Erickson, G.F., and Yen, S.S. (1978) Sensitisation of pituitary cells to luteinising hormone releasing hormone by clomiphene citrate *in vitro*. *Nature*, **273**, 57–59.
20 Dickey, R.P., Vorys, N., Stevens, V.C., Besch, P.K. *et al.* (1965) Observations on the mechanism of action of clomiphene (MRL-41). *Fertil. Steril.*, **16**, 485–494.
21 Bryant, H.U. (2002) Selective estrogen receptor modulators. *Rev. Endocr. Metab. Disord.*, **3**, 231–241.
22 Fang, H., Tong, W., Shi, L.M., Blair, R. *et al.* (2001) Structure–activity relationships for a large diverse set of natural, synthetic, and environmental estrogens. *Chem. Res. Toxicol.*, **14**, 280–294.

23 Jordan, V.C. (1994) *Long-Term Tamoxifen Treatment for Breast Cancer* (ed. V.C. Jordan), University of Wisconsin Press, Madison, WI, pp. 3–26.
24 Kuiper, G.G., Lemmen, J.G., Carlsson, B., Corton, J.C. *et al.* (1998) Interaction of estrogenic chemicals and phytoestrogens with estrogen receptor beta. *Endocrinology*, **139**, 4252–4263.
25 Pettersson, K. and Gustafsson, J.A. (2001) Role of estrogen receptor beta in estrogen action. *Annu. Rev. Physiol.*, **63**, 165–192.
26 Sutherland, R.L. and Jordan, V.C. (eds) (1981) *Non-Steroidal Antiestrogens: Molecular Pharmacology and Antitumor Activity*, Academic Press, Sydney, Australia.
27 Zhao, C., Dahlman-Wright, K., and Gustafsson, J.A. (2008) Estrogen receptor beta: an overview and update. *Nucl. Recept. Signal.*, **6**, e003.
28 Agatonovic-Kustrin, S. and Turner, J.V. (2008) Molecular structural characteristics of estrogen receptor modulators as determinants of estrogen receptor selectivity. *Mini-Rev. Med. Chem.*, **8**, 943–951.
29 Blizzard, T.A. (2008) Selective estrogen receptor modulator medicinal chemistry at Merck. A review. *Curr. Top. Med. Chem. (Sharjah, United Arab Emirates)*, **8**, 792–812.
30 Henke, B.R. and Heyer, D. (2005) Recent advances in estrogen receptor modulators. *Curr. Opin. Drug Discov. Dev.*, **8**, 437–448.
31 Jordan, V.C. (2003) Antiestrogens and selective estrogen receptor modulators as multifunctional medicines. 2. Clinical considerations and new agents. *J. Med. Chem.*, **46**, 1081–1111.
32 Meegan, M.J. and Lloyd, D.G. (2003) Advances in the science of estrogen receptor modulation. *Curr. Med. Chem.*, **10**, 181–210.
33 Redden, P.R. (2004) Selective estrogen receptor modulators, pure antiestrogens and related estrogen receptor ligands. *Expert Opin. Ther. Pat.*, **14**, 337–353.
34 Ullrich, J.W. and Miller, C.P. (2006) Estrogen receptor modulator review. *Expert Opin. Ther. Pat.*, **16**, 559–572.
35 Veeneman, G.H. (2005) Non-steroidal subtype selective estrogens. *Curr. Med. Chem.*, **12**, 1077–1136.
36 Richardson, D.N. (1988) The history of Nolvadex. *Drug Des. Deliv.*, **3**, 1–14.
37 Bedford, G.R. and Richardson, D.N. (1966) Preparation and identification of *cis* and *trans* isomers of a substituted triarylethylene. *Nature (London)*, **212**, 733–734.
38 Harper, M.J.K. and Walpole, A.L. (1966) Contrasting endocrine activities of *cis* and *trans* isomers in a series of substituted triphenylethylenes. *Nature*, **212**, 87.
39 Kilbourn, B.T. and Owston, P.G. (1970) Crystal structure of the hydrobromide of 1-[*p*-[2-(dimethylamino)ethoxy]phenyl]-1,2-*cis*-diphenyl-1-butene, a compound with estrogenic activity. *J. Chem. Soc. B*, **1**, 1–5.
40 Holtkamp, D.E., Greslin, J.G., Root, C.A., and Lerner, L.J. (1960) Gonadotrophin inhibiting and anti-fecundity effects of chloramiphene. *Proc. Soc. Exp. Biol. Med.*, **105**, 197–201.
41 Beatson, G.T. (1896) On the treatment of inoperable cases of carcinoma of the mamma: suggestions for a new method of treatment, with illustrative cases. *Lancet*, **2**, 104–107.
42 Huggins, C.B. and Bergenstal, D.M. (1952) Inhibition of human mammary and prostatic cancers by adrenalectomy. *Cancer Res.*, **12**, 134–141.
43 Furr, B.J., Patterson, J.S., Richardson, D.N., Slater, S.R., and Wakeling, A.E. (1979) Tamoxifen. *Pharmacol. Biochem. Prop. Drug Subst.*, **2**, 355–399.
44 Lunan, C.B. and Klopper, A. (1975) Antioestrogens. A review. *Clin. Endocrinol.*, **4**, 551–572.
45 Brzozowski, A.M., Pike, A.C., Dauter, Z., Hubbard, R.E. *et al.* (1997) Molecular basis of agonism and antagonism in the oestrogen receptor. *Nature*, **389**, 753–758.
46 Shiau, A.K., Barstad, D., Loria, P.M., Cheng, L. *et al.* (1998) The structural basis of estrogen receptor/coactivator recognition and the antagonism of this interaction by tamoxifen. *Cell*, **95**, 927–937.
47 Pickar, J.H., MacNeil, T., and Ohleth, K. (2010) SERMs: progress and future perspectives. *Maturitas*, **67**, 129–138.
48 Ahmad, A., Shahabuddin, S., Sheikh, S., Kale, P. *et al.* (2010) Endoxifen, a new cornerstone of breast cancer therapy: demonstration of safety, tolerability, and systemic bioavailability in healthy human

subjects. *Clin. Pharmacol. Ther.*, **88**, 814–817.

49 Beverage, J.N., Sissung, T.M., Sion, A.M., Danesi, R., and Figg, W.D. (2007) CYP2D6 polymorphisms and the impact on tamoxifen therapy. *J. Pharm. Sci.*, **96**, 2224–2231.

50 Lim, Y.C., Desta, Z., Flockhart, D.A., and Skaar, T.C. (2005) Endoxifen (4-hydroxy-*N*-desmethyl-tamoxifen) has anti-estrogenic effects in breast cancer cells with potency similar to 4-hydroxy-tamoxifen. *Cancer Chemother. Pharmacol.*, **55**, 471–478.

51 Wu, X., Hawse, J.R., Subramaniam, M., Goetz, M.P. *et al.* (2009) The tamoxifen metabolite, endoxifen, is a potent antiestrogen that targets estrogen receptor alpha for degradation in breast cancer cells. *Cancer Res.*, **69**, 1722–1727.

52 Adam, H.K., Patterson, J.S., and Kemp, J.V. (1980) Studies on the metabolism and pharmacokinetics of tamoxifen in normal volunteers. *Cancer Treat. Rep.*, **64**, 761–764.

53 Desta, Z., Ward, B.A., Soukhova, N.V., and Flockhart, D.A. (2004) Comprehensive evaluation of tamoxifen sequential biotransformation by the human cytochrome P450 system *in vitro*: prominent roles for CYP3A and CYP2D6. *J. Pharmacol. Exp. Ther.*, **310**, 1062–1075.

54 Stearns, V., Johnson, M.D., Rae, J.M., Morocho, A. *et al.* (2003) Active tamoxifen metabolite plasma concentrations after coadministration of tamoxifen and the selective serotonin reuptake inhibitor paroxetine. *J. Natl. Cancer Inst.*, **95**, 1758–1764.

55 White, I.N. (2003) Tamoxifen: is it safe? Comparison of activation and detoxication mechanisms in rodents and in humans. *Curr. Drug Metab.*, **4**, 223–239.

56 Kellen, J.A. (ed.) (1996) *Tamoxifen: Beyond the Antiestrogen*, Birkhaeuser, Boston, MA.

57 Mani, C., Hodgson, E., and Kupfer, D. (1993) Metabolism of the antimammary cancer antiestrogenic agent tamoxifen. II. Flavin-containing monooxygenase-mediated N-oxidation. *Drug Metab. Dispos.*, **21**, 657–661.

58 Jordan, V.C. (1982) Metabolites of tamoxifen in animals and man: identification, pharmacology, and significance. *Breast Cancer Res. Treat.*, **2**, 123–138.

59 Fornander, T., Rutqvist, L.E., Cedermark, B., Glas, U. *et al.* (1989) Adjuvant tamoxifen in early breast cancer: occurrence of new primary cancers. *Lancet*, **1**, 117–120.

60 Han, X.L. and Liehr, J.G. (1992) Induction of covalent DNA adducts in rodents by tamoxifen. *Cancer Res.*, **52**, 1360–1363.

61 Nilsson, S., Koehler, K.F., and Gustafsson, J.A. (2011) Development of subtype-selective oestrogen receptor-based therapeutics. *Nat. Rev. Drug Discov.*, **10**, 778–792.

62 Hard, G.C., Iatropoulos, M.J., Jordan, K., Radi, L. *et al.* (1993) Major difference in the hepatocarcinogenicity and DNA adduct forming ability between toremifene and tamoxifen in female Crl: CD(BR) rats. *Cancer Res.*, **53**, 4534–4541.

63 Mansel, R., Goyal, A., Nestour, E.L., Masini-Eteve, V., and O'Connell, K. (2007) A phase II trial of Afimoxifene (4-hydroxytamoxifen gel) for cyclical mastalgia in premenopausal women. *Breast Cancer Res. Treat.*, **106**, 389–397.

64 Gennari, L., Merlotti, D., Valleggi, F., and Nuti, R. (2009) Ospemifene use in postmenopausal women. *Expert Opin. Invest. Drugs*, **18**, 839–849.

65 Jones, C.D., Jevnikar, M.G., Pike, A.J., Peters, M.K., Black, L.J., Thompson, A.R., Falcone, J.F., and Clemens, J.A. (1984) Antiestrogens. 2. Structure–activity studies in a series of 3-aroyl-2-arylbenzo[*b*] thiophene derivatives leading to [6-hydroxy-2-(4-hydroxyphenyl)benzo[*b*] thien-3-yl][4-[2-(1-piperidiny1)ethoxyl] phenyl]methanone hydrochloride (LY 156758), a remarkably effective estrogen antagonist with only minimal intrinsic estrogenicity. *J. Med. Chem.*, **27**, 1057–1066.

66 Shang, Y. (2006) Molecular mechanisms of oestrogen and SERMs in endometrial carcinogenesis. *Nature*, **6**, 360–368.

67 Jordan, V.C. (2001) Selective estrogen receptor modulation: a personal perspective. *Cancer Res.*, **61**, 5683–5687.

68 Vogel, V.G., Costantino, J.P., Wickerham, D.L., Cronin, W.M. *et al.* (2006) Effects of tamoxifen vs. raloxifene

on the risk of developing invasive breast cancer and other disease outcomes: the NSABP Study of Tamoxifen and Raloxifene (STAR) P-2 trial. *J. Am. Med. Assoc.*, **295**, 2727–2741.

69 Barrett-Connor, E., Mosca, L., Collins, P., Geiger, M.J. *et al.* (2006) Effects of raloxifene on cardiovascular events and breast cancer in postmenopausal women. *N. Engl. J. Med.*, **355**, 125–137.

70 National Cancer Institute (2006) Study of Tamoxifen and Raloxifene (STAR) Trial, http://www.cancer.gov/clinicaltrials/digestpage/STAR (accessed September 9, 2011).

71 Crenshaw, R.R., Jeffries, A.T., Luke, G.M., Cheney, L.C., and Bialy, G. (1971) Potential antifertility agents. 1. Substituted diaryl derivatives of benzo[*b*]thiophenes, benzo[*b*]furans, 1*H*-2-benzothiapyrans, and 2*H*-1-benzothiapyrans. *J. Med. Chem.*, **14**, 1185–1190.

72 Jones, C.D., Suarez, T., Massey, E.H., Black, L.J., and Tinsley, F.C. (1979) Synthesis and antiestrogenic activity of [3,4-dihydro-2-(4-methoxyphenyl)-1-naphthalenyl][4-[2-(1-pyrrolidinyl)ethoxy]-phenyl]methanone, methanesulfonic acid salt. *J. Med. Chem.*, **22**, 962–966.

73 Black, L.J., Jones, C.D., and Falcone, J.F. (1982) Antagonism of estrogen action with a new benzothiophene derived antiestrogen. *Life Sci.*, **32**, 1031–1036.

74 Gottardis, M. and Jordan, C. (1987) Antitumor actions of keoxifene and tamoxifen in the *N*-nitrosomethylurea-induced rat mammary carcinoma model. *Cancer Res.*, **47**, 4020–4024.

75 Jordan, V.C. (2003) Tamoxifen: a most unlikely pioneering medicine. *Nat. Rev.*, **2**, 205–213.

76 Lewis, J.S. and Jordan, V.C. (2005) Selective estrogen receptor modulators (SERMs): mechanism of anticarcinogenesis and drug resistance. *Mutat. Res.*, **591**, 247–263.

77 US Food and Drug Administration (2007) FDA News Release.

78 Deroo, B.J. and Korach, K.S. (2006) Estrogen receptors and human disease. *J. Clin. Invest.*, **116**, 561–570.

79 Lui, H., Park, W.-C., Bentrem, D.J., McKain, K.P. *et al.* (2002) Structure–function relationships of the raloxifene–estrogen receptor-alpha complex for regulating transforming growth factors-alpha expression in breast cancer cells. *J. Biol. Chem.*, **277**, 9189–9198.

80 Heringa, M. (2003) Review on raloxifene: profile of a selective estrogen receptor modulator. *Int. J. Clin. Pharmacol. Ther.*, **41**, 331–345.

81 Jeong, E.J., Liu, Y., Lin, H., and Hu, M. (2005) Species- and disposition model-dependent metabolism of raloxifene in gut and liver: role of UGT1A10. *Drug Metab. Dispos.*, **33**, 785–784.

82 Lindstrom, T.D., Whitaker, N.G., and Whitaker, G.W. (1984) Disposition and metabolism of a new benzothiophene antiestrogens in rats, dogs and monkey. *Xenobiotica*, **14** (11), 841–847.

83 Miller, C.P., Harris, H.A., and Komm, B.S. (2002) Bazedoxifene acetate. *Drugs Future*, **27**, 117–121.

84 Miller, C.P., Collini, M.D., Tran, B.D., Harris, H.A. *et al.* (2001) Design, synthesis, and preclinical characterization of novel, highly selective indole estrogens. *J. Med. Chem.*, **44**, 1654–1657.

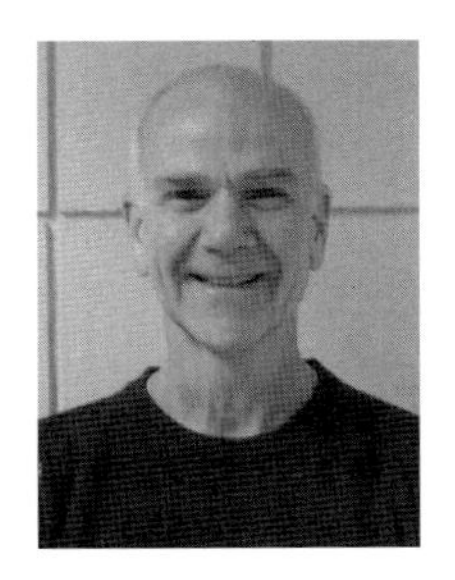

Paul W. Erhardt received a Ph.D. in Medicinal Chemistry from the University of Minnesota and carried out postdoctoral research at the University of Texas at Austin. He then spent several years within the pharmaceutical industry, where he is credited with the discovery and chemical development of esmolol. For the past several years, he has been at the University of Toledo (UT) where he is a Professor of Medicinal and Biological Chemistry within the College of Pharmacy and Pharmaceutical Sciences, a Joint Professor of Biochemistry and Cancer Biology within the College of Medicine and Life Sciences, and additionally serves as Director of UT's Center for Drug Design and Development (CD3).

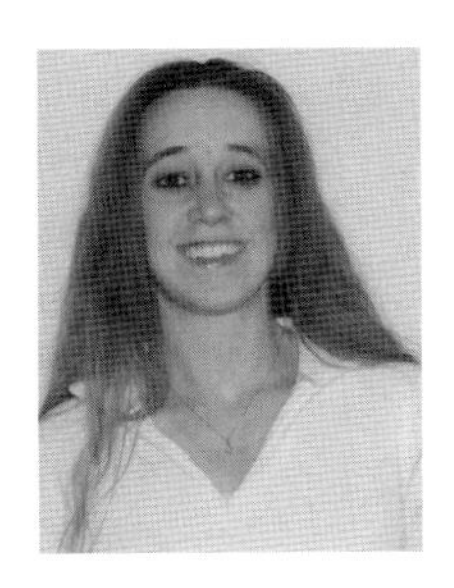

Rachael Jetson received a Bachelor of Science in Chemistry from The South Dakota School of Mines and Technology in May 2005. She then received a Master of Science in Material Science and Engineering in 2008 under the supervision of Dr. Zhengato Zhu, in which she worked on polymer/ZnO nanocomposites. In August 2008, Rachael started a Ph.D. program in Medicinal and Biological Chemistry at the University of Toledo. Since September 2009, Rachael has been conducting thesis work under Dr. Paul W. Erhardt within the Center for Drug Design and Development. Her thesis is directed toward the discovery of novel SERM compounds.

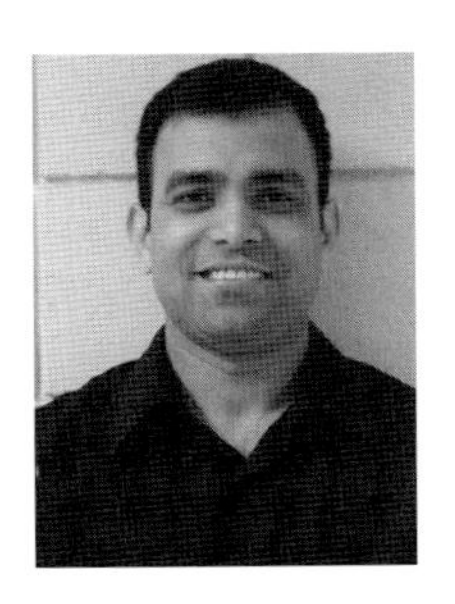

Amarjit Luniwal obtained his Bachelor of Pharmacy degree from Maharshi Dayanand University (MDU) and is a registered pharmacist in India. After obtaining his Master of Pharmacy degree from the State Technical University of Madhya Pradesh, India, he joined the Center for Drug Design and Development (CD3) at the University of Toledo to conduct Ph.D. studies in medicinal chemistry. His Ph.D. work mainly involved natural product synthesis and computer-aided molecular modeling. He completed his Ph.D. dissertation in November 2010 and presently holds a postdoctoral position in the Department of Chemistry at the University of Toledo. His postdoctoral work involves design and development of lead compounds for selective antibiotic development along with research in molecular biology and protein chemistry.

8
Discovery of Nonpeptide Vasopressin V2 Receptor Antagonists

Kazumi Kondo and Hidenori Ogawa

List of Abbreviations

ACTH	adrenocorticotropic hormone
ADH	antidiuretic hormone
AVP	arginine vasopressin
cAMP	cyclic adenosine monophosphate
EDG	electron-donating group
ED_3	the dose (mg/kg) required for a threefold increase in the 2 h urine volume over the control rats
EWG	electron-withdrawing group
FDA	the US Food and Drug Administration
GPCR	G-protein-coupled receptor
MHLW	the Japanese Ministry of Health, Labour and Welfare
MOE	molecular operating environment is a drug discovery software package developed by CCG (Chemical Computing Group Inc., Canada)

8.1
Introduction

Arginine vasopressin (AVP, Figure 8.1), also called antidiuretic hormone (ADH), is a cyclic nonapeptide hormone that is secreted from the posterior pituitary. AVP production and secretion are initiated when plasma osmolality increases and/or blood pressure decreases.

AVP mediates its action through three receptors: V_{1a}, V_{1b}, and V_2. The V_{1a} receptors are mainly expressed in the liver, vascular smooth muscle cells, platelets, uterus, and brain. The V_{1b} receptors are mainly expressed in the anterior pituitary as well as pancreatic β-cells. V_2 receptors are exclusively expressed in the kidney collecting ducts.

AVP receptors are members of the G-protein-coupled membrane receptor (GPCR) superfamily. The V_{1a} and V_{1b} receptors are linked to the phospholipase C

Analogue-based Drug Discovery III, First Edition. Edited by János Fischer, C. Robin Ganellin, and David P. Rotella.
© 2013 Wiley-VCH Verlag GmbH & Co. KGaA. Published 2013 by Wiley-VCH Verlag GmbH & Co. KGaA.

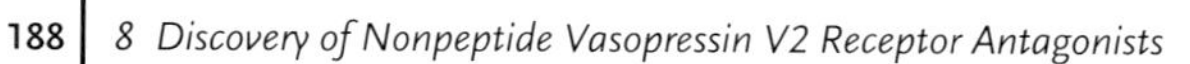

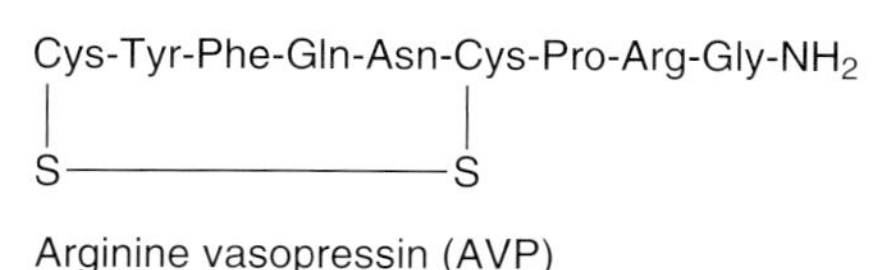

Figure 8.1 Amino acid sequence of arginine vasopressin.

activation via Gq/11, which in turn stimulates phosphatidylinositol turnover, thereby increasing the intracellular calcium ion level. The V_2 receptor is linked to the activation of adenylyl cyclase by interaction with Gs, which leads to an increase in the intracellular cAMP.

AVP plays important roles in the cardiovascular system. Vasoconstriction is mediated by the V_{1a} receptor. A relatively large amount of AVP is necessary to raise blood pressure. The activation of V_{1a} receptors is also associated with myocyte hypertrophy, glycogenolysis, and platelet aggregation.

The activation of the V_2 receptor on renal collecting ducts induces an increase in the osmotic water permeability of the apical membrane and causes water reabsorption. This effect is known as the antidiuretic activity of AVP.

The cardiovascular and renal effects of AVP mediated by V_{1a} as well as V_2 receptors are reasonably well characterized. On the other hand, the pharmacological profile of the V_{1b} receptor is somewhat complicated. The V_{1b} receptor activation stimulates the secretion of ACTH and β-endorphin from the anterior pituitary and influences blood pressure, memory, body temperature control, and social behavior. Insulin release also modulates V_{1b} receptor activation.

8.2
Peptide AVP Agonists and Antagonists

Du Vigneaud *et al.* reported the original synthesis of oxytocin and AVP in 1954 [1, 2]. Numerous analogues of AVP have been synthesized and evaluated to identify the structural features responsible for their respective biological features.

Diuretic vasopressin antagonists were first described in 1981 by Manning *et al.* [3–5] and Sawyer *et al.* [6]. These compounds were reported to inhibit vasopressin binding to renal receptors and vasopressin stimulation of renal adenylyl cyclase in a competitive fashion. However, Stassen *et al.* [7–10] and Kinter *et al.* [11, 12] reported that these compounds did not cause diuresis in dogs or squirrel monkeys.

Further studies identified vasopressin antagonists with D-Tyr-*O*-alkyl residues at position 2 as active water diuretic agents in rats, dogs, and squirrel monkeys [13, 14]. SK&F 101926 was identified as a potent vasopressin antagonist in human tissues (Figure 8.2). However, Dubb *et al.* reported that SK&F 101926 did not show diuretic activity or antagonism of the antidiuretic activity of AVP in humans, and it acted as a potent full antidiuretic agonist [15]. Brooks *et al.* reported that i.v. administration of SK&F 101926 to a hydrated rhesus monkey resulted in a full antidiuretic agonist

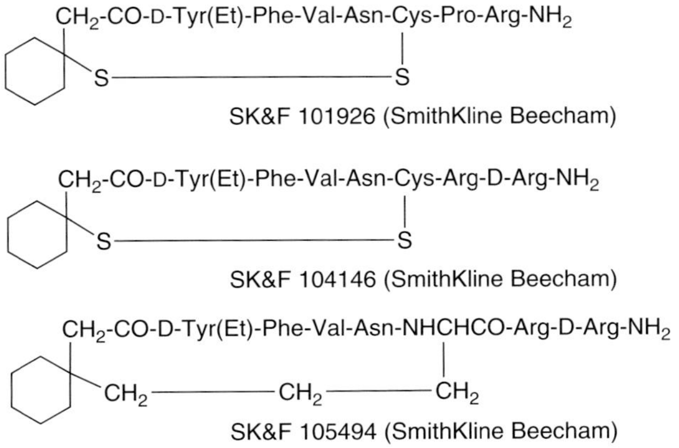

CH2-CO-D-Tyr(Et)-Phe-Val-Asn-Cys-Pro-Arg-NH2
S —— S

SK&F 101926 (SmithKline Beecham)

CH2-CO-D-Tyr(Et)-Phe-Val-Asn-Cys-Arg-D-Arg-NH2
S —— S

SK&F 104146 (SmithKline Beecham)

CH2-CO-D-Tyr(Et)-Phe-Val-Asn-NHCHCO-Arg-D-Arg-NH2
CH2 —— CH2 —— CH2

SK&F 105494 (SmithKline Beecham)

Figure 8.2 Some efforts on peptide compounds.

response, as observed in humans [16]. Modification of the terminal amino acids from Pro^7, Arg^8 to Arg^7, D-Arg^8 led to a compound (SK&F 104146) that was a less potent agonist than SK&F 101926. Further modification in SK&F 104146 of a disulfide group with methylene groups in the peptide ring to form a "dicarba bridge" resulted in a compound (SK&F 105494) that shows minimal agonist activity in hydrated monkeys. Unfortunately, marked species differences and inconsistencies were revealed between the *in vivo* and *in vitro* assay systems as reported in the case of SK&F 105494. This compound again showed a full antidiuretic response in humans [17–19].

8.3 Lead Generation Strategies [20, 21]

Further investigations focused on the discovery of nonpeptide compounds with structures distinct from AVP itself, because it is difficult to predict antagonistic activity to the human vasopressin V_2 receptor with peptide compounds. Another potential drawback in the development of peptide compounds as V_2 receptor antagonists is the poor bioavailability of peptides by oral administration.

OPC-18549 was found during in-house compound library screening using ^{3}H-AVP as a natural ligand with rat V_{1a} and rat V_2 receptors (Figure 8.3). This compound showed moderate affinity for the rat V_{1a} receptor, $IC_{50} = 2.5\,\mu M$, while the affinity to the rat V_2 receptor was very weak, $IC_{50} > 100\,\mu M$ [20].

Initial SAR studies of OPC-18549 focused on the terminal thiophene carboxamide moiety. Replacement of the thiophene ring with a phenyl ring (compound **1**) retained affinity for the V_{1a} receptor. The insertion of a methylene group between the carbonyl and the phenyl ring (compound **2**) reduced V_{1a} affinity. Replacement of the thiophene ring with a furan ring (compound **3**) also reduced binding affinity. It was therefore very interesting to note that the carbonyl group on a piperidine ring plays an important role in the affinity for the V_{1a} receptor (compound **4**).

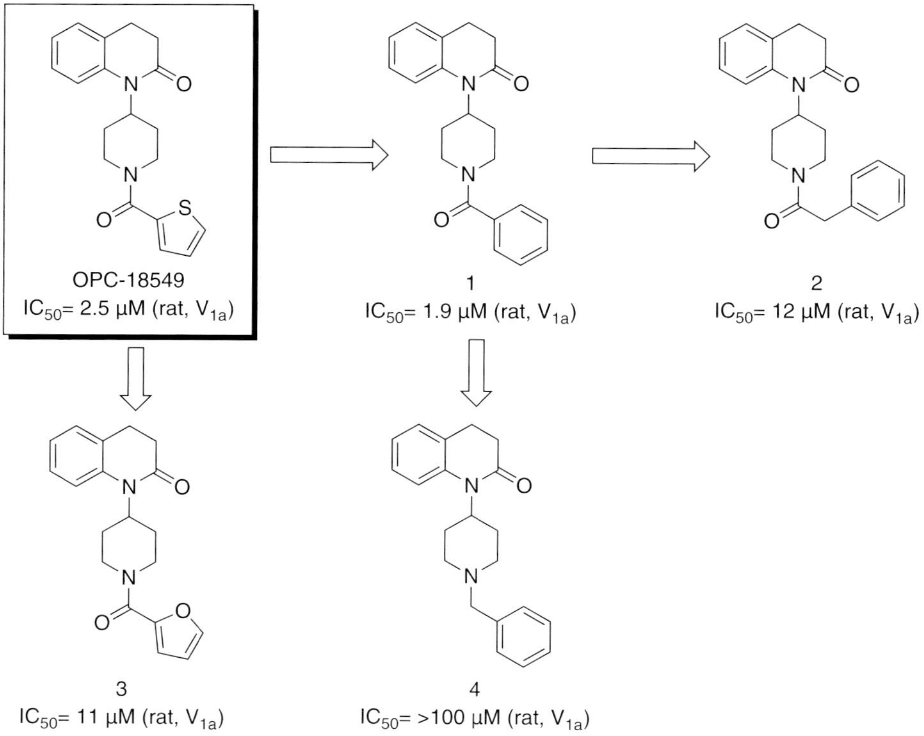

OPC-18549
IC_{50}= 2.5 μM (rat, V_{1a})

1
IC_{50}= 1.9 μM (rat, V_{1a})

2
IC_{50}= 12 μM (rat, V_{1a})

3
IC_{50}= 11 μM (rat, V_{1a})

4
IC_{50}= >100 μM (rat, V_{1a})

Figure 8.3 Initial SAR on terminal thiophene carbonyl moiety.

Further SAR evaluations investigated substituents on the terminal phenyl ring of compound **1** (Table 8.1). Substitution of either an electron-donating group (EDG) or electron-withdrawing group (EWG) was done on the phenyl ring. There was no clear correlation between the presence of an EDG or EWG on the binding affinity at the rat V_{1a} receptor. Substituents including 4-methoxy (**16**), 4-methyl (**10**), and 4-chloro (**7**) enhanced the binding affinity for the V_{1a} receptor, while a *para*-nitro group (**13**) did not show any enhancement in binding affinity. A methoxy group (**14**) only showed potent affinity for the V_{1a} receptor as a *meta*-substituent on the terminal phenyl ring and showed moderate affinity for the V_2 receptor.

Elongation on the terminal alkoxy group was examined because a *para*-methoxy substituent (**16**) enhanced the binding affinity for the V_{1a} receptor. An ethoxy compound (**17**) showed the most potent affinity for the V_{1a} receptor with moderate *in vivo* efficacy by oral administration (30 mg/kg) (Table 8.2). Tolerability in binding affinity of a substituent in the longitudinal direction looked very high (**18–20**). These results were encouraging, hence a heteroatom was introduced at the end of the alkoxy group to enhance oral efficacy.

OPC-21268 (Figure 8.4) was selected for further evaluation. This compound showed binding affinity for rat V_{1a} and rat V_2 receptors with $IC_{50}=0.44$

Table 8.1 SAR studies based on compound **1**.

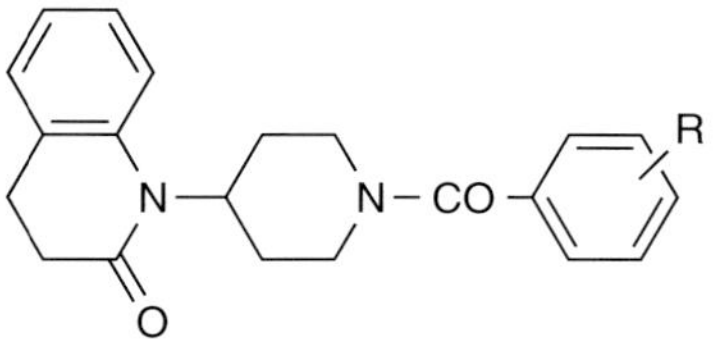

No.	R	Receptor affinity IC_{50} (μM)		Antipressor activity
		V_{1a}	V2	% Inhibition[a)]
5	2-Cl	9.9	>100	
6	3-Cl	4.4	>100	
7	4-Cl	1.2	78	
8	2-Me	8.4	>100	
9	3-Me	1.3	>100	
10	4-Me	0.5	>100	23 ± 8.9 (100)
11	2-NO_2	8.4	>100	
12	3-NO_2	3.1	>100	
13	4-NO_2	2.0	>100	
14	2-OMe	0.65	36	
15	3-OMe	2.6	>100	
16	4-OMe	0.49	>100	

a) The inhibition was expressed as percentage change in diastolic blood pressure increased by AVP (30 mU/kg, i.v.) before and after test compounds p.o. administration. Except where indicated, the number of determinations was four. Dosage in parentheses (mg/kg).

Table 8.2 SAR studies based on compound **16**.

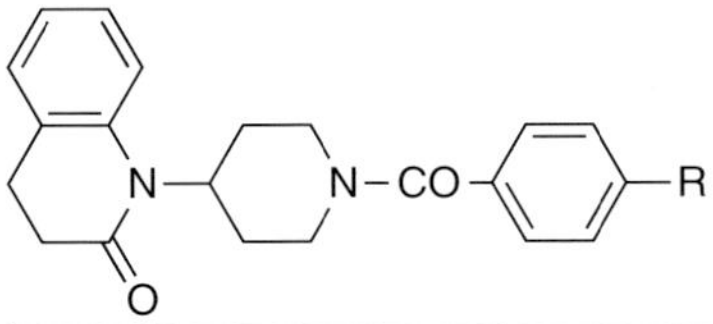

No.	R	Receptor affinity IC_{50} (μM)		Antipressor activity
		V_{1a}	V_2	% Inhibition[a)]
17	OEt	0.21	>100	75 ± 3.4 (30)
18	O-*n*Pr	0.32	>100	65 ± 6.1 (30)
19	O-*n*Bu	0.42	>100	
20	O-*n*Hex	1.5	54	

a) The inhibition was expressed as percentage change in diastolic blood pressure increased by AVP (30 mU/kg, i.v.) before and after test compounds p.o. administration. Except where indicated, the number of determinations was four. Dosage in parentheses (mg/kg).

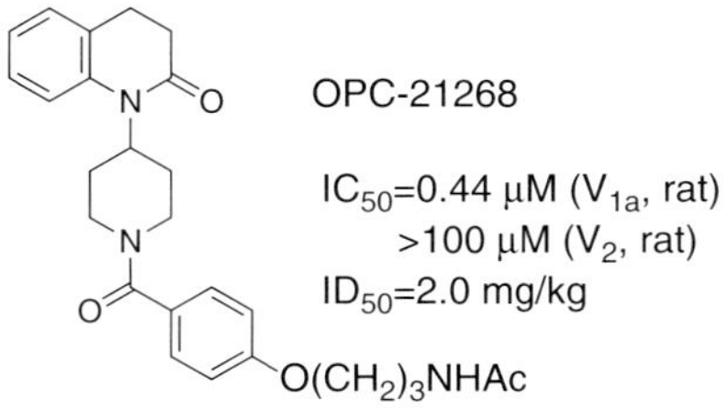

OPC-21268

IC_{50}=0.44 μM (V_{1a}, rat)
>100 μM (V_2, rat)
ID_{50}=2.0 mg/kg

Figure 8.4 Chemical structure of OPC-21268.

and >100 μM, respectively. Oral efficacy was confirmed to inhibit vasoconstriction caused by AVP (30 mU/kg, i.v.) and ID_{50} = 2.0 mg/kg [22].

OPC-21268 was reported to be an orally effective nonpeptide vasopressin V_{1a} receptor antagonist in 1991, and a marked species difference between rats and humans was reported by several groups [23–27]. Molecular cloning of human V_{1a} receptor was reported in 1994.

8.4
Lead Generation Strategy-2, V_2 Receptor Affinity [28]

Although the drug discovery program was initiated to find nonpeptide vasopressin V_2 receptor antagonists, binding affinity to the V_2 receptor was not enhanced in 2-quinolinone derivatives by modifying the terminal phenyl ring.

Intensive efforts to enhance V_2 receptor affinity were continued by replacement of the piperidine ring of compound **7** with the 4-aminophenyl group, followed by rearrangement of the carbonyl group of 2-quinolinone to the carbonyl between the quinoline and the phenyl ring to create compound **21** (Figure 8.5) [28]. Compound **21** showed binding affinity for rat V_{1a} and rat V_2 with IC_{50} = 5.1 and 1.9 μM, respectively.

Three-dimensional stable structures of compounds **7** and **21** are shown in Figure 8.6. These structures were generated using MOE [29] as modeling software

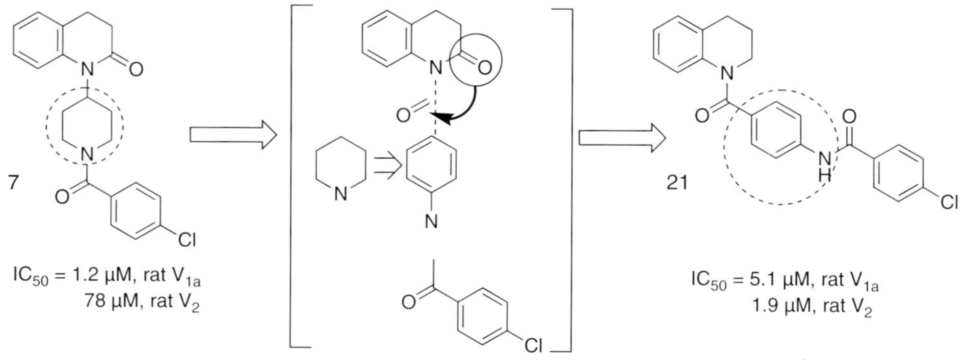

7: IC_{50} = 1.2 μM, rat V_{1a}; 78 μM, rat V_2

21: IC_{50} = 5.1 μM, rat V_{1a}; 1.9 μM, rat V_2

Figure 8.5 Structural modification of quinolinone.

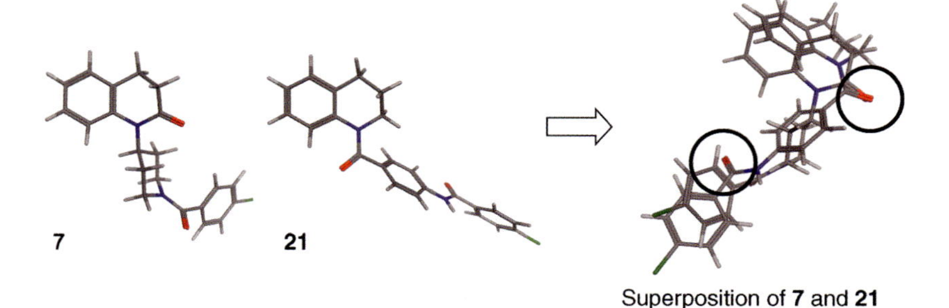

Figure 8.6 3D structures of **7** and **21**.

to examine the structure–activity relationships in a three-dimensional manner. Structural alignment was also examined with **7** and **21** (Figure 8.6). The structures of **7** and **21** (Figure 8.5) look quite different, but some pharmacophores such as phenyl rings and carbonyl groups, shown in circles, are superposed in 3D (Figure 8.6). These pharmacophores seemed to show affinity for the rat V_{1a} receptor.

A small set of SAR on substituents at the terminal phenyl ring of the tetrahydroquinoline derivative is shown in Table 8.3. A substitution at the 4-position reduced the affinity for both V_{1a} and V_2 receptors (**22** versus **21**, **23**, **24**, and **25**). While a substitution at the 2-position did not alter the binding affinity for the V_{1a} receptor, 2-Cl (**26**) and 2-Me (**28**) enhanced the binding affinity for the V_2 receptor. A substitution at the 3-position slightly reduced the binding affinity for the V_{1a} receptor, but it enhanced the binding affinity for the V_2 receptor (**29** and **30**). Substitution of an

Table 8.3 SAR studies based on compound **21**.

N-CO–(phenyl)–NHCO–(phenyl, positions 2, 3, 4)–R

No.	R	Receptor affinity IC_{50} (μM)	
		V_{1a}	V_2
22	H	1.6	0.98
21	4-Cl	5.1	1.9
23	4-OMe	2.2	1.8
24	4-Me	10	1.4
25	4-NO_2	>100	6.5
26	2-Cl	1.6	0.42
27	2-OMe	1.9	2.1
28	2-Me	1.4	0.20
29	3-Cl	6.4	0.20
30	3-OMe	2.8	0.40
31	3-Me	3.1	0.68

EDG or an EWG did not affect the binding affinity, but the steric size seemed to affect the binding affinity for the V_2 receptor (**26** versus **27**) [28].

The SAR of substituents on the terminal phenyl ring of this series had a completely different effect on V_{1a} receptor affinity in comparison to those in Table 8.1. It means that the binding mode of the terminal phenyl ring at the receptor is probably different between each series of compounds.

The head group was also examined during the evaluation of substituents on the terminal phenyl ring, shown in Table 8.3. Some examples are shown in Table 8.4.

The replacement of the tetrahydroquinoline ring (**28**) with a tetrahydrobenzazepine ring (**32**) enhanced the binding affinity for both V_{1a} and V_2 receptors. There is no substantial difference in the binding affinity between 2-Me and 2-Cl (**32** and **33**) on the terminal phenyl ring. The introduction of a nitrogen atom at the 5-position of the tetrahydrobenzazepine ring (**34**) did not alter the binding affinity for the V_2 receptor, but slightly lowered that for the V_{1a} receptor. The introduction of a nitrogen atom at the 4-position (**35**) lowered the binding affinity for both V_{1a} and V_2 receptors. The difference in binding affinity by introducing a nitrogen atom on the

Table 8.4 SAR studies of the heteroaromatic ring of compound **28**.

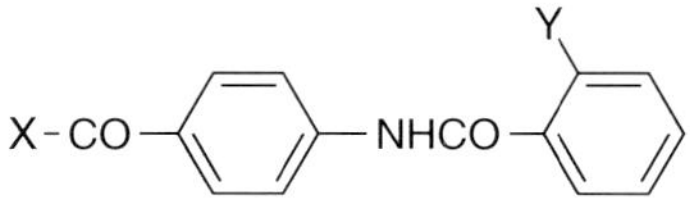

No.	X	Y	Receptor affinity IC_{50} (μM)	
			V_{1a}	V_2
28	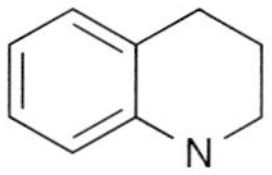	Me	1.4	0.20
32	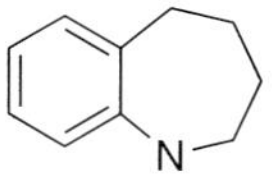	Me	0.056	0.018
33	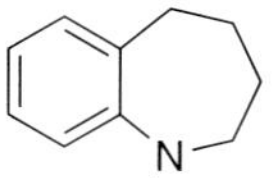	Cl	0.045	0.029
34	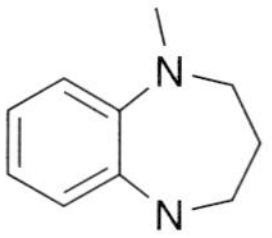	Me	0.38	0.014
35	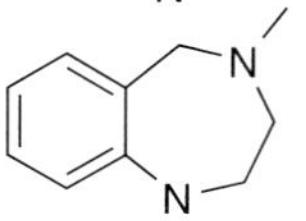	Me	1.8	0.17
36	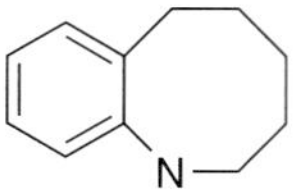	Me	0.41	0.028

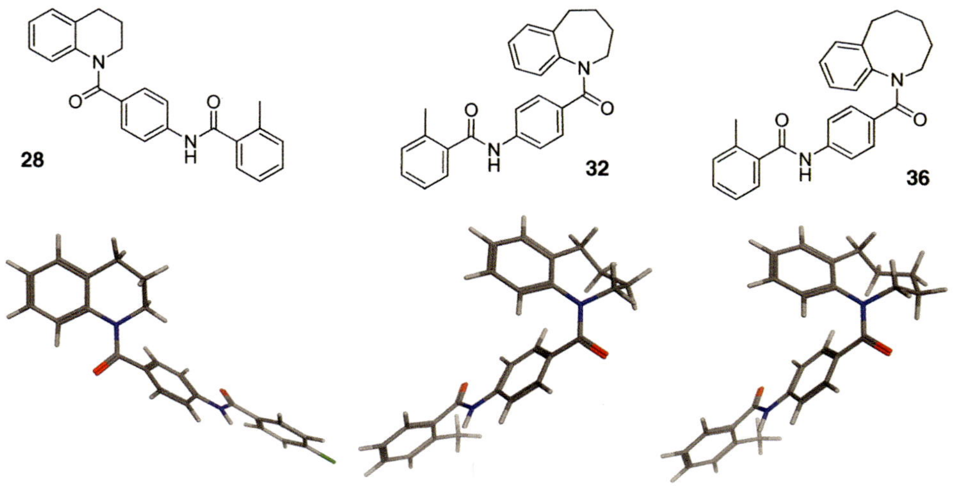

Figure 8.7 3D structures of **28**, **32**, and **36**.

benzazepine ring either at the 4- or at the 5-position is due to the difference in steric size of a substituent at the 4- or 5-position or as a difference in basicity of a nitrogen atom. The replacement of the tetrahydroquinoline ring with a hexahydrobenzazocine ring (**36**) enhanced the binding affinity for both V_{1a} and V_2 receptors [28].

3D structures of compounds **28**, **32**, and **36** were generated using MOE [29] as a stable conformation with the default setting (Figure 8.7). The only difference among these three structures was the dihedral angle of the amide linkage between the heteroaromatic ring and the benzoyl C=O moiety. Two phenyl rings beside the amide linkage in **28** are in a *trans* conformation; however, those in **32** and **36** are in a *cis* conformation. Therefore, this *cis* conformation of two phenyl rings seems to be important to show potent affinity for both V_{1a} and V_2 receptors. Furthermore, the superposed structure of compounds **7** and **21** (Figure 8.6) appeared to show a *cis* conformation in the two phenyl rings of compound **21** and these are similar to the 3D structure of compound **32**.

Although compounds **32**, **33**, **34**, and **36** showed potent binding affinity for the V_2 receptor, these compounds failed to demonstrate oral diuretic activity. On the other hand, at a dose of 100 mg/kg compound **35** showed weak oral diuretic activity, with a five- to sixfold increase in urine volume observed for 4 h in normally hydrated conscious rats over the control rats, while the binding affinity for the V_2 receptor was moderate. These results suggested that a basic amino group at the 4-position in the 1,4-benzodiazepine ring (**35**) helped to increase oral bioavailability [28].

Based on this finding, a series of compounds were designed with a basic amino group at the 5-position of the benzazepine scaffold to enhance oral bioavailability (Figure 8.8).

The introduction of an NH_2 group at the 5-position (**37**) gave only a slight reduction in the binding affinity for the V_2 receptor, and the introduction of an NH-methyl group (**38**) gave a binding affinity similar to that of compound **37**

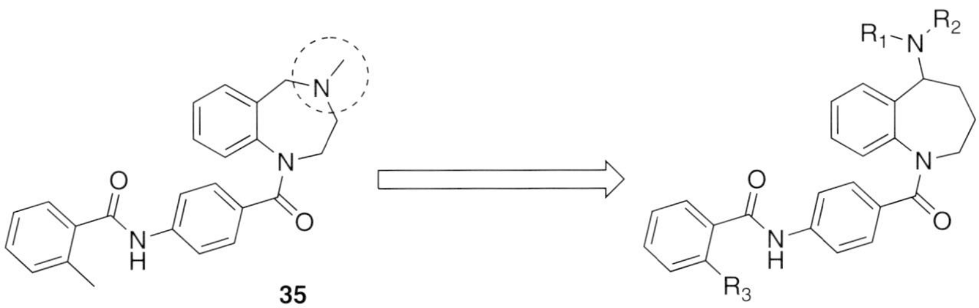

Figure 8.8 Design of orally active compounds.

(Table 8.5). This single methyl group dramatically enhanced *in vivo* efficacy, and an eightfold increase in urinary output was observed relative to the control rats. NH-ethyl (**39**) and NH-propyl (**40**) groups showed the same magnitude of binding affinity for the V_2 receptor with moderate diuretic activity by oral administration, though these showed a slight reduction in the V_{1a} binding affinity. While the introduction of an *N,N*-dimethyl group (**42**) did not alter the binding affinity for V_{1a} and V_2 receptors relative to NH-methyl (**38**), it provided very potent diuretic efficacy by oral administration ($ED_3 = 3.8$ mg/kg). The *in vivo* efficacy and the binding affinity

Table 8.5 SAR studies of the substituent at the 5-position.

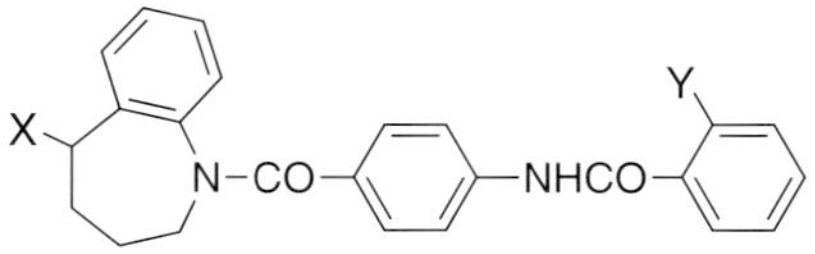

No.	X	Y	IC_{50} (μM)		*In vivo*
			V_{1a}	V_2	UV (ml)
37	NH_2	2-Me	0.39	0.032	
38	NHMe	2-Me	0.72	0.024	8.3 ± 2.5 (4.6)
39	NHEt	2-Me	1.6	0.029	5.4 ± 0.6 (8.0)
40	NH*n*Pr	2-Me	0.89	0.050	5.6 ± 1.0 (6.6)
41	NMe_2	H	3.0	0.027	(>30)
42	NMe_2	2-Me	1.4	0.012	12.3 ± 2.3 ($ED_3 = 3.8$)
43	NMe_2	3-Me	2.4	0.014	(>30)
44	NMe_2	4-Me	26	0.044	
45	NMe_2	2-Cl	3.0	0.027	7.0 ± 0.5 (4.2)
46	N(Me)*n*Pr	2-Me	1.2	0.022	8.3 ± 1.8 (4.9)
47	OH	2-Me	0.14	0.029	3.6 ± 0.8

UV values mean 2 h urine volume (ml) when the test compounds were administrated orally at a dose of 10 mg/kg and are expressed as mean ± SEM ($n = 4$). The mean value of 2 h urine volume of control rats was 1.1 ± 0.2 ml ($n = 4$). Values in parentheses indicate the ED_3 value. ED_3 represents the dose (mg/kg) required for a threefold increase in the 2 h urine volume over the control rats. Values such as >30 designate that at this dose (mg/kg) a threefold increase in the 2 h urine volume was not observed when compared with that of the control rats.

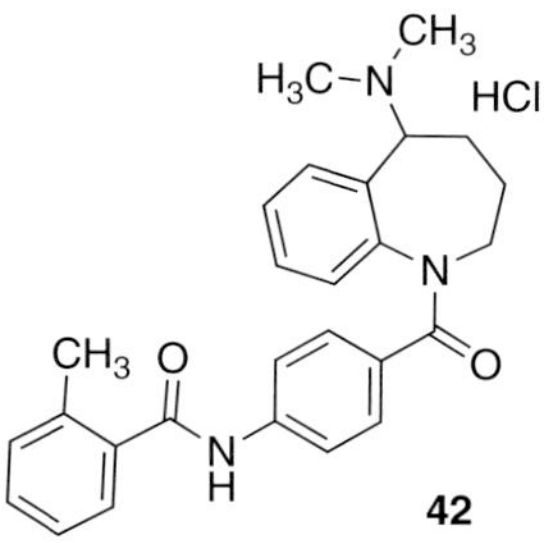

Physuline® (mozavaptan hydrochloride)
(OPC-31260)

42

Figure 8.9 Chemical structure of physuline.

for the V_{1a} receptor were dramatically influenced by substitution on the terminal phenyl ring (**41**, **43**, **44**, and **45**). *N*-Methyl-*N*-propyl derivative (**46**) showed better *in vivo* efficacy than NH-propyl derivative (**40**). The introduction of a hydroxyl group at the 5-position (**47**) did not alter the binding affinity, but it did not provide the potent *in vivo* efficacy of the 5-amino derivatives [28].

Compound **42** (Figure 8.9) was selected for further evaluation. This compound increased urine flow and decreased urine osmolality after oral administration (1–30 mg/kg) in normal conscious rats [30–32]. Compound **42** (mozavaptan, OPC-31260) is a selective V_2 receptor antagonist that acts as an aquaretic agent. The binding affinities of **42** at V_{1a} and V_2 receptors are as follows: $K_i = 9.42 \pm 0.90$ nM (human V_2), 150 ± 15 nM (human V_{1a}), 6.36 ± 1.56 nM (rat V_2), and 524 ± 119 nM (rat V_{1a}). No meaningful differences were found in the binding affinities between human and rat receptors.

Physuline® (mozavaptan hydrochloride) was approved in Japan in October 2006 to treat paraneoplastic SIADH (the syndrome of inappropriate antidiuretic hormone).

8.5
Lead Optimization [33]

Further optimization was performed on R_1, R_2, and R_3 to enhance *in vitro* and *in vivo* efficacy (Table 8.6). The introduction of a 7-Cl group (**48** versus **42**) enhanced V_{1a} affinity and also enhanced *in vivo* efficacy. Replacement of the 5-dimethylamino group with a 5-monomethylamino group slightly enhanced the binding affinity for both V_{1a} and V_2 receptors (**48** versus **49**). 5-OH (**50**) and 5-OMe (**51**) showed potent affinity for both the V_{1a} and V_2 receptors. The steric size at the 5-position of the benzazepine ring might affect binding affinity at V_{1a} as well as V_2 receptor. Replacement of the 5-amino group with 5-OH reduced the *in vivo* efficacy.

It was very interesting that the introduction of a 2-Cl group as R_3 potentiated the oral efficacy (**52**), while water solubility was poor. The same enhancement was seen with a 2-Me group (**54**) as well as a 2-OMe group (**55**) at R_3. A 3-OMe group (**56**) enhanced the binding affinity to both V_{1a} and V_2 receptors, but the oral efficacy appeared to be weak [33].

Table 8.6 Optimization of benzazepine analogues.

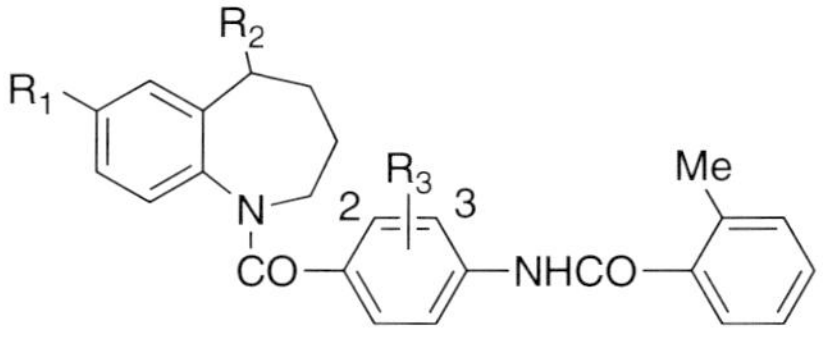

No.	R_1	R_2	R_3	Receptor affinity IC_{50} (μM)		*In vivo*	
				V_{1a}	V_2	UV (ml)	ED_3
42	H	NMe_2	H	1.4	0.012	12.3	3.8
48	Cl	NMe_2	H	0.19	0.025	14.6	1.5
49	Cl	NHMe	H	0.064	0.007	15.5	1.4
50	Cl	OH	H	0.017	0.003	7.2	
51	Cl	OMe	H	0.034	0.005	6.3	
52	Cl	OH	2-Cl	0.29	0.008	16.8	1.6
53	Cl	OH	3-Cl	0.031	0.028	3.0	
54	Cl	OH	2-Me	0.58	0.003	17.3	0.54
55	Cl	OH	2-OMe	0.039	0.013	15.2	1.4
56	Cl	OH	3-OMe	0.007	0.005	3.5	

Compound **54** (tolvaptan, Figure 8.10) was selected for advanced *in vivo* studies and clinical trials, and it showed a selective V_2 receptor affinity relative to the V_{1a} receptor and a potent *in vivo* efficacy.

Binding affinities for both V_{1a} and V_2 receptors are as follows: $K_i = 0.43 \pm 0.06$ nM (human V_2), 12.3 ± 0.8 nM (human V_{1a}), 1.33 ± 0.30 nM (rat V_2), and 325 ± 41 nM (rat V_{1a}) [34]. Tolvaptan showed potent water diuretic activity in various animal models as well as in clinical trials [35, 36].

The US Food and Drug Administration (FDA) approved Samsca® (tolvaptan) as the only oral selective vasopressin antagonist for the treatment of hypervolemic and euvolemic hyponatremia on May 21, 2009, in patients with heart failure, cirrhosis, and the syndrome of inappropriate antidiuretic hormone. The European

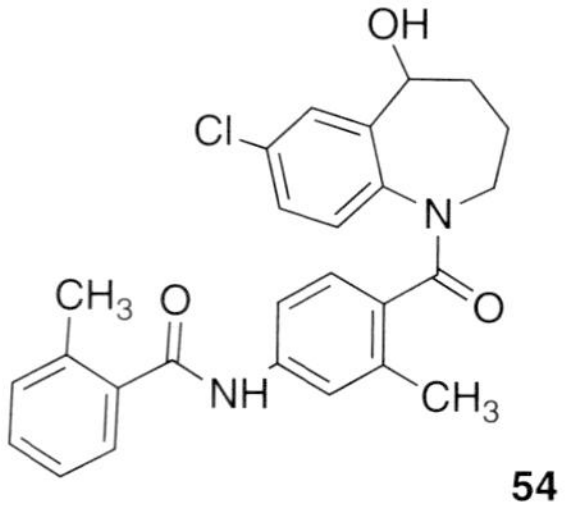

Samsca® (tolvaptan)
(OPC-41061)

54

Figure 8.10 Chemical structure of samsca.

Commission approved the Marketing Authorization Application for the oral once-daily medication Samsca® for the treatment of hyponatremia secondary to SIADH in adults in August 2009, and the Japanese Ministry of Health, Labour and Welfare (MHLW) approved Samsca® for the treatment of excess water retention in patients with cardiac failure, when the treatment by other diuretics including loop diuretics is ineffective, in October 2010.

8.6 Reported Nonpeptide Vasopressin V_2 Receptor Antagonist Compounds

8.6.1 Sanofi

Sanofi reported the nonpeptide V_{1a} receptor selective antagonist, SR 49059 (relcovaptan, Figure 8.11), in 1993 [37]. They intensively modified a dihydroindole as an original scaffold and reported SR 121463 (satavaptan) as a nonpeptide V_2 receptor selective antagonist in 1996 [38], and SSR 149415 (nelivaptan) was reported as a nonpeptide V_{1b} receptor antagonist in 2002 [39].

8.6.2 Astellas (Yamanouchi)

OPC-31260 was reported to be an orally active nonpeptide V_2 receptor antagonist in 1992 and in 1996, and Yamanouchi reported nonselective V_{1a} and V_2 receptor antagonists with tetrahydrobenzazepine as a scaffold (Figure 8.12, **57**) in 1997 [40]. The benzodiazepine analogues (**58** and **59**) [41], 5-*exo*-olefin-substituted tetrahydrobenzazepine derivative (**60**) [42], 4,5-imidazole-substituted analogue (**61**, YM 087, conivaptan) [43], and 4,4-difluoro-5-*exo*-olefin-

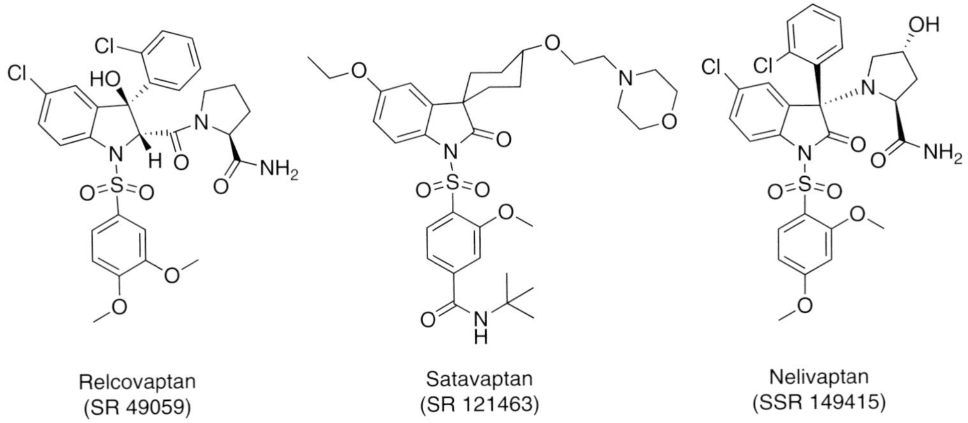

Relcovaptan (SR 49059)

Satavaptan (SR 121463)

Nelivaptan (SSR 149415)

Figure 8.11 Reported compounds from Sanofi.

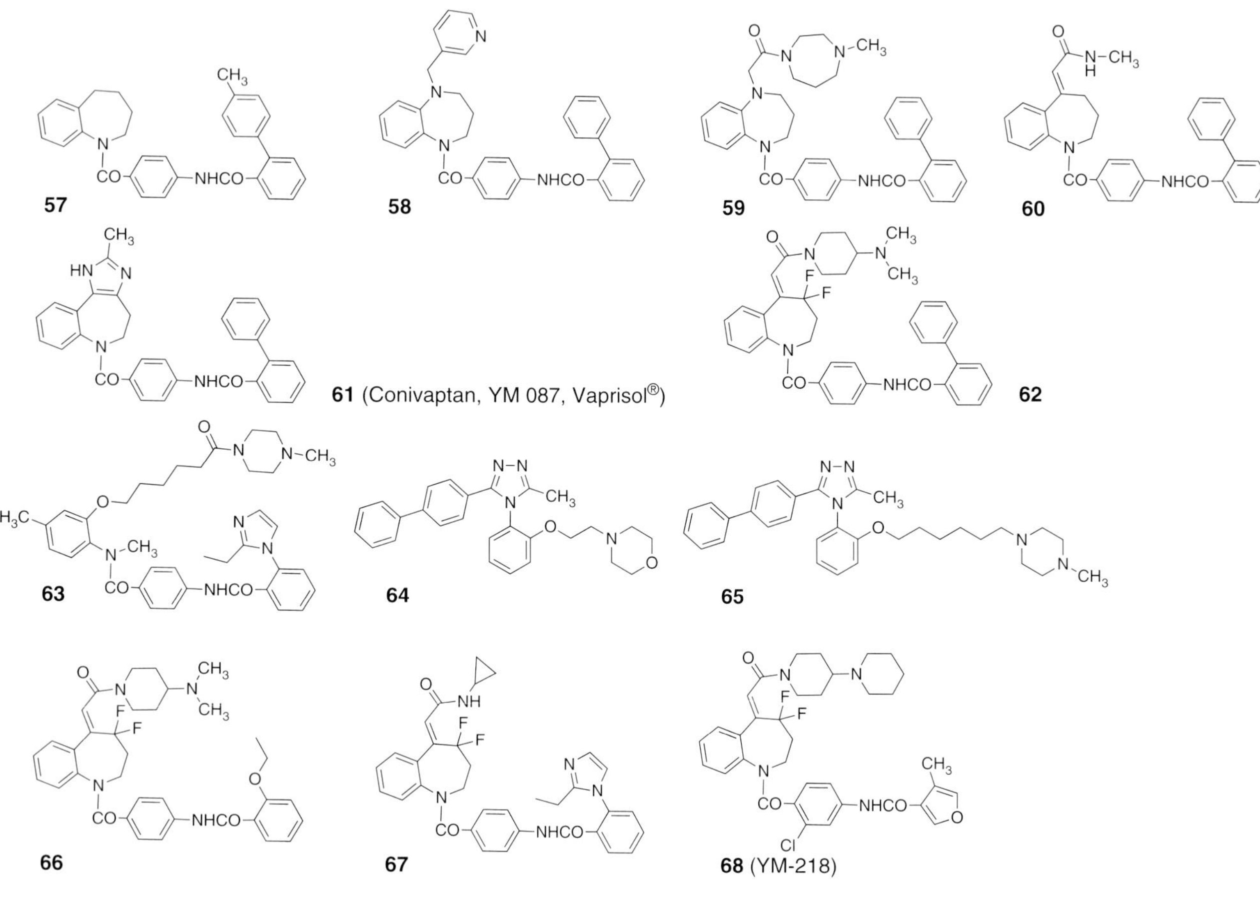

Figure 8.12 Reported compounds from Astellas.

substituted analogue (**62**) [44] were reported as nonselective antagonists. Non-cyclized benzamide derivative (**63**) [45] was derived from reported compounds and reported to show potent V_{1a} receptor affinity. Yamanouchi reported triazole derivatives (**64** and **65**) [46, 47] to show potent V_{1a} receptor affinity in 2002, and these compounds were derived from a compound identified by internal high-throughput screening efforts. Some modifications of the amino group at the 5-position of the benzazepine ring as well as terminal benzoyl or heteroaromatic carbonyl groups were reported to show potent V_{1a} receptor antagonist activity (**66**, **67**, and **68**) [48–50]. Vaprisol® (conivaptan hydrochloride injection) was approved by the FDA in 2005 for the treatment of euvolemic hyponatremia in hospitalized patients.

8.6.3 Wyeth

Wyeth reported benzopyrrolo[1,4]diazepine derivatives as a nonpeptide V_2 receptor selective antagonist (Figure 8.13, **69**, lixivaptan) in 1998 [51]. In addition, some combinations of the end group, middle aromatic ring, and terminal phenyl ring were reported (**70**, **71**, and **72**) [52–54]. Compound **73** (WAY-140288) was reported in 2000 to show a good profile in parenteral formulation [55].

8.6.4 Johnson & Johnson

Johnson & Johnson also intensively reported modification of the top benzohetero ring (Figure 8.14; **74**, **75**, and **76**) [56–58]. An optically pure analogue with a substituted oxazine ring was reported to show a potent affinity to the V_2 receptor in 2004 (**77**, RWJ-351647) [59]. Another group in Johnson & Johnson reported compounds

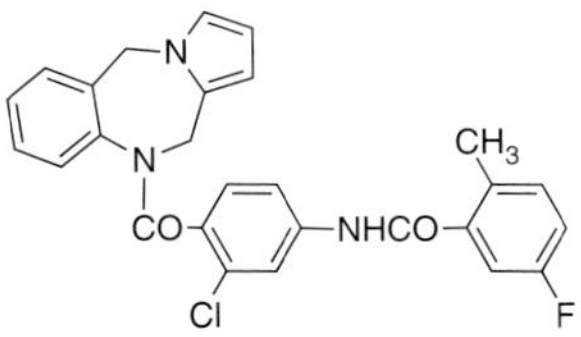

69 (VPA-985, Lixivaptan) 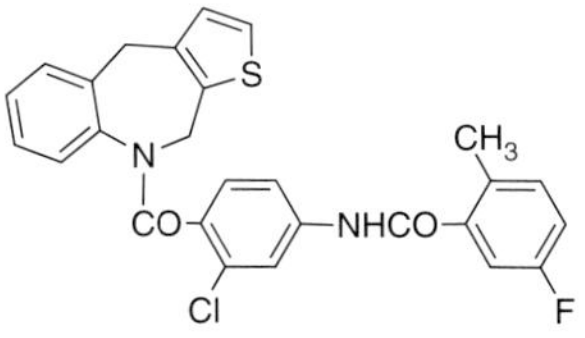 **70** 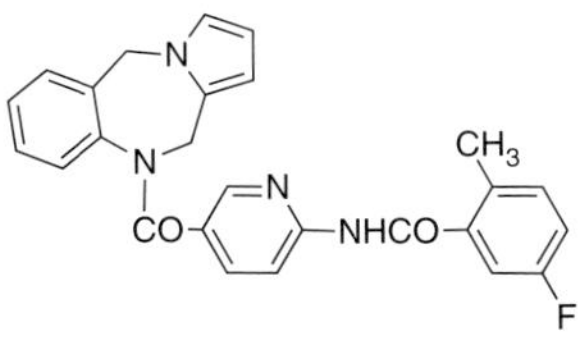 **71** (CL-385004) 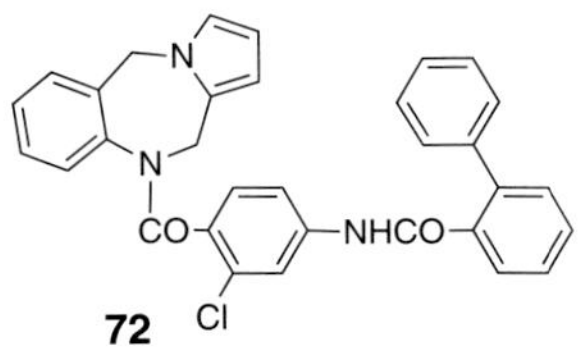 **72** 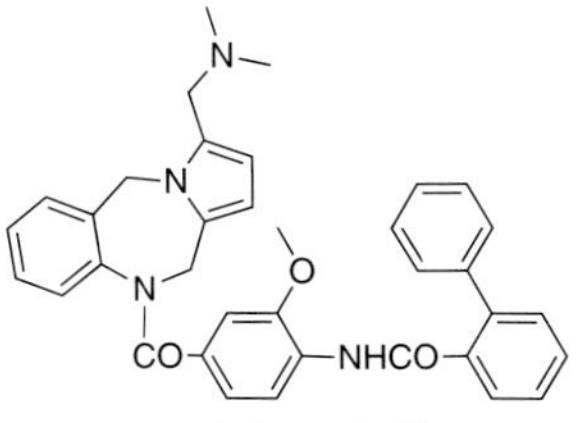 **73** (WAY-140288)

Figure 8.13 Reported compounds from Wyeth.

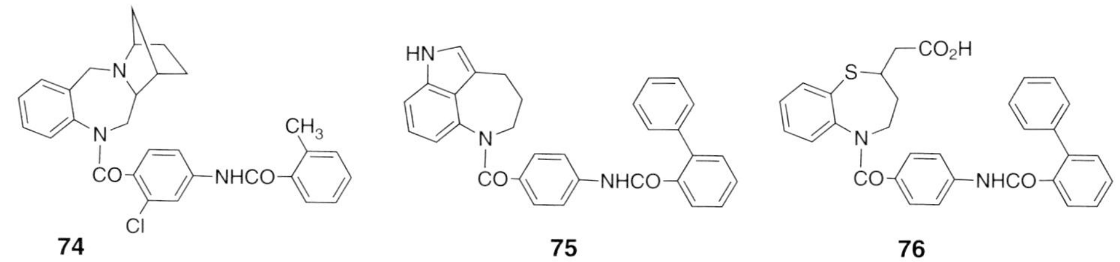

74

75

76

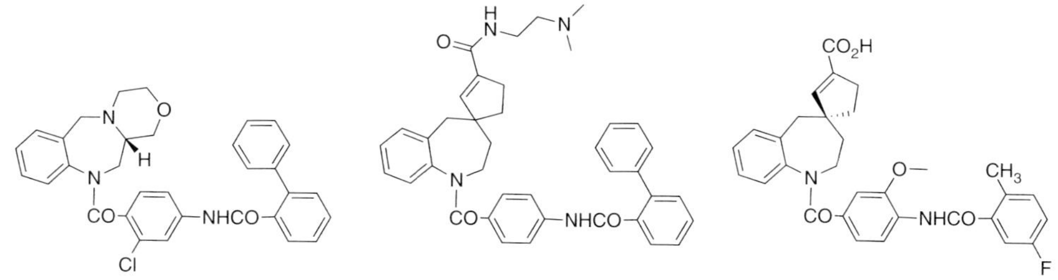

77 (RWJ-351647)

78

79 (RWJ-676070)

Figure 8.14 Reported compounds from Johnson & Johnson.

having a spirocyclopentene ring at the 4-position of the benzazepine ring (**78**) in 2004 [60]. This compound showed potent affinity for both V_{1a} and V_2 receptors. They reported the same class of compound in optically pure form in 2007 (**79**, RWJ-676070) as a balanced vasopressin V_{1a}/V_2 antagonist [61].

8.6.5 Wakamoto Pharmaceutical Co. Ltd [62]

Some analogues with a benzohetero ring as an end group were reported in 1999 as V_2 receptor selective antagonists (Figure 8.15).

8.6.6 Japan Tobacco Inc.

Japan Tobacco reported a thienoazepine derivative (**83**, JTV-605) as a potent V_{1a} and V_2 antagonist with a long duration of action in 2004 (Figure 8.16) [63].

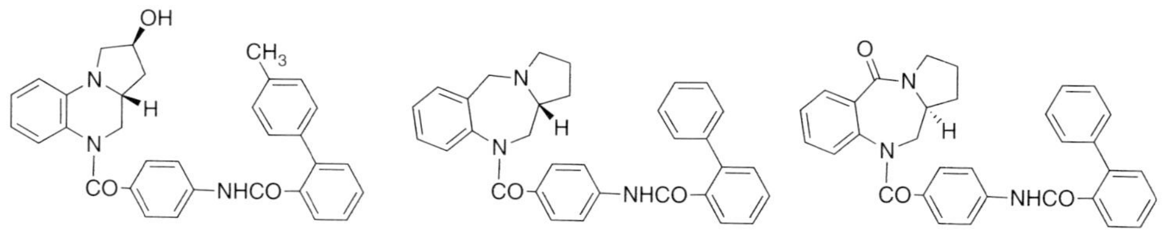

80 (VP-343)

81 (VP-365)

82 (VP-339)

Figure 8.15 Reported compounds from Wakamoto.

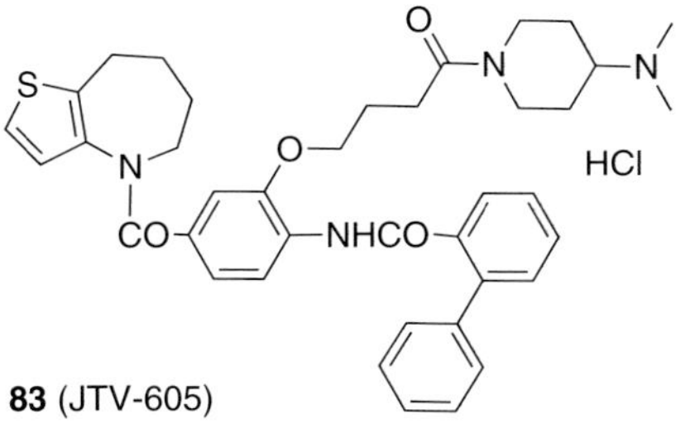

83 (JTV-605)

Figure 8.16 Reported compound from Japan Tabacco.

8.7 Conclusions

The discovery of aquaretics, water diuretics, to treat chronic heart failure has led to numerous findings demonstrating that the biological effects of AVPs are mediated through three receptor subtypes. A major contribution was the discovery of nonpeptide compounds that show high selectivity to receptors, and good oral bioavailability to permit repeated administration. In addition, the discovery of orally effective nonpeptide AVP receptor antagonists led to the discovery of nonpeptide oxytocin receptor antagonists and agonists [64].

X-ray analyses of some G-protein-coupled receptors have been reported [65–67]. More detailed consideration of the receptor–ligand interactions will be conducted using the 3D structures of receptors, and this will lead to the discovery of ligands with higher diversity in structure.

The efforts to discover nonpeptide vasopressin receptor modulators are still not finished, because the physiological roles of AVP are still under investigation. These efforts to find better compounds are therefore expected to be beneficial for patients.

References

1 Du Vigneaud, V., Ressler, C., Swan, J.M., Roberts, C.W., and Katsoyannis, P.G. (1954) The synthesis of oxytocin. *J. Am. Chem. Soc.*, **76**, 3115–3121.

2 Du Vigneaud, V., Gish, D.T., and Katsoyannis, P.G. (1954) A synthetic preparation possessing biological properties associated with arginine-vasopressin. *J. Am. Chem. Soc.*, **76**, 4751–4752.

3 Manning, M., Lammek, B., Kolodziejczyk, A.M., Seto, J., and Sawyer, W.H. (1981) Synthetic antagonists of *in vivo* antidiuretic and vasopressor responses to arginine-vasopressin. *J. Med. Chem.*, **24**, 701–706.

4 Manning, M., Olma, A., Klis, W.A., Kolodziejczyk, A.M., Seto, J., and Sawyer, W.H. (1982) Design of more potent antagonists of the antidiuretic responses to arginine-vasopressin. *J. Med. Chem.*, **25**, 45–50.

5 Manning, M., Klis, W.A., Olma, A., Seto, J., and Sawyer, W.H. (1982) Design of more potent and selective antagonists of the antidiuretic responses to arginine-vasopressin devoid of antidiuretic agonism. *J. Med. Chem.*, **25**, 414–419.

6 Sawyer, W.H., Pang, P.K.T., Seto, J., McEnroe, M., Lammek, B., and Manning, M. (1981) Vasopressin analogs that antagonize antidiuretic responses by rats to the antidiuretic hormone. *Science*, **212**, 49–51.

7 Stassen, F.L., Erickson, R.W., Huffman, W.F., Stefankiewicz, J., Sulat, L., and Wiebelhaus, V.D. (1982) Molecular mechanisms of novel antidiuretic antagonists: analysis of the effects on vasopressin binding and adenylate cyclase activation in animal and human kidney. *J. Pharmacol. Exp. Ther.*, **223**, 50–54.

8 Stassen, F.L., Bryan, W., Gross, M., Kavanagh, B., Shue, D., Sulat, L., Wiebelhaus, V.D., Yim, N., and Kinter, L.B. (1983) Critical differences between species in *in vivo* and *in vitro* responses to antidiuretic hormone antagonists. *Prog. Brain Res.*, **60**, 395–403.

9 Stassen, F.L., Berkowitz, B.B., Huffman, W.F., Wiebelhaus, V.D., and Kinter, L.B. (1984) Molecular pharmacology and mechanisms of action of aquaretic agents, in *Diuretics* (ed. J.B. Puschett), Elsevier Science Publishing Co., Inc., New York, pp. 64–71.

10 Stassen, F.L., Heckman, G.D., Schmidt, D.B., Stefankiewicz, J., Sulat, L., Huffman, W.F., Moore, M.M., and Kinter, L.B. (1985) Actions of vasopressin antagonists: molecular mechanisms, in *Vasopressin* (ed. R.W. Schrier), Raven Press, New York, pp. 145–154.

11 Kinter, L.B., Dubb, J., Huffman, F.L., Brennan, F., and Stassen, F.L. (1985) Potential role of vasopressin antagonists in treatment of water-retaining disorders, in *Vasopressin* (ed. R.W. Schrier), Raven Press, New York, pp. 553–561.

12 Kinter, L.B., Churchill, S., Stassen, F.L., Moore, M., and Huffman, W. (1987) Characterization and mechanism of action of vasopressin antagonists in squirrel monkeys (*Saimiri sciureus*). *J. Pharmacol. Exp. Ther.*, **241**, 797–803.

13 Manning, M., Olma, A., Klis, W., Kolodziejczyk, A.M., Nawrocka, E., Misicka, A., Seto, J., and Sawyer, W.H. (1984) Carboxy terminus of vasopressin required for activity but not binding. *Nature*, **308**, 652–653.

14 Kinter, L.B., Mann, W.A., Woodward, P., DePalma, D., and Brennan, F. (1987) The vasopressin antagonist SK&F 101926 is a selective aquaretic agent in dogs, in *Diuretics: Basic, Pharmacological, and Clinical Aspects* (eds V.E. Andreucci and A. Dal Canton), Proceedings of the International Meeting on Diuretics, Martinus Nijhoff, Boston, MA, pp. 218–221.

15 Dubb, J., Allison, N., Tatoian, D., Blumberg, A., Lee, K., and Stote, R. (1987) SK&F 101926 is antidiuretic in man. *Kidney Int.*, **31**, 267.

16 Brooks, D.P., Koster, P.F., Albrightson-Winslow, C.R., Stassen, F.L., Huffman, W.F., and Kinter, L.B. (1988) SK&F 105494 is a antidiuretic hormone antagonist in the rhesus monkey (*Macaca mulatta*). *J. Pharmacol. Exp. Ther.*, **245**, 211–215.

17 Caldwell, N., Brickson, B., Kinter, L.B., Brooks, D.P., Huffman., W.F., Stassen, F.L., and Albrightson-Winslow, C. (1988) SK&F 105494: a potent antidiuretic hormone antagonist devoid of partial agonist activity in dogs. *J. Pharmacol. Exp. Ther.*, **247**, 897–901.

18 Brooks, D.P., Koster, P.F., Albrightson, C.R., Huffman, W.F., Moore, M.L., Stassen, F.L., Schmidt, D.B., and Kinter, L.B. (1989) Vasopressin receptor antagonism in rhesus monkey and man: stereochemical requirements. *Eur. J. Pharmacol.*, **160**, 159–162.

19 Ruffolo, R.R., Jr., Brooks, D.P., Huffman, W.F., and Poste, G. (1991) From vasopressin antagonist to agonist: a saga of surprise! *Drug News Perspect.*, **4**, 217–222.

20 Ogawa, H., Yamamura, Y., Miyamoto, H., Kondo, K., Yamashita, H., Nakaya, K., Chihara, T., Mori, T., Tominaga, M., and Yabuuchi, Y. (1993) Orally active, nonpeptide vasopressin V1 antagonists. A novel series of 1-(1-substituted 4-piperidyl)-3,4-dihydro-2(1*H*)-quinolinone. *J. Med. Chem.*, **36**, 2011–2017.

21 Kondo, K., Ogawa, H., Nakaya, K., Tominaga, M., and Yabuuchi, Y. (1996) Structure–activity relationships of non-peptide vasopressin V_{1a} antagonists: 1-(1-multi-substituted benzoyl 4-piperidyl)-3,4-dihydro-2(1*H*)-

quinolinones. *Chem. Pharm. Bull.*, **44**, 725–733.

22 Yamamura, Y., Ogawa, H., Chihara, T., Kondo, K., Onogawa, T., Nakamura, S., Mori, T., Tominaga, M., and Yabuuchi, Y. (1991) OPC-21268, an orally effective, nonpeptide vasopressin V1 receptor antagonist. *Science*, **252**, 572–574.

23 Pettibone, D.J., Kishel, M.T., Woyden, C.J., Clineschmidt, B.V., Bock, M.G., Freidinger, R.M., Veber, D.F., and Williams, P.D. (1992) Radioligand binding studies reveal marked species differences in the vasopressin V_1 receptor of rat, rhesus and human tissues. *Life Sci.*, **50**, 1953–1958.

24 Serradeil-Le Gal, C., Wagnon, J., Garcia, C., Lacour, C., Guiraudou, P., Christophe, B., Villanova, G., Nisato, D., Maffrand, J.P., and Le Fur, G. (1993) Biochemical and pharmacological properties of SR 49059, a new, potent, nonpeptide antagonist of rat and human vasopressin V_{1a} receptors. *J. Clin. Invest.*, **92**, 224–231.

25 Serradeil-Le Gal, C., Raufaste, D., Marty, E., Garcia, C., Maffrand, J.P., and Le Fur, G. (1994) Binding of [^{3}H] SR 49059, a potent nonpeptide vasopressin V_{1a} antagonist, to rat and human liver membranes. *Biochem. Biophys. Res. Commun.*, **199**, 353–360.

26 Hirasawa, A., Shibata, K., Kotosai, K., and Tsujimoto, G. (1994) Cloning, functional expression and tissue distribution of human cDNA for the vascular-type vasopressin receptor. *Biochem. Biophys. Res. Commun.*, **203**, 72–79.

27 Shinoura, H., Take, H., Itoh, S., Hirasawa, A., Inoue, K., Ohno, Y., Hashimoto, K., and Tsujimoto, G. (2000) Key amino acids of vasopressin V_{1a} receptor responsible for the species difference in the affinity of OPC-21268. *FEBS Lett.*, **466**, 255–258. Erratum in *FEBS Lett.*, **474**, 257 (2000).

28 Ogawa, H., Yamashita, H., Kondo, K., Yamamura, Y., Miyamoto, H., Kan, K., Kitano, K., Tanaka, M., Nakaya, K., Nakamura, S., Mori, T., Tominaga, M., and Yabuuchi, Y. (1996) Orally active, nonpeptide vasopressin V_2 receptor antagonists: a novel series of 1-[4-(benzoylamino)benzoyl]-2,3,4,5-tetrahydro-1*H*-benzazepines and related compounds. *J. Med. Chem.*, **39**, 3547–3555.

29 Chemical Computing Group, *MOE: Molecular Operating Environment*, Chemical Computing Group, Montreal, Canada, current version, MOE2011.10.

30 Yamamura, Y., Ogawa, H., Yamashita, H., Chihara, T., Miyamoto, H., Nakamura, S., Onogawa, T., Yamashita, T., Hosokawa, T., Mori, T., Tominaga, M., and Yabuuchi, Y. (1992) Characterization of a novel aquaretic agent, OPC-31260, as an orally effective, nonpeptide vasopressin V_2 receptor antagonist. *Br. J. Pharmacol.*, **105**, 787–791.

31 Ohnishi, A., Orita, Y., Okahara, R., Fujihara, H., Inoue, T., Yamamura, Y., Yabuuchi, Y., and Tanaka, T. (1993) Potent aquaretic agent. *J. Clin. Invest.*, **92**, 2653–2659.

32 Ohnishi, A., Orita, Y., Takagi, N., Fujita, T., Toyoki, T., Ihara, Y., Yamamura, Y., Inoue, T., and Tanaka, T. (1995) Aquaretic effect of a potent, orally active, nonpeptide V_2 antagonist in men. *J. Pharmacol. Exp. Ther.*, **272**, 546–551.

33 Kondo, K., Ogawa, H., Yamashita, H., Miyamoto, H., Tanaka, M., Nakaya, K., Kitano, K., Yamamura, Y., Nakamura, S., Onogawa, T., Mori, T., and Tominaga, M. (1999) 7-Chloro-5-hydroxy-1-[2-methyl-4-(2-methylbenzoylamino)benzoyl]-2,3,4,5-tetrahydro-1*H*-1-benzazepine (OPC-41061): a potent, orally active nonpeptide arginine vasopressin V_2 receptor antagonist. *Bioorg. Med. Chem.*, **7**, 1743–1754.

34 Yamamura, Y., Nakamura, S., Ito, S., Hirano, T., Onogawa, T., Yamashita, T., Yamada, Y., Tsujimae, K., Aoyama, M., Kotosai, K., Ogawa, H., Yamashita, H., Kondo, K., Tominaga, M., Tsujimoto, G., and Mori, T. (1998) OPC-41061, a potent human vasopressin V_2-receptor antagonist: pharmacological profile and aquaretic effect by single and multiple oral dosing in rats. *J. Pharmacol. Exp. Ther.*, **287**, 860–867.

35 Ohnishi, A., Orita, Y., Okahara, R., Fujihara, H., Inoue, T., Yamamura, Y., Yabuuchi, Y., and Tanaka, T. (1993) Potent aquaretic agent. *J. Clin. Invest.*, **92**, 2653–2659.

36 Ohnishi, A., Orita, Y., Takagi, N., Fujita, T., Toyoki, T., Ihara, Y., Yamamura, Y., Inoue, T., and Tanaka, T. (1995) Aquaretic effect of a potent, orally active, nonpeptide V_2 antagonist in men. *J. Pharmacol. Exp. Ther.*, **272**, 546–551.

37 Serradeil-Le Gal, C., Wagnon, J., Garcia, C., Lacour, C., Guiraudou, P., Christophe, B., Villanova, G., Nisato, D., Maffrand, J.P., Le Fur, G., Guillon, G., Cantau, B., Barberis, C., Trueba, M., Ala, Y., and Jard, S. (1993) Biochemical and pharmacological properties of SR 49059, a new, potent, nonpeptide antagonist of rat and human vasopressin V_{1a} receptors. *J. Clin. Invest.*, **92**, 224–231.

38 Serradeil-Le Gal, C., Lacour, C., Valette, G., Garcia, G., Foulon, L., Galindo, G., Bankir, L., Pouzet, B., Guillon, G., Barberis, C., Chicot, D., Jard, S., Vilain, P., Garcia, C., Marty, E., Raufaste, D., Brossard, G., Nisato, D., Maffrand, J.P., and Le Fur, G. (1996) Characterization of SR 121463A, a highly potent and selective, orally active vasopressin V_2 receptor antagonist. *J. Clin. Invest.*, **98**, 2729–2738.

39 Serradeil-Le Gal, C., Wagnon, J., Simiand, J., Griebel, G., Lacour, C., Guillon, G., Barberis, C., Brossard, G., Soubrié, P., Nisato, D., Pascal, M., Pruss, R., Scatton, B., Maffrand, J.P., and Le Fur, G. (2002) Characterization of (2*S*,4*R*)-1-[5-chloro-1-[(2,4-dimethoxyphenyl)sulfonyl]-3-(2-methoxy-phenyl)-2-oxo-2,3-dihydro-1*H*-indol-3-yl]-4-hydroxy-*N*,*N*-dimethyl-2-pyrrolidine carboxamide (SSR149415), a selective and orally active vasopressin V_{1b} receptor antagonist. *J. Pharmacol. Exp. Ther.*, **300**, 1122–1130.

40 Matsuhisa, A., Tanaka, A., Kukuchi, K., Shimada, Y., Yatsu, T., and Yanagisawa, I. (1997) Nonpeptide arginine vasopressin antagonists for both V_{1a} and V_2 receptors: synthesis and pharmacological properties of 2-phenyl-4′-[(2,3,4,5-tetrahydro-1*H*-1-benzazepin-1-yl) carbonyl]benzanilide derivatives. *Chem. Pharm. Bull.*, **45**, 1870–1874.

41 Matsuhisa, A., Koshio, H., Sakamoto, K., Taniguchi, N., Yatsu, T., and Tanaka, A. (1998) Nonpeptide arginine vasopressin antagonists for both V_{1a} and V_2 receptors: synthesis and pharmacological properties of 2-phenyl-4′-(2,3,4,5-tetrahydro-1*H*-1,5-benzodiazepine-1-carbonyl)benzanilide derivatives. *Chem. Pharm. Bull.*, **46**, 1566–1579.

42 Matsuhisa, A., Kikuchi, K., Sakamoto, K., Yatsu, T., and Tanaka, A. (1999) Nonpeptide arginine vasopressin antagonists for both V_{1a} and V_2 receptors: synthesis and pharmacological properties of 4′-[5-(substituted methylidene)-2,3,4,5-tetrahydro-1*H*-1-benzoazepine-1-carbonyl] benzanilide and 4′-[5-(substituted methyl)-2,3-dihydro-1*H*-1-benzoazepine-1-carbonyl]benzanilide derivatives. *Chem. Pharm. Bull.*, **47**, 329–339.

43 Matsuhisa, A., Taniguchi, N., Koshio, H., Yatsu, T., and Tanaka, A. (2000) Nonpeptide arginine vasopressin antagonists for both V_{1a} and V_2 receptors: synthesis and pharmacological properties of 4′-(1,4,5,6-tetrahydroimidazo[4,5-*d*][1] benzoazepine-6-carbonyl)benzanilide derivatives and 4′-(5,6-dihydro-4*H*-thiazolo[5,4-*d*][1]benzoazepine-6-carbonyl) benzanilide derivatives. *Chem. Pharm. Bull.*, **48**, 21–31.

44 Shimada, Y., Taniguchi, N., Matsuhisa, A., Sakamoto, K., Yatsu, T., and Tanaka, A. (2000) Highly potent and orally active non-peptide arginine vasopressin antagonists for both V_{1a} and V_2 receptors: synthesis and pharmacological properties of 4′-[(4,4-difluoro-5-methylidene-2,3,4,5-tetrahydro-1*H*-1-benzoazepin-1-yl)carbonyl]-2-phenylbenzanilide derivatives. *Chem. Pharm. Bull.*, **48**, 1644–1651.

45 Kakefuda, A., Tsukada, J., Kusayama, T., Tahara, A., and Tsukamoto, S. (2002) *N*-Methylbenzanilide derivatives as a novel class of selective V_{1a} receptor antagonists. *Bioorg. Med. Chem. Lett.*, **12**, 229–232.

46 Kakefuda, A., Suzuki, T., Tobe, T., Tahara, A., Sakamoto, S., and Tsukamoto, S. (2002) Discovery of 4,5-diphenyl-1,2,4-triazole derivatives as a novel class of selective antagonists for the human V_{1a} receptor. *Bioorg. Med. Chem.*, **10**, 1905–1912.

47 Kakefuda, A., Suzuki, T., Tobe, T., Tsukada, J., Tahara, A., Sakamoto, S., and Tsukamoto, S. (2002) Synthesis and pharmacological evaluation of 5-(4-

biphenyl)-3-methyl-4-phenyl-1,2,4-triazole derivatives as a novel class of selective antagonists for the human vasopressin V_{1a} receptor. *J. Med. Chem.*, **45**, 2589–2598.

48 Shimada, Y., Taniguchi, N., Matsuhisa, A., Yatsu, T., Tahara, A., and Tanaka, A. (2003) Preparation of non-peptide, highly potent and selective antagonists of arginine vasopressin V_{1a} receptor by introduction of alkoxy groups. *Chem. Pharm. Bull.*, **51**, 1075–1080.

49 Shimada, Y., Akane, H., Taniguchi, N., Matsuhisa, A., Kawano, N., Kikuchi, K., Yatsu, T., Tahara, A., Tomura, Y., Kusayama, T., Wada, K., Tsukada, J., Tsunoda, T., and Tanaka, A. (2005) Preparation of highly potent and selective non-peptide antagonists of the arginine vasopressin V_{1a} receptor by introduction of a 2-ethyl-1*H*-1-imidazolyl group. *Chem. Pharm. Bull.*, **53**, 764–769.

50 Shimada, Y., Taniguchi, N., Matsuhisa, A., Akane, H., Kawano, N., Suzuki, T., Tobe, T., Kakefuda, A., Yatsu, T., Tahara, A., Tomura, Y., Kusayama, T., Wada, K., Tsukada, J., Orita, M., Tsunoda, T., and Tanaka, A. (2006) Synthesis and biological activity of novel 4,4-difluorobenzazepine derivatives as non-peptide antagonists of the arginine vasopressin V_{1a} receptor. *Bioorg. Med. Chem.*, **14**, 1827–1837.

51 Albright, J.D., Reich, M.F., Delos Santos, E.G., Dusza, J.P., Sum, F.-W., Venkatesan, A.M., Coupet, J., Chan, P.S., Ru, X., Mazandarani, H., and Bailey, T. (1998) 5-Fluoro-2-methyl-*N*-[4-(5*H*-pyrrolo[2,1-*c*]-[1,4]benzodiazepin-10(11*H*)-ylcarbonyl)-3-chlorophenyl]benzamide (VPA-985): an orally active arginine vasopressin antagonist with selectivity for V_2 receptors. *J. Med. Chem.*, **41**, 2442–2444.

52 Aranapakam, V., Albright, J.D., Grosu, G. T., Chan, P.S., Coupet, J., Saunders, T., Ru, X., and Mazandarani, H. (1999) 4,10-Dihydro-5*H*-thieno[3,2-*c*][1]benzazepine derivatives and 9,10-dihydro-4*H*-thieno [2,3-*c*][1]benzazepine derivatives as orally active arginine vasopressin receptor antagonists. *Bioorg. Med. Chem. Lett.*, **9**, 1733–1736.

53 Aranapakam, V., Albright, J.D., Grosu, G.T., Delos Santos, E.G., Chan, P.S., Coupet, J., Ru, X., Saunders, T., and Mazandarani, H. (1999) 5-Fluoro-2-methyl-*N*-[5-(5*H*-pyrrolo[2,1-*c*][1,4] benzodiazepine-10(11*H*)-yl carbonyl)-2-pyridinyl]benzamide (CL-385004) and analogs as orally active arginine vasopressin receptor antagonists. *Bioorg. Med. Chem. Lett.*, **9**, 1737–1740.

54 Albright, J.D., Delos Santos, E.G., Dusza, J.P., Chan, P.S., Coupet, J., Ru, X., and Mazandarani, H. (2000) The synthesis and vasopressin (AVP) antagonist activity of a novel series of *N*-aroyl-2,4,5,6-tetrahydropyrazolo[3,4-*d*]thieno[3,2-*b*] azepines. *Bioorg. Med. Chem. Lett.*, **10**, 695–698.

55 Ashwell, M.A., Bagli, J.F., Caggiano, T.J., Chan, P.S., Molinari, A.J., Palka, C., Park, C.H., Rogers, J.F., Sherman, M., Trybulski, E.J., and Williams, D.K. (2000) The design, synthesis and physical chemical properties of novel human vasopressin V_2-receptor antagonists optimized for parenteral delivery. *Bioorg. Med. Chem. Lett.*, **10**, 783–786.

56 Dyatkin, A.B., Hoekstra, W.J., Hlasta, D.J., Andrade-Gordon, P., de Garavilla, L., Demarest, K.T., Gunnet, J.W., Hageman, W., Look, R., and Maryanoff, B.E. (2002) Bridged bicyclic vasopressin receptor antagonists with V_2-selective or dual V_{1a}/V_2 activity. *Bioorg. Med. Chem. Lett.*, **12**, 3081–3084.

57 Matthews, J.M., Greco, M.N., Hecker, L.R., Hoekstra, W.J., Andrade-Gordon, P., de Garavilla, L., Demarest, K.T., Ericson, E., Gunnet, J.W., Hageman, W., Look, R., Moore, J.B., and Maryanoff, B.E. (2003) Synthesis and biological evaluation of novel indoloazepine derivatives as non-peptide vasopressin V_2 receptor antagonists. *Bioorg. Med. Chem. Lett.*, **13**, 753–756.

58 Urbanski, M.J., Chen, R.H., Demarest, K.T., Gunnet, J., Look, R., Ericson, E., Murray, W.V., Rybczynski, P.J., and Zhang, X. (2003) 2,5-Disubstituted 3,4-dihydro-2*H*-benzo[*b*][1,4]thiazepines as potent and selective V_2 arginine vasopressin receptor antagonists. *Bioorg. Med. Chem. Lett.*, **13**, 4031–4034.

59 Matthews, J.M., Hoekstra, W.J., Dyatkin, A.B., Hecker, L.R., Hlasta, D.J., Poulter,

B.L., Andrade-Gordon, P., de Garavilla, L., Demarest, K.T., Ericson, E., Gunnet, J.W., Hageman, W., Look, R., Moore, J.B., Reynolds, C.H., and Maryanoff, B.E. (2004) Potent nonpeptide vasopressin receptor antagonists based on oxazino- and thiazinobenzodiazepine templates. *Bioorg. Med. Chem. Lett.*, **14**, 2747–2752.

60 Xiang, M.A., Chen, R.H., Demarest, K.T., Gunnet, J., Look, R., Hageman, W., Murray, W.V., Combs, D.W., Rybczynski, P.J., and Patel, M. (2004) Synthesis and evaluation of nonpeptide substituted spirobenzazepines as potent vasopressin antagonists. *Bioorg. Med. Chem. Lett.*, **14**, 3143–3146.

61 Xiang, M.A., Rybczynski, P.J., Patel, M., Chen, R.H., McComsey, D.F., Zhang, H.C., Gunnet, J.W., Look, R., Wang, Y., Minor, L.K., Zhong, H.M., Villani, F.J., Demarest, K.T., Damiano, B.P., and Maryanoff, B.E. (2007) Next-generation spirobenzazepines: identification of RWJ-676070 as a balanced vasopressin V_{1a}/V_2 receptor antagonist for human clinical studies. *Bioorg. Med. Chem. Lett.*, **17**, 6623–6628.

62 Ohtake, Y., Naito, A., Hasegawa, H., Kawano, K., Morizono, D., Taniguchi, M., Tanaka, Y., Matsukawa, H., Naito, K., Oguma, T., Ezure, Y., and Tsuriya, Y. (1999) Novel vasopressin V_2 receptor-selective antagonists, pyrrolo[2,1-*a*] quinoxaline and pyrrolo[2,1-*c*][1,4] benzodiazepine derivatives. *Bioorg. Med. Chem.*, **7**, 247–254.

63 Cho, H., Murakami, K., Nakanishi, H., Fujisawa, A., Isoshima, H., Niwa, M., Hayakawa, K., Hase, Y., Uchida, I., Watanabe, H., Wakitani, K., and Aisaka, K. (2004) Synthesis and structure–activity relationships of 5,6,7,8-tetrahydro-4*H*-thieno[3,2-*b*]azepine derivatives: novel arginine vasopressin antagonists. *J. Med. Chem.*, **47**, 101–109.

64 Bell, I.M., Erb, J.M., Freidinger, R.M., Gallicchio, S.N., Guare, J.P., Guidotti, M.T., Halpin, R.A., Hobbs, D.W., Homnick, C.F., Kuo, M.S., Lis, E.V., Mathre, D.J., Michelson, S.R., Pawluczyk, J.M., Pettibone, D.J., Reiss, D.R., Vickers, S., Williams, P.D., and Woyden, C.J. (1998) Development of orally active oxytocin antagonists: studies on 1-(1-[4-[1-(2-methyl-1-oxidopyridin-3-ylmethyl) piperidin-4-yloxy]-2-methoxybenzoyl] piperidin-4-yl)-1,4-dihydrobenz [*d*][1,3] oxazin-2-one (L-372,662) and related pyridines. *J. Med. Chem.*, **41**, 2146–2163.

65 Palczewski, K., Kumasaka, T., Hori, T., Behnke, C.A., Motoshima, H., Fox, B.A., Le Trong, I., Teller, D.C., Okada, T., Stenkamp, R.E., Yamamoto, M., and Miyano, M. (2000) Crystal structure of rhodopsin: a G protein-coupled receptor. *Science*, **289**, 739–745.

66 Rasmussen, S.G., Choi, H.J., Fung, J.J., Pardon, E., Casarosa, P., Chae, P.S., Devree, B.T., Rosenbaum, D.M., Thian, F.S., Kobilka, T.S., Schnapp, A., Konetzki, I., Sunahara, R.K., Gellman, S.H., Pautsch, A., Steyaert, J., Weis, W.I., and Kobilka, B.K. (2011) Structure of a nanobody-stabilized active state of the β_2 adrenoceptor. *Nature*, **469**, 175–180.

67 Rosenbaum, D.M., Zhang, C., Lyons, J.A., Holl, R., Aragao, D., Arlow, D.H., Rasmussen, S.G., Choi, H.J., Devree, B.T., Sunahara, R.K., Chae, P.S., Gellman, S.H., Dror, R.O., Shaw, D.E., Weis, W.I., Caffrey, M., Gmeiner, P., and Kobilka, B.K. (2011) Structure and function of an irreversible agonist–$\beta(2)$ adrenoceptor complex. *Nature*, **469**, 236–240.

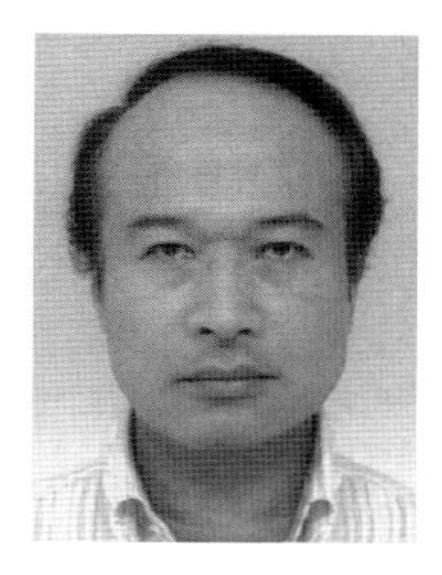

Kazumi Kondo is a Senior Researcher at Otsuka Pharmaceutical Co., Ltd. He was born in Ehime Prefecture (Japan) in 1959. He obtained his B.S. degree (1982) and M.S. degree (1985) in the field of Synthetic Organic Chemistry from Okayama University under the supervision of Prof. Dr. Shigeru Torii. Before his graduation from Okayama University, he spent 1 year (1983–1984) at Lausanne University (Switzerland) in the laboratory of Prof. Dr. Manfred Schlosser. In 1999, he received his Ph.D. degree (Pharmaceutical Science) from the Tokyo University under the supervision of Prof. Dr. Koichi Shudo. After he joined Otsuka in 1985, he contributed to a number of projects to discover cardiovascular drugs as well as CNS drugs. He is an author of over 30 publications and a co-inventor on over 20 small-molecule patents.

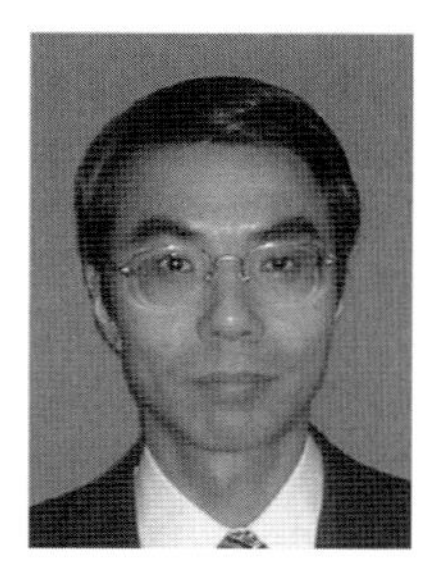

Hidenori Ogawa is an Associate Director for Qs' Research Institute of Otsuka Pharmaceutical Co., Ltd. He received his B.Eng. degree (1976) in Chemistry from Okayama University. He earned his Ph.D. (1988) in Medicinal Chemistry from Osaka University, working on design and synthesis of positive inotropic agents. He has worked at Otsuka for 32 years and has been responsible for several inventions and publications in the various therapeutic areas, including vasopressin receptor V_{1a} and/or V_2 antagonists and V_2 agonists.

9
The Development of Cysteinyl Leukotriene Receptor Antagonists

Peter R. Bernstein

List of Abbreviations

5-LO	5-lipoxygenase
b.i.d.	dosed two times/day
CSS	Churg–Strauss syndrome
CysLT	cysteinyl leukotriene
$CysLT_1R$	cysteinyl leukotriene 1 receptor
$CysLT_2R$	cysteinyl leukotriene 2 receptor
$CysLT_3R$	cysteinyl leukotriene 3 receptor
DMPK	distribution, metabolism, and pharmacokinetics
FLAP	5-lipoxygenase activating protein
gp	guinea pig
HAP	hydroxyacetophenone
HSA	human serum albumin
ID	intraduodenal
IP	intraperitoneal
IV	intravenous
LT	leukotriene
MW	molecular weight
PO	per oral
q.d.	dosed once/day
SAR	structure–activity relationship
SRS-A	slow-reacting substance of anaphylaxis

The development of the $CysLT_1R$ antagonists will be reviewed with a focus on the three agents used clinically: montelukast, zafirlukast, and pranlukast. In addition to describing the path that each company followed to their clinical agent, an effort will be made to show how the interim results obtained by these and other groups (those

Analogue-based Drug Discovery III, First Edition. Edited by János Fischer, C. Robin Ganellin, and David P. Rotella.
© 2013 Wiley-VCH Verlag GmbH & Co. KGaA. Published 2013 by Wiley-VCH Verlag GmbH & Co. KGaA.

that did not achieve a clinically available agent) influenced the competing teams' efforts.

9.1 Introduction

At the time of its approval in 1996, zafirlukast represented the fruition of a decade's long effort and the dawning of a new treatment for asthma. As a selective $CysLT_1$ receptor ($CysLT_1R$) antagonist, it exemplified the first new class of medications approved for treating asthma, in the United States in over 30 years [1]. Asthma is one of the most common medical conditions that is, as defined by the Global Initiative for Asthma, "a chronic inflammatory disorder of the airways in which many cells and cellular elements play a role".[1)] It is characterized by variable and reversible airway obstruction and hypersensitivity and had been treated by a wide variety of agents including oral and inhaled corticosteroids, oral and inhaled β-agonists, oral xanthines, and inhaled inhibitors of mediator release [2].

Due to asthma's widespread nature and the fact that in spite of this broad array of agents, it remained only partially controlled, there was a great deal of interest in the development of new treatment paradigms. The clinical effectiveness of the $CysLT_1R$ antagonists (e.g., zafirlukast, montelukast, and pranlukast) in preventing asthmatic-type responses has been demonstrated in multiple challenge studies involving allergens, aspirin, exercise, and cold air [3]. In asthmatic patients, the response to these agents is variable. However, in those who respond these medicines improve the patient's general condition and reduce the need for other medications such as β-agonists and steroids [4].

The path leading to the development of the $CysLT_1R$ antagonists as effective treatments for asthma began during the period 1938–1940 when the slow-reacting substance of anaphylaxis (SRS-A) was identified by Kellaway and Trethewie as a potent smooth muscle constrictor [5]. SRS-A, unlike histamine, induced a slowly developing and long-lasting contraction of guinea pig ileum. Initial efforts to develop agents that would either block the formation of SRS-A (biosynthesis inhibitors) or antagonize its actions (receptor antagonists) were hampered by the fact that SRS-A was (1) very unstable, (2) only available in small amounts via a complicated isolation following biological generation, and (3) its biosynthetic pathway, structure, and biological target all remained unknown.

The next breakthrough in the development of $CysLT_1R$ antagonists came in 1973 with the discovery of FPL-55712, by Augstein *et al.* [6]. This archetypical antagonist was discovered at Fisons by screening of compounds related to a chromone (cromolyn sodium [7]), used to treat asthma, against extracts containing SRS-A. Although FPL-55712 suffered from a short half-life and poor bioavailability [8], it was very important both as a starting point from which other analogous antagonists would be developed and because it played a key role in the structural elucidation of

1) http://www.ginasthma.org/ (accessed October 24, 2011).

SRS-A. Using biological extracts isolated from multiple cell types and species, research groups fractionated (purified) and concentrated the samples of SRS-A. Antagonism by FPL-55712, of the contraction induced in a tissue strip by a fraction, was the key assay to show which fractions were the ones containing SRS-A and also that different biological systems were producing the same agonist [9].

The key discoveries that unlocked the floodgates of broad and sustained drug discovery efforts occurred in 1979 and 1980. First, Bengt Samuelsson *et al.* (Karolinska Institute) determined that SRS-A was comprised of a cysteine-containing derivative of 5-hydroxy-7,9,11,14-eicosatetraenoic acid [10]. This compound was a product of the 5-lipoxygenase pathway of the arachidonic acid cascade and he proposed the name leukotriene for this family of compounds, a name that was derived from their cell source (*leukocytes*) and their unusual conjugated *triene* chemical structure (Figure 9.1). Then working with E.J. Corey (Harvard University), Samuelsson confirmed its exact structure and determined that three members of the leukotriene family, known as LTC_4, LTD_4, and LTE_4, and collectively as cysteinyl leukotrienes (CysLTs, because although they contained different peptides they all incorporated the amino acid cysteine), accounted for the original biological activity of SRS-A [11].

The belief that modulators (antagonists or inhibitors) of this biological pathway could become novel, effective antiasthma drugs was based on the finding that SRS-A and synthetic CysLTs were able to cause or potentiate many of the hallmarks of asthma, specifically induce bronchoconstriction via contraction of airway smooth muscle, enhance vascular permeability, induce migration of inflammatory cells, and stimulate mucous secretion [12, 13].

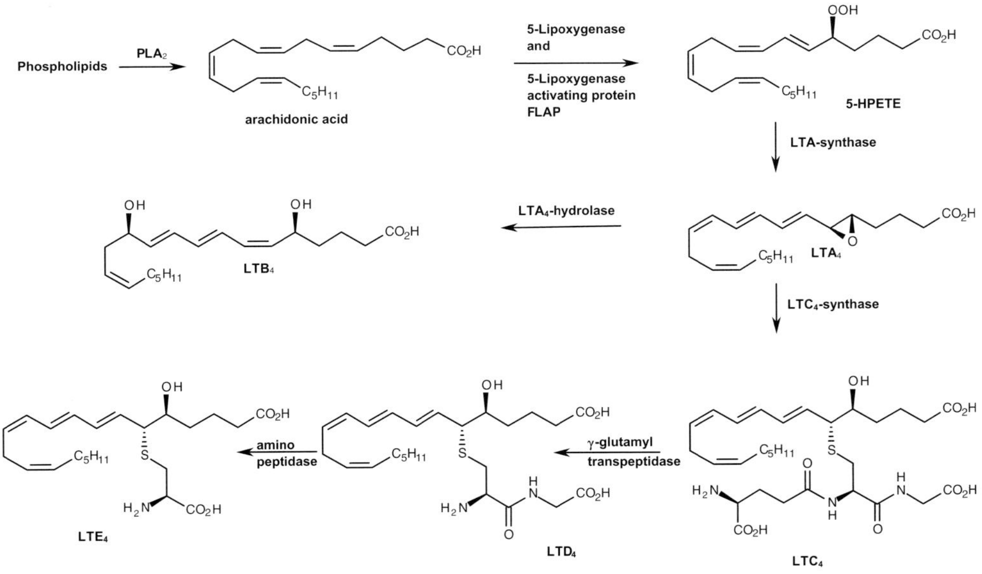

Figure 9.1 Biosynthetic pathway for LT production.

9.2
Scope of the Drug Discovery Effort on Leukotriene Modulators

Inspired by these discoveries, many pharmaceutical companies participated in the race to develop specific leukotriene modulators. Also since the leukotrienes seem to have limited, if any, physiological role and most of their pathophysiology appeared restricted to the lung, it was the goal of most groups to develop orally effective agents. The oral approach would provide a big advantage to patients over existing asthma agents that were given by inhalation, to either limit systemic side effects or because the compounds were not orally bioavailable. Oral dosing would eliminate the complicated parallel development track for the devices (nebulizers or inhalers) needed to deliver inhaled agents. In addition, an oral pill would alleviate the complicated and difficult to learn (patients have to be trained not to swallow the dose) regimens required for the inhaled agents (e.g., x number of puffs/y times per day).

Research focused on biosynthesis inhibitors (either 5-lipoxygenase inhibitors or 5-lipoxygenase activating protein inhibitors) and specific receptor antagonists (either for the cysteinyl leukotrienes or for leukotriene B_4) [14]. Just in the field of cysteinyl leukotriene antagonists, those efforts led to the preparation of tens of thousands of compounds and to dozens of clinical candidates [15–17]. Discussing all of these efforts, even just all of the clinically evaluated antagonists, is beyond the scope of this chapter. However, an excellent review on modulators of leukotriene biosynthesis and receptor activation that had been under clinical evaluation was published by Brooks and Summers [18], just before the approval of zafirlukast for the US market.[2] It is noteworthy that in the area of cysteinyl (or peptidyl as they are also known) leukotriene antagonists, of the 19 compounds for which clinical results are reported in that review only 3 made it to the market. These three compounds, pranlukast (**1**), zafirlukast (**2**), and montelukast (**3**), will be the focus of this chapter (see Figure 9.2).

A cursory examination shows that these compounds do not look at all alike. They were designed independently from each other, so they are not analogues in a chemical sense. However, all of them have a lipophilic region, an acidic group, and have been modeled back to a common cysteinyl leukotriene receptor pharmacophore.

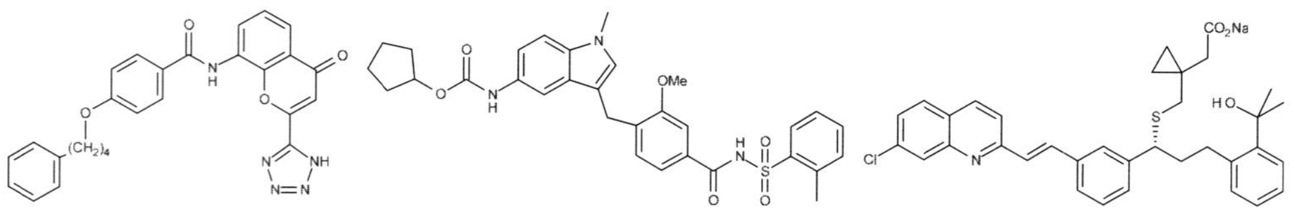

1: ONO-1078, pranlukast

2: ICI 204219, zafirlukast

3: MK-0476, montelukast

Figure 9.2 Clinically registered $CysLT_1R$ antagonists.

2) NME approval date: September 26, 1996.

Since they also share a selective $CysLT_1R$ antagonist profile, they can be considered as pharmacological analogues.

9.3 Synthetic Leukotriene Production and Benefits Derived from this Effort

Just as the effort to clarify the mysteries surrounding SRS-A (its structure, biosynthetic pathway, and molecular targets) had required FPL-55712, the newer effort to develop modulators that would be effective drugs required synthetic leukotrienes. They were needed since preparation and isolation of SRS-A from biogenic sources (primarily chopped sensitized guinea pig lung [19] or rat peritoneal cavity [20]) was inadequate to support the drug discovery and development efforts. As a result of this need, teams at many companies including Merck-Frosst [21], SmithKline [22], Ciba-Geigy [23], Hoffmann-La Roche [24], and Fisons [25] reported alternate syntheses to Corey's original approach.

Some drug discovery teams, such as the ones at SmithKline, Merck-Frosst, and Stuart Pharmaceuticals (Division of ICI Americas Inc.), in addition to developing leukotriene syntheses leveraged their internal chemical success. The team at Merck-Frosst provided many academic labs with synthetic leukotrienes, identified and synthesized metabolites of leukotrienes [26], identified and characterized leukotriene receptors [27], played a key role in the cloning, expression, and characterization of the 5-lipoxygenase enzyme [28], and were the first to identify 5-lipoxygenase activating protein (FLAP) [29, 30], a cofactor necessary for leukotriene synthesis in cells.

The group at ICI determined the relative potencies of leukotriene isomers [31], deduced the solution conformation of the leukotrienes [32], broadly characterized the nature of the leukotriene receptors in animals and humans [33, 34], and collaborated with academic teams on clinical studies of the effects of synthetic leukotrienes in humans [35, 36].

Although the overall scope of these synthetic efforts is not known, the team at ICI alone prepared over 10 g of synthetic leukotrienes, and given the Merck team's provision of material to many labs they too may have prepared equally large or even larger amounts. These stockpiles represented large resource commitment by their companies. Also, since in the early 1980s the going rate to buy samples of the leukotrienes from an academic group was $5000/mg, the commercial value of these reserves was in the many millions of dollars. The per mg price is remarkably consistent with the current commercial price of €3495/mg by Cayman Chemical (quote on 12/04/11).

Utilization of synthetic leukotrienes in humans in the United States required that they be prepared to exacting standards, and that detailed characterization, control, and stability data be generated. In the case of ICI, the synthetic leukotrienes were stored in liquid nitrogen cooled cryogenic storage systems. Although the intermediate LTA_4-methyl ester or protected CysLTs could be stored as oils or as solutions, the final leukotrienes were best stored as lyophilized powders that were reconstituted into a standard strength solution prior to use. Since the CysLTs are naturally amphiphilic substances and since their chemically unstable triene is in the hydrophobic tail, it was critical that transformation of dilute solutions to dry powder be done under conditions that minimized globular micelle formation. Shipment of the powder to the various testing facilities was usually achieved under dry ice cooling.

All of these data were supplied to the FDA in a "Drug Master File" that was submitted by ICI on behalf of the clinical investigators who were doing these studies. Initially, the leukotriene D_4 produced by the chemistry team at ICI was the only source covered by such a Drug Master File. This led to multiple requests for access to their leukotrienes, to support other companies' clinical studies in which LTD_4 would be used as a specific challenge.[3] Although broadly supplying LTD_4 was beyond the ability of the ICI team, the sharing of some experimental protocols was supported[4] and this eventually led to the commercial availability of high-quality synthetic leukotrienes.

The sharing of protocols and data exemplified how, at the time this work was done, the competition between the different research groups was relatively "friendly." Unlike now, when the value of multiple ("me too") drugs working at the same target has been called into question, in the early 1980s the view existed that more than one group could be successful and that there was value to the patient and the physician from them having multiple drugs from which to choose. The apparent lead group (closest to a registered drug) was frequently changing and as will be evident from the discovery story herein the different teams benefited from, and were spurred on by the results published by their competitors. It is hoped that the growing concept of "personalized medicine" that describes at a molecular (genomic) level why patients respond differently to, for example, a specific receptor antagonist will both inspire and support the value of developing multiple similarly targeted drugs, each, however, focused to a more specific subpopulation.

9.4
Bioassays and General Drug Discovery Testing Cascade

The period during which the cysteinyl leukotriene antagonists were developed corresponds to one during which drug discovery testing cascades were rapidly changing. At the beginning of this era, cloned LT receptors (either human or animal) did not exist and isolated tissue binding studies were just being introduced.

As their primary *in vitro* screen, some research teams initially relied on inhibiting the contraction induced in isolated tissues (usually guinea pig ileum strips or

3) Peter Bernstein, Ph.D., personal communication, exemplified by letter from Dr. W.S. Hitchings, Director Control & Manufacturing Data Registration, Merck Sharp & Dohme Research Laboratories to Dr. Bernstein, Stuart Pharmaceuticals, dated June 12, 1985.

4) Tony Kreft, Ph.D., personal communication, exemplified by letter and experimental procedures from Dr. P.R. Bernstein, Stuart Pharmaceuticals to Dr. Tony Kreft, Wyeth Laboratories, dated July 19, 1982.

guinea pig tracheal spirals) by a standardized unit of "SRS-A" that was isolated from a biogenic source. After pure synthetic leukotrienes became available, assays were developed that reported, for example, the % inhibition of the contraction induced by 8 nM LTD_4 on guinea pig tracheal spirals at a specific concentration of drug. For compounds that warranted further evaluation, either IC_{50} values or the calculated pK_B values could be determined in an array of animal and/or human tissues. Comparison of the compound's ability to block the LTD_4- or LTE_4-induced response and its ability to block the response in the same tissue of a different spasmogen (e.g., 1.5 mM $BaCl_2$ on guinea pig tracheal spirals) provided a measure of its specificity as a LT antagonist.

Later, LTD_4 binding assays were developed that measured the displacement of $[^3H]LTD_4$ from tissue membranes [37]. These assays were first done utilizing tissue that naturally included the LT receptors (e.g., guinea pig lung). The Merck efforts discussed in this chapter exemplify this approach as they report inhibition of $[^3H]LTD_4$ binding to guinea pig lung membranes. After cells expressing cloned receptors [38] became available, those were utilized. Studies coincident with the drug development efforts demonstrated the existence of two CysLT receptors designated as $CysLT_1R$ and $CysLT_2R$ both in animals and in humans [39, 40]. The order of binding affinity to the $CysLT_1R$ is $LTD_4 > LTC_4 \gg LTE_4$, whereas the rank order to $CysLT_2R$ is $LTD_4 \sim LTC_4 \gg LTE_4$. The two receptors are distinguished by the fact that the actions of LTD_4 and LTE_4 on $CysLT_1R$ are blocked by FPL-55712, whereas the effect of LTC_4 on $CysLT_2R$ is not blocked by FPL-55712. The antagonists covered in this chapter are all specific $CysLT_1R$ antagonist.

The complexity of this field is such that our understanding of the leukotriene receptors, their distribution, and pathophysiological functions continues to evolve [41]. Exemplifying this, a third CysLT receptor ($CysLT_3R$) was recently proposed [42], to explain biological effects by LTE_4 that are not mediated via the two well-characterized receptors.

The existence of multiple receptors and multiple ligands led to potentially confusing screening cascades. Although all groups did not use the same cascade, the group at ICI chose to use the effect of LTE_4 on guinea pig trachea as their initial primary screen. This was because LTE_4 was selective for one of the two receptors found in that tissue [43] and that receptor had high pharmacological similarity to the single receptor ($CysLT_1R$) found in human bronchus. The role of the human $CysLT_2R$ remains undefined and awaits the clarifying impact that would occur from discovery and development of a selective $CysLT_2R$ antagonist. That these compounds are selective may in part be explained by the fact that there is only 38% amino acid identity between the two receptors [44]. Furthermore, localization studies of the $hCysLT_2R$ show that the highest receptor expression levels occur in adrenal glands, heart, and placenta, indicating that whatever its role is, it is probably not linked to asthma [45].

Initial *in vivo* evaluation of $CysLT_1R$ antagonists was most commonly done in guinea pigs by evaluating their ability to block a leukotriene challenge. The leukotriene could be administered either i.v. or by aerosol and pretreatment by the drug (PO, IP, ID, or IV) would cause a delay in the bronchoconstriction induced by the leukotriene. At first, pulmonary mechanics parameters were measured in anesthetized animals. This model, while very precise, was very labor intensive and required surgically prepared animals. Therefore, to create a higher throughput *in vivo* assay, a "dyspnea" model was developed that measured the ability of compounds to block the induction of "labored abdominal breathing" in conscious guinea pigs by LTD_4 [46].

While being very intensive in the use of both manpower and precious leukotrienes, these *in vivo* assays proved invaluable for the progression of antagonist structure–activity work. Also, as will be discussed in detail later, they helped to bridge gaps in pharmacokinetic knowledge now routinely filled by *in vitro* and *in vivo* DMPK assays.

9.5 Development of Antagonists – General Approaches

In the early 1980s when much of the discovery research on cysteinyl leukotriene antagonists was done, there was little information on the structure of G-protein-coupled receptors such as $CysLT_1R$, the biological target of the cysteinyl leukotrienes. As a result, some modern approaches, such as the building of a model of the receptor and the *de novo* design of ligands to it, were not possible. Similarly, this was before the advent of high-throughput screening or combinatorial (high-throughput or robot-assisted) synthesis. This left chemistry teams with three starting points: synthesizing analogues of FPL-55712, using the structure of the natural leukotrienes as starting points, and the screening of selected compounds in a bioassay. This could be either a binding assay or a functional assay formatted in a way to provide higher throughput, for example, determining if 10 μM compound significantly blocks the contraction induced by 8 nM LTE_4 on guinea pig tracheal spirals.

Although all of these approaches were utilized, structural analogues of FPL-55712 represented the greatest percentage of clinically evaluated compounds [18]. However, none of the three successful products discussed below has much structural resemblance to FPL-55712 (see Figure 9.3).

9.6 Discovery of Zafirlukast

The discovery of zafirlukast has been described in many prior papers and presentations that expand upon the summary given here [14, 47–49]. The team at ICI explored all three possible starting points; however, their efforts on selected screening did not yield useful leads, and it was the combination of output from making analogues of FPL-55712 and of the natural leukotrienes that led to zafirlukast.

In the early 1980s, the newly reinvigorated efforts to prepare improved analogues of FPL-55712 benefited from the researchers knowing the structure of the cysteinyl leukotrienes. At ICI, the team viewed LTD_4 as being made up of three regions:

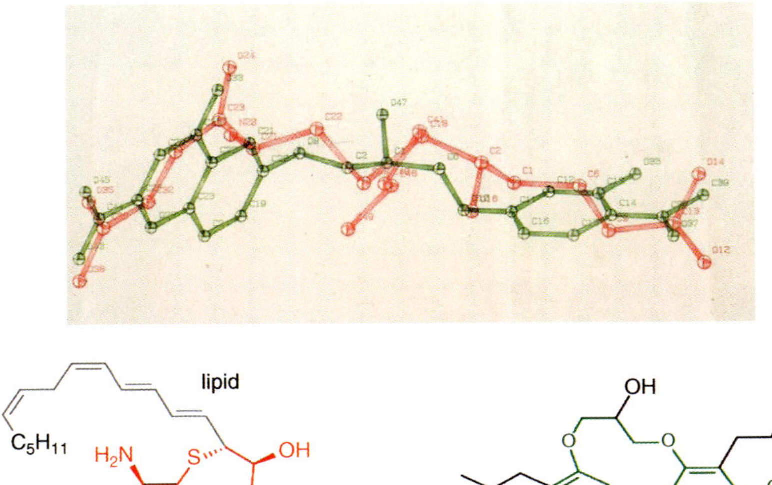

Figure 9.3 Molecular modeling of FPL-55712 and LTD_4.

lipophilic lipid, polar C1 acid, and peptide areas, and that FPL-55712 incorporated two regions: the chromone carboxylic acid and hydroxyacetophenone (HAP). They hypothesized that FPL-55712 was mimicking two of the three regions of LTD_4 with the chromone being a surrogate for the peptide region and that the HAP was mimicking either the lipid backbone or the C1 acid [50]. Early molecular modeling efforts (~1981) were undertaken to illustrate these overlaps (Figure 9.3) [48].

This hypothesis led them to prepare a small set of compounds that linked *either* the chromone carboxylic acid *or* the hydroxyacetophenone portions of FPL-55712 with fragments exemplifying the different regions of LTD_4. That effort led to the discovery that linkage of simple aliphatic acids of six to eight atoms in length to the hydroxyacetophenone afforded leukotriene antagonists of modest potency, for example, **4** (Figure 9.4). Given the well-exemplified path of improving potency by introducing structural constraints that preorganize a compound into an orientation preferred at a receptor [51], a series of aryl groups were explored as replacements for the aliphatic chain. This led to the discovery that a *para*-toluic acid analogue **5** was slightly more potent. Further SAR exploration in this aryl series led to the discovery that a 3-methoxy substituent **6** yielded greater *in vitro* potency and selectivity, and demonstrated *in vivo* activity when administered i.p.

Simultaneously, the ICI team also explored preparation of antagonists using the structure of LTC_4 as their starting point (Figure 9.5). Support for this approach was provided by the success of many efforts to prepare receptor antagonists by starting

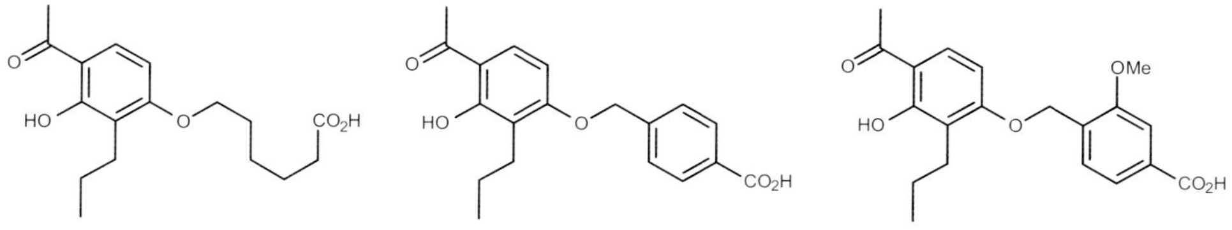

4: Inhibition 52% at 10 μM

5: Inhibition 100% at 10 μM

6: Inhibition 57% at 1 μM
Selectivity vs. $BaCl_2$: 50
Active *in vivo:* when administered intraperitoneally 50 mg/kg, 60 min before LTD_4 challenge

Figure 9.4 FPL-55712-derived compounds at ICI.

with the structure of their natural ligand, for example, H_2 antagonists from histamine or β-adrenergic blockers from epinephrine. However, unlike those earlier examples the teams trying to develop CysLT receptor antagonists also had to address the extreme biological and chemical lability of the leukotrienes.

Since ^{1}H-nuclear magnetic resonance studies done as part of their leukotriene synthesis and characterization efforts [32] had indicated that the triene region of the lipid backbone preferred a coplanar conformation, the ICI team explored replacement of the unstable triene with a series of aryl groups. This led to the discovery of potent (nM level) agonists, for example, **7**, with much greater chemical stability [52]. Detailed pharmacological studies showed that the effects induced by these compounds were specifically antagonized by FPL-55712, affirming that they were acting at the cysteinyl leukotriene receptor [53]. Replacement of the peptide

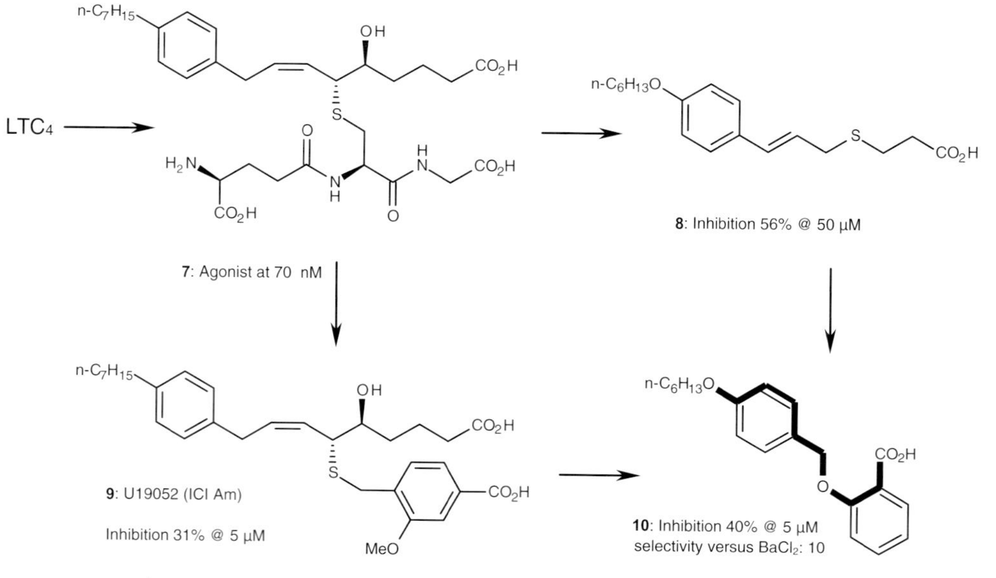

LTC_4 →

7: Agonist at 70 nM

8: Inhibition 56% @ 50 μM

9: U19052 (ICI Am)

Inhibition 31% @ 5 μM

10: Inhibition 40% @ 5 μM
selectivity versus $BaCl_2$: 10

Figure 9.5 Leukotriene D_4-derived compounds.

region in these analogues with the aliphatic and aryl acidic groups that had been found in the hydroxyacetophenone effort [50] led to compounds that had a range of agonist and antagonist properties [54]. One of the more potent antagonists **9**, U19052, was broadly characterized as a specific antagonist of LTC_4, LTD_4, and LTE_4: it had a pK_B value of 7.2 against LTD_4- or LTE_4-induced contraction of isolated guinea pig ileum. However, these compounds demonstrated a very delicate balance between agonist and antagonist activity. Minor changes in their structures, for example, replacement of the n-C_7H_{15}-aryl substituent in U19052 with n-$C_6H_{13}O$-, resulted in agonist activity. Weaker but consistent antagonist activity was found upon removal of one of the two acidic regions [49]. The SAR of this simpler bis-aromatic series, exemplified by **8**, was broadly explored and optimal potency was found when the two ether groups were *para* to one another and the carboxylic acid was *ortho* to the ether linkage, for example, **10**. For example, moving the carboxylic acid in **10** to the *para*-position resulted in ~10-fold decrease in potency.

Although these bis-aryl antagonists represented great structural simplification and improvement in stability compared to the starting leukotrienes, they were also several orders of magnitude weaker at the leukotriene receptor than LTC_4. As had been demonstrated previously in the effort on FPL-55712-derived compounds, one way to enhance potency is by decreasing flexibility and locking the compound into an orientation preferred by the receptor. To achieve this in this series, various bicyclic frameworks were considered, and due to a combination of synthetic considerations and commercial availability nitroindazole was chosen as the starting material (Figure 9.6). To explore this concept, eight regioisomeric indazoles **11** were prepared, with the linkage positions indicated by the asterisks. Of these compounds only one, the *para*-benzoic acid **12**, was an antagonist at 10 μM. This was both surprising and perplexing since the bis-aryl series that was the starting point for them had demonstrated a clear preference for the *ortho*-benzoic acid. However, such *para*-benzoic acid derivatives had been optimal both in the original leukotriene analogues (those with three regions) and in the HAP series. Consideration of this fact and comparison of potential overlaps between the series led to the suggestion to add back in the methoxy substituent that had been beneficial in those earlier series. Since only the N_1-alkylated indazole had been active, this modification was done in the corresponding indole series. This was to avoid having to separate the mixture of N_1- and N_2-substituted compounds that were formed during the alkylation step

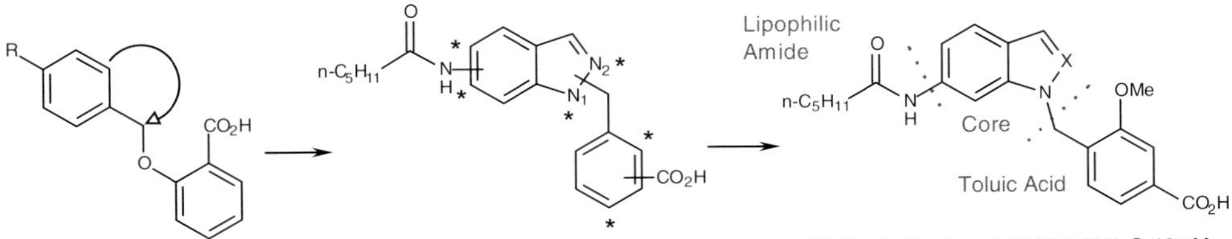

10: R = $_nC_6H_{13}O$-

11

Lipophilic Amide, Core, Toluic Acid

12: X = N R = H Inhibition 60% @ 10 μM
13: X = CH R = OMe Inhibition 70% @ 5 μM
Selectivity vs. $BaCl_2$: 100

Figure 9.6 Discovery of the indazole/indole series by imposing structural rigidity.

in the indazoles. The resultant compound **13**, although slightly weaker than the most potent HAP derivative **6**, was surprisingly more selective for the leukotriene receptor (100 versus 50).

At this point, the team concentrated its efforts on this indole series. In addition to the improved selectivity of the indoles, efforts to improve potency in either of the earlier series were not efficiently progressing and the indoles represented a novel structural type of leukotriene antagonist. In contrast, both FPL-55712- and LT-derived antagonists were being worked on by many other groups.

Consideration of what needed to be achieved in their exploration of structure–activity relationships, in combination with a synthetic analysis, led to the indole antagonist being viewed as composed of three regions: the lipophilic amide, the core heterocycle, and the toluic acid.

Exploration of the amide substituent (Figure 9.7) revealed that branching of the aliphatic chain resulted in increased *in vitro* potency, with the α-ethyl-hexanamide **14** also demonstrating oral activity at 100 mg/kg in the guinea pig labored abdominal breathing model [55]. However, β-branched amides with cyclic end cap groups proved the most potent. The exploration also revealed that the carbon α to the amide carbonyl could be replaced with either O or N resulting in carbamates or ureas that retained excellent *in vitro* activity. Such β-cyclic compounds, for example, **16** and **17**, were almost 100-fold more potent *in vitro* than the initial hexanamide. At ICI Pharmaceuticals, this was an exciting find, breaking the plateau of 1 μM antagonism, after having worked in the area for several years.

Simultaneous to the exploration of the amide substituents, a second set of explorations was underway on the acid region of the molecule [56]. Those efforts were in part inspired by efforts at Lilly that had shown in a set of HAP-derived leukotriene

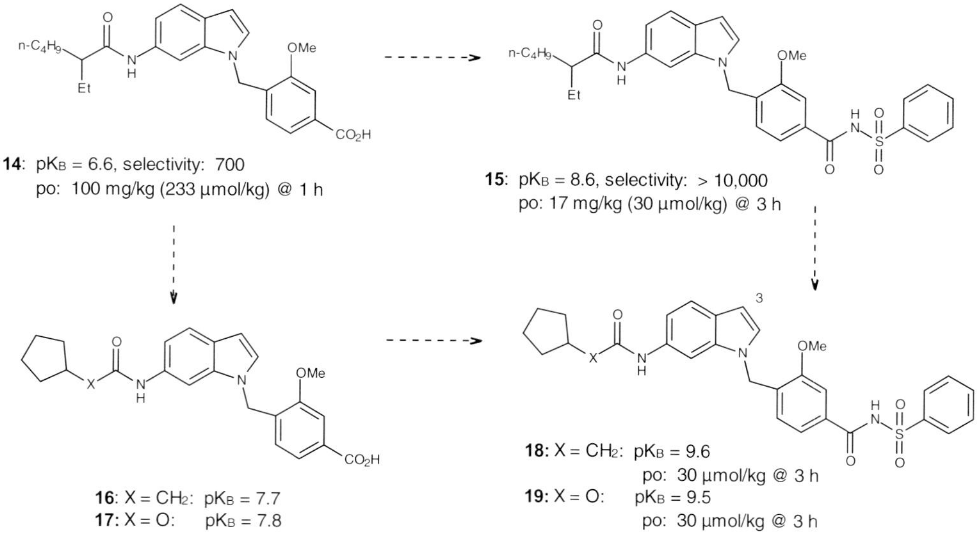

14: pK_B = 6.6, selectivity: 700
po: 100 mg/kg (233 μmol/kg) @ 1 h

15: pK_B = 8.6, selectivity: > 10,000
po: 17 mg/kg (30 μmol/kg) @ 3 h

16: X = CH_2: pK_B = 7.7
17: X = O: pK_B = 7.8

18: X = CH_2: pK_B = 9.6
po: 30 μmol/kg @ 3 h
19: X = O: pK_B = 9.5
po: 30 μmol/kg @ 3 h

Figure 9.7 Exploration of the acid and amide regions.

antagonists that replacement of a carboxylic acid with a tetrazole resulted in a 30-fold increase in potency, *in vitro*, and led to the clinical candidate LY-171883 [57]. The importance of the discovery and development of this compound by J. Fleisch, W. Marshall, and their colleagues is hard to overstate. It was the first major improvement over FPL-55712 and highlighted the importance of the nature of the acid group to activity. The ICI team confirmed that the 3-methoxy-*p*-toluic acid was the optimal aryl acid in this indole series and discovered that while the impact of replacing the acid with tetrazole or most other carboxylic acid mimetics was small, the use of phenylsulfonimide mimetics afforded an additional 100-fold increase in potency, *in vitro*, for example, **15**. The results also demonstrated a consistent cross-over of the impact on potency of changes in the different regions of the molecules. Specifically, acid replacements that improved *in vitro* or *in vivo* potency in compounds with one amide substituent had a similar effect with a different amide substituent, **18** and **19**. Simultaneous to this, the team noted that these compounds were only mimicking two of the three regions of the natural leukotrienes. They postulated that addition of a second polar group would increase potency [58]. Substitution at the 3-position of the 1,6-substituted indole of **18** did result in increased *in vitro* potency, but not an equivalent increase in oral potency (compound not shown). This provided support for how these compounds were being recognized by the receptor, but was not a route to a better oral drug.

Turning back to the core heterocyclic structure, it was shown that variation of the core resulted in significant changes in potency both *in vitro* and *in vivo* (Figure 9.8) [59]. However, a disconnect existed between the results in that the cores that were most potent *in vitro*, for example, **20** and **21**, were not the most potent when given orally, for example, **22**. At the time, the reason for this disconnect was not understood and an indazole **20** (ICI-198615) was initially considered a potential clinical candidate because of its *in vitro* potency and its robust oral efficacy. Subsequent detailed pharmacokinetic studies with ICI-198615 demonstrated less than 0.3% oral bioavailability, demonstrating an issue in spite of its oral efficacy. In the absence of routine DMPK assays, the team chose to use the PO/IV ratio in the dyspnea model as a surrogate for oral bioavailability and focused on obtaining compounds with low PO/IV ratios. Analysis of the data indicated that the

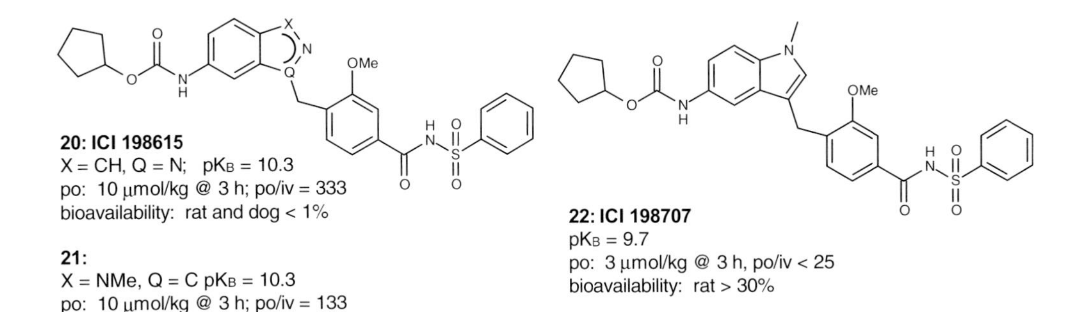

Figure 9.8 Comparison of different core structures.

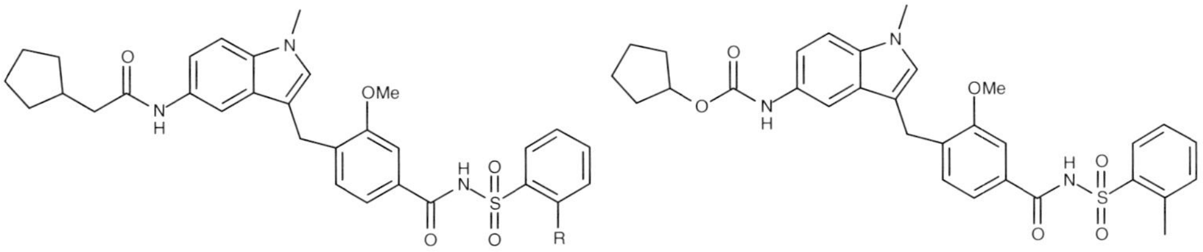

23: R = H; pK_B = 9.6, po: 30 μmol/kg @ 3 h
24: R = CH_3: pK_B = 9.9, po: 1 μmol/kg @ 3 h
25: R = Cl: pK_B = 9.8, po: 3 μmol/kg @ 3 h

26: ICI 204219; zafirlukast
pK_B = 9.7, po: 0.52 μmol/kg @ 3 h
bioavailability: rat (68%), dog (67%)

Figure 9.9 Optimization of the sulfonamide and discovery of zafirlukast.

"inverted" indole core was more effective than the other cores in translating *in vitro* potency into *in vivo* efficacy.

Further studies on variation of the substitution pattern of the phenylsulfonimide (Figure 9.9) showed that although potency *in vitro* was largely unchanged by substituents on the phenyl ring, for example, **23**, **24**, and **25**, there was a marked effect on oral potency. In the amide-linked series, the 2-methylphenyl-substituted analogue **24** was approximately 30 times more potent orally than the parent phenyl **23** despite being less than twofold more potent *in vitro*. Application of this finding in the carbamate-linked series led to **26** (ICI 204219, zafirlukast) [60]. Zafirlukast was confirmed to have high bioavailability in the rats (68%) and dogs (67%).

Although the total number of compounds prepared and/or tested in the development of zafirlukast is not available, some statistics have been reported. The ICI LT antagonist effort started in September 1980 and ICI 204219 was nominated for development in early 1986. The chemistry team that did both the LT synthesis effort and the LT antagonist SAR studies ranged from 3 to 10 chemists in size. During its most rapid progress, the team increased potency by five orders of magnitude, from the first indazole **12** to picomolar antagonists such as **20** and **22**, in approximately 15 months. This too was exciting and quite remarkable, given the 1 μM potency plateau that the team had struggled to surmount for several years!

9.7 Discovery of Montelukast

The discovery and development of montelukast sodium has been summarized in many prior presentations and papers [14, 61, 62].[5] The Merck-Frosst team also used all three of the previously listed approaches for lead generation. In their case, in spite of their extensive synthetic leukotriene efforts, little is known about the work they did to develop antagonists starting directly from the structure of the natural leukotrienes. However, starting from FPL-77512 they developed several agents

5) For a series of video presentations by Merck-Frosst scientists on the discovery and development of montelukast sodium, see http://aboutdrugdiscovery.ca/en/main_ENG_short.html (accessed October 29, 2011).

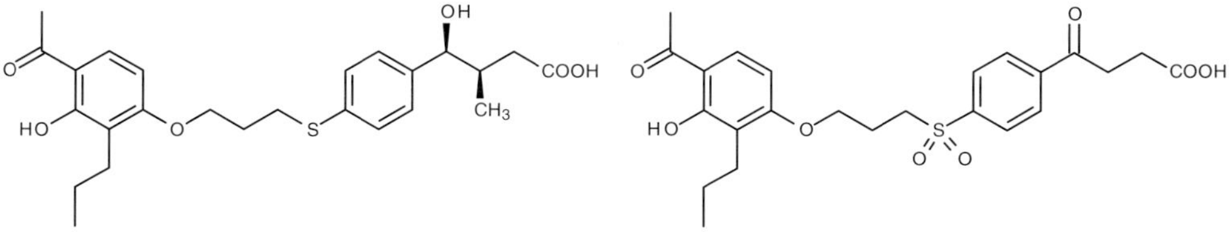

27: L-649923 K_i = 400 nM vs LTD_4

28: L-648051 K_i = 6200 nM vs LTD_4

Figure 9.10 FPL-derived clinical candidates developed at Merck-Frosst.

(Figure 9.10) that entered development and were evaluated in humans, including **27** (L-649923) and **28** (L-648051) [63, 64]. Although progression of these compounds was terminated and they do not appear to have provided SAR data used in the montelukast series, they provided limited support to the hypothesis linking leukotrienes to asthma. (*Note*: All Merck activity data are reported as binding of $[^3H]LTD_4$ to guinea pig lung membranes.)

As a second starting point (Figure 9.11), the team used a broad screening effort that found a styryl quinoline **29** [65]. It is not clear how many compounds were evaluated to come up with this lead, but it is safe to presume that this included many of 15 000 compounds that were reported as being evaluated at Merck as $CysLT_1R$ antagonists over the course of their research program.[5)] In trying to understand how this lead might be binding to the $CysLT_1$ receptor, the Merck team applied an analysis they had done of leukotriene receptor structure–activity studies. That analysis had led to a hypothetical model for the LTD_4 receptor that had three regions: a planar hydrophilic region for the triene, an ionic hydrophilic site for one of the carboxylates of LTD_4, and a second hydrophilic (polar) binding site [66]. Fitting this compound **29** to this model implied that it was binding to the part of the receptor that recognized the flat triene region of LTD_4, and that polar substitution at the 3-position would be beneficial. Independent support for the compound binding in such a way was provided by the greater potency of a related compound, **30** (REV-5901) [67]. REV-5901 exemplified a second series of quinoline-based LTD_4 antagonists [68] that had been independently discovered and that were eventually abandoned. Furthermore, it is not known if the data on these quinolines played any role in selecting what sets of compounds were included in the Merck-Frosst screening efforts.

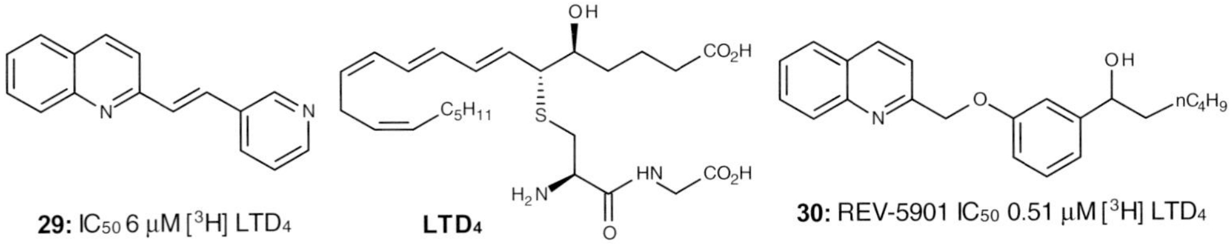

29: IC_{50} 6 μM $[^3H]$ LTD_4

LTD4

30: REV-5901 IC_{50} 0.51 μM $[^3H]$ LTD_4

Figure 9.11 Quinolinyl hits and comparison to the structure of LTD_4.

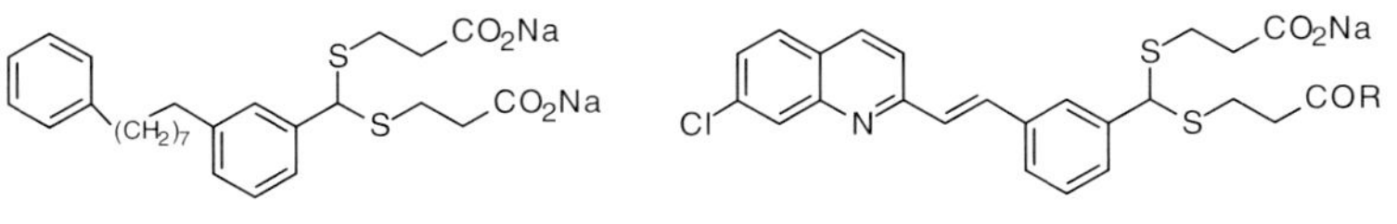

31: SK&F 102922
K_i = 225 nM vs. [^{3}H] LTD_4

32: R = ONa IC_{50} = 3.0 ± 1.4 nM
33: MK-0571, R = NMe_2 IC_{50} = 0.8 ± 0.6 nM

Figure 9.12 Genesis of the aryl acid substituent.

As a polar substituent, the Merck team added two acidic groups to their styryl quinoline core via a dithioacetal linker (Figure 9.12). This unit was based on SK&F 102922 (**31**), a compound that had been discovered at SmithKline during their development of antagonists starting from the structure of LTD_4 [69]. Extensive SAR studies on this series at Merck-Frosst showed that the styryl linker [–CH=CH–] could be replaced with the CH_2O linker found in the Revlon series with only a slight decrease in potency and highlighted the importance of the quinoline group. Replacement of the quinoline with a naphthalene led to almost complete loss of binding (not illustrated), whereas incorporation of a 7-chloro substituent led to **32**, a compound that displayed a further 10-fold increase in activity in the *in vitro* binding assay. Unfortunately, the increased *in vivo* efficacy of **32** did not equal the degree of increase seen *in vitro*. The Merck team postulated that this was due to poor physicochemical and DMPK properties by **32** and that this diacid might be too polar. Based on work done on LTD_4 that had shown that activity was retained if one of the acids was replaced with an amide [70], they explored monoamide derivatives and discovered **33** (MK-0571), which was nominated for further development.

During toxicological studies, this racemic compound was found to be a potent inducer of liver peroxisomal enzymes. It was then determined that its *R*-enantiomer **34** (MK-0679, verlukast) retained most of the LT antagonist activity (Figure 9.13) and had an improved safety profile (liver weight increase of

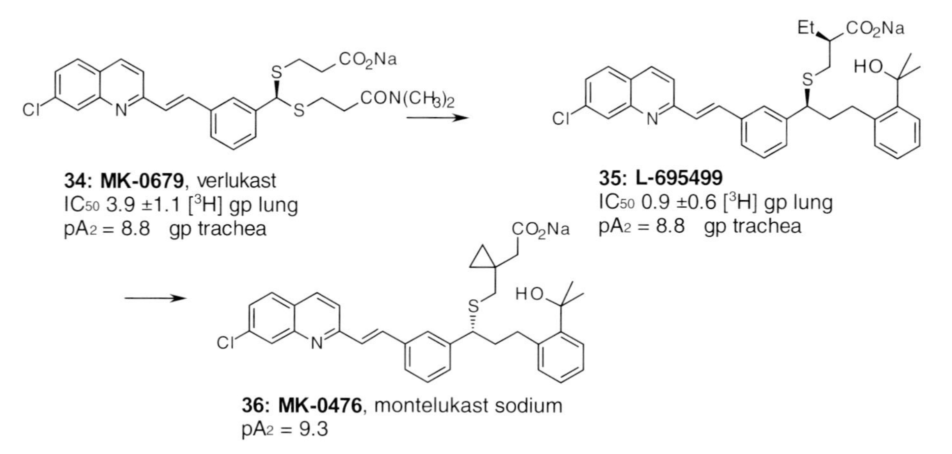

Figure 9.13 Verlukast to montelukast.

0% versus 38%) [71]. Development of MK-0679 was also terminated when extended studies showed that it too induced liver function abnormalities. Efforts to retain the leukotriene antagonist activity while separating out the liver effects focused on replacement of one of the thioether chains. In addition, since peroxisomes recognize and β-oxidize fatty acids, substituents blocking the acid chain metabolism were explored and those studies led to **35** (L-695499) [72]. This compound unfortunately had acute toxicity in mice at high doses [73]. Further studies on the impact of the thioether stereochemistry to both toxicity and LT efficacy along with additional acid chain substituents led to the discovery that extending the aliphatic acid chain length and blocking the carboxylate β-position via either dimethyl substitution or cyclopropanation afforded potent orally active leukotriene D_4 antagonists that were devoid of peroxisomal enzyme induction. The choice of **36** (MK-0476) for clinical development was due to its superior DMPK parameters [71, 74].

9.8 Discovery of Pranlukast

The effort to develop pranlukast has been reported to start with **37** (Figure 9.14) [75, 76]. How this weak antagonist was found at Ono, whether it was specifically prepared or was a hit in a screen, is not clear. The team has reported that they used both the structure of the leukotrienes and results found in other series of leukotriene antagonists in their effort to improve the potency of this lead. Notably, they felt that both the cysteinyl leukotrienes and **37** each had hydrophobic and hydrophilic regions. They postulated that in **37** the *p*-*n*-pentyl-cinnamyl and the anthranilate regions were, respectively, mimicking the lipophilic triene and the combined C_1 carboxylic acid–peptide region of the CysLTs.

Exploration of the carboxylate region (varying linker length and type) in **37** did not yield significant improvements in activity until a carboxylate **38** was replaced with tetrazole **39** (Figure 9.15). Then, as had been precedented by the work leading to LY-171883 [57], potency of **39** versus **38** increased, both *in vitro* and *in vivo*. Simultaneous to this (and similar to the reasoning at ICI), the team chose to preorganize

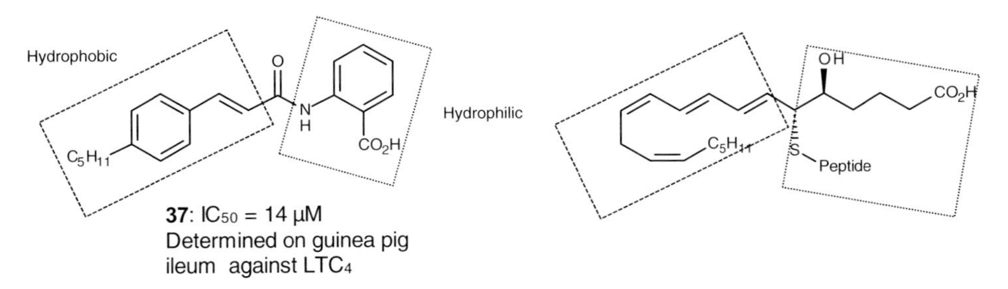

Figure 9.14 Ono screening hit and its comparison to the cysteinyl leukotrienes.

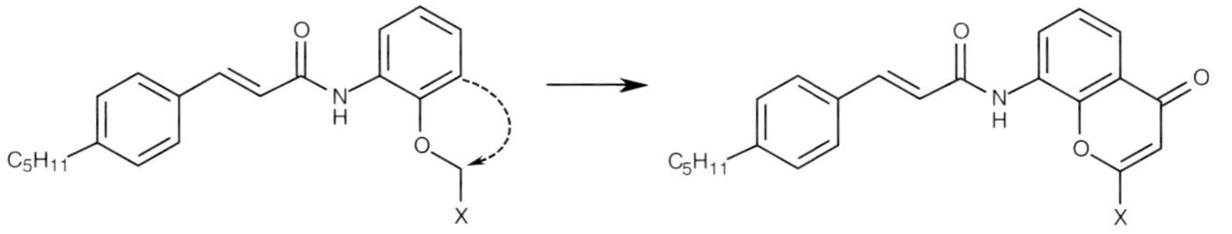

38: X = CO_2H IC_{50} = 9 μM
39: X = Tetrazole IC_{50} = 3 μM

40: X = CO_2H IC_{50} = 0.1 μM
41: X = Tetrazole IC_{50} = 0.03 μM

Figure 9.15 The impact of structural preorganization on potency for the Ono lead.

the orientation of the aliphatic acid chain by locking it into various ring systems. This led to the discovery that a chromone ring (similar to that found in FPL-55712) was the optimal group and that the increased potency of tetrazole versus carboxylic acid carried over to the cyclic system, **41** versus **40**. Given the multiple ring systems explored by the Ono team, it is not clear whether the choice of a chromone was inspired by FPL-55712.

Next variations of the lipophilic region were explored (Figure 9.16) and it was confirmed that *para*-substitution of the aryl group was best, but that alkoxy chains were more potent than the corresponding alkyl chain. Furthermore, deleting the styryl link between the aryl group and the carboxamide combined with increasing the length of the *para* chain resulted in maximum antagonism, **42** and **43**. Then, replacement of the terminal part of the chain with a phenyl ring combined with varying the length of the linker to optimize activity afforded **44** (ON-RS 411, ONO-1078, pranlukast).

Support for the original design hypothesis was provided by a detailed QSAR analysis of the benzamide series (Figure 9.17) by an academic group [77]. Their modeling suggested the overlap of LTE_4 and ONO-1078 shown in Figure 9.1. They suggested that much like had been found in the SKF (and ICI) work on LT analogues that agonist activity required two acidic groups and that this was why YM-17690 (**45**), a related compound reported by a team at Yamanouchi, was an agonist.

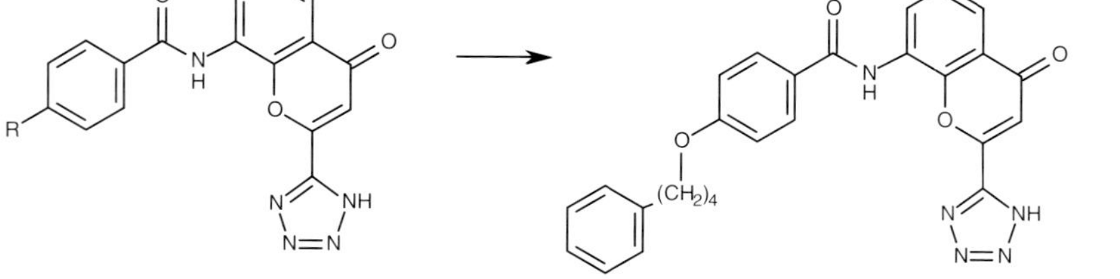

42: R = $_nC_7H_{15}$- IC_{50} = 4.2 nM
43: R = $_nC_7H_{15}O$- IC_{50} = 0.5 nM

44: ONO-1078, pranlukast IC_{50} = 0.044 nM

Figure 9.16 Impact of varying the amide region.

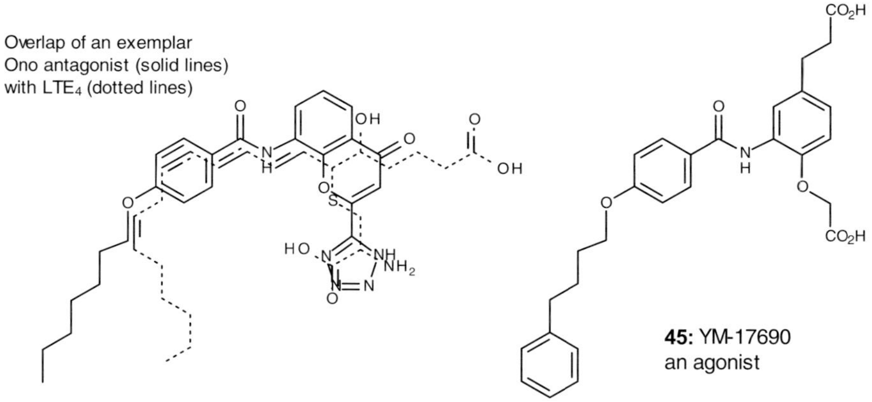

Figure 9.17 Postulated overlap of the amino-chromone series and LTE_4. Figure adapted from illustration in Ref. [77].

9.9
Comparative Analysis and Crossover Impact

All three of the marketed agents are potent, selective, orally active, $CysLT_1R$ antagonists that, since they neither look like – nor were derived from – each other, are pharmacological and not chemical analogues. However, they are all amphiphilic compounds with distinct lipophilic and acidic regions.

Their rank order of potency (see Table 9.1) varies depending on which criteria are used. For functional *in vitro* efficacy (inhibition of Ca^{2+} mobilization), the order is pranlukast > zafirlukast ≫ montelukast; for *in vitro* binding to the $hCysLT_1R$, it is zafirlukast ≥ pranlukast ~ montelukast, whereas for clinical efficacy [daily dose] it is montelukast > zafirlukast ≫ pranlukast. These results indicate that

Table 9.1 Comparison of clinical agents.

	Montelukast sodium	Zafirlukast	Pranlukast
IC_{50} (nM) inh. of LTD_4-induced Ca^{2+} in HEK-293-CysLTR cells [38]	2.3	0.26	0.1
IC_{50} (nM) inh. of LTD_4 binding in HEK-293-CysLTR cells [38]	4.9 ± 1.2	1.8 ± 0.7	4.4 ± 0.9
Recommended adult dose	10 mg q.d.	20 mg b.i.d.	225 mg b.i.d.
Food interaction in label	No	Yes	Yes
MW	585 (as free acid)	575	480
clogP (ACD)	7.8	6.15	3.77
Plasma protein binding	>99 [80]	>99 [80]	>98.9 [81]
Rule of 5 violations	2	2	0

a disconnection exists between *in vitro* and *in vivo* potency. This can be fully explained only by a detailed DMPK analysis that is beyond the scope of this work. In part, this differential translation may be explained by their protein binding. The impact of plasma protein binding (PPB) on relative *in vivo* efficacy had been underappreciated at the time of the $CysLT_1R$ discovery effort, but has since been highlighted [78]. Since all three are $>\sim 99\%$ bound, differences in the reported PPB values do not explain the divergence. However, it is possible that *M* is $\sim 99.1\%$ bound, whereas the other two agents are $>99.9\%$ bound and this would then impact their relative potency. Support for this possibility is provided by a second set of $hCysLT_1R$ binding studies that described the impact of the addition of 0.06% human serum albumin (HSA) [79]. In that study, the IC_{50} (nM) values for montelukast/pranlukast/zafirlukast change upon addition of HSA from 3.3/5.6/2.2 to 1.9/72/5.4. The latter numbers roughly approximate the ratios of their orally efficacious doses in humans.

In contrast to montelukast and zafirlukast, only pranlukast, which is by far the least potent orally, meets Lipinski's "rule of 5" for orally efficacious agents [82]. Both montelukast and zafirlukast fail due to their MW and extremely high lipophilicity. Given that "rule of 5" violations do not preclude oral efficacy but rather indicate it is less likely, and that most of the other clinically tested but failed $CysLT_1R$ antagonists reported in the review by Brooks and Summers [18] do fail, these two compounds are "exceptions" for unknown reasons.

Montelukast, unlike zafirlukast or pranlukast, is indicated for once-daily dosing. However, it should be noted that the full prescribing information states "once daily in the evening".[6] This is an important distinction because asthma is a diurnal disease and many individuals suffer from nocturnal asthma, or asthma worsening overnight. The importance of the time of dose for asthma medications was first demonstrated in a key study on oral corticosteroid treatment [83]. Oral corticosteroids are considered the most effective antiasthmatic agents, used for the most difficult cases. This study showed that oral prednisolone was only effective once daily when taken at 15:00 h. When it was taken at either 08:00 or 20:00 h, it was not effective once daily.

Although the three agents discussed in this chapter are pharmacological and not chemical analogues, the efforts by each of the teams and also by groups that did not produce a clinically registered compound did impact their development. Following the limited clinical efficacy demonstrated by LY-171883 and L-648051 (**28**), doubts about the role of cysteinyl leukotrienes in asthma slowed the development of ICI-204219 (**26**). Then, the clinical results with MK-0571 (**33**) showed clear efficacy for a $CysLT_1R$ antagonist in asthma. Since by many measures ICI-204219 was superior to MK-0571 (intrinsic potency and projected clinical dose), this reinvigorated its development program. Similarly, when first MK-0571 and

6) Singulair® (montelukast sodium) prescribing information. Available at http://www.accessdata.fda.gov/drugsatfda_docs/label/2011/020829s057,020830s059,021409s034lbl.pdf (accessed November 9, 2011).

then its single isomer MK-0679 (**34**) both raised liver safety concerns in late-stage studies, there was concern at Merck over whether the "right compound" could be found. Then, the results of ICI-204219 clinical studies became available and they inspired Merck to continue to seek an agent that could be superior by needing only once-daily dosing.

That only 3 of the 19 clinical candidates reported in the review by Brooks made it to the market illustrates how difficult it was to successfully develop $CysLT_1R$ antagonists. The lack of information on why many compounds were stopped in development precludes a detailed analysis of the causes. However, the fact that two of the three registered compounds violate the "rule of 5" implies that competitive antagonists of the $CysLT_1R$ may populate the region of medicinal chemistry that is relatively "unfriendly" to orally active agents. Also, several of the compounds reported were being developed via aerosol administration, so the success of the oral agents would have negatively impacted the commercial viability of this subset.

9.10 Postmarketing Issues

In February 1998, a report described eosinophilia following corticosteroid withdrawal in patients with asthma receiving zafirlukast [84]. The report proposed that the eosinophilia represented a type of Churg–Strauss syndrome (CSS) that might be linked to antileukotriene therapy and/or zafirlukast specifically. CSS is a rare but serious vasculitis that is considered to develop in a phasic pattern over time, which can initially present as asthma [85]. Because of the seriousness of this disease and the potential for rare side effects to be uncovered only after a drug has gone out to a larger population, significant effort has gone into clarifying the relationship between $CysLT_1R$ antagonist therapy and CSS.[7] Following this initial report, there have been numerous additional reports associating not only zafirlukast, but also montelukast and pranlukast to CSS [86]. By 2002, the data appeared to be most consistent with the association being the unmasking of a previously contained condition, or that it was part of the natural progression of the disease that had occurred because the use of $CysLT_1R$ antagonists allowed the avoidance of systemic steroids [86]. This viewpoint was strengthened by the association of newer high-potency inhaled corticosteroids (e.g., fluticasone), that also allowed for reduction in systemic corticosteroids, with cases of CSS [86]. By 2005, the data had swung back to being suggestive of a causal linkage, but not a definitive association, between $CysLT_1R$ antagonist therapy and development of CSS [85]. The complexity of the question is indicated by the fact that at this time, more than 10 years since the first report, the potential association remains unclear [87]. FDA approved

7) A search of the PubMed database for "Churg–Strauss and leukotriene" on November 9, 2011, resulted in 129 publications.

prescribing information for the two agents available in the United States, zafirlukast[8] and montelukast;[6] both cite the presentation of eosinophilia consistent with Churg–Strauss in their "warnings" sections.

More perplexing, both zafirlukast and montelukast have been associated with neuropsychiatric events (e.g., depression) and list this in the "warnings" sections of their prescribing information. The linkage between $CysLT_1R$ antagonist therapy and neuropsychiatric events is even less clear than that for CSS. This is because neither agent is thought to cross the blood–brain barrier and therefore any effect would need to be indirectly mediated. However, the potential linkage to leukotriene modulation is indicated by the fact that when the FDA asked for this warning it also asked for a similar change in the label for zileuton,[9] the only clinically approved LT biosynthesis inhibitor (a 5-LO inhibitor).

While the labels for both zafirlukast and montelukast list liver injury in their "adverse reactions" sections, zafirlukast also includes hepatoxicity in its "warnings" section.

9.11 Conclusions

Multiple studies have concluded that introduction of the $CysLT_1R$ antagonist class of medications has been of significant benefit to the treatment of asthma. Like all other antiasthma treatments, there is variability of response to them, across broad patient groups. Despite efforts to more accurately define good responders, the only definitive conclusion is that individuals with aspirin-induced asthma tend to be very strong responders. Exploration of the potential utility of these agents in other diseases has led to the licensing of montelukast for the treatment of rhinitis. The potential role for antagonists of the $CysLT_2R$ and the potential role for a $CysLT_3R$ remain areas of active research.

Acknowledgment

The author thanks Dr. Fred J. Brown (AstraZeneca, retired) for his careful proofreading of this chapter.

Disclaimer

The opinions expressed are those of the author alone based on the listed citations. They do not represent the opinion of, or an endorsement by, his former employer, AstraZeneca Pharmaceuticals.

8) Accolate® (zafirlukast) prescribing information. Available at http://www.accessdata.fda.gov/drugsatfda_docs/label/2011/020547s031lbl.pdf (accessed November, 2011).
9) FDA warning update. Available at http://www.fda.gov/drugs/drugsafety/postmarketdrugsafetyinformationforpatientsandproviders/drugsafetyinformationforheathcareprofessionals/ucm165489.htm (accessed November 10, 2011).

References

1. Jones, T.R. and Rodger, I.W. (1999) Role of leukotrienes and leukotriene receptor antagonists in asthma. *Pulm. Pharmacol. Ther.*, **12**, 107–110.
2. Bernstein, P.R. (1992) Antiasthmatic agents, in *Kirk-Othmer's Encyclopedia of Chemical Technology*, vol. **2**, 4th edn, John Wiley & Sons, Inc., New York, pp. 830–854.
3. Montuschi, P. (2008) Leukotrienes, antileukotrienes and asthma. *Mini-Rev. Med. Chem.*, **8**, 1–10.
4. Montuschi, P. and Peters-Golden, M.L. (2010) Leukotriene modifiers for asthma treatment. *Clin. Exp. Allergy*, **40**, 1732–1741.
5. Kellaway, C.H. and Trethewie, E.R. (1940) The liberation of a slow reacting substance, smooth muscle stimulating substance in anaphylaxis. *Q. J. Exp. Physiol.*, **30**, 121–145.
6. Augstein, J., Farmer, J.B., Lee, T.B., Sheard, P., and Tattersall, M.L. (1973) Selective inhibitor of slow-reacting substance of anaphylaxis. *Nat. New Biol.*, **245**, 215–217.
7. Shapiro, G.G. and Konig, P. (1985) Cromolyn sodium: a review. *Pharmacotherapy*, **5** (3), 156–170.
8. Sheard, P., Lee, T.B., and Tattersall, M.L. (1977) Further studies on the SRS-A antagonist FPL 55712. *Monographs in Allergy: Mediators of Immediate Type Inflammatory Reaction, 11th Symposium of the Collegium Internationale Allergologicum*, vol. 12, pp. 245–249.
9. Piper, P.J. (1984) Biological actions of the leukotrienes, in *The Leukotrienes Chemistry and Biology* (eds L.W. Chakrin and D.M. Bailey), Academic Press, New York, pp. 215–230.
10. Murphy, R.C., Hammarström, S., and Samuelsson, B. (1979) Leukotriene C: a slow reacting substance from murine mastocytoma cells. *Proc. Natl. Acad. Sci. USA*, **76**, 4275–4279.
11. Drazen, J.M., Austen, K.F., Lewis, R.A., Clark, D.A., Goto, G., Marfat, A., and Corey, E.J. (1980) Comparative airway and vascular activity of leukotriene C-1 and D *in vivo* and *in vitro*. *Proc. Natl. Acad. Sci. USA*, **77**, 4345–4358.
12. Marom, Z., Shelhamer, J.H., Bach, M.K., Morton, D.R., and Kaliner, M. (1982) Slow-reacting substances, leukotriene C4and D4 increase the release of mucus from human airways. *Am. Rev. Respir. Dis.*, **126**, 449–451.
13. Barnes, N.C., Piper, P.J., and Costello, J.F. (1984) Comparative actions of inhaled leukotriene C4, leukotriene D4 and histamine in normal human subjects. *Thorax*, **39**, 500–504.
14. Bernstein, P.R., Bird, T.G., and Brewster, A.G. (1997) Agents affecting the actions of leukotrienes and thromboxanes, in *Burger's Medicinal Chemistry and Drug Discovery, vol. 5: Therapeutic Agents*, 5th edn (ed. M.E. Woff), John Wiley & Sons, Inc., New York, pp. 405–493.
15. Musser, J.H. (1989) Leukotriene D_4 receptor antagonists. *Drug News Perspect.*, **2**, 202–213.
16. von Sprecher, A., Beck, A., Gerspacher, M., and Bray, M.A. (1992) Peptidoleukotriene antagonists: state of the art. *Chimia*, **46**, 304–311.
17. Ford-Hutchison, A., Young, R., and Gillard, J. (1991) Leukotriene blockers, novel therapeutic strategies for the treatment of asthma. *Drug News Perspect.*, **4**, 264–271.
18. Brooks, C.D.W. and Summers, J.B. (1996) Modulators of leukotriene biosynthesis and receptor activation. *J. Med. Chem.*, **39**, 2629–2654.
19. Piper, P.J. and Seale, J.P. (1979) Non-immunological release of slow-reacting substance from guinea-pig lungs. *Br. J. Pharmacol.*, **67**, 67–72.
20. Orange, R.P., Murphy, R.C., Karnovsky, M.L., and Austen, K.F. (1973) The physicochemical characteristics and purification of slow reacting substance of anaphylaxis. *J. Immunol.*, **110**, 760–770.
21. Rokach, J., Zamboni, R., Lau, C.K., and Guindon, Y. (1981) A C-gycloside route to leukotrienes. *Tetrahedron Lett.*, **22**, 2759–2762.
22. Gleason, J.G., Bryan, D.B., and Kinzig, C. M. (1980) Convergent synthesis of leukotriene A methyl ester. *Tetrahedron Lett.*, **21**, 1129–1132.

23 Ernest, I., Main, A.J., and Menasse, R. (1982) Synthesis of the 7-*cis* isomer of the natural leukotriene D4. *Tetrahedron Lett.*, **23**, 167–170.

24 Cohen, N., Banner, B.L., and Lopresti, R.C. (1980) Synthesis of optically active leukotriene (SRS-A) intermediates. *Tetrahedron Lett.*, **21**, 4163–4166.

25 Marriott, D.P. and Bantick, J.R. (1981) 5(*S*),6(*R*)-5,7-Dibenzoyloxy-6-hydroxyheptanoate ester: improved synthesis of a leukotriene intermediate. *Tetrahedron Lett.*, **22**, 3657–3658.

26 Foster, A., Fitzsimmons, B., Rokach, J., and Letts, L.G. (1987) Metabolism and excretion of peptide leukotrienes in the anesthetized rat. *Biochim. Biophys. Acta*, **921**, 486–493.

27 Lynch, K.R., O'Neill, G.P., Liu, Q., Im, D.S., Sawyer, N., Metters, K.M., Coulombe, N., Abramovitz, M., Figueroa, D.J., Zeng, Z., Connolly, B.M., Bai, C., Austin, C.P., Chateauneu, A., Stocco, R., Greig, G.M., Kargman, S., Hooks, S.B., Hosfield, E., Williams, D.L., Jr., Ford-Hutchinson, A.W., Caskey, C.T., and Evans, J.F. (1999) Characterization of the human cysteinyl leukotriene CysLT1 receptor. *Nature*, **399** (6738), 789–793.

28 Dixon, R.A.F., Jones, R.E., Diehl, R.E., Bennett, C.D., Kargman, S., and Rouzer, C.A. (1988) Cloning of the cDNA for human 5-lipoxygenase. *Proc. Natl. Acad. Sci. USA*, **85**, 416–420.

29 Miller, D.K., Gillard, J.W., Vickers, P.J., Sadowski, S., Léveillé, C., Mancini, J.A., Charleston, P., Dixon, R.A.F., Ford-Hutchinson, A.W., Fortin, R., Gauthier, J.Y., Rodkey, J., Rosen, R., Rouzer, C.A., Sigal, I.S., Strader, C.D., and Evans, J.F. (1990) Identification and isolation of a membrane protein necessary for leukotriene production. *Nature*, **343**, 278–281.

30 Dixon, R.A.F., Diehl, R.E., Opas, E., Rands, E., Vickers, P.J., Evans, J.F., Gillard, J.W., and Miller, D.K. (1990) Requirement of a 5-lipoxygenase-activating protein for leukotriene synthesis. *Nature*, **343**, 282–284.

31 Tsai, B.S., Bernstein, P.R., Macia, R.A., Conaty, J., and Krell, R.D. (1982) Comparative potency and pharmacology of isomers of leukotriene D4 on guinea pig trachea: requirement for a 5(*S*),6(*R*) configuration. *Prostaglandins*, **23**, 489–506.

32 Loftus, P. and Bernstein, P.R. (1983) A study of some leukotriene A4 and D4 analogues by proton NMR spectroscopy. *J. Org. Chem.*, **48**, 40–44.

33 Patterson, R., Harris, K.E., Smith, L.J., Greenberger, P.A., Shaughnessy, M.A., Bernstein, P.R., and Krell, R.D. (1983) Airway response to leukotriene D4 in rhesus monkeys. *Int. Arch. Allergy Appl. Immunol.*, **71**, 156–160.

34 Buckner, C.K., Krell, R.D., Laravuso, R.B., Coursin, D.B., Bernstein, P.R., and Will, J.A. (1986) Pharmacological evidence that human intralobar airways do not contain different receptors that mediate contractions to leukotriene C4 and leukotriene D4. *J. Pharmacol. Exp. Ther.*, **237**, 558–562.

35 Smith, L.J., Greenberger, P.A., Patterson, R., Krell, R.D., and Bernstein, P.R. (1985) The effect of inhaled leukotriene D4 in humans. *Am. Rev. Respir. Dis.*, **131**, 368–372.

36 Kern, R., Smith, L.J., Patterson, R., Krell, R.D., and Bernstein, P.R. (1986) Characterization of the airway response to inhaled LTD_4 in normal subjects. *Am. Rev. Respir. Dis.*, **133**, 1127–1132.

37 Aharony, D., Falcone, R.C., and Krell, R.D. (1987) Inhibition of 3*H*-leukotriene D4 binding to guinea pig lung receptors by the novel leukotriene antagonist ICI 198615. *J. Pharmacol. Exp. Ther.*, **243**, 921–926.

38 Sarau, H.M., Ames, R.S., Chambers, J., Ellis, C., Elshourbagy, N., Foley, J.J., Schmidt, D.B., Muccitelli, R.M., Jenkins, O., Murdock, P.R., Herrity, N.C., Halsey, W., Sathe, G., Muir, A.I., Nuthulaganti, P., Dytko, G.M., Buckley, P.T., Wilson, S., Bergsma, D.J., and Hay, D.W.P. (1999) Identification, molecular cloning, expression, and characterization of a cysteinyl leukotriene receptor. *Mol. Pharmacol.*, **56**, 657–663.

39 Krell, R.D., Tsai, B.-S., Berdoulay, A., Barone, M., and Giles, R.E. (1983) Heterogeneity of leukotriene receptors in guinea-pig trachea. *Prostaglandins*, **25**, 171–178.

40 Nicosia, S., Capra, V., Ravasi, S., and Rovati, G.E. (2000) Binding to cysteinyl-leukotriene receptors. *Am. J. Respir. Crit. Care Med.*, **161**, S46–S50.

41 Back, M., Dahlen, S.-E., Drazen, J.M., Evans, J.F., Serhan, C.N., Shimizu, T., and Yokomizo, T., and Rovati, G.E. (2011) International union of basic and clinical pharmacology. LXXXIV. Leukotriene receptor nomenclature, distribution, and pathophysiological functions. *Pharmacol. Rev.*, **63**, 539–584.

42 Austen, K.F., Maekawa, A., Kanaoka, Y., and Boyce, J.A. (2009) The leukotriene E4 puzzle: finding the missing pieces and revealing the pathobiologic implications. *J. Allergy Clin. Immunol.*, **124** (3), 406–414.

43 Snyder, D.W. and Krell, R.D. (1984) Pharmacological evidence for a distinct leukotriene C_4 receptor in guinea-pig trachea. *J. Pharmacol. Exp. Ther.*, **231**, 616–622.

44 Heise, C.E., O'Dowd, B.F., Figueroa, D.J., Sawyer, N., Nguyen, T., Im, D.S., Stocco, R., Bellefeuille, J.N., Abramovitz, M., Cheng, R., Williams, D.L., Jr., Zeng, Z., Liu, Q., Ma, L., Clements, M.K., Coulombe, N., Liu, Y., Austin, C.P., George, S.R., O'Neill, G.P., Metters, K.M., Lynch, K.R., and Evans, J.F. (2000) Characterization of the human cysteinyl leukotriene 2 receptor. *J. Biol. Chem.*, **275**, 30531–30536.

45 Nothacker, H.P., Wang, Z., Zhu, Y., Reinscheid, R.K., Lin, S.H., and Civelli, O. (2000) Molecular cloning and characterization of a second human cysteinyl leukotriene receptor: discovery of a subtype selective agonist. *Mol. Pharmacol.*, **58** (6), 1601–1608.

46 Snyder, D.W., Liberati, N.J., and McCarthy, M.M. (1988) Conscious guinea-pig aerosol model for evaluation of peptide leukotriene antagonists. *J. Pharmacol. Methods*, **19** (3), 219–231.

47 Bernstein, P.R. (1997) The challenge of drug discovery: developing leukotriene antagonists, in *SRS-A to Leukotrienes: The Dawning of a new treatment* (eds S. Holgate and S.-E. Dahlén), Blackwell Science, Oxford, UK, pp. 171–186.

48 Bernstein, P.R. (1998) The Development of Accolate: A Peptide Leukotriene Antagonist for the Treatment of Asthma. Course Handouts, Residential School on Medicinal Chemistry, Drew University, Madison, NJ.

49 Brown, F.J. (1995) Discovery of Accolate^{TM} (ICI 204, 219), a peptide leukotriene antagonist for asthma, in *The Search for Anti-inflammatory Drugs* (eds V.J. Merluzzi and J. Adams), Birkhauser, Boston, MA, pp. 161–189.

50 Brown, F.J., Bernstein, P.R., Cronk, L.A., Dosset, L.L., Hebbel, K.C., Maduskuie, T.P., Shapiro, H.S., Vacek, E.P., Yee, Y.K., Willard, A.K., Krell, R.D., and Snyder, D.W. (1989) Hydroxyacetophenone-derived antagonists of the peptidoleukotrienes. *J. Med. Chem.*, **32**, 807–826.

51 Mann., A. (2003) Conformational restrictions and/or steric hindrance in medicinal chemistry, in *The Practice of Medicinal Chemistry*, 2nd edn (ed. C.G. Wermuth), Academic Press, London, UK, pp. 233–250.

52 Bernstein, P.R., Snyder, D.W., Adams, E.J., Krell, R.D., Vacek, E.P., and Willard, A.K. (1986) Chemically stable homo-cinnamyl analogs of the leukotrienes; synthesis and preliminary biological evaluation. *J. Med. Chem.*, **29**, 2477–2483.

53 Snyder, D.W. and Bernstein, P.R. (1987) Pharmacologic profile of chemically stable analogs of peptide leukotrienes. *Eur. J. Pharm.*, **138**, 397–405.

54 Bernstein, P.R., Vacek, E.P., Adams, E.J., Snyder, D.W., and Krell, R.D. (1988) The synthesis and pharmacological characterization of a series of leukotriene analogues with antagonist and agonist activities. *J. Med. Chem.*, **31**, 692–696.

55 Brown, F.J., Yee, Y.K., Hebbel, K.C., Cronk, L.A., Krell, R.D., and Snyder, D.W. (1990) Evolution of a series of peptidoleukotriene antagonists: synthesis and structure–activity relationships of 1,6-disubstituted indoles and indazoles. *J. Med. Chem.*, **33**, 2437–2351, 1771–1781.

56 Yee, Y.K., Bernstein, P.R., Adams, E.J., Brown, F.J., Cronk, L.A., Hebbel, K.C., Vacek, E.P., Krell, R.D., and Snyder, D.W. (1990) A novel series of leukotriene antagonists: exploration and optimization of the acidic region in 1,6-disubstituted

indoles and indazoles. *J. Med. Chem.*, **33**, 2437–2351.

57 Fleisch, J.H., Rinkema, L.E., Haisch, K.D., Swanson-Bean, D., Goodson, T., Ho., P.P.K., and Marshall, W.S. (1985) 1-[2-Hydroxy-3-propyl-4-([4-(1*H*-tetrazol-5-ylmethyl)phenoxy]methyl)phenyl] ethanone, an orally active leukotriene D4 antagonist. *J. Pharmacol. Exp. Ther.*, **233** (1), 148–157.

58 Brown, F.J., Cronk, L.A., Aharony, D., and Snyder, D.W. (1992) 1,3,6-Trisubstituted indoles as peptidoleukotriene antagonists: benefits of a second, polar, pyrrole substituent. *J. Med. Chem.*, **35**, 2419–2439.

59 Matassa, V.G., Brown, F.J., Bernstein, P.R., Shapiro, H.S., Maduskuie, T.P., Jr., Cronk, L.A., Vacek, E.P., Yee, Y.K., Snyder, D.W., Krell, R.D., Lerman, C.L., and Maloney, J.J. (1990) Synthesis and *in vitro* LTD4 antagonist activity of bicyclic and monocyclic cyclopentylurethane and cyclopentylacetamide *N*-arylsulfonyl amides. *J. Med. Chem.*, **33**, 2621–2629.

60 Matassa, V.G., Maduskuie, T.P., Jr., Shapiro, H.S., Hesp, B., Snyder, D.W., Aharony, D., Krell, R.D., and Keith, R.A. (1990) Evolution of a series of peptidoleukotriene antagonists: synthesis and structure/activity relationships of 1,3,5-substituted indoles and indazoles. *J. Med. Chem.*, **33**, 1781–1790.

61 Young, R.N. (2007) Discovery of Singulair[R] and its impact on treatment of asthma in children and adults. Book of Abstracts. The 234th ACS National Meeting, Boston, MA, August 19–23, 2007, MEDI 214.

62 Rodger, I.W. (2000) From bench to bedside: the hurdles of discovering a new leukotriene receptor antagonist. *Am. J. Respir. Crit. Care Med.*, **161**, S7–S10.

63 Jones, T.R., Young, R., Champion, E., Charette, L., Denis, D., Ford-Hutchinson, A.W., Frenette, R., Gauthier, J.Y., Guindon, Y., Kakushima, M., Masson, P., McFarlane, C., Piechuta, H., Rokach, J., and Zamboni, R. (1986) L-649,923, sodium (beta S^*, gamma R^*)-4-(3-(4-acetyl-3-hydroxy-2-propylphenoxy) propylthio)-gamma-hydroxy-beta-methylbenzenebutanoate, a selective, orally active leukotriene receptor antagonist. *Can. J. Physiol. Pharmacol.*, **64**, 1068–1075.

64 Jones, T.R., Guindon, Y., Champion, E., Charette, L., De Haven, R.N., Denis, D., Ethier, D., Ford-Hutchinson, A.W., Fortin, R., Frenette, R. *et al.* (1987) L-648,051: an aerosol active leukotriene D4 receptor antagonist. *Adv. Prostaglandin Thromboxane Res.*, **17**, 1012–1017.

65 Zamboni, R., Belley, M., Champion, E., Charette, L., DeHaven, R., Frenette, R., Gauthier, J.Y., Jones, T.R., Leger, S., Masson, P., McFarlane, C.S., Metters, K., Pong, S.S., Piechuta, H., Rokach, J., Thérien, M., Williams, H.W.R., and Young, R.N. (1992) Development of a novel series of styrylquinoline compounds as high-affinity leukotriene D4 receptor antagonists: synthetic and structure–activity studies leading to the discovery of (±)-3-[[[3[2-(7-chloro-2-quinolinyl)-(*E*)-ethenyl]phenyl][[3-(dimethylamino)3-oxopropyl]thio]methyl]thio]propionic acid. *J. Med. Chem.*, **35**, 3832–3844.

66 Young, R.N. (1989) The development of new anti-leukotriene drugs L-648,501 and L-649,923 specific leukotriene D4 antagonists. *Drugs Future*, **13**, 745–759.

67 (a) Van Inwegen, R.G., Khandwala, A., Gordon, R., Sonnino, P., Coutta, S., and Jolly, S., (1987) REV 5901: an orally effective peptidoleukotriene antagonist, detailed biochemical/pharmacological profile. *J. Pharmacol. Exp. Ther.*, **241**, 117–124. (b) Musser, J.H., Kubrak, D.M., Chang, J., and Lewis, J. (1986) Synthesis of [[(naphthalenylmethoxy)- and [[(quinolinylmethoxy)phenyl]amino] oxoalkanoic acid esters. A novel series of leukotriene D4 antagonists and 5-lipoxygenase inhibitors. *J. Med. Chem.*, **29**, 1429–1435.

68 Musser, J.H., Chakraborty, U.R., Sciortino, S., Gordon, R.J., Khandwala, A., Neiss, E.S., Pruss, T.P., Van Inwegen, R., Weinryb, I., and Coutta, S.M. (1987) Substituted arylmethyl phenyl ethers. 1. A novel series of 5-lipoxygenase inhibitors and leukotriene antagonists. *J. Med. Chem.*, **30**, 96–104.

69 Perchonock, C.D., McCarthy, M.E., Erhard, K.F., Gleason, J.G., Wasserman, M.A., Muccitelli, R.M., DeVan, J.F.,

Tucker, S.S., Vickery, L.M., Kirchner, T., Weichman, B.M., Mong, S., Crooke, S.T., and Newton, J.F. (1986) Synthesis and pharmacological characterization of 5-(2-dodecylphenyl)-4,6-dithianonanedioic acid and 5-[2-(8-phenyloctyl)-phenyl-4,6-dithianonanedioic acid: prototypes of a novel class of leukotriene antagonists. *J. Med. Chem.*, **28**, 1145–1147.

70 Lewis, R.A., Drazen, J.M., Austen, K.F., Toda, M., Brion, F., Marfat, A., and Corey, E.J. (1981) Contractile activities of structural analogs of leukotriene C and D: role of the polar substituents. *Proc. Natl. Acad. Sci. USA*, **78**, 4579–4583.

71 Labelle, M., Belley, M., Gareau, Y., Gauthier, J.Y., Guay, D., Gordon, R., Grossman, S.G., Jones, T.R., LeBlanc, Y., McAuliffe, M., McFarlane, C., Masson, P., Metters, K.M., Ouimet, N., Patrick, D.H., Piechuta, H., Rochette, C., Sawyer, N., Xiang, Y.B., Pickett, C.B., Ford-Hutchinson, A.W., Zamboni, R.J., and Young, R.N. (1995) Discovery of MK-0476, a potent and orally active leukotriene D4 receptor antagonist devoid of peroxisomal enzyme induction. *Bioorg. Med. Chem. Lett.*, **5**, 283–288.

72 Labelle, M., Prasit, P., Belley, M., Blouin, M., Champion, E., Charette, L., DeLuca, J.G., Dufresne, C., Frenette, R., Gauthier, J.Y., Grimm, E., Grossman, S.G., Guay, D., Herold, E.G., Jones, T.R., Lau, C.K., Leblanc, Y., Leger, S., Lord, A., McAuliffe, M., McFarlane, C., Masson, P., Metters, K.M., Ouimet, N., Patrick, D.H., Perrier, H., Pickett, C.B., Piechuta, H., Roy, P., Williams, H., Wang, Z., Xiang, Y.B., Zamboni, R.J., Ford-Hutchinson, A.W., and Young, R.N. (1992) The discovery of a new structural class of potent orally active leukotriene D4 antagonists. *Bioorg. Med. Chem. Lett.*, **2**, 1141–1146.

73 Labelle, M., Belley, M., Champion, E., Gordon, R., Jones, T.R., Leblanc, Y., McAuliffe, M., McFarlane, C., Masson, P., Metters, K.M., Nicoll-Griffith, D., Ouimet, N., Piechuta, H., Rochette, C., Sawyer, N., Xiang, Y.B., Yergey, J., Ford-Hutchinson, A.W., Pickett, C.B., Zamboni, R.J., and Young, R.N. (1994) The discovery of L-699,392, a novel potent and orally active leukotriene D4 receptor antagonist. *Bioorg. Med. Chem. Lett.*, **4**, 463–468.

74 Jones, T.R., Labelle, M., Belley, M., Champion, E., Charette, L., Evans, J., Ford-Hutchinson, A.W., Gauthier, J.-Y., Lord, A., Masson, P., McAuliffe, M., McFarlane, C.S., Metters, K.M., Pickett, C., Piechuta, H., Rochette, C., Rodger, I.W., Sawyer, N., Young, R.N., Zamboni, R., and Abraham, W.M. (1995) Pharmacology of montelukast sodium (Singulair^{TM}), a potent and selective leukotriene D4 receptor antagonist. *Can. J. Physiol. Pharmacol.*, **73** (2), 191–201.

75 Toda, M., Nakai, H., Kosuge, S., Konno, M., Arai, Y., Miyam-oto, T., Obata, T., Katsube, A., and Kawasaki, A. (1985) A potent antagonist of the slow-reacting substance of anaphylaxis. *Adv. Prostaglandin Thromboxane Leukot. Res.*, **15**, 307–308.

76 Nakai, H., Konno, M., Kosuge, S., Sakuyama, S., Toda, M., Arai, Y., Obata, T., Katsube, N., Miyamoto, T., Okegawa, T., and Kawasaki, A. (1988) New potent antagonists of leukotriene C4 and D4 1. Synthesis and structure–activity relationships. *J. Med. Chem.*, **31**, 84–91.

77 Goto, S., Guo, Z., Futatsuishi, Y., Hori, H., Taira, Z., and Terada, H. (1992) Quantitative structure–activity relationships of benzamide derivatives for anti-leukotriene activities. *J. Med. Chem.*, **35**, 2440–2445.

78 Trainor, G.L. (2007) Plasma protein binding and the free drug principle: recent developments and applications. *Annu. Rep. Med. Chem.*, **42**, 489–502.

79 Lynch, K.R., O'Neill, G.P., Liu, Q., Im, D.S., Sawyer, N., Metters, K.M., Coulombe, N., Abramovitz, M., Figueroa, D.J., Zeng, Z., Connolly, B.M., Bai, C., Austin, C.P., Chateauneuf, A., Stocco, R., Greig, G.M., Kargman, S., Hooks, S.B., Hosfield, E., Williams, D.L., Jr., Ford-Hutchinson, A.W., Caskey, C.T., and Evans, J.F. (1999) Characterization of the human cysteinyl leukotriene CysLT1 receptor. *Nature*, **399**, 789–793.

80 Thummel, K.E. and Shen, D.D. (2001) Plasma protein binding, in *Goodman & Gilman's The Pharmacological Basis of Therapeutics*, 10th edn (eds J.G. Hardman,

L.E. Limbird, and A.G. Gilman), McGraw-Hill, New York, pp. 1917–2023.

81 Ishido, M., Shibakawa, K., Takamoto, M., Kajiwara, I., Sawada, M., and Aishita, H. (1993) Studies on the metabolic fate of leukotriene antagonist ONO-1078 (4): metabolism and protein binding. *Yakubutsudoutai*, **8**, 49–66.

82 Lipinski, C.A., Lombardo, F., Dominy, B.W., and Feeney, P.J. (1997) Experimental and computational approaches to estimate solubility and permeability in drug discovery and development settings. *Adv. Drug Deliv. Rev.*, **23**, 3–25.

83 Beam, W.R., Weiner, D.E., and Martin, R.J. (1992) Timing of prednisone and alterations of airways inflammation in nocturnal asthma. *Am. Rev. Respir. Dis.*, **146** (6), 1524–1530.

84 Wechsler, M.E., Garpestad, E., Flier, S.R., Kocher, O., Weiland, D.A., Polito, A.J., Klinek, M.M., Bigby, T.D., Wong, G.A., Helmers, R.A., and Drazen, J.M. (1998) Pulmonary infiltrates, eosinophilia, and cardiomyopathy following corticosteroid withdrawal in patients with asthma receiving zafirlukast. *J. Am. Med. Assoc.*, **279** (6), 455–7.

85 McDanel, D.L. and Muller, B.A. (2005) The linkage between Churg–Strauss syndrome and leukotriene receptor antagonists: fact or fiction? *Ther. Clin. Risk Manage.*, **1** (2), 125–40.

86 Lilly, C.M., Churg, A., Lazarovich, M., Pauwels, R., Hendeles, L., Rosenwasser, L.J., Ledford, D., and Wechsler, M.E. (2002) Asthma therapies and Churg-Strauss syndrome. *J. Allergy Clin. Immunol.*, **109** (1), 1–19.

87 Bibby, S., Healy, B., Steele, R., Kumareswaran, K., Nelson, H., and Beasley, R. (2010) Association between leukotriene receptor antagonist therapy and Churg–Strauss syndrome: an analysis of the FDA AERS database. *Thorax*, **65** (2), 132–138.

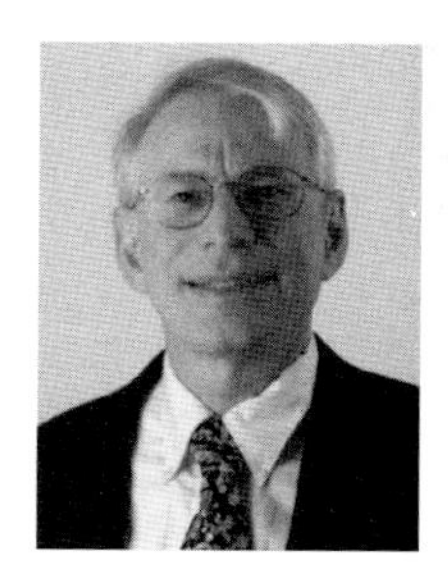

Peter R. Bernstein received a B.S. degree in Chemistry from the University of Rochester, a Ph.D. degree in Organic Chemistry from Columbia University (advisor Prof. Gilbert Stork), and was a postdoctoral fellow at the University of Wisconsin, Madison, with Prof. Barry Trost. He then joined ICI Pharmaceuticals, Wilmington, DE, and worked, for over 30 years in the pharmaceutical industry, there and at its successor companies, Zeneca and AstraZeneca. He is the co-inventor of zafirlukast and is recognized for his work, on many different targets, that has led to more than 10 clinical candidates. Upon his retirement in 2010, he formed PhaRmaB LLC as a platform to provide consulting and training in medicinal chemistry and drug discovery. He now holds several editorial appointments including Digests Editor for *Bioorganic Medicinal Chemistry Letter* and Section Editor for Topics in Drug Design and Discovery for *Annual Reports in Medicinal Chemistry*. He has received several honors and awards and most recently, in 2011, was inducted into the *Hall of Fame* of the ACS Division of Medicinal Chemistry.

Part III
Case Studies

Analogue-based Drug Discovery III, First Edition. Edited by János Fischer, C. Robin Ganellin, and David P. Rotella.
© 2013 Wiley-VCH Verlag GmbH & Co. KGaA. Published 2013 by Wiley-VCH Verlag GmbH & Co. KGaA.

10
The Discovery of Dabigatran Etexilate

Norbert Hauel, Andreas Clemens, Herbert Nar, Henning Priepke, Joanne van Ryn, and Wolfgang Wienen

List of Abbreviations

aPTT	activated partial thromboplastin time
ASA	acetylsalicylic acid
AT	antithrombin
bid	*bis in die* (twice daily)
CrCl	creatine clearance
DVT	deep venous thrombosis
ECT	ecarin clotting time
FDA	US Food and Drug Administration
FXa	coagulation factor Xa
INR	international normalized ratio
LMWH	low molecular weight heparin
PAR	protease-activated receptor
Pgp	permeability glycoprotein
PT	prothrombin time
SPAF	stroke prevention in patients with atrial fibrillation
TAFI	thrombin activatable fibrinolysis inhibitor
THR	total hip replacement
TKR	total knee replacement
TM	thrombomodulin
VKA	vitamin K antagonist
VTE	venous thromboembolism

10.1
Introduction

Thrombin is a serine protease that plays a central role in thrombosis and hemostasis. It is a key enzyme in the blood coagulation cascade, exhibiting both pro- and

Analogue-based Drug Discovery III, First Edition. Edited by János Fischer, C. Robin Ganellin, and David P. Rotella.
© 2013 Wiley-VCH Verlag GmbH & Co. KGaA. Published 2013 by Wiley-VCH Verlag GmbH & Co. KGaA.

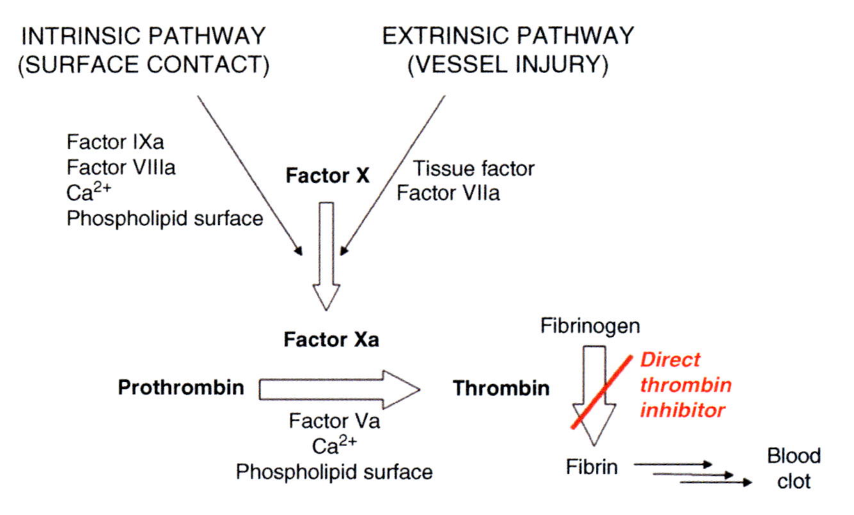

Scheme 10.1 Simplified version of coagulation cascade.

anticoagulant properties [1, 2]. It is generated via proteolytic cleavage from inactive prothrombin by the serine protease factor Xa (FXa, see Scheme 10.1) in the prothrombinase complex. Thrombin plays a major role in the initiation and propagation of thrombotic disease by catalyzing fibrinogen conversion into fibrin and reinforcing the clot structure by FXIII activation. It also feeds back and activates the factors V, VIII, and XI of the coagulation cascade, thereby amplifying the coagulation response. Its activity is downregulated by inhibition via antithrombin (AT). Thrombin is a very potent agonist of platelet activation and further promotes clot stabilization by activating thrombin activatable fibrinolysis inhibitor (TAFI), thereby reducing endogenous fibrinolytic capacities [3]. By activating protein C, thrombin also prevents unnecessary progression of a thrombus once intact endothelium in vessels is encountered [2].

In addition, thrombin induces many cellular effects, including cell proliferation, cytokine release, and tissue remodeling [4–6]. These cellular effects of thrombin are mediated via a family of G-protein-coupled protease-activated receptors (PARs) PAR1, PAR3, and PAR4 [6–8]. The expression of PAR1 on the endothelium and vasculature, in both physiological and disease states, suggests that thrombin may play a role in these pathologies.

For more than 50 years, established anticoagulation therapy has also targeted thrombin. Heparin has been the mainstay of anticoagulation in both the prophylaxis and treatment of venous thromboembolism (VTE) [9]. It mainly reduces thrombin activity by catalyzing the inhibition of thrombin by AT activity. Though replaced by the low molecular weight heparins (LMWH) in many indications today, both of these compounds are limited by their parenteral route of administration for long-term therapy. The use of more targeted direct thrombin inhibition has been approved with two other parenteral therapies, both argatroban (**1**) for predominantly heparin-induced thrombocytopenia [10] and the oligopeptide bivalirudin in percutaneous coronary interventions [11]. As the only available oral therapy, warfarin (**2**) and its derivatives have been used for over 50 years in long-term anticoagulation treatment [12]. Warfarin, a vitamin K antagonist (VKA), that blocks the biosynthesis of thrombin and other coagulation factors has proven a very effective therapy in inhibiting thrombosis. However, administration is problematic due to its slow onset and offset of activity and the large number of drug–drug and drug–food interactions, which require frequent monitoring and dose adjustment in patients to ensure that appropriate anticoagulation is maintained [13].

Due to the central position of thrombin in the coagulation cascade, research activities in many pharmaceutical companies have been focused on the identification of inhibitors of this enzyme. In 2004, ximelagatran (**3**, AstraZeneca) [14] gained approval in a number of countries for short-term anticoagulation treatment after orthopedic surgery. However, in 2006 the drug was withdrawn from the market due to reports of hepatotoxicity after long-term application.

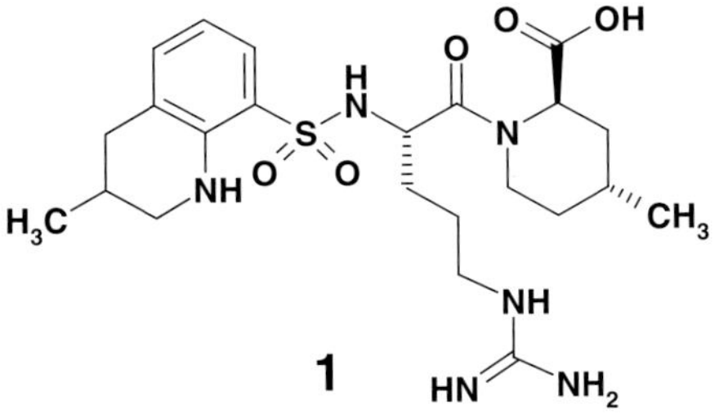

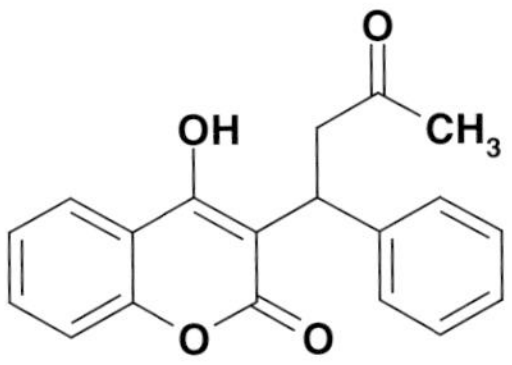

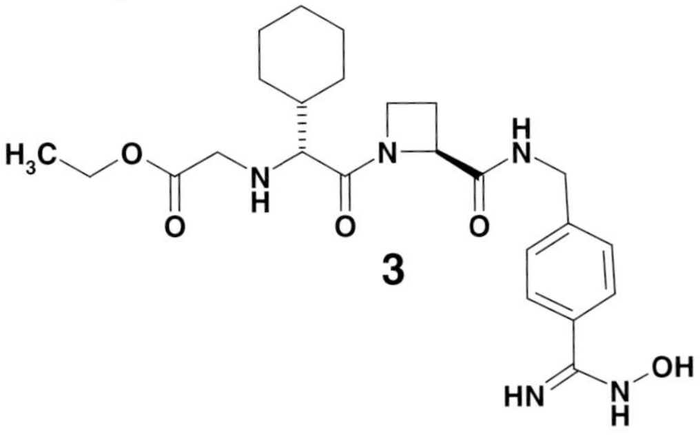

Furthermore, a number of companies concentrated their research activities on the inhibition of FXa [15], thereby blocking the conversion of prothrombin to thrombin, and recently, three FXa inhibitors – rivaroxaban [16] (**4**), apixaban [17] (**5**), and edoxaban [18] (**6**) – were approved in different countries.

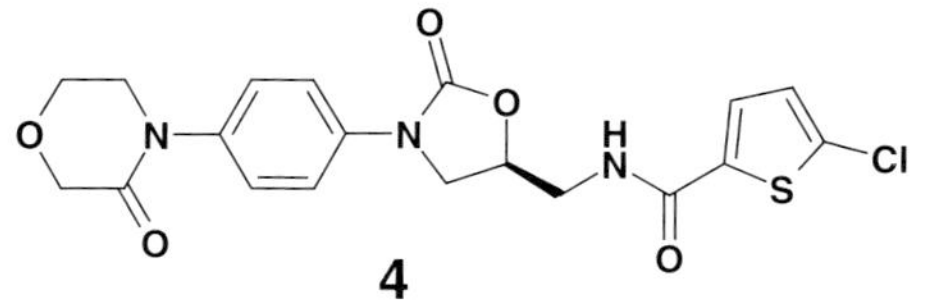

This chapter will focus on the design and development of dabigatran (**34**, Table 10.3) [19], the first new oral anticoagulant that gained market approval for long-term indications after introduction of warfarin 50 years ago. Dabigatran is a potent, reversible, and direct inhibitor of thrombin, with a good efficacy, safety, and tolerability profile as compared to both warfarin and low molecular weight heparin [20]. We will discuss its *in vitro* and *in vivo* pharmacology and summarize the clinical development. Dabigatran has now been approved in many countries around the world, including the United States, Canada, Japan, and Europe, for stroke prevention in patients with atrial fibrillation and in over 73 countries for the prevention of thrombosis after orthopedic hip and knee surgery.

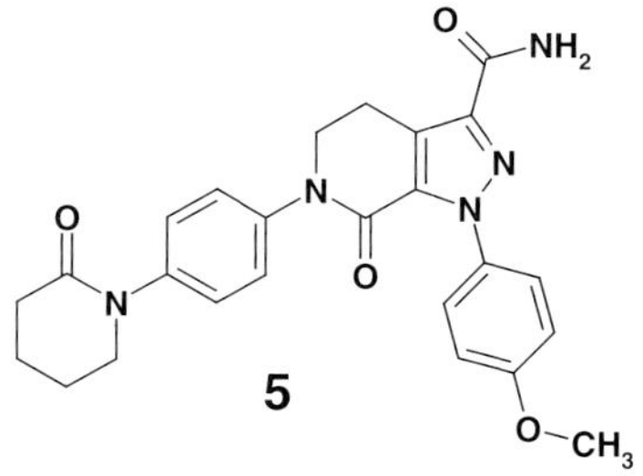

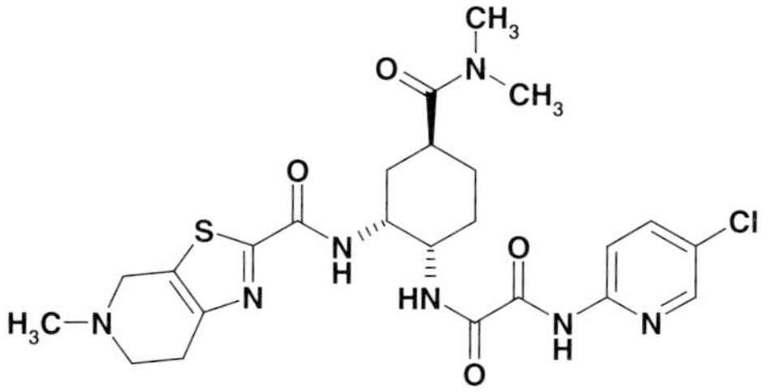

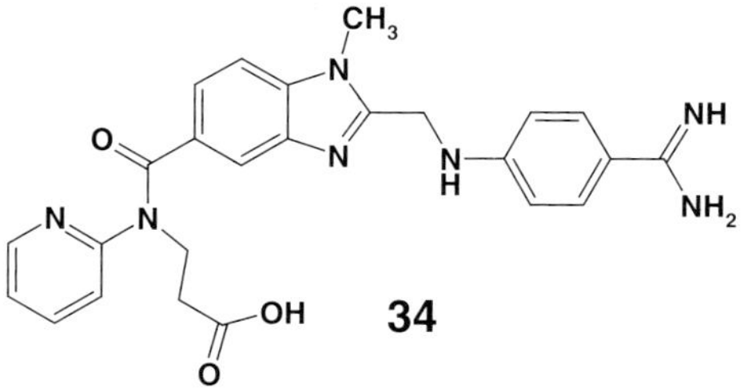

10.2 Dabigatran Design Story

In 1992, Brandstetter *et al.* published the X-ray crystal structure of a bovine thrombin complex formed with the peptide-like benzamidine-based inhibitor NAPAP (7) [21]. The analysis revealed, for the first time, the conformation of a noncovalent, enzyme-bound thrombin inhibitor and its interactions with the residues of the active site cleft. In this complex, the amidine group of the inhibitor forms a bidentate salt bridge with the carboxylate of Asp189. Hydrophobic interactions are formed by the piperidine ring and the naphthyl moiety with the S2 and S4 pockets of the thrombin active site, respectively. In addition, the bridging glycine moiety of NAPAP forms the canonical hydrogen bonding pattern with residues Trp215 and Gly216 at the rim of the specificity (S1) pocket that was previously observed with peptidic serine protease inhibitors.

Based on this structural information, we designed a very simple acylated diaminophenyl scaffold (exemplified in compound **8**) as a surrogate for the central glycine in the NAPAP molecule. The aim was to avoid the peptidic structure elements and eventually develop a new chemotype with improved metabolic stability.

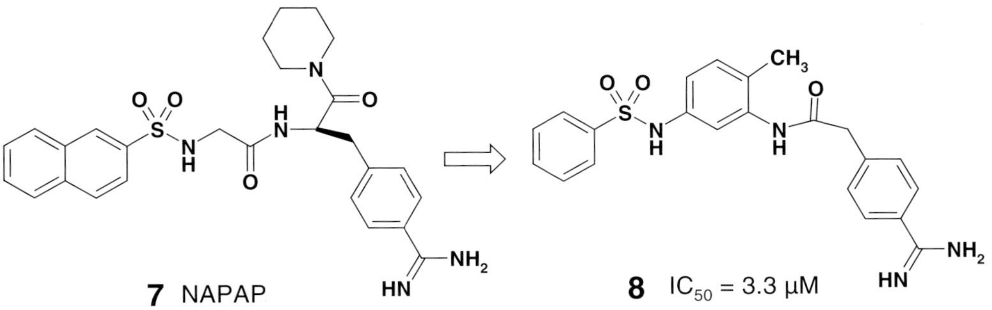

7 NAPAP

8 IC_{50} = 3.3 μM

Our efforts to improve the rather weak activity of **8** through variations of substituents were not successful. With about 30 derivatives, no substantial improvement in potency could be achieved (Hauel, N.H., unpublished work).

Further progress could only be achieved when we designed the bicyclic compound **9** that was derived from structure **8** by ring closure of the central part (Hauel, N.H., unpublished work). This turned out to be the most important change in the core structure.

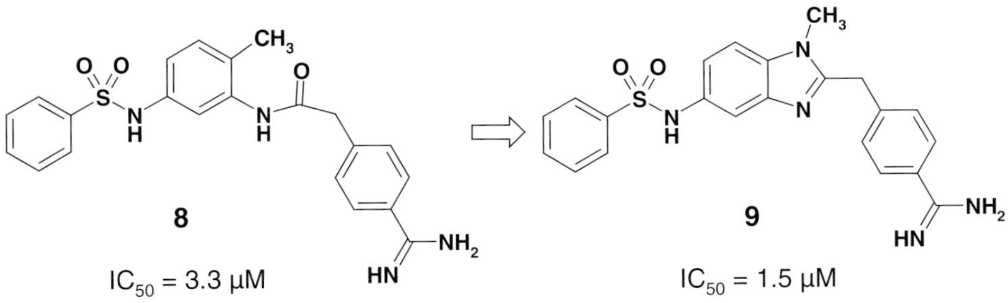

8 IC_{50} = 3.3 μM

9 IC_{50} = 1.5 μM

Although only twofold more potent than compound **8**, this new benzimidazole core was a real breakthrough for the whole optimization program. In order to analyze in detail the exact binding mode of inhibitor **9**, we determined a crystal structure of its complex with human α-thrombin. This analysis revealed that the benzimidazole core appeared to be a most favorable template to place the three essential substituents into the right positions (Figure 10.1).

Like with NAPAP, the amidine portion of compound **9** interacts via a salt bridge with Asp189 in the thrombin active site. The terminal phenyl ring is bound by a hydrophobic interaction in the S4 pocket, and the *N*-methyl group nicely fits into the S2 pocket. There is no additional hydrogen bond between the benzimidazole moiety of the inhibitor and enzyme, which in part may explain why in our test

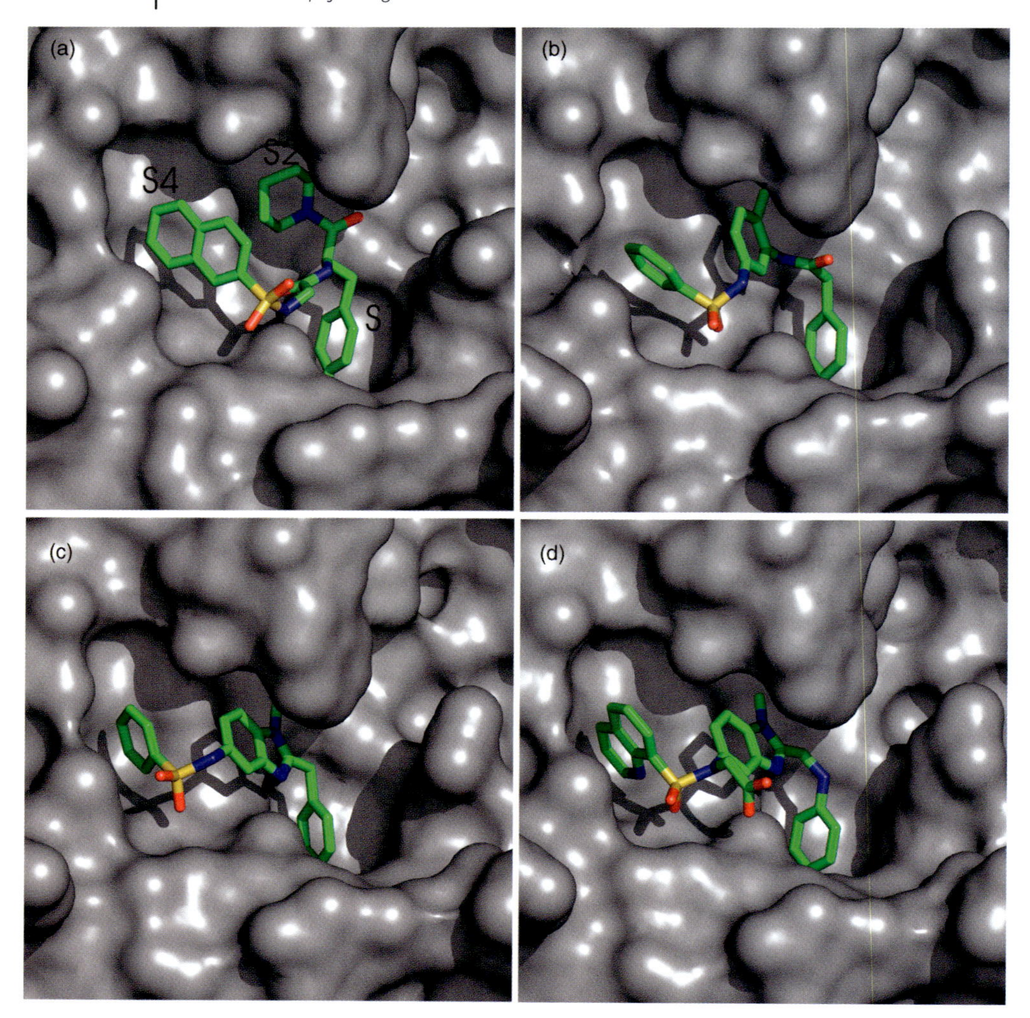

Figure 10.1 Evolution of thrombin inhibitor structural classes and their binding modes starting from NAPAP (compound **7**). Costructures of NAPAP (a), compound **8** (b), compound **9** (c), and compound **26** (d) in complex with thrombin. Thrombin is shown as a surface representation; the compounds are shown as stick models. The dominant common motif of inhibitor binding is the interaction of the conserved benzamidine moiety in the S1 pocket (lower right in each image) with the Asp189 residue forming a bidentate salt bridge (hidden). The hydrophobic S2 pocket (residues Trp60D, His57, Tyr60B, and Leu99) is occupied by methyl groups anchored at aromatic ring systems in each of the three lead classes. The S4 pocket above residue Trp215 (plus residues) is filled by mono- or bicyclic (hetero-)aromatic ring systems that are in edge-on position relative to Trp215.

system compound **9** was about one order of magnitude less active ($IC_{50} = 1.5\ \mu M$) than NAPAP ($IC_{50} = 0.2\ \mu M$).

Intrigued and stimulated by the binding mode of **9**, we now focused our efforts on the optimization of this new class of inhibitors, as described by the general formula **10**.

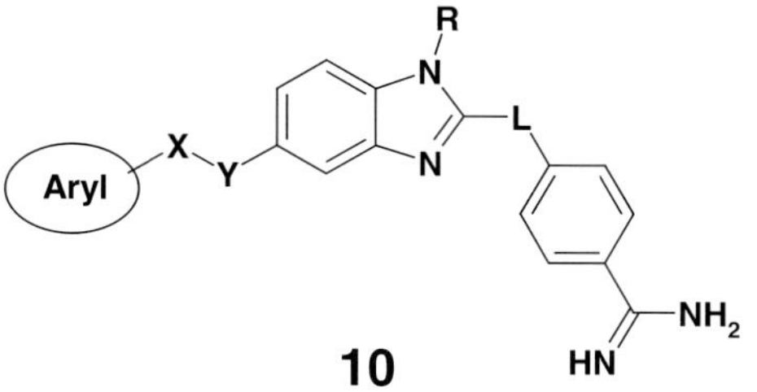

10

Our goal was to refine this structure class in order to increase the inhibitory potency and to achieve acceptable metabolic stability and pharmacokinetic properties.

Table 10.1 shows a selection of sulfonamides with variations in three positions. Starting from lead structure **9**, we synthesized analogues **11–13** (Table 10.1) with

Table 10.1 Structural variations of lead compound **9** [19].

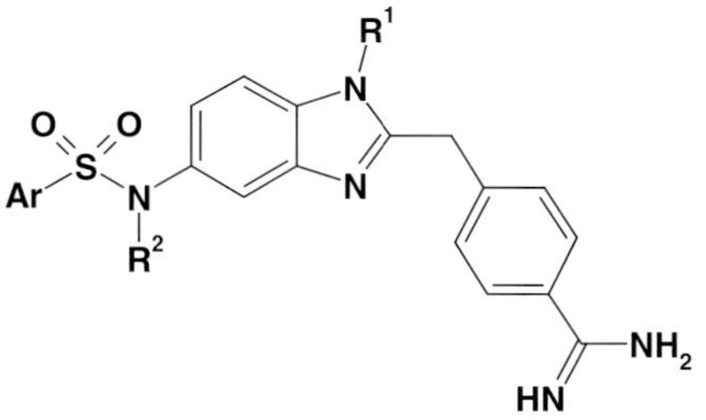

Compound	R^1	R^2	Ar	IC_{50} (μM)
9	$-CH_3$	$-H$	Phenyl	1.5
11	$-H$	$-H$	Phenyl	19
12	—Ethyl	$-H$	Phenyl	2.4
13	—*n*-Propyl	$-H$	Phenyl	4.0
14	$-CH_3$	$-CH_3$	Phenyl	1.3
15	$-CH_3$	$-H$	3-Pyridyl	1.6
16	$-CH_3$	$-H$	1-Naphthyl	0.6
17	$-CH_3$	$-H$	2-Naphthyl	24
18	$-CH_3$	$-H$	5-Isoquinolyl	0.51
19	$-CH_3$	$-H$	8-Quinolyl	0.26
20	$-CH_3$	$-CH_2-COOH$	8-Quinolyl	0.12
21	$-CH_3$	$-(CH_2)_3-COOH$	8-Quinolyl	0.13

alkyl substituents R^1 of different sizes at the benzimidazole N-1, in order to explore their relative contributions to the binding energy and to identify the optimum alkyl chain length. Compound **11** ($R^1 = H$) turned out to be one order of magnitude less potent than **9**, which clearly demonstrates the importance of the lipophilic/hydrophobic interaction of the methyl group of **9** with the lipophilic P pocket formed by the residues His57, Tyr60A, Leu99, and Trp60D of thrombin. This finding was not a surprise because it was part of our design concept to make use of this hydrophobic interaction and because we had already information about the localization of the methyl group in the enzyme active site from the X-ray structure (Figure 10.1). We did, however, not expect that an increase in the alkyl chain length (compounds **12** and **13**) would result in a decrease in potency. We had hoped, instead, that a larger buried hydrophobic surface area (and therefore a stronger van der Waals interaction) would result in stronger ligand binding. The observed decrease in affinity, albeit very small, may best be explained by a decrease of entropy due to a loss of rotational degrees of freedom during formation of the enzyme–inhibitor complex [22].

The X-ray structure (Figure 10.1) clearly shows that the sulfonamide hydrogen of compound **9** does not take part in a hydrogen bond with the protein. The N—H bond is directed out of the binding site into the solvent phase; *N*-alkylation should therefore have no influence on affinity, as was proven with the *N*-methyl derivative **14**.

The inhibitor interaction with the so-called thrombin S4 pocket, formed by residues Leu99, Ile174, and Trp215, was explored by variations of the terminal aryl substituent. A selection of some derivatives is listed in Table 10.1 (compounds **15–19**). Substitution of the phenyl group by 3-pyridyl (compound **15**) did not influence affinity. A small increase in potency compared to compound **9** was achieved with the 1-naphthyl residue (compound **16**), whereas activity dropped 40-fold with the 2-naphthyl group (compound **17**), probably caused by a repulsive interaction with Asn98 at the back of the S4 pocket. The 5-isoquinolyl and 8-quinolyl groups (compounds **18** and **19**) were as effective as the 1-naphthyl.

As was reported by others with a different class of thrombin inhibitors [23], the lipophilicity of the molecules influences their inhibitory activity when measured in the presence of blood plasma: the more lipophilic the inhibitor, the more pronounced the reduction in activity will be. The reason for this phenomenon most probably is plasma protein binding that reduces the inhibitor free concentration. We therefore planned to introduce polar groups into the molecules in order to increase their hydrophilicity, thereby hopefully reducing protein binding and optimizing *in vivo* activity. To this end, we synthesized the zwitterionic compounds **20** and **21** by adding acetic acid and butyric acid, respectively, to the sulfonamide nitrogen. As inferred from the crystal structure of the thrombin–**9** complex, the carboxylate groups are located outside the active site in the solvent phase and do not interfere with inhibitor binding. The inhibitory activity of both compounds was not reduced in the presence of plasma proteins (data not shown).

From X-ray structure analyses of this class of inhibitors in complex with thrombin, we reasoned that elongation of the linker L between the benzimidazole template and the benzamidine moiety (general structure **4**) by an additional atom

Table 10.2 Variations of the linker L in lead structure **10**.

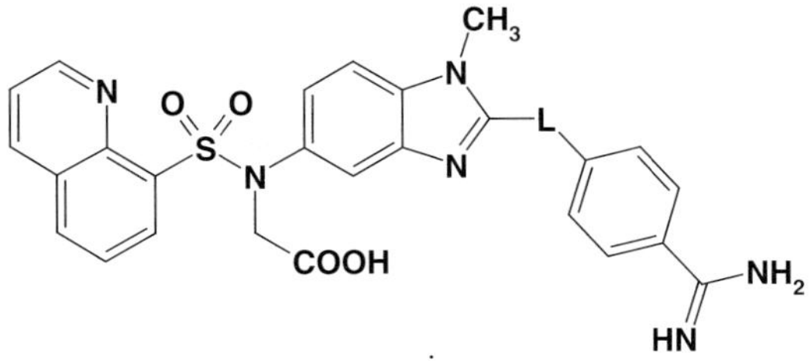

Compound	L	IC_{50} (μM)
22	$-CH_2-CH_2-$	0.032[a)]
23	$-S-CH_2-$	0.102[b)]
24	$-CH_2-S-$	0.041[b)]
25	$-CH_2-O-$	0.058[a)]
26	$-CH_2-NH-$	0.011[a)]
27	$-CH_2-NH-CH_2$-	1.31[b)]

a) Ref. [19].
b) Ref. (Hauel, N.H., unpublished work).

should generate molecules that fit equally well into the active site. This was proven by compounds **22–26** (Table 10.2).

One of the diatomic linkers, the aminomethyl group, turned out to be especially favorable: to our surprise, the potency of compound **26** was one order of magnitude stronger than that of **20**.

Based on various X-ray structures (one example shown in Figure 10.1d), our hypothesis at this point was that the diatomic linker facilitates a better positioning of the benzamidine group in the S1 pocket, whereas further elongation of the linker (compound **27**) resulted in a decrease of potency.

In the molecules of Tables 10.1 and 10.2, the position of the terminal aryl residue Ar in relation to the central benzimidazole scaffold is determined by the torsion angles of the sulfonamide spacer between them. Having obtained detailed information about enzyme-bound conformations of a number of inhibitors, we reasoned that utilizing a carboxamide instead of the sulfonamide spacer the aryl group should also be placed in a favorable position for strong S4 pocket interaction. This hypothesis was verified by the carboxamide analogues listed in Table 10.3.

From three variations of the linker $-CH_2-A-$ (compounds **28–30**), again the amino derivative **30** was the most potent, as was the case in the sulfonamide series in Table 10.2. Compounds **30**, **31**, and **32** demonstrate that the chain length *n* (up to three methylene groups) between the carboxylate and the amide nitrogen has only a minor influence on the *in vitro* activity. Substitution of the terminal phenyl by a 3-pyridyl residue (compound **33**) reduced potency by a factor of 10, whereas a 2-pyridyl group could be introduced without substantial loss of activity (compound **34**).

Table 10.3 Carboxamide analogues.

Compound	A	*n*	X	Y	IC_{50} (μM)
28	$-CH_2-$	1	CH	CH	0.054[a]
29	—O—	1	CH	CH	0.33[a]
30	—NH—	1	CH	CH	0.010[a]
31	—NH—	2	CH	CH	0.0054[a]
32	—NH—	3	CH	CH	0.010[a]
33	—NH—	2	CH	N	0.054[b]
34	—NH—	2	N	CH	0.0093[a]

a) Ref. [19].
b) Ref. (Hauel, N.H., unpublished work).

The X-ray structure of **34** in complex with thrombin is shown in Figure 10.2. It demonstrates that dabigatran (**34**) and our starting point, compound **9**, share a similar binding mode: the amidine group interacts with Asp189 via a bidentate salt bridge, the central template is bound to thrombin by a hydrophobic interaction with the S2 pocket, and the pyridine ring is positioned between Leu99 and Ile174 in the S4 pocket. As predicted, there is no interaction between the enzyme and the carboxylate group that is directed out of the binding site into bulk solvent. It is one of the most remarkable characteristics of this inhibitor that it does not make use of the canonical hydrogen bonding pattern with the enzyme, which is a common feature of most high-affinity thrombin inhibitors reported so far. Apart from the salt bridge with Asp189, the binding energy of **34** solely results from hydrophobic interactions, which underscores the general importance of this binding force in drug–receptor interactions [24].

Compound **34** was investigated biologically in depth because of its strong *in vitro* activity and its favorable selectivity profile versus related serine proteases (Table 10.4).

It turned out to be a very potent anticoagulant also *in vivo*. Among all inhibitors of this structural class, it exhibited the strongest activity and the longest duration of action in anaesthetized rats after i.v. administration. It was well tolerated in these animals up to the highest given dose of 10 mg/kg. However, it was not orally active, which is not a surprise considering that it is a very polar, permanently charged, hydrophilic molecule ($\log P < -0.6$ in *n*-octanol/buffer).

In principle, compounds with physicochemical characteristics like this can be converted into orally active prodrugs by turning the carboxylate into an ester group

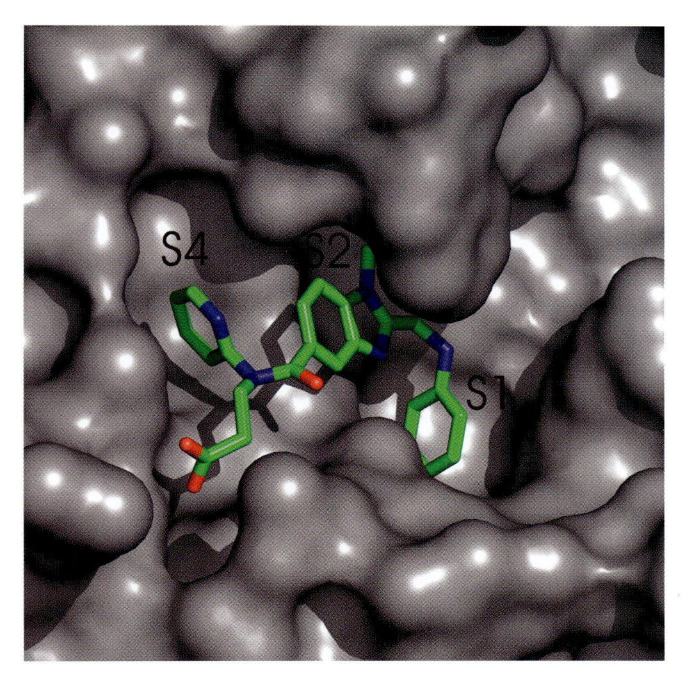

Figure 10.2 X-ray crystal structure of dabigatran (compound **34**) in complex with thrombin in a surface representation. The ligand interacts in a similar fashion as compound **8** with thrombin residues of the specificity pocket and the S2 pocket. The S4 pocket is occupied by the pyridine ring, while the propionic acid substituent on the amide nitrogen projects into bulk solvent without forming further interactions with the protein.

and by masking the amidinium moiety as a carbamate ester [25], provided that both the carboxylate and the amidinium will be restored *in vivo* by hydrolytic cleavage of the prodrug. Accordingly, we synthesized a series of double prodrugs of this type as exemplified by **35** (Scheme 10.2), which is a rather lipophilic compound with a log P value of > 2.5 (n-octanol/buffer).

Given orally to rhesus monkeys, this prodrug **35** exhibited strong and long-lasting anticoagulant effects as measured by the activated partial thromboplastin time (aPTT) *ex vivo* (Figure 10.3) [26].

Table 10.4 Selectivity profile of dabigatran (**34**).

Human enzymes	K_i **(nM)**
Thrombin	4.5
Factor Xa	3760
Trypsin	50
Plasmin	1695
tPA	45 360
Activated protein C	20 930
aPTT (human plasma): $ED_2 = 230 \pm 21$ nM	

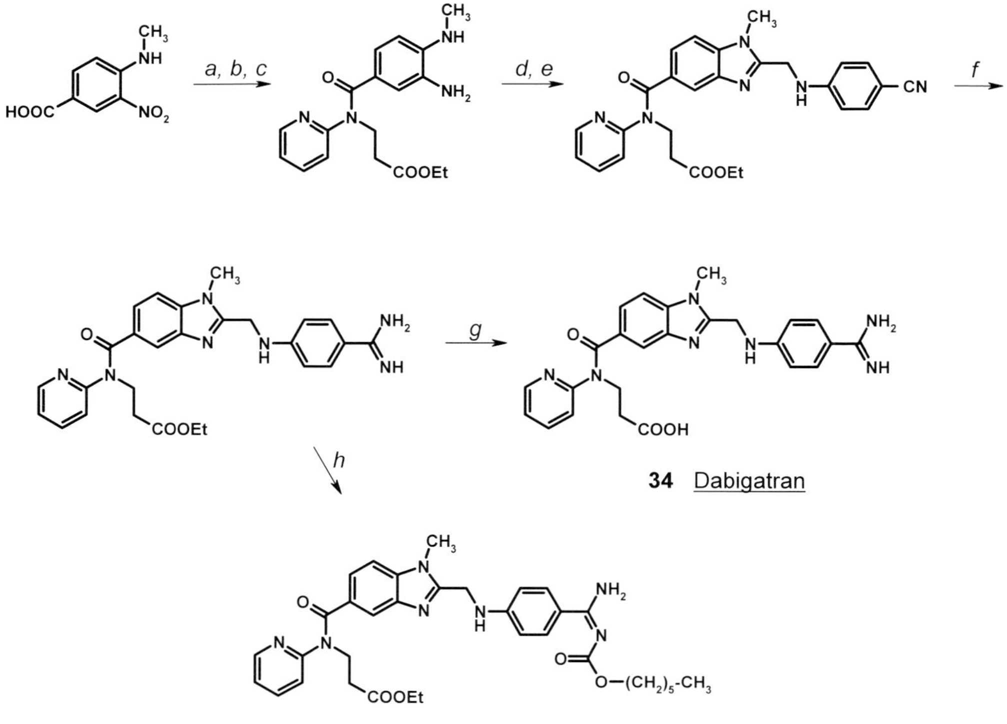

34 Dabigatran

35 Dabigatran Etexilate

Scheme 10.2 Synthesis of dabigatran and dabigatran etexilate. (a) $SOCl_2$/DMF, reflux; (b) 2-pyridylamino-propionic acid ethyl ester, THF, triethylamine, rt; (c) H_2, 10% Pd/C, methanol/CH_2Cl_2, rt; (d) 4-cyanophenyl-glycine, CDI, THF, 50 °C; (e) acetic acid, reflux; (f) HCl (gas), ethanol 0 °C, $(NH_4)_2CO_3$/ethanol, rt; (g) NaOH, H_2O/ethanol, rt; (h) *n*-hexyl chloroformate, K_2CO_3, THF/H_2O, rt.

Based on the overall profile and promising *in vivo* activity, compound **35** was selected for clinical development.

10.3 Preclinical Pharmacology Molecular Mechanism of Action of Dabigatran

Dabigatran inhibits human thrombin in a concentration-dependent and competitive fashion, with a K_i of 4.5 nM. This inhibition is rapid and reversible as shown by real-time binding kinetics using surface plasmon resonance techniques. IC_{50} values for other proteases involved in the coagulation and fibrinolytic pathway are >700-fold and up to >10,000-fold compared to thrombin, demonstrating the high selectivity of dabigatran for thrombin (Table 10.4).

Thrombin generated on the platelet surface in response to a hemostatic challenge also mediates platelet activation and aggregation as one of the most potent

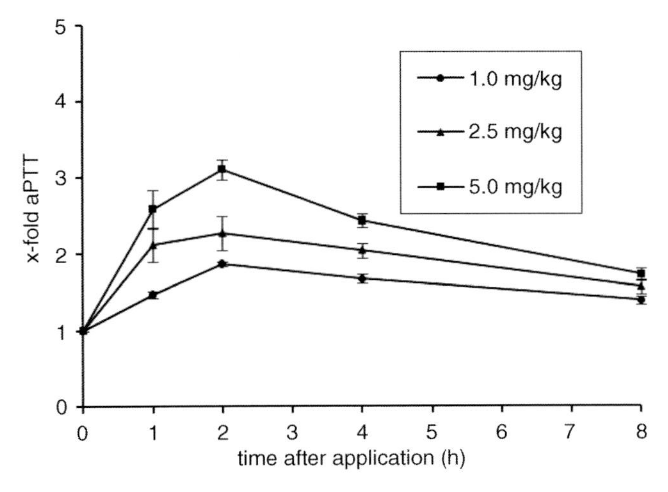

Figure 10.3 The dose- and time-dependent effects on aPTT after oral administration of compound **35** (dabigatran etexilate) to rhesus monkeys. Data represent mean ± SEM.

physiological agonists. Dabigatran inhibits thrombin-induced platelet aggregation with an IC_{50} of 10 nM, but has no inhibitory effect on platelet aggregation induced by arachidonic acid, collagen, or adenosine 2′,5′-diphosphate at concentrations of up to 1×10^{-4} M [26].

Dabigatran also effectively inhibits tissue factor-induced thrombin generation in human platelet poor plasma in a concentration-dependent manner with an IC_{50} of 0.56 μM as shown by the concentration-dependent decrease in the endogenous thrombin potential. Thus, in addition to its direct inhibition of thrombin activity, dabigatran is also able to inhibit thrombin generation.

Thrombin bound to fibrin, either in an existing thrombus or on an artificial surface, is thought to be protected from inhibition by the high molecular weight complex between heparin and antithrombin. This surface could therefore remain "active" despite heparin therapy. Dabigatran inhibits both clot-bound and fluid-phase thrombin to a similar degree with IC_{50} values of 128 and 113 nM, respectively, consistent with direct inhibition of the active site of thrombin by a small molecule. This binding appears independent of whether thrombin is bound via the exosite to fibrin or is present as free enzyme in plasma [27].

10.3.1
In Vitro Antihemostatic Effects of Dabigatran

Consistent and potent anticoagulant activity of dabigatran *in vitro* in platelet-poor plasma has been demonstrated using common clotting assays across several species (human, rhesus monkeys, dog, rabbit, and rat) [26]. A doubling of the aPTT, prothrombin time (PT), and ecarin clotting time (ECT) is observed at concentrations ranging from as low as 0.1 up to 4.6 μM of dabigatran with the ECT being the most sensitive parameter for anticoagulant activity.

10.3.2 *Ex Vivo* Antihemostatic Effects of Dabigatran/Dabigatran Etexilate

Dose- and time-dependent, significant anticoagulant efficacy *ex vivo* has also been demonstrated after intravenous administration of dabigatran to rats and rhesus monkeys. In rats, doses of 0.3, 1, and 3 mg/kg i.v. produce a maximum prolongation of the *ex vivo* aPTT to 29, 159, and 582 s, respectively, 5 min after administration. aPTT remains significantly elevated at all doses within the first hour after administration and decreases gradually thereafter.

In rhesus monkeys, intravenous administration (0.15, 0.3, or 0.6 mg/kg) of dabigatran prolongs the aPTT to 47.3, 70.1, and 98.9 s, respectively, 5 min after administration. This effect is long lasting with a significant prolongation still observed at >8 h after administration of the highest dose. Dabigatran etexilate also shows dose- and time-dependent anticoagulant effects in these species. Of note, single oral doses of 1, 2.5, and 5 mg/kg, administered to conscious rhesus monkeys, revealed a significant and long-lasting (>8 h) prolongation of the aPTT at all doses (Figure 10.3) [26].

10.3.3 Venous and Arterial Antithrombotic Effects of Dabigatran/Dabigatran Etexilate

The antithrombotic effects of dabigatran have been tested in a rat model of tissue factor/stasis-induced venous thrombosis. Dabigatran, administered intravenously as a slow bolus infusion, inhibited clot formation dose dependently and completely with an ED_{50} of 0.033 mg/kg [28]. Of note, no significant increase in bleeding time was observed at the maximum effective antithrombotic dose of 0.1 mg/kg. Using the same model, the prodrug dabigatran etexilate was administered orally (5–30 mg/kg) between 0.5 and 7 h prior to thrombus induction. Pretreatment resulted in a dose- and time-dependent inhibition of thrombus formation with significant inhibition lasting for >3 h for all doses tested.

Furthermore, both compounds have been examined in a rabbit arteriovenous shunt model of thrombosis. Intravenous administration of dabigatran revealed a dose-dependent inhibition of clot formation with a corresponding ED_{50} of 0.066 mg/kg [29]. Oral administration of dabigatran etexilate, in doses of 1–20 mg/kg, inhibited clot formation dose dependently, and with the highest dose completely. In both the rat and rabbit thrombosis models, the observed antithrombotic effects were inversely correlated with a prolongation of the *ex vivo* aPTT in a dose- and time-dependent manner.

Dabigatran, either alone or in combination with ASA, has also been tested in a Folts model of arterial thrombosis in pigs. The model is characterized by acute and severe arterial thrombus formation and a cyclic reduction of blood flow in response to a mechanical injurious stimulus and a concomitant partial stenosis of the carotid artery. ASA treatment alone reduced cyclic flow reductions by 40% and dabigatran alone by 44%. When the two compounds were given together, closures were reduced by 88%. In addition, a complete closure of the injured vessels was not observed in the dabigatran-treated and the dabigatran–aspirin-treated animals. Both compounds were shown to be effective and safe in this model of arterial thrombosis. These effects were achieved at clinically relevant plasma levels and show that dabigatran can effectively be used in an arterial thrombosis setting [30].

10.3.4 Mechanical Heart Valves

Thromboprophylaxis after mechanical heart valve implantation with warfarin therapy is required for the lifetime of the patient; this may be an area where direct thrombin inhibition could provide alternative therapy. This concept was tested in several preclinical studies. *In vitro,* a thrombosis tester was used that circulates human blood only anticoagulated with the agent being tested over a mechanical heart valve in a closed circuit. Thrombus formation on the valve after adding various antithrombotic regimens versus control was tested. In this study, it was shown that dabigatran was an effective inhibitor of fibrin deposition *in vitro* [31].

In vivo, dabigatran was tested in an experimental model in pigs, with an aortic heart valve placed as a graft in the descending aorta [32]. Dabigatran was administered postimplantation in pigs for 30 days versus LMWH, and a significant reduction in thrombus and platelet deposition onto the valve was seen.

10.3.5 Cancer

A link between cancer and thrombosis has long been recognized [33]. Whether this is due to prothrombotic mediators from the tumor, chemotherapy interventions, or both is unknown. In addition, there is a great deal of experimental evidence implicating PAR1-mediated events with tumor growth and metastasis. There is a correlation between expression of PAR1 on tumor cells and invasiveness of the cancer [33]. Upon activation in tumor cells, PAR1 is not internalized as in normal cells [34]. In addition, when metastatic breast cancer tumor cells (MDA-231) are genetically modified to express an inactive form of PAR1, they were no longer as tumorigenic as wild type in a xenograft model [35]. Studies testing the effects of chronic dabigatran treatment (4 weeks) in a syngeneic mouse model of breast cancer demonstrated a reduction in both primary tumor growth and metastasis in dabigatran-treated mice as compared to control [36].

10.3.6 Fibrosis

One chronic hallmark of atrial fibrillation and many other degenerative diseases is the extent of fibrosis, or the conversion of the normal cell type into a collagen secreting, fibroblastic phenotype [4]. This is present in myocardium of patients with atrial fibrillation, in renal tissue of patients with renal impairment, and in pulmonary tissue of patients with idiopathic pulmonary fibrosis. Activation of coagulation following tissue injury is one of the earliest responses, resulting in the deposition of fibrin. In addition, activation of PAR1 by thrombin can differentiate normal lung fibroblasts into a myofibroblast phenotype and induces fibrogenic cytokine release, such as transforming growth factor β, and increased expression of extracellular matrix proteins, such as collagen [37]. These effects are all inhibited *in vitro* by dabigatran. In addition, a recent study looking at chronic dabigatran etexilate treatment in mice with bleomycin-induced pulmonary injury showed a reduction in the extent of fibrosis and collagen release [38].

10.3.7 Atherosclerosis

There is increasing evidence in experimental atherosclerosis that inflammation and coagulation may play an important role in atherosclerotic development [5, 39]. Thus, it was tested whether direct thrombin inhibition with dabigatran can mitigate the progression of plaque formation. In an $ApoE^{-/-}$ mouse model of atherosclerosis, mice were fed a normal diet supplemented with dabigatran etexilate for up to 20 weeks. Lesion size of forming but not advanced atherosclerotic plaque was reduced in the dabigatran-fed mice and plaque stability, measured as fibrous cap thickness, was also increased [40].

A separate study in a procoagulant/atherosclerotic mouse model ($ApoE^{-/-}$:$TM^{pro/pro}$) also tested the effects of dabigatran etexilate-supplemented high-fat diet versus placebo. These $ApoE^{-/-}$:$TM^{pro/pro}$ mice have elevated plasma fibrinogen, prothrombin, factor X, and thrombin–antithrombin levels and develop extensive plaque formation due to their atherosclerotic backgrounds crossed with mice with a mutation in thrombomodulin (TM), resulting in loss of activity. The administration of dabigatran etexilate significantly reduced plaque area and the degree of stenosis after a carotid cuff injury [41].

10.4 Clinical Studies and Indications

For over 50 years, vitamin K antagonists have been the gold standard in chronic anticoagulation treatment. While they provide significant benefit when used properly as compared to no treatment, there are also significant drawbacks (e.g., frequent laboratory monitoring and dose adjustments, large number of drug interactions, and risk of bleeding). This translates in clinical practice into an underuse of treatment with VKAs in a substantial proportion of patients with atrial fibrillation. Therefore, there is a significant unmet medical need to develop anticoagulation treatment that is easy to use, predictable, effective, and safe. Dabigatran etexilate represents the first broadly approved new oral anticoagulant with these attributes.

Dabigatran has a fast onset of action (peak plasma concentrations 2–3 h after ingestion of dabigatran etexilate). The half-life is 12–14 h [42]. It does not require routine coagulation monitoring and has no drug–food interactions. Cytochrome P450 enzymes are not involved in the metabolism, but it is a substrate for the Pgp transporter, so there is the potential for drug interactions with agents using this transporter that in some indications results in a dose adaptation. Dabigatran is 80% renally excreted; thus, caution needs to be executed when prescribing to patients with kidney disease. In the United States, the FDA recommends a lower therapeutic dose (75 mg bid) in patients with a creatine clearance (CrCl) between 15 and 30 ml/min and no use in patients with CrCl under 15 ml/min for the prevention of strokes in patients with atrial fibrillation. In Europe, dabigatran is contraindicated in patients with a CrCl below 30 ml/min. However, no dose adjustment is needed for moderate liver disease [42, 43].

10.4.1 Prevention of Deep Venous Thrombosis

Dabigatran has been studied in more than 10 000 patients in four phase III trials of DVT prophylaxis in lower extremity orthopedic surgery [44–48]. In a study in total knee replacement (TKR), when compared to enoxaparin 30 mg bid, dabigatran etexilate at 150 and 220 mg daily was inferior due to a greater number of distal thromboses (dabigatran etexilate 220 mg – 27.6%, dabigatran etexilate 150 mg – 30.5%, and enoxaparin – 23.0%) [44]. In studies comparing dabigatran to 40 mg enoxaparin (European dosing regimen), equivalence was shown for both thrombosis prevention and bleeding in total hip replacement (THR) and TKR [45, 46]. The result of the THR trial was reproduced in the RE-NOVATE II trial, where dabigatran additionally showed a superior reduction of major venous thromboembolism with a same rate of major bleeding [48]. A pooled analysis of the THR trials demonstrated the superiority in the prevention of major VTE [49]. In the countries where dabigatran etexilate is approved for DVT prophylaxis, it is recommended at a dose of 220 mg daily (110 mg first dose after surgery) and at 150 mg (75 mg first dose after surgery) daily for patients with renal impairment or concomitant treatment with verapamil (a Pgp inhibitor).

10.4.2 Therapy of Venous Thromboembolism

In the treatment of VTE (includes DVT or pulmonary embolism), 150 mg dabigatran etexilate twice daily was compared to standard warfarin (INR 2.0–3.0) treatment [50]. All patients received heparin or low molecular weight heparin for a median of 9 days following one of the oral anticoagulants. Dabigatran demonstrated the same efficacy in the prevention of thrombosis with significantly less minor bleeding and similar major bleeding. The extension study RE-MEDY (versus warfarin) and RE-SONATE (versus placebo) showed in the warfarin comparison again the same efficacy and a better bleeding profile and in the placebo comparison a 92% relative risk reduction of recurrent VTE with statistically no difference in major bleeding, but as to be expected against placebo, elevated clinical relevant non-major bleeding (5.3% dabigatran versus 1.8% placebo) [51, 52]. These indications have not yet been registered.

10.4.3
Stroke Prevention in Patients with Atrial Fibrillation

In the RE-LY study, 18 234 patients with atrial fibrillation and at least one risk factor for stroke were randomized between warfarin INR 2–3, 110 mg of dabigatran twice daily, and 150 mg of dabigatran twice daily [53, 54]. The RE-LY trial was the only major phase 3 study that evaluated two different doses and had enough power for each dose, to define the most appropriate patient population. This resulted in the opportunity to tailor the dose according to the patient profile/population. The 150 mg bid dabigatran etexilate dose showed superior efficacy with the same major bleeding rate as warfarin, and the 110 mg bid dose had a significantly lower major bleeding rate and the same efficacy as warfarin. Both doses had a significant, up to 70%, reduction of intracranial hemorrhage and also a reduction in life-threatening bleeding. There was a nonsignificant 12% mortality benefit ($p = 0.051$) with the 150 mg bid dose [53, 54]. These results were consistent across all patient groups, such as those with a previous history of stroke or transient ischemic attack [55], or patients previously taking warfarin or those new to oral anticoagulation [56].

10.4.4
Prevention of Recurrent Myocardial Infarction in Patients with Acute Coronary Syndrome

In a phase II dose identification study, RE-DEEM, with a treatment time of 6 months, dabigatran in addition to dual antiplatelet therapy showed an expected dose-dependent increase in bleeding and significantly reduced coagulation activity. In the dose groups of 150 and 110 mg bid, the composite of cardiovascular death, nonfatal myocardial infarction, hemorrhagic stroke, cardiovascular death, and all-cause death was numerically lower compared to placebo (dual antiplatelet therapy) [57].

10.5
Summary

Based on a NAPAP–thrombin X-ray crystal structure, we designed a new structural class of inhibitors employing benzimidazole as a central scaffold. Supported by a series of X-ray structure analyses, we optimized the potency of these compounds in a number of iterative steps. During this process, enzyme inhibition in the lower nanomolar range could be achieved by gaining binding energy mainly from hydrophobic interactions. In order to reduce plasma protein binding, we increased the hydrophilicity of the inhibitors by introducing a carboxylate group at a position of the molecules, where it does not interfere with the thrombin binding site interaction. One of these inhibitors, dabigatran, showed very strong *in vivo* activity after i.v. administration; however, due to its highly polar nature, its oral absorption was insufficient. We therefore synthesized a number of prodrugs, from which dabigatran etexilate emerged as a clinical candidate due to its strong and long-lasting oral activity.

In-depth preclinical pharmacological investigations illustrated that dabigatran is an effective antithrombotic agent in both venous and arterial models. Furthermore, since thrombin has been shown to play a central role in many disease processes, dabigatran was investigated in additional biochemical pathways showing beneficial effects, for example, in fibrotic and atherosclerotic animal models.

In four clinical studies, this new drug has been shown to be as effective as enoxaparin in the prevention of venous thrombosis after orthopedic surgery, and to be as effective as warfarin in the therapy of acute thrombosis with no increased risk of bleeding. In stroke prevention in patients with atrial fibrillation, it was more effective than warfarin with a lesser risk of intracranial hemorrhage. The prevention of thromboembolic events in patients with mechanical heart valves is currently under evaluation.

More than 50 years after the introduction of warfarin, the development of dabigatran can be seen as a major breakthrough for the treatment of thrombosis.

References

1 DiCera, E. (2008) Thrombin. *Mol. Aspects Med.*, **29**, 203–254.

2 Griffin, J.H. (1995) Blood coagulation. The thrombin paradox. *Nature*, **378**, 337–338.

3 Lane, D.A., Philippou, H., and Huntington, J.A. (2005) Directing thrombin. *Blood*, **106**, 2605–2612.

4 Tan, A.Y. and Zimetbaum, P. (2011) Atrial fibrillation and atrial fibrosis. *J. Cardiovasc. Pharmacol.*, **57**, 625–629.

5 Borissoff, J.I., Spronk, H.M.H., Heeneman, S., and ten Cate, H. (2009) Is thrombin a key player in the "coagulation atherogenesis" maze? *Cardiovasc. Res.*, **82**, 392–403.

6 Derian, C.K., Maryanoff, B.E., Zang, H.E., and Andrade-Gordon, P. (2003) Therapeutic potential of protease receptor-1 antagonists. *Expert Opin. Invest. Drugs*, **12**, 209–221.

7 Martorell, L., Martínez-González, J., Rodríguez, C., Gentile, M., Calvayrac, O., and Badimon, L. (2008) Thrombin and protease-activated receptors (PARs) in atherothrombosis. *Thromb. Haemost.*, **99**, 305–315.

8 Coughlin, S.R. (2005) Protease-activated receptors in hemostasis, thrombosis and vascular biology. *J. Thromb. Haemost.*, **3**, 1800–1814.

9 Hirsh, J., Bauer, K.A., Donati, M.B., Gould, M., Samama, M.M., and Weitz, J.I. (2008) Parenteral anticoagulants: American College of Chest Physicians Evidence-Based Clinical Practice Guidelines (8th edition). *Chest*, **133**, 141S–159S.

10 Yeh, R.W. and Jang, I.-K. (2006) Argatroban: update. *Am. Heart J.*, **151**, 1131–1138.

11 Warkentin, T.E., Greinacher, A., and Koster, A. (2008) Bivalirudin. *Thromb. Haemost.*, **99**, 830–839.

12 Hirsh, J., Dalen, J.E., Anderson, D.R., Poller, L., Bussey, H., Ansell, J., Deykin, D.,

and Brandt, J.T. (1998) Oral anticoagulants. Mechanism of action, clinical effectiveness, and optimal therapeutic range. *Chest*, **114**, 445S–469S.

13 Mann, K.G. (2005) The challenge of regulating anticoagulant drugs: focus on warfarin. *Am. Heart J.*, **149**, S36–S42.

14 Gustafsson, D., Bylund, R., Antonsson, T., Nilsson, I., Nystroem, J.-E., Eriksson, U., Bredberg, U., and Teger-Nilsson, A.-C. (2004) Case history: a new oral anticoagulant: the 50-year challenge. *Nat. Rev. Drug Discov.*, **3**, 649–659.

15 Pinto, D.J.P., Smallheer, J.M., Cheney, D.L., Knabb, R.M., and Wexler, R.R. (2010) Factor Xa inhibitors: next-generation antithrombotic agents. *J. Med. Chem.*, **53**, 6243–6274.

16 Perzborn, E., Roehrig, S., Straub, A., Kubitza, D., and Misselwitz, F. (2011) The discovery and development of rivaroxaban, an oral, direct factor Xa inhibitor. *Nat. Rev. Drug Discov.*, **10**, 61–75.

17 Pinto, D.J.P., Orwat, M.J., Koch, S., Rossi, K.A., Alexander, R.S., Smallwood, A., Wong, P.C., Rendina, A.R., Luettgen, J.M., Knabb, R.M., He, K., Xin, B., Wexler, R.R., and Lam, P.Y.S. (2007) Discovery of 1-(4-methoxyphenyl)-7-oxo-6-(4-(2-oxopiperidin-1-yl)phenyl)-4,5,6,7-tetrahydro-1*H*-pyrazolo[3,4-*c*]pyridine-3-carboxamide (apixaban, BMS-562247), a highly potent, selective, efficacious, and orally bioavailable inhibitor of blood coagulation factor Xa. *J. Med. Chem.*, **50**, 5339–5356.

18 Furugohri, T., Isobe, K., Honda, Y., Kamisato-Matsumoto, C., Sugiyama, N., Nagahara, T., Morishima, Y., and Shibano, T. (2008) DU-176b, a potent and orally active factor Xa inhibitor: *in vitro* and *in vivo* pharmacological profiles. *J. Thromb. Haemost.*, **6**, 1542–1549.

19 Hauel, N.H., Nar, H., Priepke, H., Ries, U., Stassen, J.M., and Wienen, W. (2002) Structure-based design of novel potent nonpeptide thrombin inhibitors. *J. Med. Chem.*, **45**, 1757–1766.

20 Hankey, G.J. and Eikelboom, J.W. (2011) Dabigatran etexilate: a new oral thrombin inhibitor. *Circulation*, **123**, 1436–1450.

21 Brandstetter, H., Turk, D., Hoeffken, H.W., Grosse, D., Stuerzebecher, J., Martin, P.D., Edwards, B.F.P., and Bode, W. (1992) Refined 2.3 Å X-ray crystal structure of bovine thrombin complexes formed with the benzamidine and arginine-based thrombin inhibitors NAPAP, 4-TAPAP and MQPA. *J. Mol. Biol.*, **226**, 1085–1099.

22 Andrews, P.R., Craik, D.J., and Martin, J.L. (1984) Functional group contributions to drug–receptor interactions. *J. Med. Chem.*, **27**, 1648–1657.

23 Tucker, T.J., Lumma, W.C., Lewis, S.D., Gardell, S.J., Lukas, B.J., Baskin, E.P., Woltmann, R., Lynch, J.J., Lyle, E.A., Appleby, S.D., Chen, I.-W., Dancheck, K.B., and Vacca, J.P. (1997) Potent noncovalent thrombin inhibitors that utilize the unique amino acid D-dicyclohexylalanine in the P3 position: implications on oral bioavailability and antithrombotic efficacy. *J. Med. Chem.*, **40**, 1565–1569.

24 Davis, A.M. and Teague, S.J. (1999) Hydrogen bonding, hydrophobic interactions, and failure of the rigid receptor hypothesis. *Angew. Chem., Int. Ed.*, **38**, 736–749.

25 (a) Himmelsbach, F., Austel, V., Guth, B., Linz, G., Mueller, T.H., Pieper, H., Seewaldt-Becker, E., and Weisenberger, H., (1995) Design of potent nonpeptidic fibrinogen receptor antagonists. *Eur. J. Med. Chem.*, **30**, 243s–254s. (b) Mueller, T.H., Weisenberger, H., Brickl, R., Narjes, H., Himmelsbach, F., and Krause, J. (1997) Profound and sustained inhibition of platelet aggregation by fradafiban, a nonpeptide platelet glycoprotein IIb/IIIa antagonist, and its orally active prodrug, lefradafiban, in men. *Circulation*, **96**, 1130–1138.

26 Wienen, W., Stassen, J.-M., Priepke, H., Ries, U.-J., and Hauel, N. (2007) *In-vitro* profile and *ex-vivo* anticoagulant activity of the direct thrombin inhibitor dabigatran and its orally active prodrug, dabigatran etexilate. *Thromb. Haemost.*, **98**, 155–162.

27 van Ryn, J., Hauel, N., Waldmann, L., and Wienen, W. (2008) Dabigatran inhibits both clot-bound and fluid-phase thrombin

in vitro: comparison to heparin and hirudin. *Arterioscler. Thromb. Vasc. Biol.*, **28**, e136–e137.

28 Wienen, W., Stassen, J.-M., Priepke, H., Ries, U.-J., and Hauel, N. (2007) Effects of the direct thrombin inhibitor dabigatran and its orally active prodrug, dabigatran etexilate, on thrombus formation and bleeding time in rats. *Thromb. Haemost.*, **98**, 333–338.

29 Wienen, W., Stassen, J.-M., Priepke, H., Ries, U.-J., and Hauel, N. (2007) Antithrombotic and anticoagulant effects of the direct thrombin inhibitor dabigatran, and its oral prodrug, dabigatran etexilate, in a rabbit model of venous thrombosis. *J. Thromb. Haemost.*, **5**, 1237–1242.

30 van Ryn, J., Dietze, T., Kuritsch, I., Kink-Eiband, M., and Wienen, W. (2009) Effect of the direct thrombin inhibitor, dabigatran, on arterial thrombosis when given in combination with aspirin (ASA) in a cyclic flow model in anesthetised pigs (Abstract). *J. Thromb. Haemost.*, **7** (Suppl. 2), 435.

31 Maegdefessel, L., Linde, T., Krapiec, F., Hamilton, K., Steinseifer, U., van Ryn, J., Raaz, U., Buerke, M., Werdan, K., and Schlitt, A. (2010) *In vitro* comparison of dabigatran, unfractionated heparin, and low-molecular-weight heparin in preventing thrombus formation on mechanical heart valves. *Thromb. Res.*, **126**, e196–e200.

32 McKellar, S.H., Abel, S., Camp, C.L., Suri, R.M., Ereth, M.H., and Schaff, H.V. (2011) Effectiveness of dabigatran etexilate for thromboprophylaxis of mechanical heart valves. *J. Thorac. Cardiovasc. Surg.*, **141**, 1410–1416.

33 Iodice, S., Gandini, S., Lohr, M., Lowenfels, A.B., and Maisonneuve, P. (2008) Venous thromboembolic events and organ-specific occult cancers: a review and meta-analysis. *J. Thromb. Haemost.*, **6**, 781–788.

34 Booden, M.A., Eckert, L.B., Der, C.J., and Trejo, J.A. (2004) Persistent signalling by dysregulated thrombin receptor trafficking promotes breast carcinoma cell invasion. *Mol. Cell. Biol.*, **24**, 1990–1999.

35 Boire, A., Covic, L., Agarwal, A., Jacques, S., Sherifi, S., and Kuliopulos, A. (2005) PAR1 is a matrix metalloprotease-1 receptor that promotes invasion and tumorigenesis of breast cancer cells. *Cell*, **120**, 303–313.

36 DeFeo, K., Hayes, C., Chernick, M., van Ryn, J., and Gilmour, S.K. (2010) Use of dabigatran etexilate to reduce breast cancer progression. *Cancer Biol. Ther.*, **10**, 1001–1008.

37 Bogatkevich, G.S. and Silver, R. (2009) Dabigatran inhibits the thrombin-induced differentiation of lung fibroblasts to a myofibroblast phenotype. *Arthritis Rheum.*, **60**, 3455–3464.

38 Bogatkevich, G.S., Ludwicka-Bradley, A., Nietert, P.J., van Ryn, J., and Silver, R.M. (2011) Antifibrotic effects of the oral, direct thrombin inhibitor dabigatran etexilate on lung injury in mice model of pulmonary fibrosis. *Arthritis Rheum.*, **63**, 1416–1425.

39 Borissoff, J.I., Spronk, H.M.H., and ten Cate, H. (2011) The haemostatic system as a modulator of atherosclerosis. *N. Engl. J. Med.*, **364**, 1746–1760.

40 Preusch, M.R., Wijelath, E.S., Cabbage, S., Ieronimakis, N., Callegari, A., Bea, F., Blessing, E., Reyes, M., van Ryn, J., and Rosenfeld, M.E. (2010) Dabigatran etexilate, a new oral thrombin inhibitor, retards the initiation and progression of atherosclerotic lesions and inhibits the expression of oncostatin M in apolipoprotein E deficient mice (Abstract). *Arterioscler. Thromb. Vasc. Biol.*, **30**, e185.

41 Borissoff, J.I., Loubele, S.T., Leenders, P., Soehnlein, O., Koenen, R.R., van Oerle, R., Hamulyak, K., Heeneman, S., Daemen, M.J., Weiler, H., van Ryn, J., Spronk, H.M., and ten Cate, H. (2010) Direct thrombin inhibition by dabigatran protects against severe atherosclerosis progression in prothrombotic mice (Abstract). *Circulation*, **122** (Suppl. 1), A19384.

42 Stangier, J. and Clemens, A. (2009) Pharmacology, pharmacokinetics, and pharmacodynamics of dabigatran etexilate, an oral direct thrombin inhibitor. *Clin. Appl. Thromb. Hemost.*, **15** (Suppl 1), 9S–16S.

43 Garnock-Jones, K.P. (2011) Dabigatran etexilate: a review of its use in the prevention of stroke and systemic embolism in patients with atrial fibrillation. *Am. J. Cardiovasc. Drugs*, **11**, 57–72.

44 Ginsberg, J.S., Davidson, B.L., Comp, P.C., Francis, C.W., Friedman, R.J., Huo, M.H., Lieberman, J.R., Muntz, J.E., Raskob, G.E., Clements, M.L., Hantel, S., Schnee, J.M., and Caprini, J.A. (2009) Oral thrombin inhibitor dabigatran etexilate vs North American enoxaparin regimen for prevention of venous thromboembolism after knee arthroplasty surgery. *J. Arthroplasty*, **24**, 1–9.

45 Eriksson, B.I., Dahl, O.E., Rosencher, N., Kurth, A.A., van Dijk, C.N., Frostick, S.P., Kalebo, P., Christiansen, A.V., Hantel, S., Hettiarachchi, R., Schnee, J., and Buller, H.R. (2007) Oral dabigatran etexilate vs. subcutaneous enoxaparin for the prevention of venous thromboembolism after total knee replacement: the RE-MODEL randomized trial. *J. Thromb. Haemost.*, **5**, 2178–2185.

46 Eriksson, B.I., Dahl, O.E., Rosencher, N., Kurth, A.A., van Dijk, C.N., Frostick, S.P., Prins, M.H., Hettiarachi, R., Hantel, S., Schnee, J., and Bueller, H.R. (2007) Dabigatran etexilate versus enoxaparin for prevention of venous thromboembolism after total hip replacement: a randomised, double-blind, non-inferiority trial. *Lancet*, **370**, 949–956.

47 Friedman, R.J., Dahl, O.E., Rosencher, N., Caprini, J.A., Kurth, A.A., Francis, C.W., Clemens, A., Hantel, S., Schnee, J.M., and Eriksson, B.I. (2010) Dabigatran versus enoxaparin for prevention of venous thromboembolism after hip or knee arthroplasty: a pooled analysis of three trials. *Thromb. Res.*, **126**, 175–182.

48 Eriksson, B.I., Dahl, O.E., Huo, M.H., Kurth, A.A., Hantel, S., Hermansson, K., Schnee, J.M., and Friedman, R.J. (2011) Oral dabigatran versus enoxaparin for thromboprophylaxis after primary total hip arthroplasty (RE-NOVATE II). *Thromb. Haemost.*, **105**, 721–729.

49 Eriksson, B.I., Kurth, A.A., Dahl, O.E., Clemens, A., Schnee, J., Hantel, S., Feuring, M., Friedman, R.J., and Huo, M. (2011) Oral dabigatran etexilate vs. enoxaparin for prevention of venous thromboembolism after total hip arthroplasty: a pooled analysis of two randomized trials. *J. Thromb. Haemost.*, **9** (Suppl. 2), 856–857.

50 Schulman, S., Kearon, C., Kakkar, A.K., Mismetti, P., Schellong, S., Eriksson, H., Baanstra, D., Schnee, J., and Goldhaber, S. Z. (2009) Dabigatran versus warfarin in the treatment of acute venous thromboembolism. *N. Engl. J. Med.*, **361**, 2342–2352.

51 Schulman, S., Eriksson, H., Goldhaber, S.Z., Kakkar, A.K.L., Kearon, C., Kvamme, A.M., Mismetti, P., Schellong, S., and Schnee, J. (2011) Dabigatran or warfarin for extended maintenance therapy of venous thromboembolism. *J. Thromb. Haemost.*, **9** (Suppl. 2), 731–732.

52 Schulman, S., Baanstra, D., Eriksson, H., Goldhaber, S., Kakkar, A., Kearon, C., Mismetti, P., Schellong, S., and Schnee, J. (2011) Dabigatran *versus* placebo for extended maintenance therapy of venous thromboembolism. *J. Thromb. Haemost.*, **9** (Suppl. 2), 22.

53 Connolly, S.J., Ezekowitz, M.D., Yusuf, S., Eikelboom, J., Oldgren, J., Parekh, A., Pogue, J., Reilly, P.A., Themeles, E., Varrone, J., Wang, S., Alings, M., Xavier, D., Zhu, J., Diaz, R., Lewis, B.S., Darius, H., Diener, H.C., Joyner, C.D., and Wallentin, L. (2009) Dabigatran versus warfarin in patients with atrial fibrillation. *N. Engl. J. Med.*, **361**, 1139–1151.

54 Connolly, S.J., Eszekowitz, M., Yusuf, S., Reilly, P.A., and Wallentin, L. (2010) Newly Identified events in the RE-LY trial. *N. Engl. J. Med.*, **363**, 1875–1876.

55 Diener, H.C., Connolly, S.J., Ezekowitz, M.D., Wallentin, L., Reilly, P.A., Yang, S., Xavier, D., di Pasquale, G., and Yusuf, S. (2010) Dabigatran compared with warfarin in patients with atrial fibrillation and previous transient ischaemic attack or stroke: a subgroup analysis of the RE-LY trial. *Lancet Neurol.*, **9**, 1157–1163.

56 Ezekowitz, M.D., Wallentin, L., Connolly, S.J., Parekh, A., Chernick,

M.R., Pogue, J., Aikens, T.H., Yang, S., Reilly, P.A., Lip, G.Y.H., and Yusuf, S. (2010) Dabigatran and warfarin in vitamin K antagonist-naive and -experienced cohorts with atrial fibrillation. *Circulation*, **122**, 2246–2253.

57 Oldgren, J., Budaj, A., Granger, C.B., Khder, Y., Roberts, J., Siegbahn, A., Tijssen, J.G.P., van de Werf, F., and Wallentin, L. (2011) Dabigatran vs. placebo in patients with acute coronary syndrome on dual antiplatelet therapy: a randomised, double blind, phase II trial. *Eur. Heart J.*, **32**, 2781–2789.

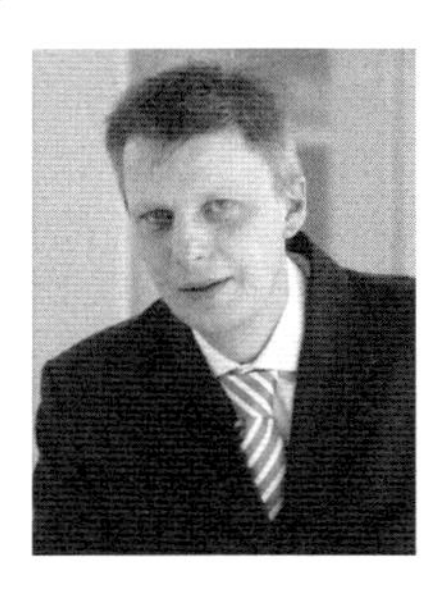

Andreas Clemens completed his graduation as Medical Doctor, Internist, and Endocrinologist in 2002 and after working for about 8 years in university hospitals from 2001 onward started his career in the pharmaceutical industry. He joined Boehringer Ingelheim in 2005 in this global position where he launched dabigatran worldwide for the primary prevention of venous thromboembolic events in patients after orthopedic surgery and recently for the prevention of stroke in patients with atrial fibrillation. He is currently the Global Senior Director Clinical Research & Medical Affairs and leads the group responsible for the further development of dabigatran etexilate beyond the clinical indications to date.

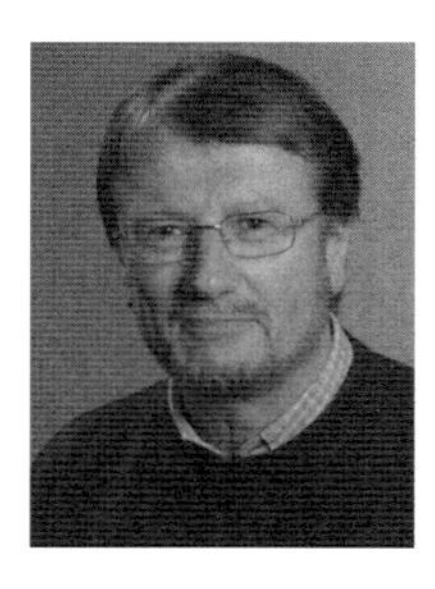

Norbert Hauel received his master's degree in Organic Chemistry and his Ph.D. from the University of Marburg, Germany (Prof. R.W. Hoffmann). In October 1979, he joined Boehringer Ingelheim and started to work as a lab head in the Department of Medicinal Chemistry. In 1988, he was promoted to become a Group Leader of four laboratories. At that time, his main area of research was cardiovascular diseases, which resulted in the invention of the angiotensin II antagonist telmisartan (Micardis®) in 1990 and dabigatran (Pradaxa®) in 1996. Since then, he has been working on numerous drug discovery projects in oncology and CNS diseases.

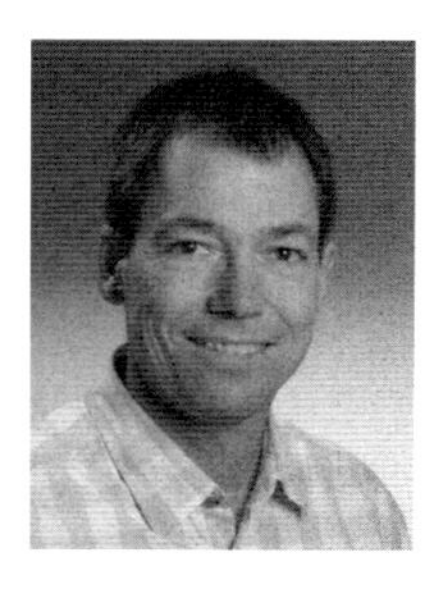

Herbert Nar graduated from the Technical University Munich in Chemistry and obtained his Ph.D. from the same institute with structural studies on blue copper electron transfer proteins. In his postdoctoral work with Robert Huber at the Max-Planck-Institute für Biochemie, he determined the 3D structures of proteins involved in pterin biosynthesis and studied their enzymatic mechanisms. He joined Boehringer Ingelheim in 1995 to establish a protein crystallography laboratory. In 2000, he took over responsibility for the Structural Research Group that comprises units for protein expression and purification, biophysics of ligand binding, and NMR and protein crystallography.

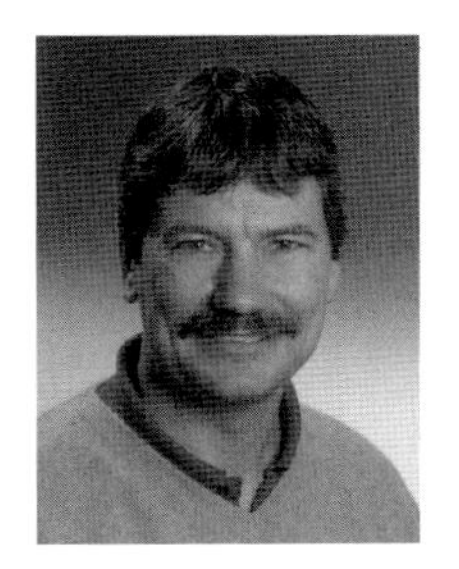

Henning Priepke received his diploma degree from the University of Marburg and his Ph.D. from the University of Würzburg (Prof. Reinhard Brückner). After two stimulating postdoctoral stays at the University of Cambridge in Prof. Steven Ley's group and in Basel at the Ciba-Geigy Central Research Unit with Prof. Beat Ernst, he joined Boehringer Ingelheim in 1995 where he has worked in different therapeutic areas including cardiovascular, CNS, and metabolic diseases.

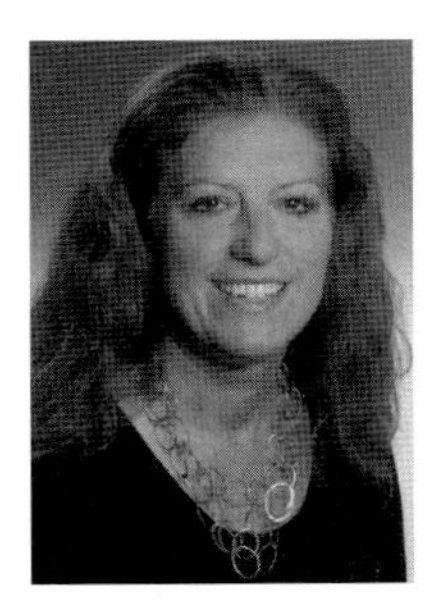

Joanne van Ryn graduated from McMaster University in Hamilton, Canada, and also obtained an M.Sc. and Ph.D. from this same institution in the Department of Medical Sciences, specializing in thrombosis and fibrinolysis research. She began her career at Boehringer in 1990, first as a Post Doc and then as head of a laboratory, focusing on translational aspects of thrombosis therapy and detection. Currently, she is the Global Head of Scientific Support for dabigatran, initiating studies investigating the role of thrombin in other disease processes and proof-of-concept studies in potential new indications.

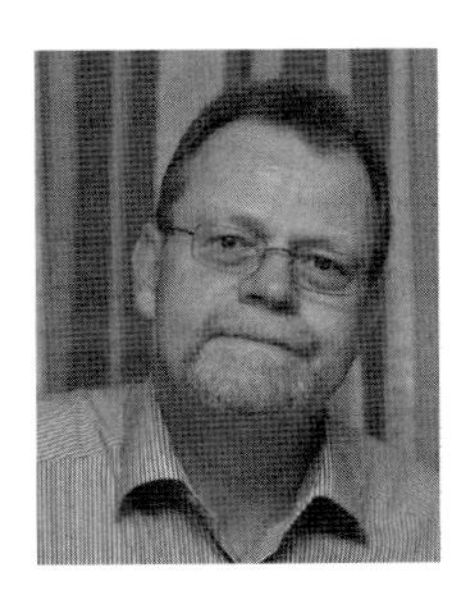

Wolfgang Wienen received his master's degree in Biology from the Technical University of Aachen, Germany. He joined the group of Professor H. Kammermeier in the Department of Physiology in the Medical Faculty of the RWTH Aachen, where he received a Ph.D. in Animal Physiology and Pharmacology. In 1987, he started to work as lab head in the Department of Cardiovascular Pharmacology at Boehringer Ingelheim, Germany. As responsible pharmacologist, he has supported the development of telmisartan (Micardis®), an angiotensin II receptor antagonist, and dabigatran etexilate (Pradaxa®). Since 2003, he has been working in various drug discovery research projects in the Department of Respiratory Diseases Research.

11
The Discovery of Citalopram and Its Refinement to Escitalopram

Klaus P. Bøgesø and Connie Sánchez

List of Abbreviations

CHO	Chinese hamster ovary
DA	dopamine
DAT	dopamine transporter
DMPK	drug metabolism and pharmacokinetics
DTTA	ditoluoyl tartaric acid
gSERT	chicken (gallus) serotonin transporter
5-HIAA	5-hydroxyindoleacetic acid
HPLC	high-pressure liquid chromatography
hSERT	human serotonin transporter
5-HT	5-hydroxytryptamin
5-HT1A	5-hydroxytryptamin 1A (receptor)
5-HTP	5-hydroxytryptophan
LeuT	leucine transporter
MAOI	monoamine oxidase inhibitor
NE	norepinephrine
NET	norepinephrine transporter
NMR	nuclear magnetic resonance
NRI	norepinephrine reuptake inhibitor
PET	positron emission tomography
PKC	protein kinase C
QSAR	quantitative structure–activity relationship
SAR	structure–activity relationship
SERT	serotonin transporter
SIP	serotonin interaction protein
SLC6	solute carrier 6
SMB	simulated moving bed
SNRI	serotonin norepinephrine reuptake inhibitor
WT SERT	wild type serotonin transporter

Analogue-based Drug Discovery III, First Edition. Edited by János Fischer, C. Robin Ganellin, and David P. Rotella.
© 2013 Wiley-VCH Verlag GmbH & Co. KGaA. Published 2013 by Wiley-VCH Verlag GmbH & Co. KGaA.

SPECT	single-photon emission computer tomography
SSRI	selective serotonin reuptake inhibitor
TCA	tricyclic antidepressants

11.1 Introduction

The serendipitous discoveries of the monoamine oxidase inhibitor (MAOI) iproniazid and the tricyclic antidepressant (TCA) imipramine in the late 1950s were major breakthroughs in the treatment of depression. The discovery of imipramine initiated a search for new tricyclic antidepressants using analogue design. Among these analogues were amitriptyline (**1**), nortriptyline (**2**), and melitracen (**3**) (Figure 11.1). Lundbeck developed new patentable syntheses of these three drugs (at that time, product patents were not obtainable, only process patents) and entered the market with these products in the early 1960s. However, the use of TCAs is associated with disturbing and serious side effects, such as dryness of the mouth, constipation, confusion, dizziness, sedation, orthostatic hypotension, tachycardia, and/or arrhythmia. Relatively narrow therapeutic indices limit the dose range in which they can be used and pose a risk in the case of overdose.

As increasing knowledge was gained about the mechanism of action of the TCAs and appropriate screening assays were developed, chemists started to look for ways to improve them. TCAs either inhibit the reuptake of serotonin

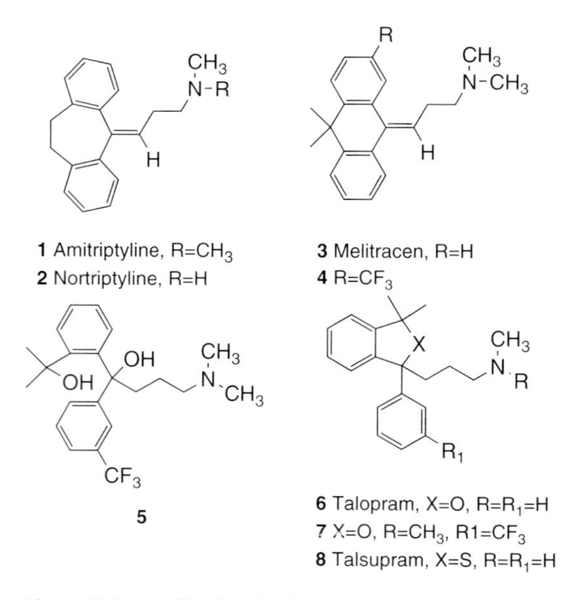

Figure 11.1 Lundbeck's tricyclic antidepressants and the selective NE uptake inhibitors talopram and talsupram.

(5-hydroxytryptamine, 5-HT) and norepinephrine (NE) (imipramine, amitriptyline), or predominantly NE (desipramine, nortriptyline). But they also block a number of postsynaptic receptors, notably those for NE, acetylcholine, and histamine. The latter effects were mainly associated with the side effects, whereas inhibition of the monoamine transporters was associated with the therapeutic effects. Two major hypothesis of depression emerged from this research, the 5-HT and the NE hypotheses, where lowered 5-HT levels in the brain were associated with lowered mood, and lowered NE levels were associated with lowered psychomotor drive. The discovery of the selective serotonin reuptake inhibitors (SSRIs) has already been described broadly in a previous volume of this series [1]. Thus, the following will focus on the discovery of citalopram and escitalopram [2–4].

11.2 Discovery of Talopram

The discoveries of both citalopram and escitalopram (*S*-citalopram) are good examples of how analogue design can lead to drugs with either totally different or greatly improved therapeutic profiles compared with the starting structure.

The discovery of citalopram started with the discovery of talopram (**6**) (Figure 11.1) in 1965. In an attempt to make a trifluoromethyl-substituted derivative of melitracen (**4**) using a precursor molecule (**5**) and reaction conditions (ring closure in concentrated sulfuric acid) similar to those used in the production of melitracen, a chemist at Lundbeck ended up with a different product, which after meticulous structural elucidation proved to be the phthalane structure **7**. This compound proved to be a surprisingly selective NE uptake inhibitor. Analogue design revealed that the unsubstituted *N*-des-methyl analogue **6** (talopram, Lu 03-010) was a highly selective and very potent NE uptake inhibitor. The sulfur analogue of talopram, called talsupram (**8**, Lu 05-003), was likewise a very potent, selective inhibitor of the NE transporter (NET). Both compounds were therefore major improvements with regard to selectivity compared with the nonselective TCAs, desipramine and nortriptyline.

Both drugs entered early clinical testing in the late 1960s, but were stopped in phase II for various reasons, among which was a rather activating profile. This observation was supportive of the hypothesis proposed by Professor Arvid Carlsson that NE uptake inhibition would mainly increase psychomotor drive. Carlsson had noticed that the tertiary amine drugs, which were mixed 5-HT and NE reuptake inhibitors, were “mood elevating,” while the secondary amines, being primarily NE reuptake inhibitors, increased the psychomotor drive in the depressed patients [5]. Carlsson advocated the development of selective 5-HT uptake inhibitors to treat the lowered mood state and avoid the potential suicide risk associated with an increased psychomotor drive in a depressed patient. Carlsson presented his theory at Lundbeck, and in 1971 it was decided to start a search for a selective serotonin reuptake inhibitor.

Although it may seem paradoxical, it was decided to use talopram as template for designing an SSRI. However, the reason was that there were already a few analogues of talopram available in-house that had dual 5-HT/NE uptake inhibition [2]. In particular, derivatives lacking the 3,3-dimethyl substituents of talopram, but with a chlorine either at the 5-position or at the 4′-position (see the structure in Table 11.1), were more potent as 5-HT uptake inhibitors than NE uptake inhibitors. Like their tricyclic dual-acting counterparts, these compounds also had a dimethylamino group, instead of the monomethylamino group found in the selective NE uptake inhibitors.

We, therefore, decided to use the structure at the top of Table 11.1 as the core structure for a program investigating the structure–activity relationships (SARs) of aromatic substitution in the two benzene rings.

11.3
Discovery of Citalopram

We published our initial SAR study (actually a quantitative structure–activity relationship (QSAR) study) in 1977 [7]. At that time, *in vitro* assays measuring inhibition of neuronal 5-HT and NE uptake were not available at Lundbeck, so 5-HT and NE uptake inhibition was measured as inhibition of $[^3H]$-5-HT uptake into rabbit platelets and as inhibition of $[^3H]$-NE uptake into the mouse heart *ex vivo*, respectively. Although these models were not directly comparable, they were acceptable as long as the goal was to develop selective compounds. Later on, assays based on inhibition of $[^3H]$-5-HT and $[^3H]$-NE uptake into rat brain synaptosome preparations as well as recombinant cell-based assays expressing the cloned human serotonin transporter (hSERT) or NET were developed. Table 11.1 shows a number of key citalopram derivatives (**9–16**) with the original blood platelet results as well as data for inhibition of $[^3H]$-5-HT uptake in recombinant cells expressing the cloned hSERT. All citalopram derivatives are highly selective serotonin transporter (SERT) inhibitors compared to inhibition of the NET and the dopamine transporters (DATs). Thus, data for NET and DAT inhibition are not shown.

Applying the observations mentioned above regarding monosubstituted chloro derivatives led to the synthesis of the 5,4′-dichloro derivative (**10**, Table 11.1) that proved to be a very potent SSRI. SAR studies of inhibitors of SERT, NET, and DAT very often show that optimal potency is found in 3,4-dichlorophenyl derivatives [8]. This derivative (**11**) also proved to be very potent, whereas the corresponding 3′,5′-dichloro derivative (**12**) had 25–100 times weaker activity. Substitution with chlorine at the 6-, 4-, and 7-positions (compounds **13**, **14**, and **15**) was also allowed. The most potent derivatives were generally found among the 4′,5-disubstituted derivatives substituted with F, Cl, Br, or CF_3. Electron-donating groups (3′-OCH_3, 4′-OCH_3, or 4′-isopropyl) had very low activity [7].

At that time, a cyano group was not considered an obvious choice in systematic aromatic substitution SAR investigations. One reason was that a nitrile

Table 11.1 Inhibition of 5-HT uptake and allosteric effect in a series of selected citalopram derivatives.

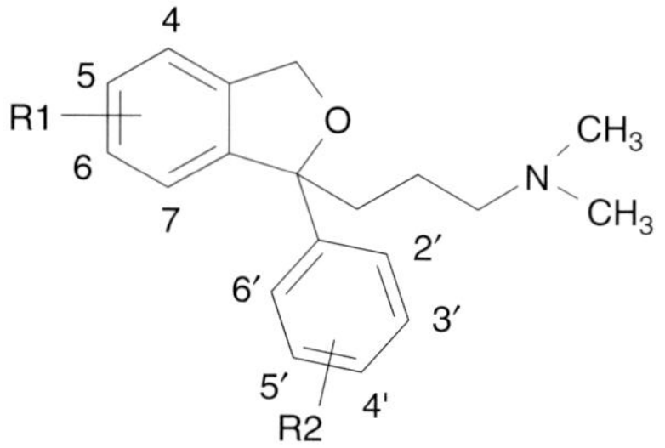

			Inhibition of uptake of $[^3H]$5-HT			
			Rat blood pl[a]	hSERT	hSERT	hSERT allosteric[b]
Compound	**R1**	**R2**	IC_{50} (nM)	IC_{50} (nM)	IC_{50} (nM)	IC_{50} (μM)
9	5-CN (citalopram)	4′-F	14	6.7		8.7
S-**9**	5-CN (escitalopram)	4′-F		2.1		5.1
R-**9**	5-CN (*R*-citalopram)	4′-F		170		25
10	5-Cl	4′-Cl	20	7.4		12.1
11	H	3′,4′-Cl_2	17		13	29.6
12	H	3′,5′-Cl_2	1600	200	340	15
12a[c]	H	3′,5′-Cl_2			350	8.8
12b[c]	H	3′,5′-Cl_2			300	20
13	6-Cl	4′-Cl	120		23	
14	4-Cl	4′-Cl	47	33	9.2	6.1
15	7-Cl	4′-Cl	63		26	
16	5-Br	4′-F	22	13		30.2
17	5-$(CH_3)_2N(CH_2)_3CO$	4′-F		1.6		714
18	5-CN	4′-(4-F-C_6H_4-S)			200	12

(continued)

Table 11.1 (*Continued*)

			Inhibition of uptake of [^{3}H]5-HT			
			Rat blood pl[a]	hSERT	hSERT	hSERT allosteric[b]
Compound	R1	R2	IC_{50} (nM)	IC_{50} (nM)	IC_{50} (nM)	IC_{50} (μM)
18a[c]	5-CN	4′-(4-F-C_6H_4-S)			310	8.3
18b[c]	5-CN	4′-(4-F-C_6H_4-S)			330	22
19	5-CN	[2-Naphthyl]			34	68
19a[c]	5-CN	[2-Naphthyl]			10	41
19b[c]	5-CN	[2-Naphthyl]			150	55
20	5-CN	[1-Naphthyl]			250	19
20a[c]	5-CN	[1-Naphthyl]			740	14
20b[c]	5-CN	[1-Naphthyl]			280	19

If not referred to in the text, data are unpublished data, H. Lundbeck A/S. Inhibition of [^{3}H]-5-HT uptake at the hSERT was performed in Chinese hamster ovary (CHO) cells stably expressing wild-type hSERT, as described by Ref. [6]. The two columns represent essentially similar assay conditions.

a) Data from Ref. [7].

b) Dissociation binding studies at the hSERT were conducted as described [6].

c) a and b refer to different enantiomeric forms.

may be metabolically labile to be transformed to an amide or carboxylic acid. However, one of the authors of this chapter (KPB) had previously worked on a project in which nitriles were key intermediates and had used the relatively new reaction where the aromatic halogen was reacted with cuprous cyanide to produce the nitrile. In August 1972, having already synthesized the potent 5-bromo-4′-fluoro-derivative **16**, he used this reaction directly on **16** and made the first sample of **9** (citalopram). The compound proved to be a very potent SSRI. It was selected together with a few other potent SSRIs from the series for further preclinical studies, proved overall to have the best safety profile, and it was selected as a clinical development candidate. Interestingly, the cyano group proved to be totally metabolically stable.

11.4 Synthesis and Production of Citalopram

The syntheses used for preparation of citalopram and derivatives are outlined in Scheme 11.1. The starting materials were phthalides (**I**). These were either made by methods published in the literature, or by improved or completely new procedures. The majority of compounds could then be produced by a "double Grignard" reaction, in which the phthalide was reacted with a substituted phenyl magnesium bromide to give the benzophenone intermediate **II**, which was further reacted with 3-(dimethylamino)propyl magnesium chloride to afford the "dicarbinol" **III**. The dicarbinols were then ring closed in strong acid to the final product **VI**.

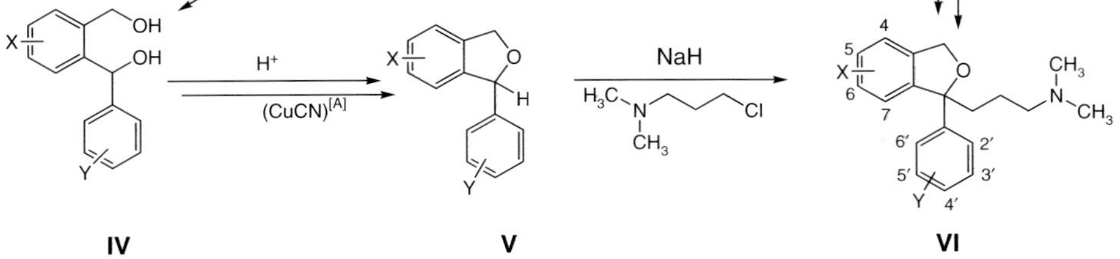

I II III IV V VI
MgBr
$LiAlH_4$
H_3C N MgCl CH_3
H^+ $(CuCN)^{[A]}$
NaH
H_3C N Cl CH_3

Scheme 11.1 The syntheses used for preparation of citalopram and derivatives. [A] represents extra step exchanging Br with CN using cuprous cyanide in DMF if the end product was a cyano-substituted derivative.

The 5-bromo derivative **16** was made by this synthesis (from 5-bromophthalide) and as mentioned above, citalopram (X = 5-CN, Y = 4′-F) was synthesized for the first time by reacting the Br in **16** with cuprous cyanide. However, it quickly turned out that this method was unsuited for the preparation of larger quantities, so an alternative method was developed. Starting again with 5-bromophthalide, the benzophenone **II** was reduced with $LiAlH_4$ to the intermediate **IV**, which was ring closed in strong acid to the phenylphthalane **V** (X = 5-Br, Y = 4′-F). By reaction with cuprous cyanide, a crystalline 5-cyano-1-(4′-fluorophenyl)phthalane was obtained. Citalopram was then obtained by metallation with NaH in dimethyl sulfoxide and subsequent reaction with 3-(dimethylamino)propyl chloride. This method was used to produce the first 5 kg. Unfortunately, this method was also unsuited for large-scale production. This was a critical point in the development of citalopram, but we made a very surprising discovery. It turned out that the cyano group in 5-cyanophthalide did not react with the Grignard reagents, contrary to expectation, and did not hydrolyze in the strong acid used in the final ring closure. We also found that the second "side chain" Grignard reagent could be added directly after the 4-fluorophenyl magnesium bromide without isolating the intermediate benzophenone. This was a major improvement, and this synthesis proved to be an excellent production method.

11.5
The Pharmacological Profile of Citalopram

The pharmacological characterization of citalopram showed that it potently inhibited the uptake of $[^3H]$-5-HT in rabbit and rat thrombocytes and rat brain synaptosomes with IC_{50} values in the nanomolar range (14 and 1.7 nM, respectively) [9, 10]. Furthermore, citalopram turned out to be the most selective 5-HT uptake inhibitor among the SSRIs in clinical use at that time, with a selectivity ratio of 3400 relative to the inhibition of $[^3H]$-NE uptake in rat brain synaptosomes compared to selectivity ratios of 840, 280, and 54 for sertraline, paroxetine, and fluoxetine, respectively, and the selectivity relative to the inhibition of $[^3H]$-dopamine (DA) uptake was even greater, that is 22 000 compared to selectivity ratios of 250, 18 000, and 740 for sertraline, paroxetine, and fluoxetine [11]. Citalopram had very low affinity for the receptors studied, the highest affinity being for the σ_1 and histamine H1 receptors (IC_{50} 200 and 350 nM, respectively) [11]. Interestingly, early binding dissociation studies of $[^3H]$-imipramine, $[^3H]$-paroxetine, and $[^3H]$-citalopram suggested that these drugs bind to different areas of the SERT [12], even though the implications of this were unclear at that time.

The available mechanistic *in vivo* assays only provided indirect measures of uptake inhibition and selectivity. For example, citalopram inhibited the uptake of the 5-HT depleting agent, H75/12, into neurons with an ED_{50} of 0.80 mg/kg and failed to inhibit NE depletion by the depleting agent H77/77 at doses as high as 160 mg/kg [9]. Similarly, studies of amine turnover showed that an acute dose of citalopram reduced 5-HT turnover in the brain (i.e., [5-HT] was unchanged and the metabolite, [5-hydroxyindoleacetic acid, 5-HIAA], was decreased) and had no effect on NE synthesis. This suggested that citalopram was the most selective of the compounds tested [13, 14]. Finally, simple behavioral screening assays, such as the potentiation of 5-hydroxytryptophan (5-HTP)-induced 5-HT syndrome (5-HT uptake inhibition), tetrabenazine-induced ptosis (NE uptake inhibition), and apomorphine-induced gnawing (DA uptake inhibition), supported a selective 5-HT uptake inhibition *in vivo* [15]. Citalopram, like other SSRIs, had limited and variable effects in validated behavioral models predictive of antidepressant effect, such as the forced swim test, which had been validated with TCAs and MAOIs [16]. It was not until after the development of citalopram had been completed that more advanced *in vivo* assays, such as microdialysis, *in vivo* electrophysiology, and more complex behavioral models, became available.

11.6 Clinical Efficacy of Citalopram

Citalopram was first launched for the treatment of major depressive disorder in 1989 in Denmark as Cipramil® and subsequently marketed worldwide, including the United States in 1998 under the trade name Celexa®. Following the approval for major depressive disorder, citalopram was also approved for the treatment of panic disorders. After only a few years on the market, the drug attained blockbuster status.

A large number of clinical short- and long-term studies of patients with major depressive disorder have been conducted with citalopram over the years, and different subsets of the clinical data have been subjected to meta-analyses as well. In general, citalopram was found to have an efficacy comparable to that of other SSRIs and, in some studies, also like other SSRIs, to be slightly less efficacious than the TCAs [17, 18]. Citalopram has also been shown to be efficacious in the treatment of other conditions, such as social phobia, obsessive compulsive disorder, post-traumatic stress disorder, mixed anxiety and depression, and poststroke depression [17, 18]. Citalopram has a favorable pharmacokinetic profile with good bioavailability and linear kinetics and a low potential for interactions with concomitant medication [17]. It is generally well tolerated with a better tolerability than the TCAs [19, 20]. These favorable properties made citalopram a good choice, particularly for depressed patients who required continuation and long-term treatment, as well as for elderly patients [17]. Overall, citalopram was on par with the other SSRIs with respect to efficacy, but has more favorable drug metabolism and pharmacokinetics (DMPK) properties (e.g., approximately 80% bioavailability and 80% protein binding, dose-proportional linear pharmacokinetics, an elimination half-life of 1.5 days, negligible pharmacological activity of metabolites, and low drug–drug interaction potential), which are the likely reasons why citalopram became such a commercial success, even though it was the fifth SSRI introduced onto the US market.

11.7 Synthesis and Production of Escitalopram

The preparation of the closest analogues of citalopram, its single enantiomers, proved to be a major challenge. Direct resolution via diastereomeric salts failed after many fruitless attempts. Different chiral acids, different solvents, and different stoichiometric ratios of citalopram and acid were tried, but the major problem was the lack of crystal formation in almost all cases. A crystalline (+)-camphor sulfonate was obtained, but no separation of enantiomers could be accomplished. Chiral high-pressure liquid chromatography (HPLC) was in its infancy, and the available analytical columns were tried with negative results. We wanted to avoid acid ring closure of resolved intermediates due to the risk of racemization. Therefore, we spent some time on various asymmetric syntheses focusing on derivatives with a partially finished side chain that after potential resolution could be transformed to the citalopram enantiomers without risk of racemization. However, these attempts were also unsuccessful.

Finally, we decided to try to resolve the intermediate diol **III** (Scheme 11.1), although we did not have a strategy for a subsequent stereoselective ring closure at hand. We made the diasteromeric esters with the enantiomers of α-methoxy-α-trifluoromethyl acetic acid (Mosher's acid, known as a shift reagent for nuclear magnetic resonance (NMR)) and tried to separate them on preparative (nonchiral) HPLC. By repeated peak shaving, we obtained small samples of the pure diastereomers. Importantly, we had noticed a seemingly spontaneous slow ring closure to citalopram of the mixture of diastereomeric esters (in the presence of triethylamine) during their synthesis. This encouraged us to try a stronger base (potassium *tert*-butoxide), and to our great surprise, this resulted in a stereoselective ring closure of the pure diastereomers to afford the very first small sample of the pure citalopram enantiomers. Later we found that the diol **III** also could be resolved by diastereomeric salt formation with di-*p*-toluoyl tartaric acid (DTTA) and, in this way, it became possible to produce larger quantities of the enantiomers (using a basic ring closure with a mesylate of the diol and triethylamine).

This method was possibly also suited for production scale, but as chromatographic separation of the diols using simulated moving bed (SMB) technology in the late 1990s proved very effective, two SMB plants (a pilot and a full scale) were built for escitalopram production. Later, production became even more cost-effective when development chemists discovered that acidic ring closure of the *R*-diol led to a mixture of approximately 30% *R*-citalopram and 70% escitalopram, which could subsequently be isolated as citalopram and pure escitalopram.

In recent years, many chemists outside Lundbeck have worked with alternative syntheses (for a recent review, see Ref. [21]) of citalopram and escitalopram. Of special interest was a publication in 2007 by researchers from Dr. Reddy's Laboratories who published a direct resolution of citalopram using DTTA [22]. At that point, we had completed a systematic study with a large number of chiral acids (including DTTA) without finding a single one that worked. So we were not surprised to find that in our hands the Dr. Reddy method did not work. Through a series of experiments, we showed that resolution of citalopram was not possible by Dr. Reddy's method [23]. In a subsequent response, Dr. Reddy researchers admitted that the method did not work as described. They then claimed success with a highly modified procedure, but in our hands that did not work either [24, 25].

In conclusion, the preparation and production of citalopram and escitalopram have been major challenges, but we finally succeeded in developing highly innovative and effective syntheses that are still the best and most cost-effective production methods.

11.8 The Pharmacological Profile of the Citalopram Enantiomers

Shortly after the citalopram enantiomers had been successfully produced in the laboratory in 1988, they were characterized *in vitro* in the rat brain synaptosome assay of [^{3}H]-5-HT uptake inhibition and *in vivo* in the mouse 5-HTP potentiation assay. Completely unexpectedly, the 5-HT uptake inhibition of citalopram turned out to reside in the *S*-enantiomer, and *R*-citalopram was found to be practically devoid of this activity in both the *in vitro* and *in vivo* assays. These initial findings were reproduced and substantiated by studies of NE and DA uptake inhibitory activity and published in 1992 [26]. Based on these studies and the fact that racemic citalopram is a highly selective inhibitor of the SERT, *R*-citalopram was thought to be pharmacologically inactive. Only very few pharmacological studies were conducted with escitalopram in the next few years. It was not until new production methods (see above) made it feasible to produce escitalopram at an industrial scale and it was decided in 1997 to develop escitalopram for major depressive disorder that there was a renewed interest in pharmacological studies of escitalopram. Based on the knowledge available then, the original expectation was that escitalopram would be comparable to citalopram with respect to efficacy, and that the tolerability would be improved by removing the presumably pharmacologically inactive *R*-enantiomer and thereby minimizing the drug load in the body.

11.9 *R*-Citalopram's Surprising Inhibition of Escitalopram

It was not until about a decade after the first characterization of the citalopram enantiomers that observations from behavioral studies made us hypothesize that *R*-citalopram counteracts the effect of escitalopram. A comparison of escitalopram and citalopram in a simple rat model predictive of anxiolytic activity, inhibition of footshock-induced ultrasonic vocalization, revealed that escitalopram dose dependently and completely abolished the vocalization, whereas citalopram only partially reduced the vocalization and reached a plateau of about 60% inhibition when the dose was increased [27]. These findings made us hypothesize that *R*-citalopram might counteract the anxiolytic-like activity of escitalopram in this model.

Knowing that the ultrasonic vocalization model is very sensitive to serotonergic mechanisms, it was a logical next step to investigate the effect of *R*-citalopram alone and in combination with escitalopram on the extracellular 5-HT levels in relevant brain regions, such as the frontal cortex and the ventral hippocampus. From pharmacokinetics studies in humans, we also knew that the citalopram enantiomers are metabolized at a different rate, which meant that the plasma level of *R*-citalopram is at least twofold higher than that of escitalopram in individuals treated with racemic citalopram [28]. Thus, these first behavioral observations were followed up by a series of microdialysis studies in freely moving rats where the effects of escitalopram and citalopram as well as ratios of escitalopram to *R*-citalopram of 1 : 1, 1 : 2, and 1 : 4 were studied. The outcome of these studies was that escitalopram produced a significantly higher increase in the level of extracellular 5-HT compared to equivalent doses of citalopram, and that *R*-citalopram antagonized the effect of escitalopram in a dose-dependent manner [29].

These observations triggered a series of experiments aimed at identifying the mechanism by which *R*-citalopram counteracts the therapeutic effect of escitalopram. Studies of brain exposure levels in rats treated with escitalopram alone versus combinations of escitalopram and *R*-citalopram quickly ruled out a pharmacokinetic interaction as the explanation [29]. A very broad receptor screening including 144 targets did not reveal any obvious target through which *R*-citalopram could exert its action [30]. A reverse dialysis study in rats dosed systemically with escitalopram showed that *R*-citalopram could exert its inhibitory action when administered at terminal areas of 5-HT neurons, such as the prefrontal cortex [29]. *In vivo* recordings of individual 5-HT neurons in the rat dorsal raphe nucleus demonstrated that desensitization of somatodendritic 5-HT_{1A} autoreceptors, a mechanism believed to be associated with the delayed clinical response of SSRIs, occurred after only 2 weeks' treatment with escitalopram, whereas 3 weeks' treatment was required for an equivalent dose of citalopram [31]. In another study using the same methodology, it was shown that *R*-citalopram delayed the recovery of 5-HT neuronal firing and the 5-HT_{1A} receptor desensitization produced by escitalopram [31–33]. The superior effect of escitalopram compared to citalopram and the inhibitory action of *R*-citalopram on the pharmacological activities of escitalopram have been confirmed in numerous animal models using acute or repeated dosing [34–36] (Table 11.2).

The mechanistic *in vivo* studies all pointed toward the SERT as the target for the interaction between escitalopram and *R*-citalopram. This and the original *in vitro* reports from Plenge *et al.* [12] that SSRIs could bind differently to the SERT made us decide to investigate the *in vitro* binding kinetics of the individual citalopram enantiomers in further detail. Kinetic studies of [^{3}H]-escitalopram binding to the SERT demonstrated that cold escitalopram slows down the dissociation rate of [^{3}H]-escitalopram from the primary (inhibitory) site of the SERT [6]. This is indicative of the existence of a secondary allosteric

Table 11.2 Superior effect of escitalopram over citalopram and inhibitory action of *R*-citalopram on the pharmacological activities of escitalopram in nonclinical models after acute or prolonged exposure.

Assay	Outcome	References
Mechanistic		
Microdialysis		
Extracellular 5-HT in prefrontal cortex and ventral hippocampus in rats	Escitalopram increases 5-HT more than citalopram	[29, 32, 37, 38]
	R-Citalopram antagonizes escitalopram-induced increase of 5-HT	
Voltammetry in rats	Escitalopram is more potent than citalopram at inhibiting 5-HT clearance	[39]
	R-Citalopram counteracts escitalopram inhibition of 5-HT clearance	
Electrophysiology	.	
5-HT neuronal firing in dorsal raphe nucleus in rats	Escitalopram is four times more potent than citalopram, acute dosing	[31–33]
	R-Citalopram antagonizes escitalopram-induced suppression of firing, acute dosing	
	Escitalopram normalizes DRN firing faster than citalopram, chronic dosing	
	R-Citalopram delays effect of escitalopram on firing	
DA neuron firing in ventral tegmental area in rats	Escitalopram increases firing rate and burst firing of DA neurons, acute dosing	[40]
	R-Citalopram antagonizes the effect of escitalopram on DA neuron firing	
NMDA-induced currents in hippocampal pyramidal neurons in rats	Escitalopram but not citalopram potentiates NMDA-induced currents in pyramidal neurons	[40]
	R-Citalopram antagonizes the effect of escitalopram	
LTP in rats	*R*-Citalopram counteracts escitalopram effect on LTP	[41]
Neurogenesis in rats	*R*-Citalopram counteracts escitalopram-induced cell proliferation in the dentate gyrus	[33]
HPA axis		
Plasma corticosterone in rat	*R*-Citalopram antagonizes escitalopram-induced increase of plasma corticosterone	[42]
Behavior		
Potentiating of 5-HTP-induced behavior, rat, mouse	*R*-Citalopram antagonizes the potentiating effect of escitalopram	[42, 43]

(continued)

Table 11.2 (*Continued*)

Assay	Outcome	References
Anxiolytic and antidepressant effects and cognitive function		
Elevated plus maze, rat	*R*-Citalopram antagonizes anxiolytic effect of escitalopram	[44]
Vogel conflict test, rat	*R*-Citalopram antagonizes anxiolytic effect of escitalopram	[44]
Separation-induced vocalization, mouse pup	*R*-Citalopram antagonizes anxiolytic effect of escitalopram	[45]
Footshock-induced ultrasonic vocalization, rat	*R*-Citalopram antagonizes anxiolytic effect of escitalopram	[27]
Conditioned fear, rat	*R*-Citalopram antagonizes anxiolytic effect of escitalopram	[46]
Resident intruder, rat	Escitalopram produces antidepressant effect earlier than citalopram *R*-Citalopram counteracts escitalopram-induced antidepressant effect	[47]
Chronic mild stress, rat	Escitalopram produces antidepressant effect earlier than citalopram *R*-Citalopram counteracts escitalopram-induced antidepressant effect	[48]
Novel object recognition, rat	Escitalopram but not citalopram improved recognition memory	[40]

binding site that modulates the binding properties of the drug at the primary site. In addition, we found that *R*-citalopram attenuated the decreased dissociation rate of [^{3}H]-escitalopram in the presence of cold escitalopram [6, 49]. Finally, we found that *R*-citalopram also slowed the association rate of [^{3}H]-escitalopram to the SERT [32, 49]. These findings were supportive of the notion that *R*-citalopram counteracts the effects of escitalopram at the SERT, and that the interaction takes place at a secondary allosteric modulator site. As described in further detail in the next section, species comparisons and site-directed mutagenesis studies have led to identification of domains on the SERT that are critical for the delayed dissociation produced by escitalopram and the negative effects of *R*-citalopram on the binding of escitalopram to the SERT [49, 50].

Using brain imaging techniques, positron emission tomography (PET), or single-photon emission computer tomography (SPECT) and appropriate radiolabeled ligands, it was demonstrated that the occupancy at the SERT in the human brain is significantly higher with escitalopram 10 mg than with the corresponding dose of citalopram (20 mg, containing 10 mg of *R*-citalopram and 10 mg of *S*-citalopram) at steady state. The mean occupancies at 6 and 54 h after last doses were 82 and 63% for escitalopram, respectively, and 64 and 49% for citalopram, respectively [51]. The results were confirmed in a pooled analysis, in which the authors concluded that the buildup of the *R*-enantiomer after repeated citalopram dosing may lead to lower SERT occupancy by the *S*-enantiomer [52].

11.10
Binding Site(s) for Escitalopram on the Serotonin Transporter

Early on in the era of antidepressant drugs, medicinal chemists started to speculate about the mode of binding of these drugs to their target, that is SERT and NET. With respect to citalopram and escitalopram, as described above, we noticed that relatively small changes in the structure could transform a selective NE uptake inhibitor such as talopram into an SSRI such as citalopram. Eli Lilly made a similar observation with the NRIs tomoxetine and nisoxetine, and the SSRI fluoxetine. However, the chiral SSRIs differed with regard to stereoselectivity. While the enantiomers of fluoxetine were equipotent as SSRIs, a high stereoselectivity was observed with the enantiomers of citalopram and with paroxetine and its enantiomers.

We worked in the 1980s with another structural class of antidepressants, the 3-phenyl-1-indanamines where the amine could be a dimethyl- or monomethylamine or a piperazine [8, 53]. We observed a moderate stereoselectivity of the enantiomers of *trans*-isomers with the small amines in favor of the 1*R*,3*S* conformation, but a high stereoselectivity of the piperazine enantiomers with 1*S*,3*R* as the active stereoisomer. We tried to rationalize this in a simple cartoon of a three-point binding model [54]. However, this model was not useful for the prediction of the stereoselectivity of citalopram.

Smith presented a three-dimensional model that he interpreted as predicting a high stereoselectivity of the *R*-enantiomer of citalopram versus the *S*-enantiomer (this was obviously later proved wrong) [55]. However, the author did not take the semisymmetrical structure of citalopram into account. If one does that, both enantiomers fit his model equally well, and the model could just as well predict no stereoselectivity.

Later on when we established computational chemistry (and citalopram had been resolved into its individual enantiomers), we developed a pharmacophore model that was used to rationalize both the structural elements determining SERT or NET selectivity and the observed stereoselectivity of citalopram and several other SSRIs [56]. When fitting *R*- and *S*-citalopram into the model, we took advantage of the semisymmetrical nature of the compound mentioned above, that is, the *p*-fluorophenyl ring of one enantiomer was superimposed onto the phthalane ring of the other enantiomer. Interestingly, these different binding modes were also the outcome of a subsequent, more comprehensive computational study of the binding of the enantiomers [57]. In order to further study the structural elements in talopram and citalopram that were important for SERT and NET selectivity, respectively, 14 derivatives of the two compounds were either selected or synthesized [58] and tested for 5-HT and NE uptake inhibition [59]. This study showed, in agreement with our previous pharmacophore model study, that the phthalane 3,3-dimethyl substituents and 5-cyano group are key determinants for inhibitory activity and selectivity toward NET and SERT, respectively.

However, the real breakthrough came with the publication of the X-ray structure of the leucine transporter (LeuT), a bacterial homologue to the mammalian solute carrier 6 (SLC6) transporters [60]. We developed a SERT homology model based on the LeuT structure with escitalopram bound to a site equivalent to the leucine binding site in LeuT [61, 62]. Subsequently, several other homology models supported by mutational studies strongly supported this site as the escitalopram binding site, despite some differences in the suggested escitalopram conformation and binding mode at the site [57, 63, 64].

Interestingly, two X-ray structures of LeuT were then published with the TCAs clomipramine and desipramine bound within the transporter [65, 66]. The TCAs bound (with low affinity) in a cavity (called the vestibule or the S2 site), located ~15 Å above the S1 site (the substrate binding site). This site had also been found in a study we made of the driving forces for migration of leucine through LeuT [67]. Subsequently, X-ray structures of LeuT with the SSRIs sertraline and *R*- and *S*-fluoxetine bound within the S2 site were published [68]. The authors of this study speculated that the equivalent site in the SERT might be the binding site for antidepressants. However, the mutational studies mentioned above showed not only a strong influence on escitalopram binding of mutations at the S1 site on escitalopram binding, but also that mutations in the S2 pocket did not influence escitalopram binding [63, 64]. Moreover, we have recently shown that mutation of just five amino acids within the S1 binding pocket of the NET to the corresponding residues in the SERT conferred affinity equivalent to WT SERT for citalopram and its enantiomers at the mutated NET. In contrast, the binding of talopram was almost unaffected by all mutations at both the SERT and the NET. The binding mode of talopram to NET is, therefore, not at the S1 site [59].

As mentioned above, escitalopram has an allosteric effect that we believe is attained through a separate allosteric binding site on the SERT. Studies on chicken SERT (gSERT) have demonstrated a low allosteric potency of escitalopram in this species. However, mutation of nine residues in transmembrane domains 10, 11, and 12 to their corresponding human residues restored the allosteric effect [50]. The location of these nine residues did not seem to comprise a cavity for a putative allosteric binding site. It has recently been proposed that the SERT allosteric site could be identical to the S2 site [57]. Accordingly, the nine residues might have an indirect effect on escitalopram binding at the S2 site (Figure 11.2).

A clear indication of the different nature of the S1 and S2 sites is that escitalopram derivatives show a different SAR toward to two sites. In Table 11.1, the effect on the hSERT S1 site (inhibition of [^{3}H]-5-HT uptake) is shown, as well as the allosteric effect (inhibition of [^{3}H]-escitalopram dissociation) of a number of escitalopram derivatives. While the 5-chloro (**10**), 5-bromo (**16**), and 3′,4′-dichloro (**11**) derivatives retain their effect at both sites, the 3′,5′-dichloro analogues (**12** and enantiomers **12a** and **12b**), which lack an effect at the S1 site, are still potent allosteric modulators. A study of naphthyl derivatives of citalopram was recently published [69]. Here we found that while the 2-naphthyl derivative of citalopram (**19** and enantiomers **19a** and **19b**) retained its effect at both sites, the 1-naphthyl

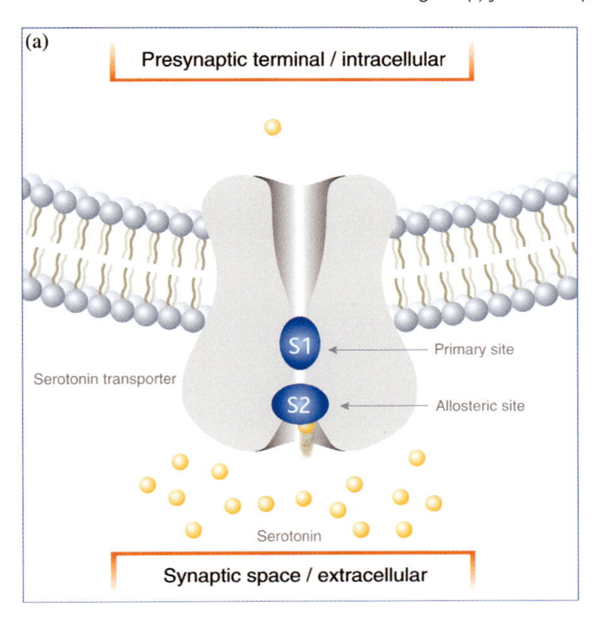

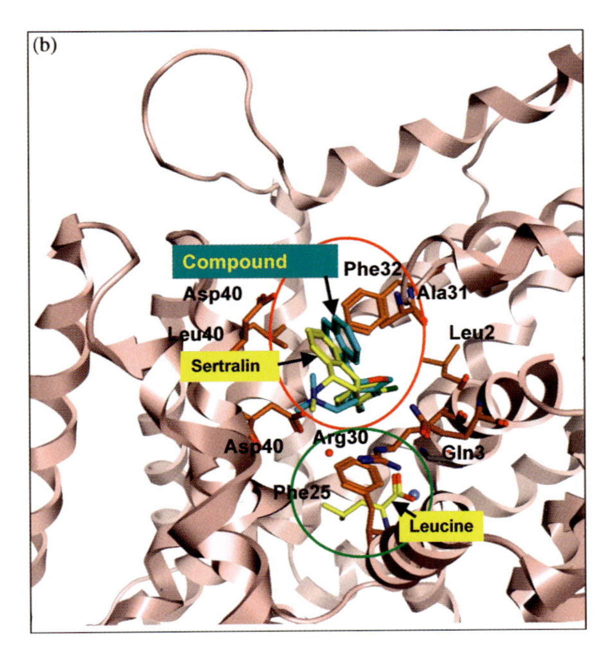

Figure 11.2 Escitalopram's two binding sites at SERT. (a) A schematic drawing of the suggested positions of escitalopram's primary binding site (S1) and allosteric binding site (S2). (b) The X-ray structure model of LeuT taken from Ref. [68]. The leucine binding pocket is encircled in green. The "vestibule" pocket is encircled in red. The corresponding ligands from the X-ray structure (leucine and sertraline, respectively) are depicted in yellow. Superimposed on these is the docked structure of escitalopram, where the additional aromatic ring of compound **20** has been sketched in.

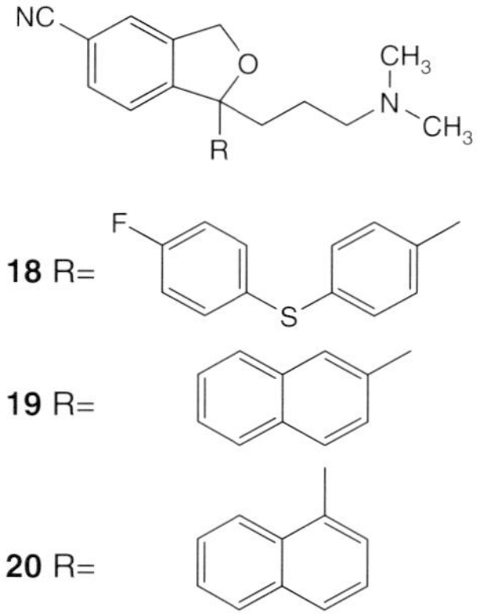

18 R=

19 R=

20 R=

Figure 11.3 Citalopram derivatives with selective (S2 site) allosteric effect (**18** and **20**) and dual (S1 and S2 sites) effect (**19**).

derivatives (**20** and enantiomers **20a** and **20b**) were selective allosteric modulators (Figure 11.3).

Compounds **17** and **18** were originally identified as impurities formed in escitalopram production. Amazingly, testing showed that **17** (citalopram with an extra side chain at the 5-position) has a very high affinity at the S1 site, but is devoid of an allosteric effect. Conversely, **18** (and enantiomers **18a** and **18b**) are selective allosteric modulators. The stereoselectivity at the S2 site is generally low as can be seen from the data on the enantiomers of **9**, **12**, **18**, **19**, and **20**.

In conclusion, analogue design of citalopram has turned out to be potentially much more complicated than originally anticipated. The insight gained in recent years into the dual effect of escitalopram and the different SARs of derivatives for the S1 and S2 sites underlines how fortunate it is that citalopram was originally selected for development. In principle, there was a risk, of which we were then unaware, of selecting a derivative such as **17**, which has no allosteric effect.

11.11
Future Perspectives on the Molecular Basis for Escitalopram's Interaction with the SERT

It has been shown that SSRIs in addition to blocking the reuptake of 5-HT also cause an internalization of the SERT [70], and that the potency ranking of SSRIs to cause internalization and to block the uptake of 5-HT appear to differ [71]. Recent research shows that *R*-citalopram antagonizes escitalopram's effect on the expression of SERT in the cell membrane and that protein kinase C (PKC) appears to be involved in this effect as the PKC inhibitor staurosporine abolished the effect of *R*-citalopram [72]. A putative interaction between the allosteric mechanism of the SERT and the so-called serotonin interaction proteins (SIPs), of which PKC is one, may potentially open up a new area of research into the function of the SERT and eventually lead to new drug targets [73].

11.12
Clinical Efficacy of Escitalopram

In 2002, escitalopram was launched as Cipralex® in Europe and as Lexapro® in the United States. Escitalopram is approved for the treatment of major depressive disorder and social anxiety disorder in the United States, and major depressive disorder, panic disorder, social anxiety disorder, generalized anxiety disorder, and obsessive compulsive disorder in Europe and elsewhere.

Four pivotal randomized placebo-controlled short-term studies were conducted for the registration file. Three of these studies had a citalopram group included as active reference. Interestingly, and surprisingly, there was a signal that escitalopram had a faster onset of acting and/or was more efficacious than an equivalent dose of citalopram [74, 75]. These studies were not designed or powered to show differences to an active reference, but subsequent studies with head-to-head comparisons of citalopram and escitalopram confirmed the original observation that escitalopram is superior to citalopram, particularly in patients with severe depression [76, 77]. In a meta-analysis of pooled data at an individual patient level, escitalopram was statistically significantly superior to citalopram, with response rates of 59.7 and 52.3%, respectively, for the complete data set, and 61.2 and 49.9%, respectively, for the subset of patients with severe depression [78]. In a meta-analysis of publicly available data [79], statistically superior response rates of 72.3% for escitalopram versus 63.9% for citalopram were reported. The efficacy of escitalopram has been further confirmed in a prospective, randomized, double-blind study against paroxetine [80], and in a post-hoc analysis of the effect of anxiety symptoms on patients with severe depression from the same study [81]. Data from this study and an analysis of data from two studies comparing escitalopram with paroxetine [82] confirmed the superior efficacy of escitalopram over another SSRI. Further comparisons of pooled data from patients with severe depression treated with escitalopram versus other antidepressants again confirm that escitalopram is superior to other comparators, including the serotonin norepinephrine reuptake inhibitors (SNRIs) venlafaxine and duloxetine [83–87]. In patients with generalized anxiety disorder, escitalopram has also shown statistically significant superiority over the comparator, paroxetine [88, 89]. Overall, the tolerability of escitalopram was very similar to that of citalopram [34], whereas toxicity in relation to overdose has been reported to be more serious for citalopram than escitalopram [90, 91]. Thus, the original expectation of similar efficacy of escitalopram and citalopram and escitalopram being better tolerated proved to be wrong, at least at therapeutic doses. Escitalopram not only resulted in being clinically superior to citalopram, but has also proven to be superior to other SSRIs and to SNRIs in several clinical studies. In 2010, it reached the status of being the most prescribed branded antidepressant globally and, by mid-2011, more than 265 million patients have been treated with the drug.

11.13 Conclusions

The development of citalopram, and subsequently of escitalopram, has not been trivial and was full of surprises, where time after time predictions based on the established rules and perceptions have been proven wrong as the data emerged. The discovery of citalopram and escitalopram underlines the point that analogue design is not trivial and can lead to drugs with either totally different or greatly improved profiles compared with the starting structure. Similarly, the complexity of the biological mechanisms we are dealing with calls for caution when making predictions and for an open mind to recognize and follow through on serendipitous findings.

References

1 Childers, W.E., Jr., and Rotella, D.P. (2011) Selective serotonin uptake inhibitors for the treatment of depression, in *Analogue-Based Drug Discovery II* (eds J. Fischer, and C.R. Ganellin), Wiley-VCH Verlag GmbH, Weinheim, pp. 269–295.

2 Bang-Andersen, B. and Bøgesø, K.P. (2010) Dopamine and serotonin, in *Textbook of Drug Design and Discovery*, 4th edn (eds P. Krogsgaard-Larsen, K. Strømgaard, and U. Madsen), CRC Press, Boca Raton, FL,, pp. 299–312.

3 H. Lundbeck A/S (2010) Cipralex®: Building a Success. H. Lundbeck A/S, Valby, Denmark.

4 Pedersen, V. and Bøgesø, K.P. (1998) Drug hunting, in *The Psychopharmacologists II* (ed. D. Healy), Chapman & Hall, London, UK, pp. 561–579.

5 Carlsson, A., Corrodi, H., Fuxe, K., and Hökfelt, T. (1969) Effect of antidepressant drugs on the depletion of intraneuronal brain 5-hydroxytryptamine stores caused by 4-methyl-α-ethyl-*meta*-tyramine. *Eur. J. Pharmacol.*, **5**, 357–366.

6 Chen, F., Larsen, M.B., Neubauer, H.A., Sanchez, C., Plenge, P., and Wiborg, O. (2005) Characterization of an allosteric citalopram-binding site at the serotonin transporter. *J. Neurochem.*, **92**, 21–28.

7 Bigler, A.J., Bøgesø, K.P., Toft, A., and Hansen, V. (1977) Quantitative structure–activity relationships in a series of selective 5-HT uptake inhibitors. *Eur. J. Med. Chem.*, **12**, 289–295.

8 Bøgesø, K.P., Christensen, A.V., Hyttel, J., and Liljefors, T. (1985) 3-Phenyl-1-indanamines. Potential antidepressant activity and potent inhibition of dopamine, norepinephrine, and serotonin uptake. *J. Med. Chem.*, **28**, 1817–1828.

9 Hyttel, J. (1977) Neurochemical characterization of a new potent and selective serotonin uptake inhibitor: Lu 10-171. *Psychopharmacology*, **51**, 225–233.

10 Hyttel, J. (1978) Effect of a specific 5-HT uptake inhibitor, citalopram (Lu 10-171), on [^{3}H]-5-HT uptake in rat brain synaptosomes *in vitro*. *Psychopharmacology*, **60**, 13–18.

11 Hyttel, J., Arnt, J., and Sanchez, C. (1995) The pharmacology of citalopram. *Rev. Contemp. Pharmacother.*, **6**, 271–285.

12 Plenge, P., Mellerup, E.T., and Laursen, H. (1991) Affinity modulation of [^{3}H]imipramine, [^{3}H]paroxetine and [^{3}H]citalopram binding to the 5-HT transporter from brain and platelets. *Eur. J. Pharmacol.*, **206**, 243–250.

13 Hyttel, J. (1977) Effect of a selective 5-HT uptake inhibitor – Lu 10-171 – on rat brain 5-HT turnover. *Acta Pharmacol. Toxicol.*, **40**, 439–446.

14 Carlsson, A. and Lindqvist, M. (1978) Effects of antidepressant agents on the synthesis of brain monoamines. *J. Neural Transm.*, **43**, 73–91.

15 Christensen, A.V., Fjalland, B., Pedersen, V., Danneskiold-Samsøe, P., and Svendsen, O. (1977) Pharmacology of a new phthalane (Lu 10-171), with specific 5-HT uptake inhibiting properties. *Eur. J. Pharmacol.*, **41**, 153–162.

16 Porsolt, R.D., Bertin, A., Blavet, N., Deniel, M., and Jalfre, M. (1979) Immobility induced by forced swimming in rats: effects of agents which modify central catecholamine and serotonin activity. *Eur. J. Pharmacol.*, **57**, 201–210.

17 Joubert, A.F., Sanchez, C., and Larsen, F. (2000) Citalopram. *Hum. Psychopharmacol.*, **15**, 439–451.

18 Bezchlibnyk-Butler, K., Aleksic, I., and Kennedy, S.H. (2000) Citalopram – a review of pharmacological and clinical effects. *J. Psychiatry Neurosci.*, **25**, 241–254.

19 Baldwin, D., and Johnson, F.N. (1995) Tolerability and safety of citalopram. *Rev. Contemp. Pharmacother.*, **6**, 315.

20 Muldoon, C. (1996) The safety and tolerability of citalopram. *Int. Clin. Psychopharmacol.*, **11** (Suppl. 1), 35–40.

21 Harrington, P.J. (2011) Lexapro® (escitalopram oxalate), in *Pharmaceutical Process Chemistry for Synthesis, Rethinking the Routes to Scale-Up*, John Wiley & Sons, Inc., Hoboken, NJ, pp. 30–91.

22 Elati, C.R., Kolla, N., Vankawala, P.J., Gangula, S., Chalamala, S., Sundaram, V., Bhattacharya, A., Vurimidi, H., and Mathad, V.T. (2007) Substrate modification approach to achieve efficient resolution: didesmethylcitalopram: a key intermediate for escitalopram. *Org. Process Res. Dev.*, **11**, 289–292.

23 Dancer, R.J., and de Diego, H.L. (2009) Attempted resolution of citalopram using (−)-*O,O'*-di-*p*-toluoyl-(*R,R*)-tartaric acid, and reflections on an alkylation reaction; comment on an article by Elati *et al.* *Org. Process Res. Dev.*, **13**, 23–33.

24 Dancer, R.J., and de Diego, H.L. (2009) Response to the comments by Elati *et al.* in response to our article examining one of their previous papers. *Org. Process Res. Dev.*, **13**, 38–43.

25 Elati, C.R., Kolla, N., and Mathad, V.T. (2009) Response to Dancer's comments on our article "Substrate modification approach to achieve efficient resolution: didesmethylcitalopram: a key intermediate for escitalopram." *Org. Process Res. Dev.*, **13**, 34–37.

26 Hyttel, J., Bogeso, K.P., Perregaard, J., and Sanchez, C. (1992) The pharmacological effect of citalopram residues in the (*S*)-(+)-enantiomer. *J. Neural Transm.*, **88**, 157–160.

27 Sanchez, C. (2003) *R*-Citalopram attenuates anxiolytic effects of escitalopram in a rat ultrasonic vocalisation model. *Eur. J. Pharmacol.*, **464**, 155–158.

28 Sidhu, J., Priskorn, M., Poulsen, M., Segonzac, A., Grollier, G., and Larsen, F. (1997) Steady-state pharmacokinetics of the enantiomers of citalopram and its metabolites in humans. *Chirality*, **9**, 686–692.

29 Mørk, A., Kreilgaard, M., and Sanchez, C. (2003) The *R*-enantiomer of citalopram counteracts escitalopram-induced increase in extracellular 5-HT in the frontal cortex of freely moving rats. *Neuropharmacology*, **45**, 167–173.

30 Sanchez, C., Bergqvist, P.B., Brennum, L.T., Gupta, S., Hogg, S., Larsen, A., and Wiborg, O. (2003) Escitalopram, the *S*-(+)-enantiomer of citalopram, is a selective serotonin reuptake inhibitor with potent effects in animal models predictive of antidepressant and anxiolytic activities. *Psychopharmacology*, **167**, 353–362.

31 El Mansari, M., Sanchez, C., Chouvet, G., Renaud, B., and Haddjeri, N. (2005) Effects of acute and long-term administration of escitalopram and citalopram on serotonin neurotransmission: an *in vivo* electrophysiological study in rat brain. *Neuropsychopharmacology*, **30**, 1269–1277.

32 El Mansari, M., Wiborg, O., Mnie-Filali, O., Benturquia, N., Sanchez, C., and Haddjeri, N. (2007) Allosteric modulation of the effect of escitalopram, paroxetine and fluoxetine: *in-vitro* and *in-vivo* studies. *Int. J. Neuropsychopharmacol.*, **10**, 31–40.

33 Mnie-Filali, O., Faure, C., Mansari, M.E., Lambas-Senas, L., Berod, A., Zimmer, L., Sanchez, C., and Haddjeri, N. (2007) *R*-Citalopram prevents the neuronal adaptive changes induced by escitalopram. *Neuroreport*, **18**, 1553–1556.

34 Sanchez, C., Bogeso, K.P., Ebert, B., Reines, E.H., and Braestrup, C. (2004) Escitalopram versus citalopram: the surprising role of the *R*-enantiomer. *Psychopharmacology*, **174**, 163–176.

35 Sanchez, C. (2006) The pharmacology of citalopram enantiomers: the antagonism by *R*-citalopram on the effect of *S*-citalopram. *Basic Clin. Pharmacol. Toxicol.*, **99**, 91–95.

36 Zhong, H., Haddjeri, N., and Sanchez, C. (2012) Escitalopram, an antidepressant with an allosteric effect at the serotonin transporter – a review of current understanding of its mechanism of action. *Psychopharmacology*, **219** (1), 1–13.

37 Cremers, T.I.F.H. and Westerink, B.H.C. (2003) Pharmacological difference between escitalopram and citalopram. *Int. J. Psychiatry Clin. Pract.*, **7**, 306..

38 Lucki, I. and Brown, K. (2003) Different roles of the enantiomers of citalopram on serotonin transmission. *Biol. Psychiatry*, **53**, 45S.

39 Altamirano, A.V., and Frazer, A. (2005) Comparison of the effects of the enantiomers of citalopram on the clearance of exogenous serotonin. Poster presented at the SoPB 2005.

40 Schilstrom, B., Konradsson-Geuken, A., Ivanov, V., Gertow, J., Feltmann, K., Marcus, M.M., Jardemark, K., and Svensson, T.H. (2011) Effects of *S*-citalopram, citalopram, and *R*-citalopram on the firing patterns of dopamine neurons in the ventral tegmental area, *N*-methyl-D-aspartate receptor-mediated transmission in the medial prefrontal cortex and cognitive function in the rat. *Synapse*, **65**, 357–367.

41 Mnie-Filali, O., El, M.M., Espana, A., Sanchez, C., and Haddjeri, N. (2006) Allosteric modulation of the effects of the 5-HT reuptake inhibitor escitalopram on the rat hippocampal synaptic plasticity. *Neurosci. Lett.*, **395**, 23–27.

42 Sanchez, C., and Kreilgaard, M. (2004) *R*-Citalopram inhibits functional and 5-HTP-evoked behavioural responses to the SSRI, escitalopram. *Pharmacol. Biochem. Behav.*, **77**, 391–398.

43 Storustovu, S., Sanchez, C., Porzgen, P., Brennum, L.T., Larsen, A.K., Pulis, M., and Ebert, B. (2004) *R*-Citalopram functionally antagonises escitalopram *in vivo* and *in vitro*: evidence for kinetic interaction at the serotonin transporter. *Br. J. Pharmacol.*, **142**, 172–180.

44 Bien, E., Gruca, P., and Papp, M. (2003) *R*-Citalopram attenuates the anxiolytic-like activity of escitalopram in two animal models. *Behav. Pharmacol.*, **14** (Suppl. 1), S37.

45 Fish, E.W., Faccidomo, S., Gupta, S., and Miczek, K.A. (2004) Anxiolytic-like effects of escitalopram, citalopram, and *R*-citalopram in maternally separated mouse pups. *J. Pharmacol. Exp. Ther.*, **308**, 474–480.

46 Sanchez, C., Gruca, P., Bien, E., and Papp, M. (2003) *R*-Citalopram counteracts the effect of escitalopram in a rat conditioned fear stress model of anxiety. *Pharmacol. Biochem. Behav.*, **75**, 903–907.

47 Mitchell, P.J., Hogg, S., and Sánchez, C. (2004) Agonistic behaviour of resident rats after acute and chronic treatment with *S*(+)- and *R*(−)-citalopram. *Int. J. Neuropsychopharmacol.*, **7**, S187. Poster presented at the 24th CINP, June 20–24, 2004, Paris, France, P01.206.

48 Sanchez, C., Gruca, P., and Papp, M. (2003) *R*-Citalopram counteracts the antidepressant-like effect of escitalopram in a rat chronic mild stress model. *Behav. Pharmacol.*, **14**, 465–470.

49 Zhong, H., Hansen, K.B., Boyle, N.J., Han, K., Muske, G., Huang, X., Egebjerg, J., and Sanchez, C. (2009) An allosteric binding site at the human serotonin transporter mediates the inhibition of escitalopram by *R*-citalopram: kinetic binding studies with the ALI/VFL-SI/TT mutant. *Neurosci. Lett.*, **462**, 207–212.

50 Neubauer, H.A., Hansen, C.G., and Wiborg, O. (2006) Dissection of an allosteric mechanism on the serotonin transporter: a cross-species study. *Mol. Pharmacol.*, **69**, 1242–1250.

51 Klein, N., Sacher, J., Geiss-Granadia, T., Mossaheb, N., Attarbaschi, T., Lanzenberger, R., Spindelegger, C., Holik, A., Asenbaum, S., Dudczak, R., Tauscher, J., and Kasper, S. (2007) Higher serotonin transporter occupancy after multiple dose administration of escitalopram compared

to citalopram: an ^{123}IADAM SPECT study. *Psychopharmacology*, **191**, 333–339.

52 Kasper, S., Sacher, J., Klein, N., Mossaheb, N., Attarbaschi-Steiner, T., Lanzenberger, R., Spindelegger, C., Asenbaum, S., Holik, A., and Dudczak, R. (2009) Differences in the dynamics of serotonin reuptake transporter occupancy may explain superior clinical efficacy of escitalopram versus citalopram. *Int. Clin. Psychopharmacol.*, **24**, 119–125.

53 Bøgesø, K.P. (1983) Neuroleptic activity and dopamine-uptake inhibition in 1-piperazino-3-phenylindans. *J. Med. Chem.*, **26**, 935–947.

54 Bøgesø, K.P., Hyttel, J., Christensen, A.V., and Arnt, J. (1986) Chirality as determinant for neuroleptic or antidepressant action of drugs, in *Innovative Approaches in Drug Research*, vol. **9** (ed. A.F. Harms), Elsevier, Amsterdam, pp. 371–392.

55 Smith, D.F. (1986) The stereoselectivity of serotonin uptake in brain tissue and blood platelets: the topography of the serotonin uptake area. *Neurosci. Biobehav. Rev.*, **10**, 37–46.

56 Gundertofte, K., Liljefors, T., and Bøgesø, K.P. (1997) A stereoselective pharmacophoric model of the serotonin reuptake site, in *Computer-Assisted Lead Finding and Optimization* (eds H. van de Waterbeemd, B. Testa, and G. Folkers), VHCA, Basel, pp. 443–459.

57 Koldso, H., Severinsen, K., Tran, T.T., Celik, L., Jensen, H.H., Wiborg, O., Schiott, B., and Sinning, S. (2010) The two enantiomers of citalopram bind to the human serotonin transporter in reversed orientations. *J. Am. Chem. Soc.*, **132**, 1311–1322.

58 Eildal, J.N., Andersen, J., Kristensen, A.S., Jorgensen, A.M., Bang-Andersen, B., Jorgensen, M., and Stromgaard, K. (2008) From the selective serotonin transporter inhibitor citalopram to the selective norepinephrine transporter inhibitor talopram: synthesis and structure–activity relationship studies. *J. Med. Chem.*, **51**, 3045–3048.

59 Andersen, J., Stuhr-Hansen, N., Zachariassen, L., Toubro, S., Hansen, S. M., Eildal, J.N., Bond, A.D., Bogeso, K.P., Bang-Andersen, B., Kristensen, A.S., and Stromgaard, K. (2011) Molecular determinants for selective recognition of antidepressants in the human serotonin and norepinephrine transporters. *Proc. Natl. Acad. Sci. USA*, **108**, 12137–12142.

60 Yamashita, A., Singh, S.K., Kawate, T., Jin, Y., and Gouaux, E. (2005) Crystal structure of a bacterial homologue of Na^+/Cl^--dependent neurotransmitter transporters. *Nature*, **437**, 215–223.

61 Jorgensen, A.M., Tagmose, L., Jorgensen, A.M., Topiol, S., Sabio, M., Gundertofte, K., Bogeso, K.P., and Peters, G.H. (2007) Homology modeling of the serotonin transporter: insights into the primary escitalopram-binding site. *ChemMedChem*, **2**, 815–826.

62 Jorgensen, A.M., Tagmose, L., Jorgensen, A.M., Bogeso, K.P., and Peters, G.H. (2007) Molecular dynamics simulations of Na^+/Cl^--dependent neurotransmitter transporters in a membrane-aqueous system. *ChemMedChem*, **2**, 827–840.

63 Andersen, J., Olsen, L., Hansen, K.B., Taboureau, O., Jorgensen, F.S., Jorgensen, A.M., Bang-Andersen, B., Egebjerg, J., Stromgaard, K., and Kristensen, A.S. (2010) Mutational mapping and modeling of the binding site for (*S*)-citalopram in the human serotonin transporter. *J. Biol. Chem.*, **285**, 2051–2063.

64 Andersen, J., Taboureau, O., Hansen, K. B., Olsen, L., Egebjerg, J., Stromgaard, K., and Kristensen, A.S. (2009) Location of the antidepressant binding site in the serotonin transporter: importance of Ser-438 in recognition of citalopram and tricyclic antidepressants. *J. Biol. Chem.*, **284**, 10276–10284.

65 Singh, S.K., Yamashita, A., and Gouaux, E. (2007) Antidepressant binding site in a bacterial homologue of neurotransmitter transporters. *Nature*, **448**, 952–956.

66 Zhou, Z., Zhen, J., Karpowich, N.K., Goetz, R.M., Law, C.J., Reith, M.E., and Wang, D.N. (2007) LeuT-desipramine structure reveals how antidepressants block neurotransmitter reuptake. *Science*, **317**, 1390–1393.

67 Jorgensen, A.M., and Topiol, S. (2008) Driving forces for ligand migration in the leucine transporter. *Chem. Biol. Drug Des.*, **72**, 265–272.

68 Zhou, Z., Zhen, J., Karpowich, N.K., Law, C.J., Reith, M.E., and Wang, D.N. (2009) Antidepressant specificity of serotonin transporter suggested by three LeuT-SSRI structures. *Nat. Struct. Mol. Biol.*, **16**, 652–657.

69 Bøgesø, K.P., Bregnedal, P., Juhl, K., Zhong, H., and Wiborg, O. (2010) New naphthalene derivatives of citalopram discriminate between the primary and the allosteric binding sites at the human serotonin transporter. *Basic Clin. Pharmacol. Toxicol.*, **107** (Suppl. 1), 210.

70 Lau, T., Horschitz, S., Berger, S., Bartsch, D., and Schloss, P. (2008) Antidepressant-induced internalization of the serotonin transporter in serotonergic neurons. *FASEB J.*, **22**, 1702–1714.

71 Kittler, K., Lau, T., and Schloss, P. (2010) Antagonists and substrates differentially regulate serotonin transporter cell surface expression in serotonergic neurons. *Eur. J. Pharmacol.*, **629**, 63–67.

72 Mnie-Filali, O., Mansari, M.E., Sanchez, C., and Haddjeri, N. (2009) Therapeutic relevance of the allosteric modulation of the 5-HT transporter. *Curr. Signal Transduct. Ther.*, **4**, 82–87.

73 Zhong, H., Sanchez, C., and Caron, M.G. (2011) Consideration of allosterism and interacting proteins in the physiological functions of the serotonin transporter. *Biochem. Pharmacol.*, **83** (4), 435–442.

74 Burke, W.J., Gergel, I., and Bose, A. (2002) Fixed-dose trial of the single isomer SSRI escitalopram in depressed outpatients *J. Clin. Psychiatry*, **63**, 331–336.

75 Lepola, U.M., Loft, H., and Reines, E.H. (2003) Escitalopram (10–20mg/day) is effective and well tolerated in a placebo-controlled study in depression in primary care. *Int. Clin. Psychopharmacol.*, **18**, 211–217.

76 Moore, N., Verdoux, H., and Fantino, B. (2005) Prospective, multicentre, randomized, double-blind study of the efficacy of escitalopram versus citalopram in outpatient treatment of major depressive disorder. *Int. Clin. Psychopharmacol.*, **20**, 131–137.

77 Yevtushenko, V.Y., Belous, A.I., Yevtushenko, Y.G., Gusinin, S.E., Buzik, O.J., and Agibalova, T.V. (2007) Efficacy and tolerability of escitalopram versus citalopram in major depressive disorder: a 6-week, multicenter, prospective, randomized, double-blind, active-controlled study in adult outpatients. *Clin. Ther.*, **29**, 2319–2332.

78 Kennedy, S.H., Andersen, H.F., and Thase, M.E. (2009) Escitalopram in the treatment of major depressive disorder: a meta-analysis. *Curr. Med. Res. Opin.*, **25**, 161–175.

79 Montgomery, S., Hansen, T., and Kasper, S. (2011) Efficacy of escitalopram compared to citalopram: a meta-analysis. *Int. J. Neuropsychopharmacol.*, **14**, 261–268.

80 Boulenger, J.P., Huusom, A.K., Florea, I., Baekdal, T., and Sarchiapone, M. (2006) A comparative study of the efficacy of long-term treatment with escitalopram and paroxetine in severely depressed patients. *Curr. Med. Res. Opin.*, **22**, 1331–1341.

81 Boulenger, J.P., Hermes, A., Huusom, A.K., and Weiller, E. (2010) Baseline anxiety effect on outcome of SSRI treatment in patients with severe depression: escitalopram vs paroxetine. *Curr. Med. Res. Opin.*, **26**, 605–614.

82 Kasper, S., Baldwin, D.S., Larsson, L.S., and Boulenger, J.P. (2009) Superiority of escitalopram to paroxetine in the treatment of depression. *Eur. Neuropsychopharmacol.*, **19**, 229–237.

83 Khan, A., Bose, A., Alexopoulos, G.S., Gommoll, C., Li, D., and Gandhi, C. (2007) Double-blind comparison of escitalopram and duloxetine in the acute treatment of major depressive disorder. *Clin. Drug Invest.*, **27**, 481–492.

84 Montgomery, S.A., and Andersen, H.F. (2006) Escitalopram versus venlafaxine XR in the treatment of depression. *Int. Clin. Psychopharmacol.*, **21**, 297–309.

85 Kennedy, S.H., Andersen, H.F., and Lam, R.W. (2006) Efficacy of escitalopram in the treatment of major depressive disorder compared with conventional selective serotonin reuptake inhibitors and venlafaxine XR: a meta-analysis. *J. Psychiatry Neurosci.*, **31**, 122–131.

86 Wade, A., Gembert, K., and Florea, I. (2007) A comparative study of the efficacy of acute and continuation treatment with escitalopram versus duloxetine in patients with major depressive disorder. *Curr. Med. Res. Opin.*, **23**, 1605–1614.

87 Cipriani, A., Furukawa, T.A., Salanti, G., Geddes, J.R., Higgins, J.P., Churchill, R., Watanabe, N., Nakagawa, A., Omori, I.M., McGuire, H., Tansella, M., and Barbui, C. (2009) Comparative efficacy and acceptability of 12 new-generation antidepressants: a multiple-treatments meta-analysis. *Lancet*, **373**, 746–758.

88 Baldwin, D.S., Huusom, A.K., and Maehlum, E. (2006) Escitalopram and paroxetine in the treatment of generalised anxiety disorder: randomised, placebo-controlled, double-blind study. *Br. J. Psychiatry*, **189**, 264–272.

89 Lader, M., Stender, K., Burger, V., and Nil, R. (2004) Efficacy and tolerability of escitalopram in 12- and 24-week treatment of social anxiety disorder: randomised, double-blind, placebo-controlled, fixed-dose study. *Depress. Anxiety*, **19**, 241–248.

90 Hayes, B.D., Klein-Schwartz, W., Clark, R.F., Muller, A.A., and Miloradovich, J.E. (2010) Comparison of toxicity of acute overdoses with citalopram and escitalopram. *J. Emerg. Med.*, **39**, 44–48.

91 Yilmaz, Z., Ceschi, A., Rauber-Luthy, C., Sauer, O., Stedtler, U., Prasa, D., Seidel, C., Hackl, E., Hoffmann-Walbeck, P., Gerber-Zupan, G., Bauer, K., Kupferschmidt, H., Kullak-Ublick, G.A., and Wilks, M. (2010) Escitalopram causes fewer seizures in human overdose than citalopram. *Clin. Toxicol.*, **48**, 207–212.

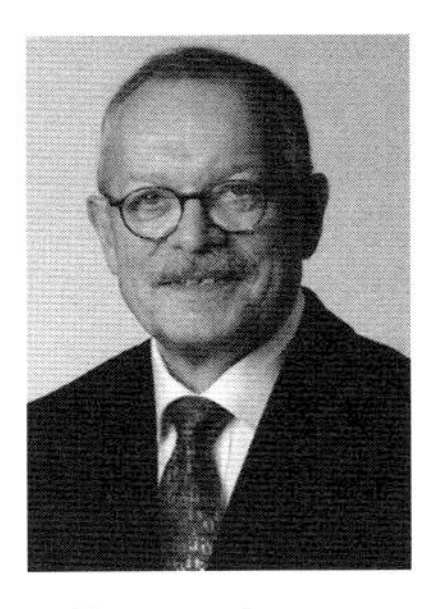

Klaus P. Bøgesø, B.Sc., D.Sc., has been working at H. Lundbeck A/S with drug discovery within the CNS field for more than 40 years. Klaus P. Bøgesø started at Lundbeck as a Research Chemist in 1971. In 1986, he became Director of Medicinal Chemistry and in 1999 he became Vice President of Medicinal Chemistry Research. In 2006, he became Vice President of Research, Denmark. In 2008, he became Vice President of External Affairs, Lundbeck Research Management. In 2011, he became Vice President, External Scientific Affairs and Patents.

The research activities of Klaus P. Bøgesø have focused on drug design and development within psychiatric and neurological diseases, such as schizophrenia, depression, anxiety, Alzheimer's disease, Parkinson's disease, and epilepsy. Primary targets have been serotonin, norepinephrine, and dopamine receptors and transporters, muscarinic receptors, and glutamate receptors. Klaus P. Bøgesø is inventor of the selective serotonin reuptake inhibitor citalopram (Cipramil®, Celexa®) and co-inventor of its *S*-enantiomer, escitalopram (Cipralex®, Lexapro®). Both drugs have attained blockbuster status. The differential action of stereoisomers of chiral drugs has been a focus area in many of the research projects Klaus P. Bøgesø has been involved in, and has been a major topic in several of his publications, including his doctoral thesis.

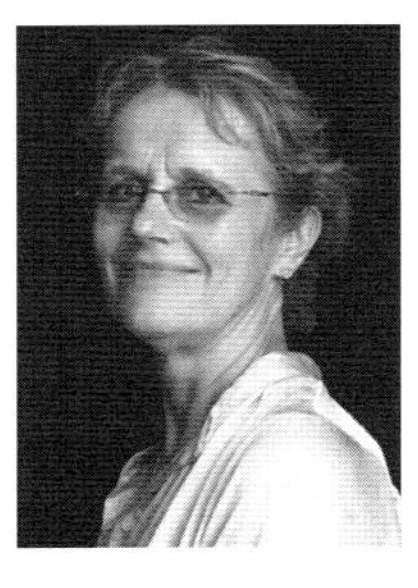

Connie Sánchez, currently at Lundbeck Research USA and before that at H. Lundbeck A/S, in Copenhagen, Denmark, has more than 25 years of drug discovery experience. She graduated from the Pharmaceutical University of Denmark and has acquired a D.Sc. degree in Pharmacology at the same institution. She has a broad experience within drug discovery and drug development for neuropsychiatric and neurological diseases, including depression, anxiety, schizophrenia, Alzheimer's disease, Parkinson's disease, epilepsy, and insomnia, and she has contributed to bringing various drug candidates into clinical development, some of which have been brought to the market. Most notably, she established and successfully led a research project aiming at uncovering the mechanism of action of the antidepressant drug escitalopram (Cipralex®). She has authored approximately 100 scientific papers and more than 20 patent publications.

12
Tapentadol – From Morphine and Tramadol to the Discovery of Tapentadol

Helmut Buschmann

List of Abbreviations

5-HT	5-hydroxytryptamine (serotonin)
COX	cyclooxygenases
CYP	cytochrome P450
DOR	delta-opioid receptor
ED_{50}	dose that produces 50% effect (*in vivo* measure of potency)
ER	extended release
FDA	US Food and Drug Administration
i.c.v.	intracerebroventricular
i.p.	intraperitoneal
i.t.	intrathecal
i.v.	intravenous
IR	immediate release
K_i	dissociation constant (measure of affinity)
KOR	kappa-opioid receptor
M-1	*O*-desmethyl metabolite of tramadol
MOR	mu-opioid receptor
NE	norepinephrine (noradrenaline)
NET	norepinephrine (noradrenaline) transporter
NOP	ORL1, or nociceptin receptor
NRI	norepinephrine (noradrenaline) reuptake inhibitor
NSAID	nonsteroidal anti-inflammatory drug
ORL1	NOP, or nociceptin receptor
p.o.	per os, oral
SERT	serotonin transporter
SNL	spinal nerve ligation
SR	sustained release
SRI	serotonin reuptake inhibitor
STZ	streptozotocin
THF	tetrahydrofuran

Analogue-based Drug Discovery III, First Edition. Edited by János Fischer, C. Robin Ganellin, and David P. Rotella.
© 2013 Wiley-VCH Verlag GmbH & Co. KGaA. Published 2013 by Wiley-VCH Verlag GmbH & Co. KGaA.

TMSCl trimethylsilyl chloride
WHO World Health Organization

12.1 Introduction

Tapentadol ((−)-(1*R*,2*R*)-3-(3-dimethylamino-1-ethyl-2-methylpropyl)phenol hydrochloride; 3-[(1*R*,2*R*)-3-(dimethylamino)-1-ethyl-2-methylpropyl]phenol hydrochloride), discovered by Grünenthal (Germany) and shown in Figure 12.1 together with morphine and tramadol, was approved in November 2008 by the US Food and Drug Administration (FDA) for the treatment of moderate to severe acute pain in adults as an immediate-release formulation (Nucynta®, Johnson & Johnson). Tapentadol is a novel, centrally acting analgesic with a dual mode of action: mu-opioid receptor (MOR) agonism and norepinephrine reuptake inhibition. Tapentadol is the first oral centrally acting analgesic to be approved in the United States in more than a decade. In the United States, tapentadol has been placed into schedule II of the Controlled Substances Act[1]. An extended-release formulation of tapentadol (Nucynta ER®) obtained FDA approval for the treatment of chronic pain in August 2011.

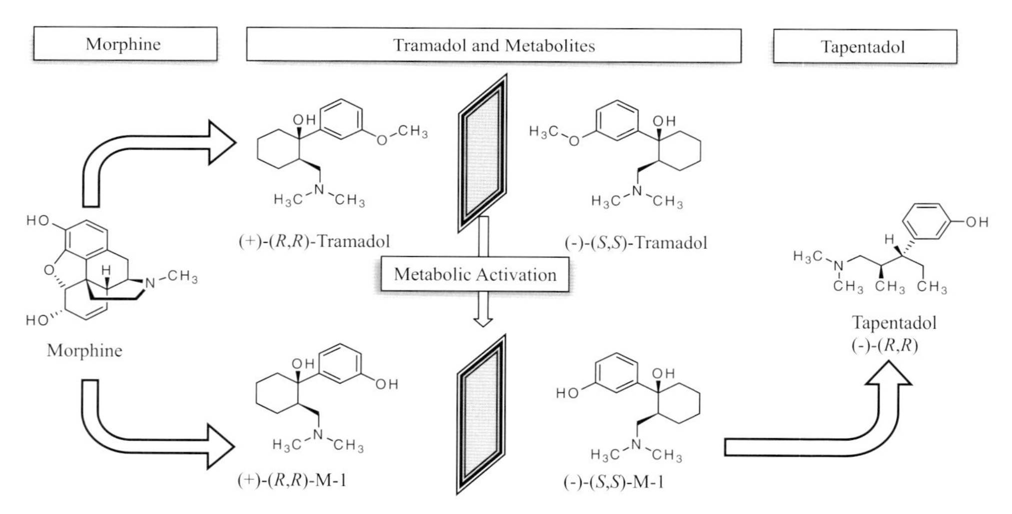

Figure 12.1 Chemical structure of tapentadol HCl, morphine, and tramadol (the absolute stereochemistry of the (−)-(*S*,*S*)-M-1 metabolite of tramadol corresponds to the stereochemistry of (−)-(*R*,*R*)-tapentadol).

1) The Controlled Substances Act (CSA) was enacted into law by the Congress of the United States as Title II of the Comprehensive Drug Abuse Prevention and Control Act of 1970. The CSA is the federal US drug policy under which the manufacture, importation, possession, use, and distribution of certain substances is regulated. Schedule II includes drugs that may have a high potential for abuse. Further examples of schedule II drugs are morphine, oxycodone, fentanyl, cocaine, methylphenidate, or methamphetamine.

On August 10, 2010, the European decentralized procedure regarding tapentadol concluded positively and the granting of national marketing authorizations in 26 European markets is expected. Tapentadol will then be available as an oral, solid, immediate-release formulation (tablets) for the relief of moderate to severe acute pain in adults, and an oral, solid, prolonged-release formulation (tablets) for the management of severe chronic pain in adults. Since October 2010, tapentadol is available on the German market as Palexia® retard for the treatment of nociceptive and neuropathic pain types. Tapentadol has been clinically tested in multiple pain models and found to combine opioid efficacy with favorable gastrointestinal tolerability. Tapentadol as a centrally acting opioid analgesic has a potency between morphine and tramadol.

12.1.1
Pain and Current Pain Treatment Options

Pain is defined as "an unpleasant sensory and emotional experience associated with actual or potential tissue damage, or described in terms of such damage" [1]. Pain is the most common reason that patients seek medical care. The experience of physical pain is familiar to everyone; however, the intensity, character, and tolerability of each person's pain are subjective. How patients perceive and react to pain is influenced by social, cultural, and psychological factors [2]. Thus, detailed examination as to the character (e.g., dull, throbbing, and stabbing), location, and intensity of pain, how and when it occurs, and the effects of pain is needed in order to recommend appropriate interventions. Pain may be acute or chronic [3]. Acute pain is generally associated with an identifiable cause, resolves after the removal of the cause, responds to treatment, and lasts less than 1–3 months [4]. *Acute* pain is defined as that associated with a sudden stimulus (e.g., accident or surgery [5]) and is generally expected to resolve as the injury heals. Clinical examples of acute pain include pain following surgery and pain associated with injury. Pain that does not have a clear cause or that lasts longer than 1–3 months after the initial injury heals is considered chronic pain. It is estimated that neuropathic pain affects over 6 million patients in the United States and Europe and over 26 million patients worldwide.

Neuropathic pain is a pain associated with a functional abnormality of the nervous system. Pain severity, however, is not correlated with the amount of damage and symptoms can persist long after tissue damage from an antecedent injury resolves [6]. Clinical features of neuropathic pain include the presence of an abnormal, unpleasant sensation (dysesthesia) that frequently has a burning or electrical quality with an occasional paroxysmal, brief, shooting, or stabbing quality. Pain may be felt in a region of sensory deficit. Non-noxious stimuli may be painful (allodynia). Noxious stimuli may produce a greater than normal response (hyperalgesia).

Chronic noncancer pain can develop as a result of persistent stimulation of or changes to nociceptors due to localized tissue damage from an acute injury or disease (e.g., osteoarthritis), or damage to the peripheral or central nervous system, or both (e.g., painful diabetic neuropathy, poststroke pain, and spinal cord injury). There is a wide range of treatments available to physicians for neuropathic pain, some of which have specific indications, and some of which are used off-label. However, currently available treatments provide modest improvements in pain and minimum improvements in physical and emotional functioning.

Pain is further categorized according to the neural and biochemical mechanisms at work. *Nociceptive* pain is the normal physiological response to a noxious stimulus, such as injury or inflammation. The stimulus causes nociceptors to release the neurotransmitters glutamate, calcitonin gene-related peptide, and substance P, which transmit the signal to second-order neurons in the spinal cord. The second-order neurons form the ascending spinothalamic tract that leads to the thalamus,

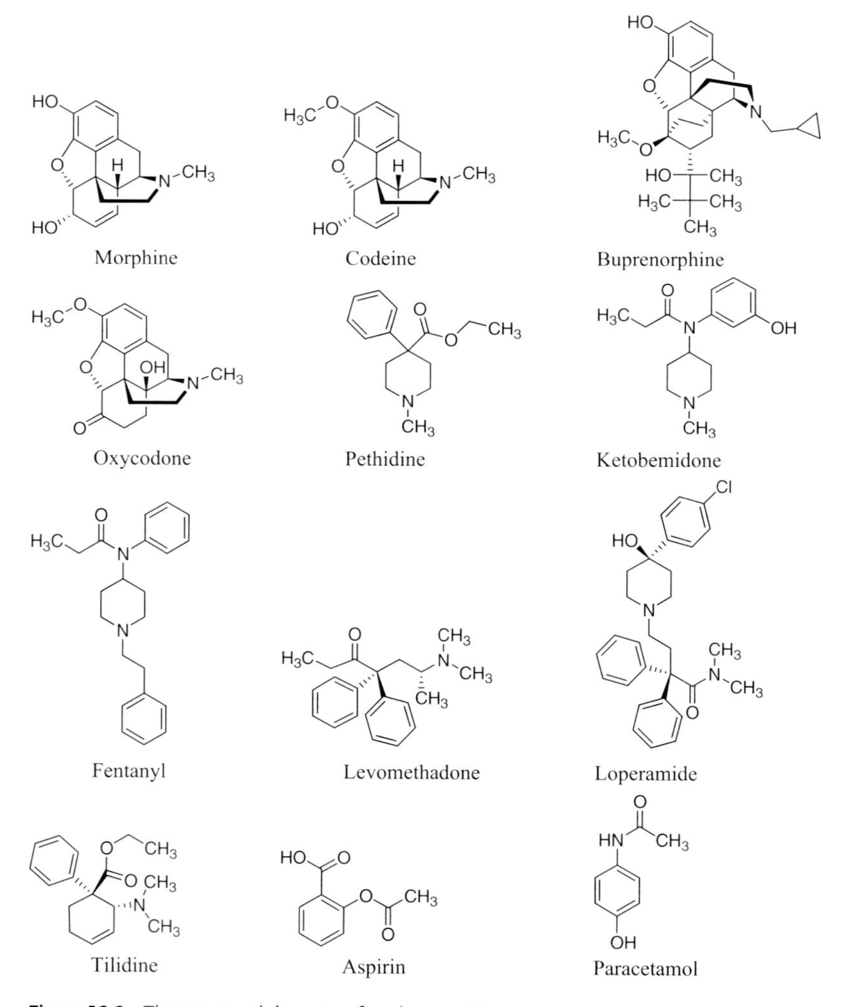

Figure 12.2 The structural diversity of analgesics [8].

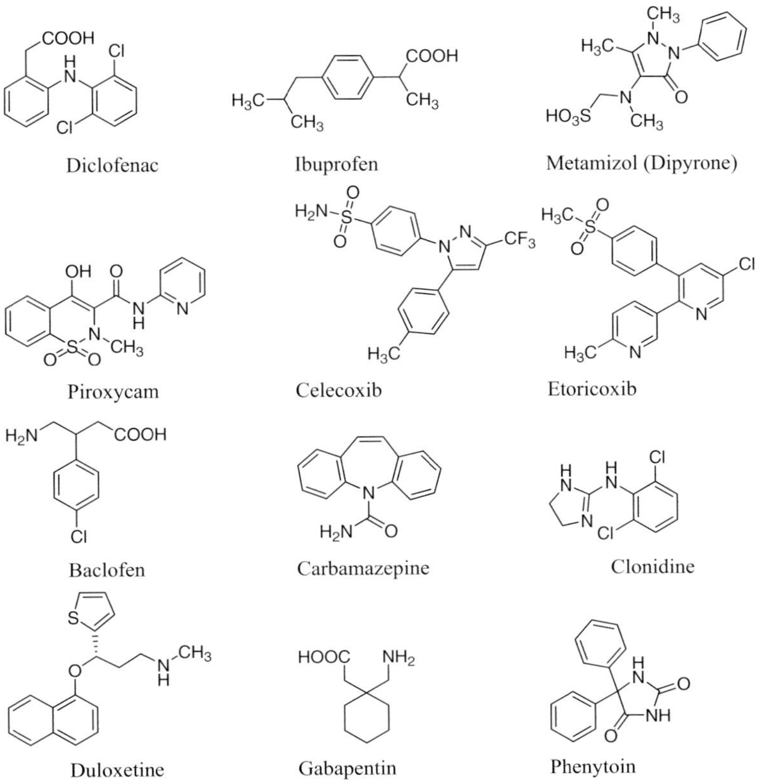

Diclofenac Ibuprofen Metamizol (Dipyrone)

Piroxycam Celecoxib Etoricoxib

Baclofen Carbamazepine Clonidine

Duloxetine Gabapentin Phenytoin

Figure 12.2 (*Continued*)

where they synapse with third-order neurons that project to the sensory cortex, where the pain is perceived [7]. Pain signals are modulated by release of endorphins and enkephalins in the midbrain. These neurotransmitters interact with specific opioid receptors in descending modulatory neurons that synapse with the primary or second-order pain transmission neurons. Descending neurons release norepinephrine and serotonin, which directly inhibit the release of pain transmitters and inhibit the activity of the second-order pain transmission neurons [7].

Pharmacological treatment for pain includes nonopioid analgesics, such as salicylates, acetaminophen, and nonsteroidal anti-inflammatory drugs (NSAIDs), opioids, and other drug classes, including antidepressants and anticonvulsants. The structural diversity of analgesics is shown in Figure 12.2 [8].

NSAIDs produce pain relief by inhibition of cyclooxygenases (COX-1 and COX-2), which catalyze the production of proinflammatory prostaglandins from arachidonic acid. The traditional NSAIDs are nonselective inhibitors of COX-1 and COX-2 [8]. Prostaglandins are important mediators of inflammation that increase pain sensations through inflammatory mechanisms [9]. Nonopioid oral medications are recommended for mild to moderate acute pain, and most are available over the counter and by prescription. Potentially serious side effects of NSAIDs include gastrointestinal effects, such as upsets, stomach ulcers, or bleeding, as well as reduced blood clotting, decreased kidney function, and cardiovascular side effects. The risk of these events is increased by higher doses and long-term use.

Opioid medications mimic the actions of endorphins by interacting with opioid receptors in the brain and spinal cord. Activation of mu-opioid receptors in ascending pathways may work to inhibit nociceptive signals [7]. An increase in the effect on ascending pathways activity of opioid receptors may activate the modulating descending neural pathways as detailed above and produce relief of pain [7]. Opioids are associated with the potential for abuse and addiction [2]. Opioids are generally indicated for moderate to severe acute pain.

12.1.2 Pain Research Today

Already in 1999, it was stated by Butera in his review about treatment options for neuropathic pain: "Despite an intensive research effort over the past two decades involving many innovative approaches in the global academic community and by the pharmaceutical industry, the latter representing an aggregate investment in excess of $2.5 billion, the only new opioid-based pain medications either in clinical development or on the market are alternative dosage forms of the classical opioids, morphine, loperamide, and fentanyl, or compounds such as tramadol" (see Figure 12.2) [10].

As physicians are faced with an increasing number of patients with numerous neuropathic pain symptoms most likely stemming from multiple etiologies, they are forced to resort to the polypharmacia approach as the mainstay therapy. Current pharmacological treatment for neuropathic pain will typically include some combination of agents from several of the following drug classes: opioids, tricyclic antidepressants, anticonvulsant agents, or nonsteroidal anti-inflammatory drugs as shown in Figure 1.2. Ironically, even with such an impressive arsenal of powerful drugs, these approaches only provide an approximate 30–50% reduction in pain in about 50% of patients. Coupled with this limited efficacy, there are low levels of compliance due to intolerable side effect profiles associated with some of these drugs. These results profoundly illustrate that treatment of neuropathic pain is a hugely unmet medical need, and they underscore the importance of considering, validating, and pursuing alternative targets to treat refractory neuropathic pain [6, 11].

Research in understanding the underlying mechanisms behind people's pain has progressed rapidly, but despite these critical advances pain remains grossly undertreated and is frequently mistreated. In the words of Jean-Marie Besson (President of the International Association for the Study of Pain) at the 9th Congress of the International Association for the Study of Pain in Vienna, Austria, in August 1999, the current treatment options are summarized as follows: "Some pain states can now be controlled, yet there are still others which are far from being treatable" [12].

12.1.3
The Complex Mode of Action of Tramadol

Since the isolation of morphine two centuries ago, numerous derivatives have been synthesized, with the primary aim of separating analgesic effects from unwanted effects, such as nausea and emesis, constipation, respiratory depression, addiction, and dependence. An alternative approach to improve the therapeutic usefulness of opioid analgesics is to combine MOR activation with an additional mechanism of action aimed at enhancing analgesic efficacy. Such an additional analgesic mechanism may result in an opiate-sparing effect, thereby attenuating the unwanted effects of MOR activation.

The concept of combined mechanisms of action was realized for the first time with the introduction of tramadol, a compound that produces MOR activation and inhibition of serotonin (5-HT) and norepinephrine reuptake.

Tramadol ((1*R*,2*R*)-*rel*-2-[(dimethylamino)methyl]-1-(3-methoxyphenyl)cyclohexanol) is a centrally acting opioid analgesic, used in treating moderate to severe pain. It is classified as a "step II" opioid analgesic in the WHO pain treatment ladder.

Tramadol was first synthesized in 1962 by Flick at Grünenthal and has been available for pain treatment in Germany since 1977. Immediate-release preparations of tramadol were introduced in the United Kingdom in 1994, in the United States in 1995, and subsequently in many other countries. Nowadays, several once-daily, sustained-release formulations of tramadol have been marketed in various countries. The drug has a wide range of applications, including treatment for restless legs syndrome and fibromyalgia.

Tramadol possesses weak agonist actions at the mu-opioid receptor, releases serotonin, and inhibits the reuptake of norepinephrine [13]. The analgesic action of tramadol has yet to be fully understood, but it is believed to work through modulation of serotonin and norepinephrine in addition to its mild agonism of the mu-opioid receptor. The contribution of nonopioid activity is demonstrated by the fact that the analgesic effect of tramadol is not fully antagonized by the mu-opioid receptor antagonist naloxone.

Tramadol is marketed as a racemic mixture of the (1*R*,2*R*)- and (1*S*,2*S*)-enantiomers with a weak affinity for the mu-opioid receptor (the affinity for the mu-opioid receptor is approximately 10 times lower than that of codeine and 6000 times lower than that of morphine). The two enantiomers of racemic tramadol function in a complementary manner to enhance the analgesic efficacy and improve the tolerability profile of tramadol. This dual mechanism of action may be attributed to the two enantiomers of racemic tramadol. The (+)-enantiomer has a higher affinity for the mu-receptor and is a more effective inhibitor of 5-HT reuptake, whereas the (−)-enantiomer is a more effective inhibitor of norepinephrine reuptake and increases its release by autoreceptor activation. The (1*R*,2*R*)-(+)-enantiomer is approximately four times more potent than the (1*S*,2*S*)-(−)-enantiomer in terms of mu-opioid receptor affinity and 5-HT reuptake, whereas the (1*S*,2*S*)-(−)-enantiomer is responsible for norepinephrine reuptake effects. These actions appear to produce a synergistic analgesic effect, with (1*R*,2*R*)-(+)-tramadol exhibiting 10-fold higher analgesic activity than (1*S*,2*S*)-(−)-tramadol [14].

Tramadol undergoes hepatic metabolism via the cytochrome P450 isozyme CYP2B6, CYP2D6, and CYP3A4, being *O*- and *N*-demethylated to five different metabolites. Of these, *O*-desmethyltramadol ((+)-M-1) is the most significant since it has 300 times the mu-affinity of (+)-tramadol, and furthermore has an elimination half-life of 9 h, compared with 6 h for tramadol itself [15]. Similarly to tramadol, *O*-desmethyltramadol (M-1) has also been shown to be a norepinephrine reuptake inhibitor [16].

The fact that these four compounds (the enantiomers of tramadol and the enantiomeric metabolites M-1) have different pharmacological properties makes tramadol an atypical opioid with a complex mechanism of action [17, 18]. This is the reason why tramadol is used as a racemate, despite known different physiological effects of the enantiomers, because the racemate has a better pharmacological profile than the single enantiomers in terms of efficacy and tolerability in animals and humans.

However, the relative contribution of the different mechanisms of action to the overall analgesic effect changes over time. As the parent molecule is metabolized, the contribution of 5-HT and NE reuptake inhibition is reduced, whereas the contribution of MOR agonism increases, resulting in a complex time- and metabolism-dependent pattern of pharmacological activities. Because tramadol is mainly metabolized via cytochrome P450 2D6 (CYP2D6), which is polymorphic in humans, approximately 5–15% of the white population are "poor metabolizers" of tramadol and do not experience satisfactory analgesia with standard doses. Furthermore, preclinical and clinical evidence, with selective 5-HT reuptake inhibitors, selective NE reuptake inhibitors, and mixed 5-HT/NE reuptake inhibitors, indicates that analgesia is more readily obtained by NE reuptake inhibition than by 5-HT reuptake inhibition. Finally, a compound without serotonergic activity would not bear the risk of producing or contributing to a serotonin syndrome.

12.2 The Discovery of Tapentadol

Based on elucidation of the favorable aspects of the multimodal analgesic mechanism of action of tramadol, a research program was initiated in the late 1980s at Grünenthal to design a new class of opioid/nonopioid analgesics that would combine MOR agonism and norepinephrine reuptake inhibition, with minimal serotonergic activity. It was also desired that both activities would reside in a single parent molecule that does not require metabolic activation via the cytochrome P450 system. Increasing evidence demonstrates that many pharmaceutically important compounds elicit their effects through binding to multiple targets. Tapentadol is an example of a rationally designed multiple ligand starting from the tramadol structure and its understanding of the complex pharmacological activity.

12.2.1 From the Tramadol Structure to Tapentadol

The discovery of tapentadol involved multiple steps of chemical innovations to become a unique drug, which may be summarizes as follows (Figure 12.3):

- **The dimethylaminomethyl fragment:** The dimethylaminomethyl moiety is a significant part of the pharmacophore that is needed for interaction with mu-opioid receptor and it seems to be relevant for interaction with the monoamine transporter system [20]. Demethylation is a metabolic pathway leading to analgesic inactive *N*-demethyl derivatives without opioid binding or transporter inhibition effect [21–23]. Increasing the size of the nitrogen substituent (e.g., ethyl or benzyl substituents) or cyclic substitution (piperidine or pyrrolidine substitution) also leads to inactive compounds. The dimethylaminomethyl fragment, therefore, appears to be essential for analgesic activity for both drugs keeping mu-opioid receptor binding and norepinephrine reuptake activity.
- **The role of absolute and relative stereochemistry:** Tramadol and tapentadol contain two chiral carbon atoms. Consequently, for both molecules, four stereoisomers exist as two diasteromeric pairs of enantiomers. However, tramadol is a racemate, whereas tapentadol is a pure enantiomer. The relative stereochemistry is critical for biological activity. In both cases, only the (*R*,*R*) and (*S*,*S*) isomers display analgesic activity, whereas the diastereomeric enantiomers are relatively inactive. In past decades, the pharmacopeia was dominated by racemates [24, 25, 23]; however, since the emergence in the 1980s of new technologies that allowed the preparation of pure enantiomers in significant quantities, the awareness and interest in the stereochemistry of drug action has increased. These factors have led to an increasing preference for selection of single

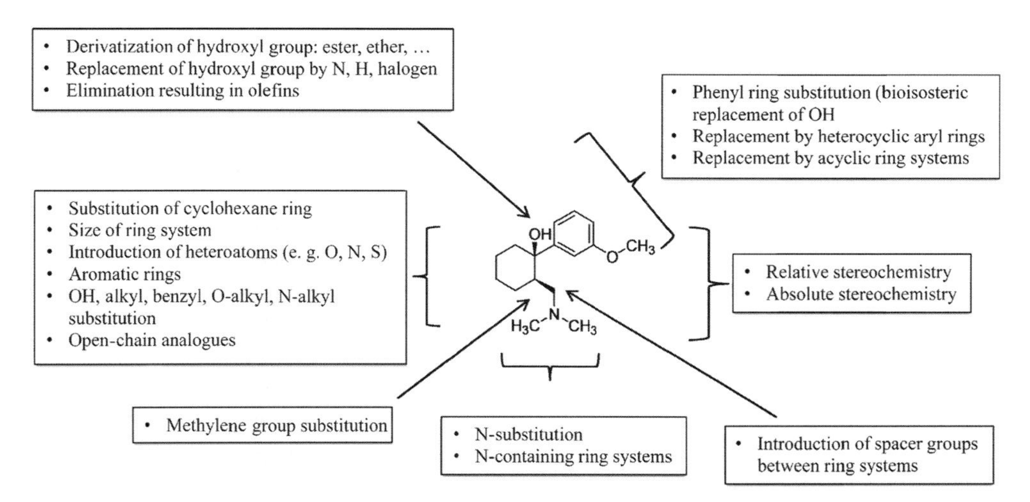

Figure 12.3 Summary of chemical modifications leading to the discovery of tapentadol [19].

enantiomers by both the pharmaceutical industry and regulatory authorities. As a consequence of this changing climate toward drug chirality, it was decided to use pure enantiomers for further optimization. The absolute stereochemistry of tapentadol corresponds to the (−)-(1*S*,2*S*)-M-1 metabolite of tramadol (Figure 1.1). Subsequently, it was found that the MOR affinity of the enantiomer acting on the norepinephrine transporter was increased, and in the following steps, modifications were made to increase this MOR affinity. In the case of the open-chain analogue, the MOR affinity is increased in comparison to the cyclic analogue without affecting the transporter inhibition effect.

- **Cyclic core structure versus open-chain molecule:** Several drugs possess cyclic aliphatic ring systems connected via linkers with other aromatic or heteroaromatic groups [26]. However, in the lead optimization phase, a cyclic ring system is typically modified by changing the ring size and introducing heteroatoms (such as nitrogen, oxygen, or sulfur) as well as introducing additional substituents in order to optimize desired hydrophobic or nonhydrophobic interactions with the biological target, thereby leading to an increase in the potency and ligand efficiency of a given lead structure. As a consequence, the cyclic structure is retained in many lead optimization programs due to the entropic and enthalpic balance of the thermodynamics of binding [27, 28]. Cyclic structures generally have the advantage of decreasing the entropic proportion of the binding energy compared with open-chain molecules, leading to more flexible derivatives with greater ligand efficiency [29]. In addition, many examples are known wherein an open-chain analogue of a given drug loses biological activity completely; for instance, the open-chain analogue of diazepam is completely inactive [30]. In the course of the development of tapentadol, it was found that opening the cyclohexane ring system led to active compounds while conserving the relative stereochemistry. However, the activity of the molecules was strongly dependent on the length of the side chain. It was found that a methyl group and an ethyl group at chiral carbon atoms were optimal in terms of analgesic potency and biochemical binding profile.
- **Replacement of the aromatic hydroxyl group:** The introduction of a phenolic hydroxy group instead of an aromatic methoxy group results in a dramatic change in pharmacological activity due to an increase of binding affinity to mu-opioid receptor [20], which is known for other opioids (e.g., morphine versus codeine). The bioisoteric replacement of the phenolic hydroxyl group by CH_2F or CHF_2 groups yielded in a significant decrease of activity. The enantiomers of open-chain phenolic structures showed increased analgesic activity compared to the cyclic tramadol-derived analogues.
- **Replacement of the aliphatic hydroxyl group:** It is known for many drugs that their aliphatic hydroxyl group is essential for pharmacological activity [31, 23]. Derivatization by introducing more bulkier groups in this position (e.g., ether or ester prodrugs) led to the complete loss of analgesic activity. However, replacement of the tertiary hydroxyl group by either fluorine or hydrogen resulted in a significant increase of MOR affinity for both enantiomers. The chlorine derivatives were also analgesically active; however, the chemical stability was decreased

(loss of chlorine). However, the fluorine derivatives were not further developed as well due to physicochemical stability issues. Critically, the hydrogen derivative was found to have both activities in one molecule. While retaining the norepinephrine reuptake inhibition (NRI) component, the MOR agonism component was increased to achieve potent analgesic activity without the prominent serotonin reuptake inhibition (SRI) effect present in tramadol.

In contrast to this serendipitous combination of mechanisms like in the tramadol case, tapentadol was designed to rationally combine two analgesic mechanisms (MOR agonism and NRI) within a single molecule. As part of this development, tapentadol was designed to have less serotonergic activity. The result is an innovative drug that retains the advantages of combining synergistic mechanisms of action, but with a significantly greater "functional" opioid component and a relatively greater inhibition of the norepinephrine reuptake than of the serotonin transporter, all in a single molecule with no analgesically active metabolites. The chemical innovations introduced in the development of tapentadol starting from the tramadol structure are summarized in Figure 12.4.

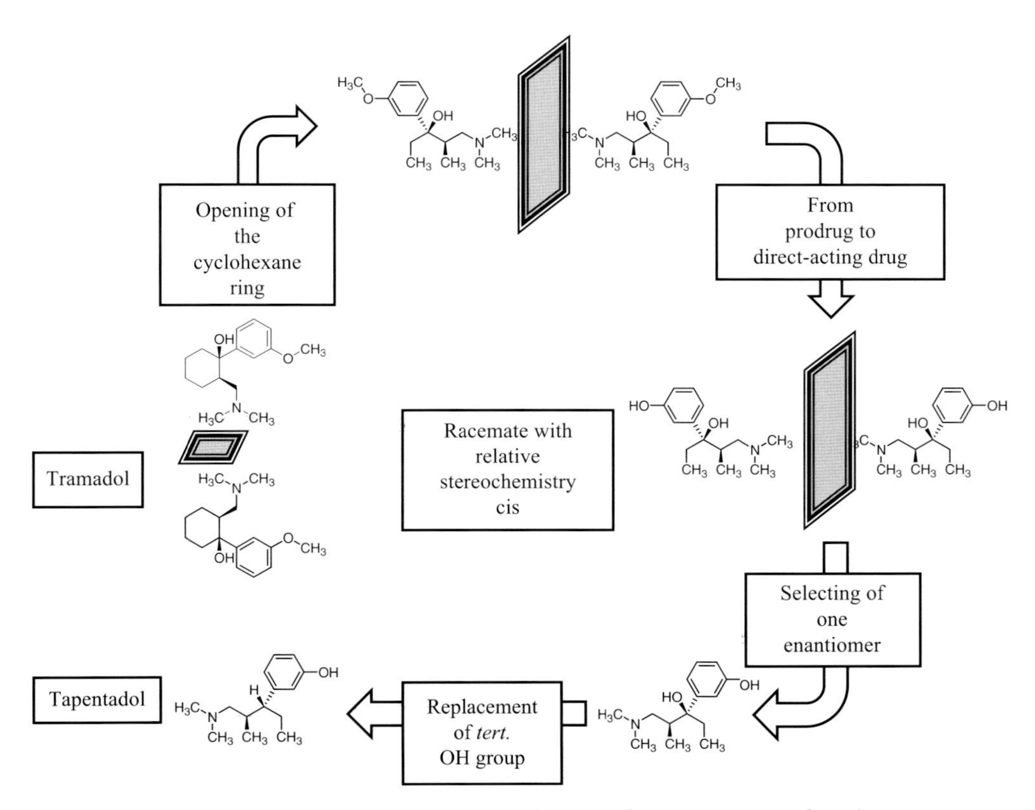

Figure 12.4 Chemical innovations introduced in the development of tapentadol starting from the tramadol structure [19].

12.2.2
Synthetic Pathways to Tapentadol

Several syntheses of tapentadol have been reported [32–34]. In the original patent, tapentadol hydrochloride is synthesized by ether cleavage (e.g., conc. HBr) from its corresponding methyl ether **1**. Compound **1** can be obtained by several methods, for example, starting from diethyl ketone, which is transformed under standard Mannich conditions to racemic **2**. The Grignard reaction with 3-bromoanisole and subsequent separation of diastereomers (crystallization as HCl salt from 2-butanone with TMSCl/H_2O) and enantiomers (HPLC) gives (−)-(*S*,*S*)- **3**. Removal of the hydroxy group can be achieved diastereoselectively (under retention) by chlorination with thionyl chloride to yield **4**, followed by treatment with zinc borohydride (from $ZnCl_2$ and $NaBH_4$), leading to tapentadol hydrochloride (Figure 12.5).

The following route developed by Hell and coworkers is described in the recent patent literature [35–37]. Ketone **5** was treated with Eschenmoser's salt in acetonitrile at room temperature and the resulting amine **6** was collected by adding ether and crystallizing the product. Amine **6** was crystallized with L-(−)-dibenzoyl tartaric acid monohydrate in ethanol at 6–8 °C to give the desired enantiomer as salt **7**. The free base of **7** was generated by reaction with aqueous sodium hydroxide and then treated with ethyl magnesium bromide in THF at 10 °C followed by stirring at

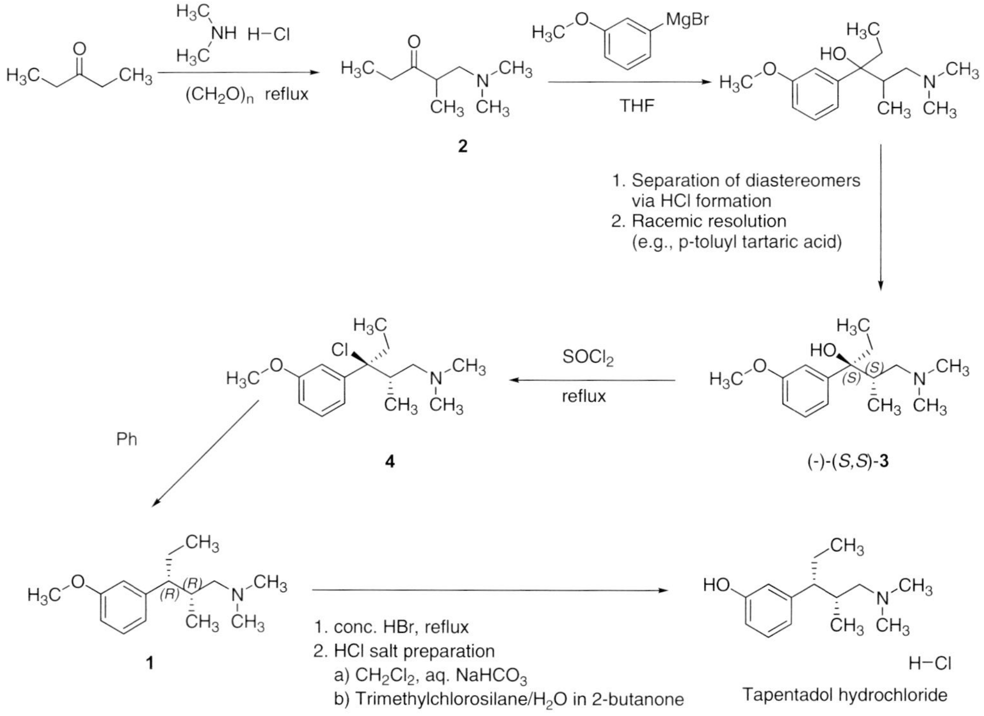

Figure 12.5 The synthesis of tapentadol hydrochloride as described in the first patent [32].

room temperature overnight to give tertiary alcohol **8**. Alcohol **8** was treated with trifluoroacetic anhydride in 2-methyl THF at 40–45 °C to give the corresponding trifluoromethyl ester that was then treated with 10% Pd/C and hydrogenated at 3 bar at ambient temperature. These hydrogenolytic conditions effected reductive cleavage of the trifluoromethyl ester and removal of the benzyl protecting group with retention of stereochemistry. Filtration of the catalyst followed by the addition of water and trimethylchlorosilane to generate HCl *in situ* and allowing the product to crystallize out at 5–8 °C gave the desired tapentadol hydrochloride with 99% purity and 96.9% ee (Figure 12.6).

Another synthetic route starts from 1-(3-methoxy-phenyl)-propan-1-one **9**[38], which reacts in a Mannich reaction to the corresponding racemic Mannich base **10**. The diastereomeric salt formation with (*R*)-(−) mandelic acid give the desired enantiomer as the mandelic acid salt in high chemical yields, because the undesired enantiomer is transformed via a keto–enol equilibrium to the desired one. Grignard reaction of the free base with ethyl magnesium bromide in tetrahydrofuran yields the corresponding tertiary alcohol **11**. Alcohol **11** was treated with trifluoroacetic anhydride in 2-methyl THF to give the corresponding trifluoromethyl ester that was then treated with 10% Pd/C and hydrogenated at ambient

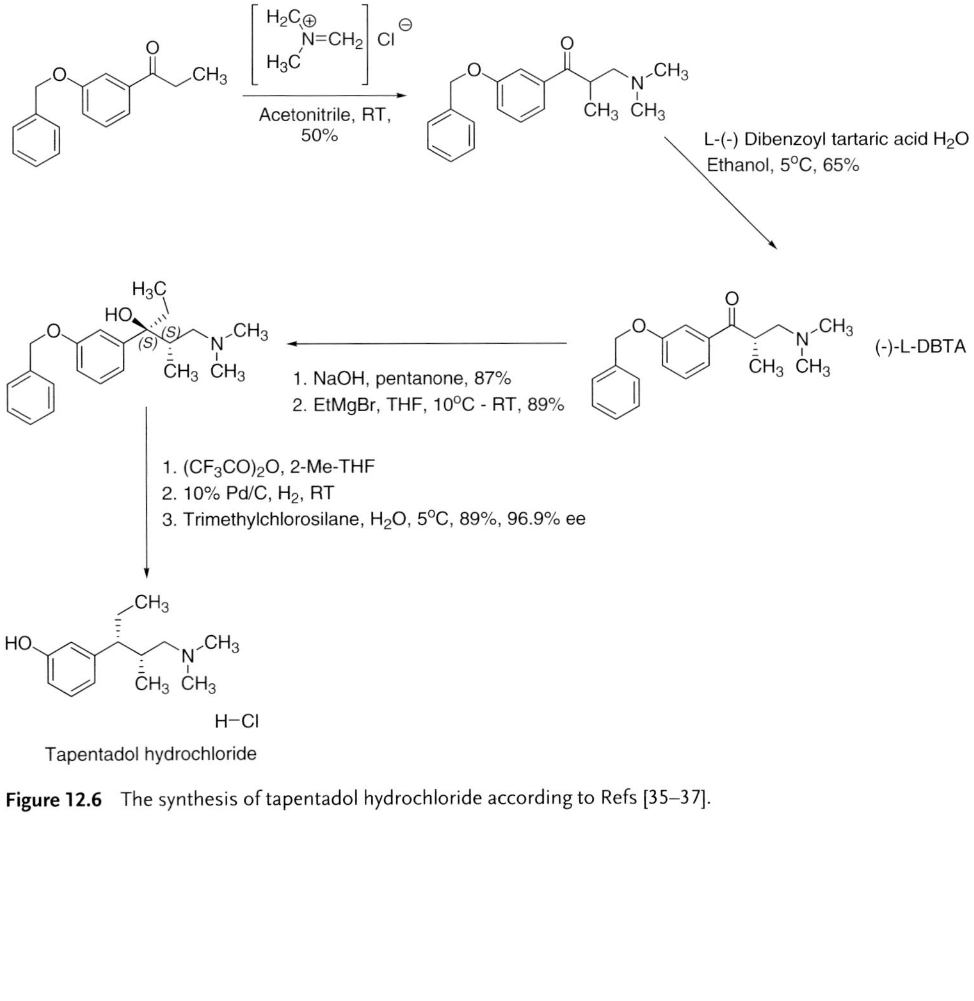

Acetonitrile, RT, 50%

L-(-) Dibenzoyl tartaric acid H_2O Ethanol, 5°C, 65%

(-)-L-DBTA

1. NaOH, pentanone, 87%
2. EtMgBr, THF, 10°C - RT, 89%

1. $(CF_3CO)_2O$, 2-Me-THF
2. 10% Pd/C, H_2, RT
3. Trimethylchlorosilane, H_2O, 5°C, 89%, 96.9% ee

H−Cl

Tapentadol hydrochloride

Figure 12.6 The synthesis of tapentadol hydrochloride according to Refs [35–37].

temperature. These hydrogenolytic conditions effected reductive cleavage of the trifluoromethyl ester and removal of the *N*-benzyl protecting group with retention of stereochemistry. Crystallization of the hydrochloride salt **12** and reductive methylation with formaldehyde in formic acid leads to the dimethyl amino derivative **13**. The methoxy ether is cleaved by methionine and methanesulfonic acid. Working up with NaOH and extraction with ethyl acetate yields the free base of tapentadol (Figure 12.7).

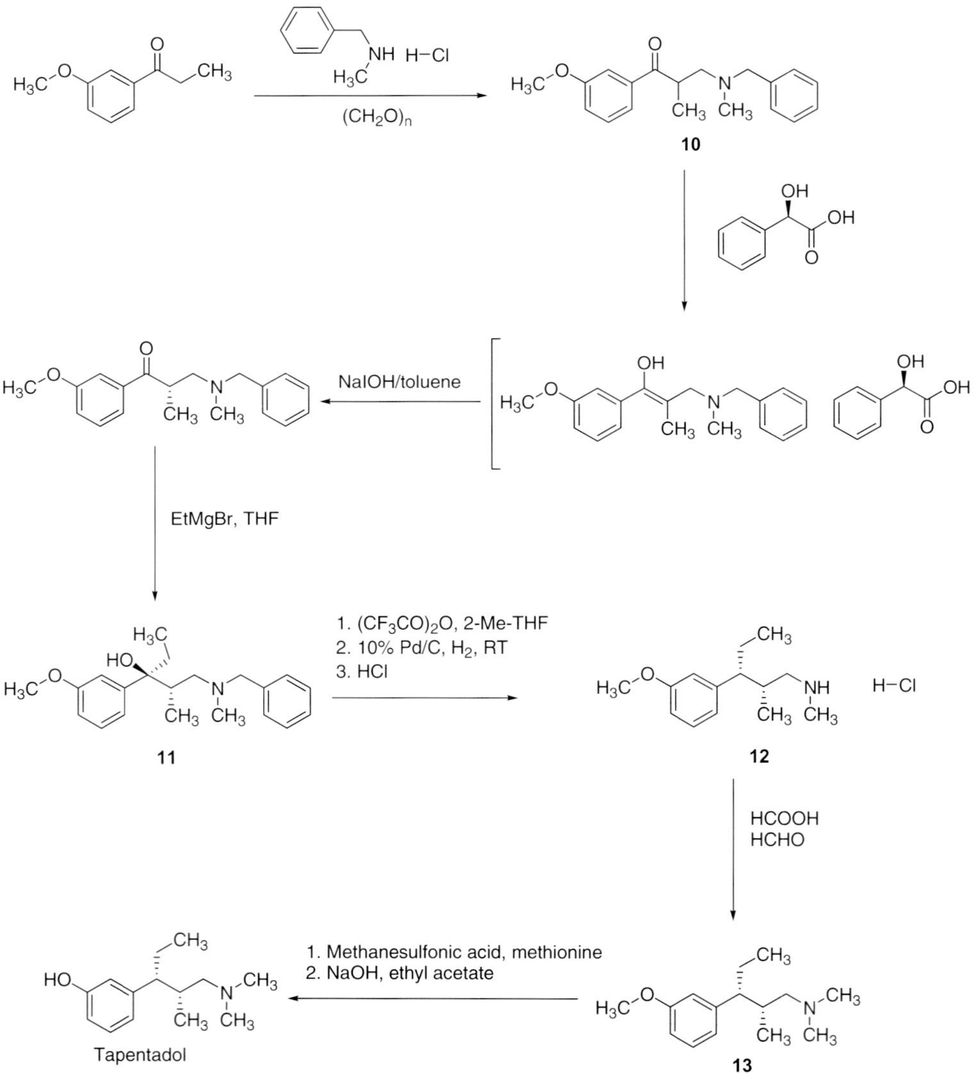

Figure 12.7 The synthesis of tapentadol hydrochloride according to Ref. [38].

Starting from *N,N*-dimethylpropionamide, a synthesis for racemic tapentadol without a Mannich reaction is described [39] as shown in Figure 12.8. *N,N*-Dimethylpropionamide is transformed to derivatives **14** and **15**. A Grignard reaction with 3-anisole magnesium bromide and ethyl magnesium bromide,

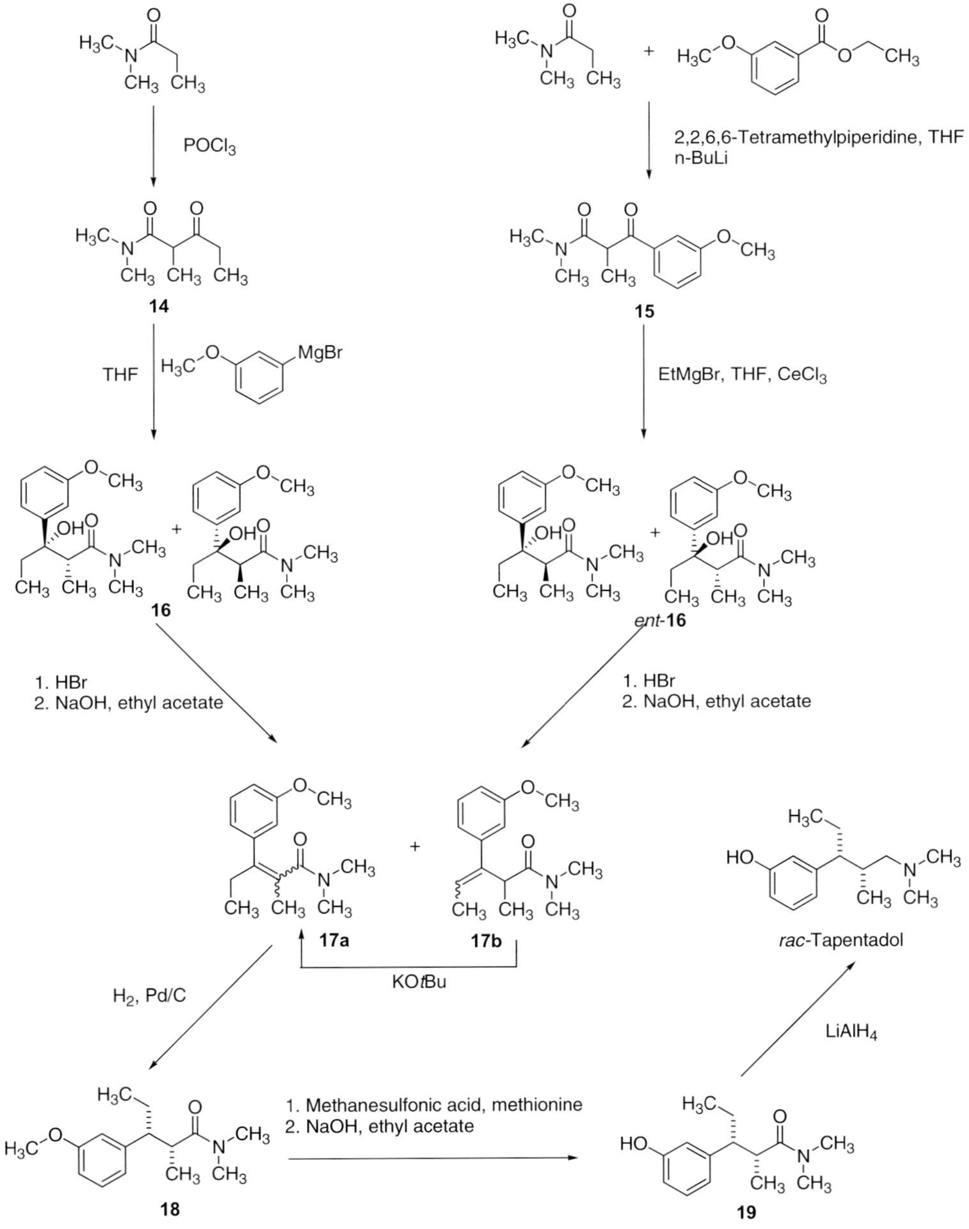

Figure 12.8 The synthesis of tapentadol hydrochloride according to Ref. [39].

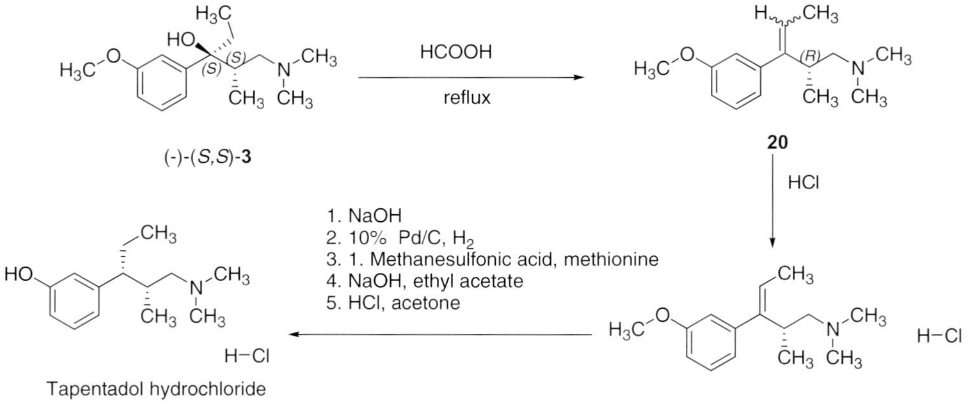

Figure 12.9 The synthesis of tapentadol hydrochloride according to Ref. [40].

respectively, gives the diasteromeric alcohols 3-hydroxy-3-(3-methoxyphenyl)-2-methylpentanoic acid dimethylamide **16** and *ent*-**16** as racemates, respectively. By elimination of the hydroxyl group with HBr, the olefins **17a** and **17b** are obtained. With a strong base such as KO*t*Bu, olefin **17b** could be isomerized to **17a**, which is hydrogenated by Pd/C to compound **18**. The methoxy ether is cleaved by methionine and methanesulfonic acid to compound **19**. The final reduction by $LiAlH_4$ gives racemic tapentadol (Figure 12.8).

Alternatively to the dehydroxylation sequence as shown in Figure 1.5, the tertiary alcohol (−)-(*S*,*S*)-**3** could be treated by formic acid to yield the olefin **20** as a diasteromeric mixture (Figure 12.9). Isolation of the *E*-olefin as hydrochloride salt and the hydrogenation of the free base yield the corresponding methoxy derivative. Chiral induction of the present chiral center creates the desired chirality of the second asymmetry carbon atom. Final ether cleavage by methionine and methanesulfonic followed by hydrochloride formation gives tapentadol hydrochloride [40].

12.3 The Preclinical and Clinical Profile of Tapentadol

Given this background, a molecule combining MOR affinity with NE reuptake inhibition in one chemical entity would be a major improvement of the combined mechanism of action approach because the full availability of MOR activity would no longer be dependent on metabolic activation, overall drug exposure would be reduced, and pharmacological activity would be limited to the two most relevant mechanisms of action. Moreover, because these two mechanisms would reside in a nonracemic molecule that does not form active metabolites, the relative contribution of the different mechanisms would not change over the course of metabolic transformation.

12.3.1
Preclinical Pharmacology of Tapentadol

Tapentadol is a novel analgesic that combines MOR agonism and norepinephrine reuptake inhibition in a single molecule and that shows potent and efficacious analgesia in various rodent models of nociceptive and neuropathic pain [34, 41, 42].

Tapentadol binds to mu, delta, and kappa opiate receptors. The compound showed K_i values of 0.1 and 0.5 μM in a rat MOR binding assay and a rat synaptosomal NE reuptake assay, respectively. Affinity for the other opioid receptor subtypes (i.e., kappa-opioid receptor (KOR), delta-opioid receptor (DOR), and ORL1 receptor (NOP)) was at least approximately one order of magnitude lower (Table 12.1). The affinity of morphine at the MOR was about 50-fold higher than that of tapentadol. At the recombinant human MOR, both tapentadol and morphine had a somewhat lower affinity than at the rat MOR ($K_i = 0.54$ and 0.023 μM, respectively). MOR agonism was confirmed in a guinea pig ileum assay [34].

Dose-dependent inhibition of norepinephrine reuptake was observed, resulting in large increases in extracellular norepinephrine levels and only a moderate increase in serotonin levels. This indicated that tapentadol's serotonergic activity was much lower than its norepinephrinergic activity. Other uptake systems, such as dopamine, adenosine, choline, and γ-aminobutyric acid, did not appear to be affected by tapentadol (Table 12.2) [34, 42].

In summary, tapentadol's MOR agonist activity is several-fold greater than tramadol's, with prominent norepinephrine reuptake inhibition and minimal serotonin effect. Preclinical studies with MOR and α_2-adrenoceptor antagonists have confirmed that both mechanisms effectively contribute to tapentadol-induced analgesia [33, 34, 42].

The two mechanisms interact in a synergistic way [21], resulting in a broad therapeutic range and high efficacy in neuropathic pain models. In non-neuropathic pain models, morphine was found only to be two to three times more potent than tapentadol, although the MOR affinity of tapentadol is 50-fold lower than that of morphine [34, 42].

Table 12.1 Comparison of the affinity of tapentadol and morphine at various opioid receptor subtypes, as assessed in binding assays using rat brain membranes (MOR, KOR, and DOR) or human recombinant receptors (NOP) [34, 42].

Compound	K_i value (μM)			
	MOR	KOR	DOR	NOP
Tapentadol	0.1	0.9	1.9	>100
Morphine	0.002	0.17	0.08	>100

MOR, mu-opioid receptor; KOR, kappa-opioid receptor; DOR, delta-opioid receptor; NOP or ORL1, nociceptin receptor.

Table 12.2 Comparison of tapentadol and desipramine with respect to neurotransmitter reuptake inhibition, as assessed in rat brain synaptosomes.

Transmitter	K_i value (μM)	
	Tapentadol	Desipramine
NE (norepinephrine)	0.5	0.001
5-HT (serotonin)	2.4	1.4
Dopamine	NE	ND
Choline	39	ND

NE, no effect <5% inhibition; ND, not determined.

In a neuropathic pain model, tapentadol is even more potent than morphine in STZ-induced heat hyperalgesia[2)], suggesting that the NRI component of tapentadol contributes significantly to its activity in this model [3].

The analgesic properties of tapentadol were investigated in various acute and chronic pain models in mice, rats, rabbits, and dogs to demonstrate the analgesic, antihyperalgesic, and antiallodynic properties of tapentadol. These experiments were performed with different routes of administration, including intravenous (i. v.), intraperitoneal (i.p.), oral (p.o.), intracerebroventricular (i.c.v.), and intrathecal (i.t.) routes, and employed a wide range of pain stimuli, including thermal, tactile, chemical, and electrical modalities. The pain tests consisted of models of acute nociceptive pain (tail flick, hot plate, tooth pulp stimulation, and phenylquinone-induced writhing models), acute and persistent inflammatory pain (yeast and formalin models), visceral pain (colorectal distension and mustard oil-induced visceral pain), and chronic mononeuropathic pain (chronic constriction injury (CCI)). The results for tapentadol in comparison to morphine and tramadol are summarized in Table 12.3[34, 42].

The animal models of pain demonstrate the substantial potency difference between tapentadol and tramadol. Across a variety of assays, tapentadol is consistently two to five times more potent than tramadol [19].

12.3.2
Clinical Trials

The pharmacological and functional differences of tramadol and tapentadol that are observed *in vitro* and *in vivo* translate into significant clinical differences. Tapentadol has demonstrated in clinical trials efficacy in both neuropathic and nociceptive pain conditions. As a result, it is expected to be prescribed for conditions involving both pain types, such as chronic lower back pain [41]. These published phase II and phase III studies used active control medications including oxycodone, morphine, or NSAIDs such as ibuprofen.

2) The streptozotocin (STZ)-induced diabetic rat is the most commonly employed animal model used to study mechanisms of painful diabetic neuropathy and to evaluate potential therapies.

Table 12.3 Overview of the analgesic activity of tapentadol, tramadol, and morphine in various animal models of acute and chronic pain[a)][34, 42].

Pain model	Route of administration	ED_{50} value (mg/kg)		
		Tapentadol	Morphine	Tramadol
Hot plate 58 °C (mouse)	i.p.	27.7	8.5	28.7
Hot plate 48 °C (mouse)	i.v.	3.3	1.3	NA
Tail flick (mouse)	i.v.	4.2	1.4	13.7
Tail flick (mouse)	p.o.	53.4	18.9	23.8
Tail flick (mouse)	i.c.v.[b)]	65.0	0.4	NA
Tail flick (rat)	i.v.	2.2	1.1	9.6
Tail flick (rat)	i.p.	10.0	5.8	10.0
Tail flick (rat)	p.o.	121	55.7	16.6
Tail flick (dog)	i.v.	4.3	0.7	NA
Phenylquinone-induced writhing (mouse)	i.v.	0.7	0.4	3.6
Phenylquinone-induced writhing (mouse)	p.o.	31.3	4.7	4.5
Phenylquinone-induced writhing (mouse)	i.c.v.[b)]	18.4	0.08	NA
Yeast model (rat)	i.v.	2.0	0.9	9.3
Yeast model (rat)	i.p.	10.1	5.6	8.6
Yeast model (rat)	i.t.[b]	56.8	1.9	NA
Formalin, phase II (rat)	i.p.	3.8	0.8	5.9
Tooth pulp stimulation (rabbit)	i.v.	3.1	2.3	NA
Colorectal distension-induced visceral pain (rat)	i.v.	5.5	3.5	18 (ND)
Spinal nerve ligation neuropathy (rat)	i.p.	8.2	2.9	4.6
Chronic constriction injury neuropathy (CCI) (rat)	i.p.	13	13.8	7.1
Vincristine polyneuropathy (rat)	i.p.	5.1	3.0	7.2
Diabetic polyneuropathy (rat)	i.p.	8.9	3.0	9.2
Mustard oil visceral pain (rat)	i.v.	1.5	1.0	9.0

ND, not determined; NA, not available.
a) All drug doses for preclinical and clinical testing are for the hydrochloride salt.
b) Dose in μg/animal.

Clinical trials have demonstrated that in patients with moderate to severe chronic pain, tapentadol as a controlled-release formulation resulted in significant pain reduction compared to placebo. Nausea, dizziness, constipation, and CNS sedation are common side effects of opioid pain medications. However, tapentadol demonstrated a marked reduction in gastrointestinal (GI) side effects such as nausea, vomiting, and constipation, and CNS side effects such as dizziness and somnolence, compared to other opioids such as oxycodone. In addition, the long-term safety and efficacy of tapentadol has been shown in two separate studies over a 12-month and 2-year period of continuous treatment.

The advantages of tapentadol over current treatment options using NSAIDs and opioids may be summarized as follows: The two categories of analgesics, that is, opioids and NSAIDs, are both effective but are associated with potentially serious side effects. Concerns regarding tolerance and dependence minimize the use of narcotics such as morphine and codeine for the treatment of acute or chronic pain. Patients on chronic NSAID therapy risk severe gastrointestinal symptoms, including ulceration and bleeding. An alternative to this dilemma is tapentadol, indicated for the management of moderate to severe pain. Its opioid-sparing effects and reduced potential for abuse will be key clinical advantages for tapentadol in neuropathic pain conditions requiring long-term management. The anticipated uptake of tapentadol controlled-release formulations in the neuropathic lower back pain market is expected to drive market growth as there are currently no treatments indicated for this prevalent condition [41].

12.3.3
Pharmacokinetics and Drug–Drug Interactions of Tapentadol

After oral administration, 32% of the drug is absorbed. It is widely distributed in the body. The plasma protein binding is low and amounts to approximately 20%. The activity of tapentadol is independent of metabolic activation and resides in a single enantiomer that readily crosses the blood–brain barrier; hence, tapentadol displays a rapid onset of action after administration. The half-life is 4 h and the peak effect is attained after 1 h. The duration of action is 4–6 h. The drug undergoes extensive first-pass hepatic metabolism, that is, 97%.

Its metabolites have no analgesic activity. The biotransformation of tapentadol by metabolic enzymes results in deactivation, that is, tapentadol has no active metabolites, and the main metabolic pathway for elimination is phase II glucuronidation. Phase I biotransformations such as hydroxylation and *N*-demethylation play only a minor role in the metabolic fate of tapentadol. Owing to the minor involvement of phase I metabolic pathways, tapentadol has a low potential for drug–drug interactions and interindividual variability. Ninety-nine percent of the drug is excreted through renal route [42].

Drug–drug interaction studies to date have documented no induction of CYP1A2, CYP2C9, or CYP3A4 activity; in addition, these studies found no significant inhibition of CYP1A2, CYP2A6, CYP2C9, CYP2C19, CYP2E1, or CYP3A4 activity. CYP2D6 activity was inhibited, but to a degree that did not appear to be clinically relevant. Tapentadol did not undergo significant protein binding. Based on these findings, it is unlikely that tapentadol will produce clinically important drug–drug interactions with agents affected by CYP activity or plasma protein binding [42].

The differences in the central nervous system functional activity of tapentadol and tramadol (based on the differences in their pharmacodynamic, pharmacokinetic, and functional activity characteristics) correlate with their clinical features and common uses.

12.4 Summary

Tapentadol is a novel centrally acting synthetic analgesic with a dual mechanism of action in one single molecule, mu-opioid agonist and norepinephrine reuptake inhibitor. It is much times less potent than morphine in binding to the human mu-opioid receptor and is two to three times less potent in producing analgesia in animal models. Tapentadol exerts its analgesic effects without a pharmacologically active metabolite. Tapentadol is effective in treating moderate to severe pain (WHO step 3). In clinical trials, tapentadol has been shown to be equiefficacious to oxycodone with fewer gastrointestinal adverse effects [19].

References

1 Merskey, H. and Bogduk, N. (eds) (2004) Part III: Pain terms, a current list with definitions and notes on usage, in *Classification of Chronic Pain*, 2nd edn, IASP Press, Seattle, WA, pp. 209–214. Available at www.iasp-pain.org (accessed February 21, 2012).

2 Waldmann, S.D. (2007) *Pain Management*, Saunders Elsevier, Philadelphia, PA.

3 Anonymous (2007) Drugs for pain. *Treat. Guidel. Med. Lett.*, **5** (56), 23–32.

4 Barkin, R.L. and Barkin, D. (2001) Pharmacologic management of acute and chronic pain: focus on drug interactions and patient-specific pharmacotherapeutic selection. *South Med. J.*, **94** (8), 756–770.

5 Wu, C.L. and Raja, S.N. (2011) Treatment of acute postoperative pain. *Lancet*, **377**, 2215–2225.

6 Turk, D.C., Wilson, H.D., and Cahana, A. (2011) Treatment of chronic non-cancer pain. *Lancet*, **377**, 2226–2235.

7 Vanderah, T.W. (2007) Pathophysiology of pain. *Med. Clin. North Am.*, **91**, 1–12.

8 Friderichs, E., Christoph, T., and Buschmann, H.H. (2007) Analgesics and antipyretics, in *Ullmann's Encyclopedia of Industrial Chemistry*, Wiley-VCH Verlag GmbH, Weinheim, pp. 1–97.

9 Rao, P.N.P. and Knaus, E.E. (2008) Evolution of nonsteroidal anti-inflammatory drugs (NSAIDs): cyclooxygenase (COX) inhibition and beyond. *J. Pharm. Pharm. Sci.*, **11**, 81–110.

10 Williams, M. *et al.* (1999) Emerging molecular approaches to pain therapy. *J. Med. Chem.*, **42**, 1481–1500.

11 Datamonitor (2007) *Pipeline Insight: Neuropathic Pain.*

12 Butera, J.A. (2007) Current and emerging targets to treat neuropathic pain. *J. Med. Chem.*, **50**, 2543–2596.

13 Reimann, W. and Schneider, F. (1998) Induction of 5-hydroxytryptamine release by tramadol. *Eur. J. Pharmacol.*, **349** (2–3), 199–203.

14 Minami, K., Uezono, Y., and Ueta, Y. (2007) Pharmacological aspects of the effects of tramadol on G-protein coupled receptors. *J. Pharmacol. Sci.*, **103**, 253–260.

15 Grond, S. and Sablotzki, A. (2004) Clinical pharmacology of tramadol. *Clin. Pharmacokinet.*, **43** (13), 879–923.

16 Valle, M., Garrido, M.J., Pavo, J.M., Calvo, R., and Troconiz, I.A. (2000) Pharmacokinetic pharmacodynamic modeling of the antinociceptive effects of main active metabolites of tramadol, (1)-*O*-desmethyltramadol and (2)-*O*-desmethyltramadol, in rats. *J. Pharmacol. Exp. Ther.*, **293**, 646–653.

17 Raffa, R.B., Friderichs, E., Reimann, W., Shank, R.P., Codd, E.E., and Vaught, J.L. (1992) Opioid and nonopioid components independently contribute to the mechanism of action of tramadol, an "atypical" opioid analgesic. *J. Pharmacol. Exp. Ther.*, **260**, 275–285.

18 Raffa, R.B., Friderichs, E., Reimann, W., Shank, R.P., Codd, E.E., Vaught, J.L., Jacoby, H.I., and Selve, N. (1993) Complementary and synergistic antinociceptive interaction between the enantiomers of tramadol. *J. Pharmacol. Exp. Ther.*, **267**, 331–340.

19 Raffa, R.B., Buschmann, H., Christoph, T., Eichenbaum, G., Englberger, W., Flores, C.W., Hertrampf, T., Kögel, B., Schiene, K., Straßburger, W., Terlinden, R., and Tzschentke, T.M. (2012) Mechanistic and functional differentiation of tapentadol and tramadol. *Expert Opin. Pharmacother.*, **13** (10), 1437–1449.

20 Casy, A.F. and Parfitt, R.T. (1986) *Opioid Analgesics – Chemistry and Receptors*, Plenum Press, New York.

21 Friderichs, E. and Buschmann, H. (2002) Opioids with clinical relevance, in *Analgesics* (eds H. Buschmann, T. Christoph, E. Friderichs, C. Maul, and B. Sundermann), Wiley-VCH Verlag GmbH, Weinheim, pp. 171–245.

22 Maul, C., Buschmann, H., and Sundermann, B. (2002) Synthetic opioids, in *Analgesics* (eds H. Buschmann, T. Christoph, E. Friderichs, C. Maul, and B. Sundermann), Wiley-VCH Verlag GmbH, Weinheim, pp. 159–169.

23 McCurdy, C.R. (2006) Development of opioid receptor ligands, in *Analogue-based Drug Discovery* (eds J. Fischer and C.R. Ganellin), John Wiley & Sons, Ltd, Chichester, pp. 259–276.

24 Agranat, I., Caner, H., and Caldwell, J. (2002) Putting chirality to work: the strategy of chiral switches. *Nat. Rev. Drug Discov.*, **1**, 753–768.

25 (a) Aboul-Enein, H.Y. and Wainer, I.W. (1997) *The Impact of Stereochemistry on Drug Development and Use*, John Wiley & Sons, Ltd, Chichester. (b)Francotte, E. and Lindner, W. (2006) *Chirality in Drug Research*, Methods and Principles in Medicinal Chemistry, vol. 33, John Wiley & Sons, Ltd, Chichester.

26 Hu, Y., Stumpfe, D., and Bajorath, J. (2011) Lessons learned from molecular scaffold analysis. *J. Chem. Inf. Model.*, **51**, 1742–1753.

27 Ferenczy, G.G. and Keserü, G.M. (2010) Thermodynamics guided lead discovery and optimization. *Drug Discov. Today*, **15**, 919–932.

28 Gleeson, M.P., Hersey, A., Montanari, D., and Overington, J. (2011) Probing the links between *in vitro* potency, ADMET and physicochemical parameters. *Nat. Rev. Drug Discov.*, **10**, 197–208.

29 Böhm, H.J., Klebe, G., and Kubinyi, H. (1996) *Wirkstoffdesign – Der Weg zum Arzneimittel*, Spektrum Akademischer Verlag.

30 Wermuth, C.G. (2008) *The Practice of Medicinal Chemistry*, 3rd edn, Academic Press.

31 Buschmann, H., Strassburger, W., and Friderichs, E. (1996) 1-Phenyl-3-dimethylaminopropane compounds with a pharmacological effect. EP 693475 A1, US Patent 6,248,737 B1.

32 Hell, W., Kegel, M., Akteries, B., Buschmann, H., Holenz, J., Loebermann, H., Heller, D., Drexler, H., and Gladow, S. (2004) Method for the preparation of 3-substituted 3-aryl-butyl amine compounds. WO 2004108658 A1.

33 Tzschentke, T.M., De Vry, J., Terlinden, R., Hennies, H.H., Lange, C., Strassburger, W., Haurand, M., Kolb, J., Schneider, J., Buschmann, H., Finkam, M., Jahnel, U., and Friderichs, E. (2006) Tapentadol hydrochloride. *Drugs Future*, **31**, 1053–1061.

34 Hell, W. (2008) Preparation of 3-[(1R,2R)-3-(dimethylamino)-1-ethyl-2-methyl-propyl]phenol. WO 2008012046 A1.

35 Hell, W., Zimmer, O., Buschmann, H.H., Holenz, J., and Gladow, S. (2008) Process for the preparation of (1R,2R)-3-(3-dimethylamino-1-ethyl-2-methyl-propyl)-phenol. WO 2008012047A1.

36 Liu, K.K.C., Subas Sakya, M., O'Donnell, C.J., Flick, A.C., and Li, J. (2011) Synthetic approaches to the 2009 new drugs. *Bioorg. Med. Chem.*, **19**, 1136–1154.

37 Motta, G., Vergani, D., and Bertolini, G. (2012) New process for the synthesis of tapentadol and intermediates thereof. WO 2012/001571 A1.

38 Reynolds, C.H. and Holloway, C.K. (2011) Thermodynamics of ligand binding and efficiency. *ACS Med. Chem. Lett.*, **2**, 433–437.

39 Buschmann, H.H. and Holenz, J. (2011) Process for the preparation of substituted

3-(1-amino-2-methylpetane-3-yl)phenyl compounds. WO 2011/157390 A2.

40 Hell, W., Kegel, M., Akteries, B., Buschmann, H.H., Holenz, J., Löbermann, H., Heller, D., and Drexler, H.J. (2004) Method for the production of substituted 3-aryl-butyl amine compounds. WO 2004/108658 A1.

41 Nightingale, S. (2012) The neuropathic pain market. *Nat. Rev. Drug Discov.*, **11**, 101–102.

42 Wade, W.E. and Spruill, W.J. (2009) Tapentadol hydrochloride: a centrally acting oral analgesic. *Clin. Ther.*, **31**, 2804–2818.

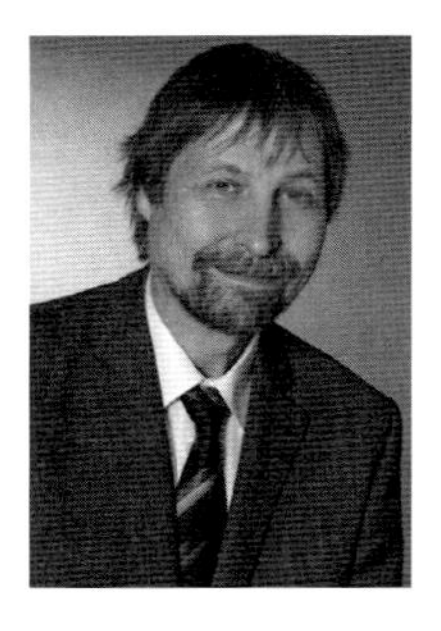

Helmut Buschmann studied chemistry at RWTH Aachen and received his Ph.D. in the group of Prof. Scharf (Isoinversion Principle). As a chemist, he started his career in pharmaceutical industry in 1992 at Grünenthal GmbH. In his final position, he was responsible for chemical research (combinatorial and medicinal chemistry, process development, and pilot plant). From 2002 to 2008, he worked as Research Director at Laboratorios Dr. Esteve (Barcelona). In this position, he managed a staff of 120 employees (more than 60 persons with university degrees) and was responsible for chemistry, pharmacology, toxicology, pharmacokinetic, and intellectual property departments. In 2009, he joined Pharma-Consulting Aachen. As a result of his research activities, more than 15 NCEs within different therapeutic areas have entered the clinical phase (e.g., rosonabant, cizolirtine, dulopetine, axomadol). Some of them have reached clinical phase III or are marketed (e.g., tapentadol: Nucynta®, Palexia®). Besides this, he is a member of several scientific advisory boards of public research institutions in Europe (Leibniz Institut für Katalyse, Rostock; Institut Català d'Investigació Quõmica, Tarragona) and gives lectures at the Universities of Aachen and Rostock. He led or coauthored more than 100 publications in major scientific journals and is listed as inventor on more than 200 patent application families. As author and editor, he has also published three books in the field of stereochemistry, analgesics, and antidepressants.

13
Novel Taxanes: Cabazitaxel Case Study

Hervé Bouchard, Dorothée Semiond, Marie-Laure Risse, and Patricia Vrignaud

List of Abbreviations

10-DAB	10-deacetylbaccatin III
AUC	area under the curve
bid	twice daily
BSA	body surface area
CAP	capecitabine
CBZ	cabazitaxel
CI	confidence interval
CL	clearance
CR	complete response
CRPC	castration-resistant prostate cancer
DLT	dose-limiting toxicity
FN	febrile neutropenia
G-CSF	granulocyte colony-stimulating factor
HNTD	highest nontoxic dose
HR	hazard ratio
IV	intravenous
mCRPC	metastatic castration-resistant prostate cancer
MDR1	multidrug resistance gene 1
mHRPC	hormone-refractory metastatic prostate cancer
MTD	maximum tolerated dose
nd	not determined
OS	overall survival
PFS	progression-free survival
P-gp	P-glycoprotein
PK	pharmacokinetics
POMA	2-(4-methoxyphenyl)-4-phenyloxazolidine-3,5-dicarboxylic acid-3-*tert*-butyl ester

Analogue-based Drug Discovery III, First Edition. Edited by János Fischer, C. Robin Ganellin, and David P. Rotella.
© 2013 Wiley-VCH Verlag GmbH & Co. KGaA. Published 2013 by Wiley-VCH Verlag GmbH & Co. KGaA.

PR	partial response
PSA	prostate-specific antigen
q3w	every 3 weeks
RD	recommended dose
SC	subcutaneous
SD	stable disease
TES-Cl	triethylsilyl chloride
TFS	tumor-free survivors
TTP	time to tumor progression
V_{ss}	volume of distribution at steady state

13.1 Introduction

Previous volumes in this series have highlighted ways in which analogue-based drug discovery (ABDD) has contributed to the discovery of new chemical entities that ultimately proved to be useful clinically [1, 2]. The application of ABDD to the modification of candidate drugs derived from natural products is an extension of this approach that was illustrated in the chapter on paclitaxel and epothilone analogues published in Volume II of this series [3]. The current chapter focuses on a novel taxane compound that was developed using ABDD from an established marketed drug that was itself derived from a natural product.

Taxoids are diterpene molecules found mainly in various yew tree species (*Taxus* spp.). They are characterized by the presence of a 20-carbon taxane core ring structure. Since the isolation and purification of the first taxane-containing molecule in the 1960s, taxanes have become an important class of cancer chemotherapeutic drugs, with proven efficacy in a wide range of human cancers.

Taxanes inhibit cell division by binding to microtubules, which are key components of the cytoskeleton and critical regulators of cell division [4]. At the onset of mitosis, microtubules assemble into a structure known as the mitotic spindle. The spindle serves as an attachment point for chromosomes prior to their segregation into the resultant daughter cells. The cycle of microtubule assembly and disassembly during cell division involves a dynamic equilibrium between microtubule polymers and a pool of intracellular tubulin, consisting of α- and β-tubulin heterodimers [5]. Research by Horwitz and colleagues [6] demonstrated that Taxol, the first taxane to be isolated, stabilizes microtubules by binding to the microtubule polymer, thereby shifting the equilibrium in favor of the microtubule and preventing depolymerization. In turn, this prevents cell division and leads to programmed cell death. The mechanism of action of taxanes is distinct from that of other microtubule inhibitors such as the vinca alkaloids, which act by inhibiting tubulin polymerization and microtubule assembly [7].

13.1.1
Isolation and Chemical Synthesis of Taxanes

Taxol (generic name paclitaxel; marketed as Taxol® (**1** in Figure 13.1)) was originally extracted from the bark of the Pacific yew tree, *Taxus brevifolia* [8]. However, purification of taxol with sufficient yield to allow testing in cancer patients required vast quantities of bark from the extremely slow-growing Pacific yew tree. As a result, significant efforts focused on finding a sustainable source of taxol and an efficient process for its isolation. Although the total synthesis of taxol has been achieved [9–11], the process, involving 40 steps with only 2% yield, is not commercially viable. An advance came with the development of a process to synthesize taxol from 10-deacetylbaccatin III (**10-DAB** in Figure 13.1), a natural precursor molecule that could be extracted easily and sustainably from the needles of the

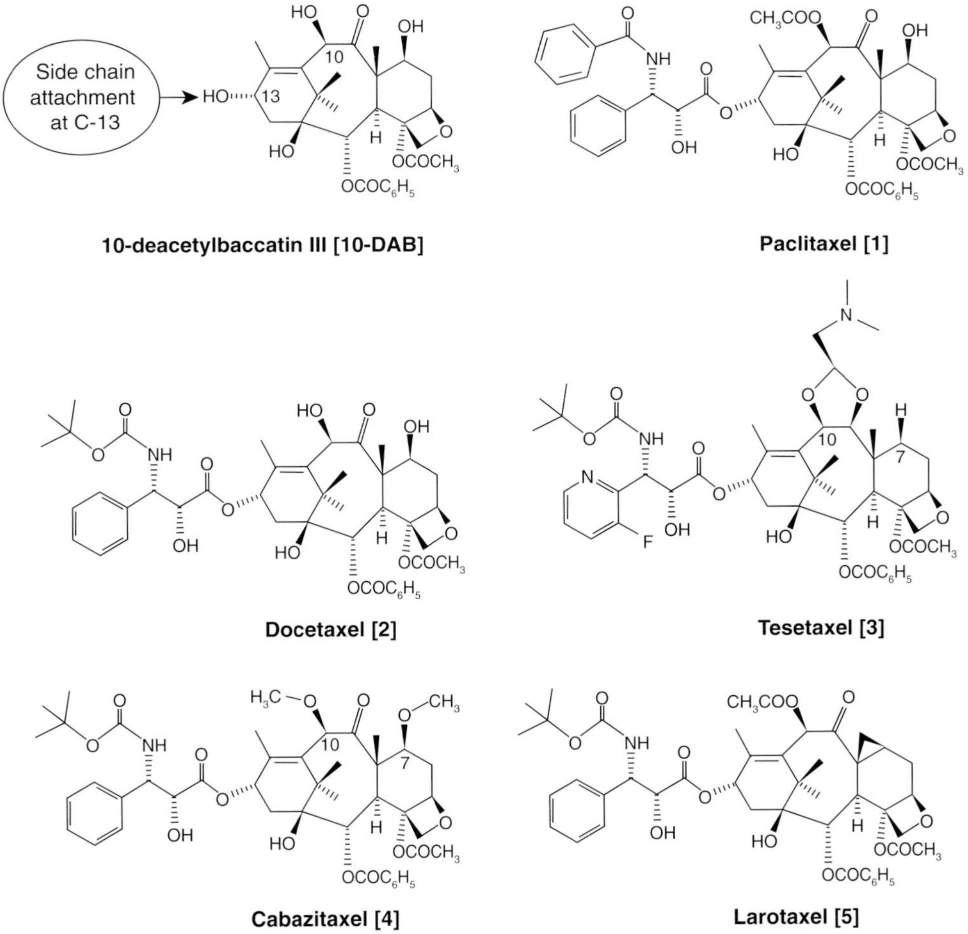

10-deacetylbaccatin III [10-DAB] **Paclitaxel [1]**

Docetaxel [2] **Tesetaxel [3]**

Cabazitaxel [4] **Larotaxel [5]**

Figure 13.1 Chemical structures of 10-deacetylbaccatin III and taxane compounds.

European yew, *Taxus baccata* [12, 13]. Taxol can now also be produced using plant cell fermentation technology [14]. A specific paclitaxel-producing *Taxus* cell line is cultured on a large scale. The paclitaxel is then extracted, purified by chromatography, and isolated by crystallization.

Other synthetic taxanes include docetaxel (Taxotere®; **2** in Figure 13.1), which is an esterified product of **10-DAB.** Docetaxel differs from paclitaxel at two positions in its chemical structure: a hydroxyl functional group at C-10 (paclitaxel has an acetate ester) and a *tert*-butyl carbamate on the phenyl propionate side chain (paclitaxel has a benzyl amide) (Figure 13.1). The change at C-10 confers greater water solubility for docetaxel compared with paclitaxel [15].

13.1.2
Drug Resistance and Novel Taxanes

Paclitaxel and docetaxel are approved for the treatment of a range of human cancers. Paclitaxel is indicated for first-line treatment of ovarian, breast, and lung cancer and for second-line treatment of AIDS-related Kaposi's sarcoma. Docetaxel is indicated for first-line treatment of breast, head and neck, gastric, lung, and prostate cancer and for second-line treatment of breast cancer. However, the utility of both paclitaxel and docetaxel as anticancer drugs is limited by the frequent development of tumor resistance [16]. Resistance to taxanes is frequently described as resulting from expression of the P-glycoprotein (P-gp) efflux pump encoded by the multidrug resistance gene *MDR1*, which leads to decreased intracellular drug levels. This mechanism of resistance was mainly observed in cell lines in which resistance was induced *in vitro*; however, the clinical significance of P-gp overexpression has yet to be validated in patients progressing after taxane therapy. Other postulated mechanisms of resistance involve changes in tubulin structure and altered intracellular signaling [7, 17].

Considerable efforts have been made toward developing novel taxanes capable of overcoming resistance to paclitaxel and docetaxel. Among several second-generation taxanes that have been developed, the two most advanced are tesetaxel (**3** in Figure 13.1) and cabazitaxel (**4** in Figure 13.1).

Tesetaxel is an orally active taxane with a similar mechanism of action to paclitaxel and docetaxel. Like docetaxel, tesetaxel has a *tert*-butyl carbamate on the propionate side chain. However, tesetaxel differs from paclitaxel and docetaxel as it includes in the propionate side chain a 3-fluoropyridine aromatic ring in place of a phenyl group. Other specific features of tesetaxel include reduced moieties at positions C-7 (CH_2) and C-9 (CH–O). Tesetaxel is currently under investigation in a variety of different human cancers [18–20].

Cabazitaxel (XRP6258, RPR 116258A, TXD258, Jevtana®) is a novel second-generation, semisynthetic taxane rationally designed to be an active anticancer treatment in both taxane-naïve and taxane-resistant tumors. Clinical activity of cabazitaxel was observed in the phase I setting and proof of concept was first achieved in a phase II study with responses obtained in patients with metastatic breast tumors resistant to previous docetaxel therapy [21–23] (see below). Clinical

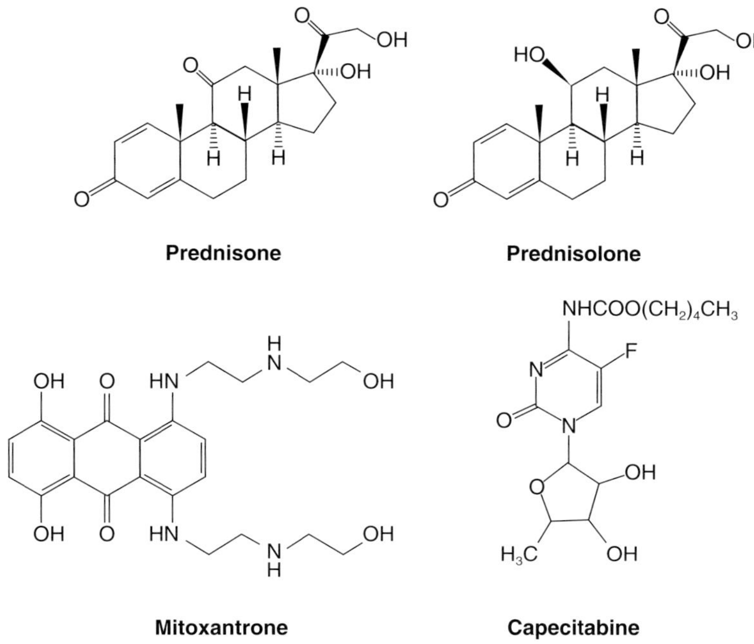

Prednisone

Prednisolone

Mitoxantrone

Capecitabine

Figure 13.2 Chemical structures of nontaxane drugs.

activity post-taxane failure was confirmed and demonstrated in a pivotal phase III study in patients with metastatic castration-resistant prostate cancer (mCRPC, also known as hormone-refractory metastatic prostate cancer (mHRPC)) previously treated with a docetaxel-containing regimen, where cabazitaxel in combination with prednisone/prednisolone (**6** and **7** in Figure 13.2) demonstrated a statistically significant benefit in overall survival compared with mitoxantrone (**8** in Figure 13.2) [24]. Cabazitaxel in combination with prednisone received regulatory approval by the US Food and Drug Administration (in 2010) and the European Medicines Agency (in 2011) for the treatment of mHRPC previously treated with a docetaxel-containing regimen. This chapter focuses on the chemical synthesis of cabazitaxel and its structure–activity relationships, including a summary of the preclinical and clinical testing of cabazitaxel.

13.2 Cabazitaxel Structure–Activity Relationships and Chemical Synthesis

13.2.1 Chemical and Physical Properties

The International Union of Pure and Applied Chemistry chemical name of cabazitaxel is (2α,5β,7β,10β,13α)-4-(acetoxy)-13-({(2*R*,3*S*)-3-[(*tert*-butoxycarbonyl)amino]-

Table 13.1 Physical and chemical properties of cabazitaxel (**4**).

Molecular formula	$C_{45}H_{57}NO_{14}{\cdot}C_3H_6O$
Relative molecular mass	894.01 g/mol for the acetone solvate
	835.93 g/mol for the solvate-free molecule
Appearance	White to almost white solid
Solubility	Lipophilic, soluble in dehydrated alcohol and insoluble in water at 25 °C

2-hydroxy-3-phenylpropanoyl}oxy)-1-hydroxy-7,10-dimethoxy-9-oxo-5,20-epoxytax-11-en-2-yl-benzoate-propan-2-one (1 : 1). Physical and chemical properties are summarized in Table 13.1.

13.2.2 Structure–Activity Relationships of Cabazitaxel

Cabazitaxel is a semisynthetic derivative of **10-DAB** and was identified through a preclinical screening process that involved the testing of approximately 450 candidate molecules. The primary objective of the screen was to select a compound as potent as docetaxel in tumor models sensitive to docetaxel and more potent than docetaxel in tumors resistant to chemotherapy, including taxanes. The main structure–activity relationships for cabazitaxel are depicted in Figure 13.3.

With initial preclinical comparative structure–activity relationships for paclitaxel and docetaxel in mind, our initial efforts with cabazitaxel were focused on changes in the side chain as it was considered that this region would be critical for potency. Attempts to replace the C-2′-Boc group of the side chain (*tert*-butyl carbamate) by other functions (e.g., ureas) or by substituted benzyl amides generally resulted in decreased *in vitro* potency when tested on cancer cell lines [25, 26]. Modulation of

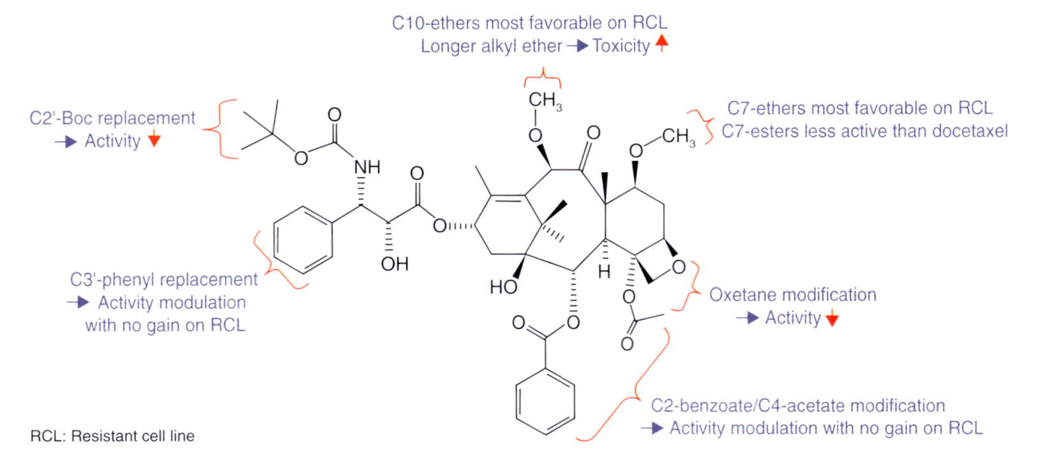

Figure 13.3 Structure–activity relationships for cabazitaxel.

activity was observed when the C-3′ phenyl group of the propionate side chain was replaced, as exemplified by the structure of the tesetaxel analogue (**3** in Figure 13.1). Substitution of this phenyl group or replacement by alkylidene groups or heteroaromatic rings (e.g., furan or thiophene) improved the *in vitro* activity but, in our hands, resulted in no relative improvement in activity against cell lines resistant to docetaxel [27].

The role of the benzoate group at position C-2 was also studied. Some *ortho*/*meta*-methoxy-substituted benzoates proved to be highly cytotoxic *in vitro*, although no significant impact was observed on docetaxel-resistant cell lines [28]. Removal of the C-4 acetate resulted in C-4 hydroxy analogues that demonstrated a large decrease in potency. Replacement of the C-4 acetate by other analogues such as propionate or methoxyacetate produced more potent analogues in *in vitro* assays, but the therapeutic index was reduced in *in vivo* models due to dose-limiting toxicities.

The oxetane ring was found to be crucial for maintaining overall activity; opening of the ring or replacement of the oxygen atom reduced *in vitro* potency.

Our efforts to better understand the structure–activity relationship in the C-7/C-10 region focused on modifications at C-7 aimed at generating new analogues of docetaxel by nucleophilic substitution at this position. We initially planned to treat a C-7 trifluoromethanesulfonate-activated derivative with different nucleophilic agents and found that 7,8,19-cyclopropanation could occur under these conditions [29]. This chemical modification in the C-7/C-10 region resulted in the larotaxel structure (**5** in Figure 13.1) and we discovered that this lipophilic modification addressed *in vitro* and *in vivo* resistance to docetaxel and issues related to P-gp. Further investigation of structure–activity relationship in the C-7/C-10 region found that C-7/C-10 ether analogues present in cabazitaxel and the 7,8,19-cyclopropane modification present in larotaxel were the most favorable modifications of the upper part of the baccatin moiety in terms of *in vitro* potency in docetaxel-sensitive and docetaxel-resistant cell lines. When compared with C-7 ethers, C-7 esters were found to be less active than docetaxel in *in vivo* models. Some longer C-10 alkyl ethers were evaluated *in vivo*; however, drug-related deaths were observed at doses equal to or lower than the maximum tolerated doses of docetaxel, thereby limiting the antitumor activity of these compounds.

13.2.3
Chemical Synthesis of Cabazitaxel

Cabazitaxel is structurally distinct from docetaxel due to the presence of two methoxy groups in positions C-7 and C-10 of the baccatin moiety (Figure 13.1). In the course of structure–activity relationship studies on analogues of docetaxel, a regioselective synthesis of C-7/C-10 ether derivatives was developed. This initial synthetic pathway allowed for the introduction of selectivity as well as for the sequential addition of substituents at C-7 and C-10. From the naturally occurring **10-DAB**, selective protection of the C-7 and C-13 hydroxy functions using triethylsilyl chloride (TES-Cl) in pyridine produced intermediate **1** (Scheme 13.1a). At this stage, only the hydroxy function at C-10 could be easily modified as the tertiary

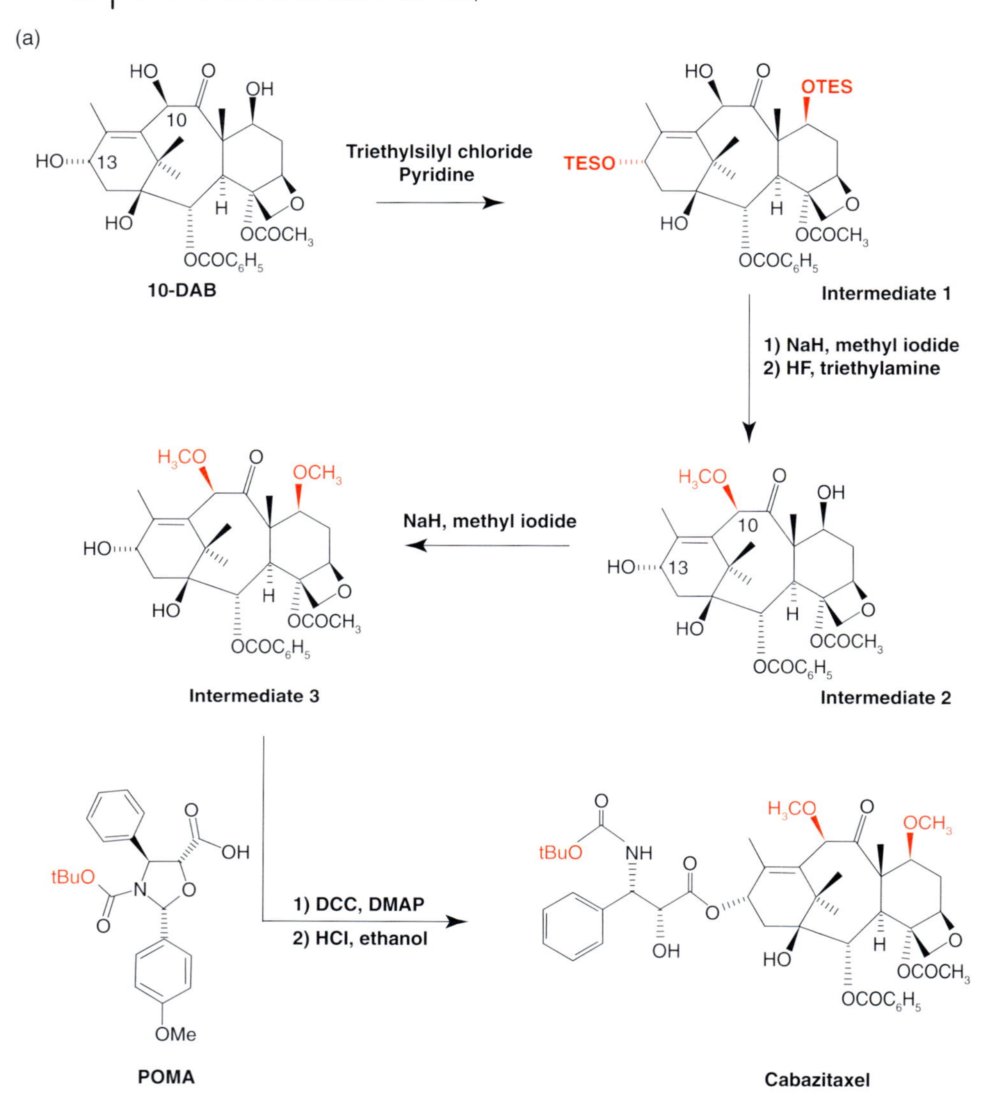

Scheme 13.1 (a) First synthetic pathway to cabazitaxel chemical entity. (b) Cabazitaxel alternative synthesis.

alcohol at C-1 was unreactive under the same conditions. Following treatment with sodium hydride and methyl iodide, intermediate **1** was converted into its methyl ether analogue. The triethylsilyl groups were then removed using hydrofluoric acid–triethylamine to give C-10 monomethoxylated baccatin (intermediate **2**). As the hydroxy function at position C-7 of the baccatin core is generally more reactive

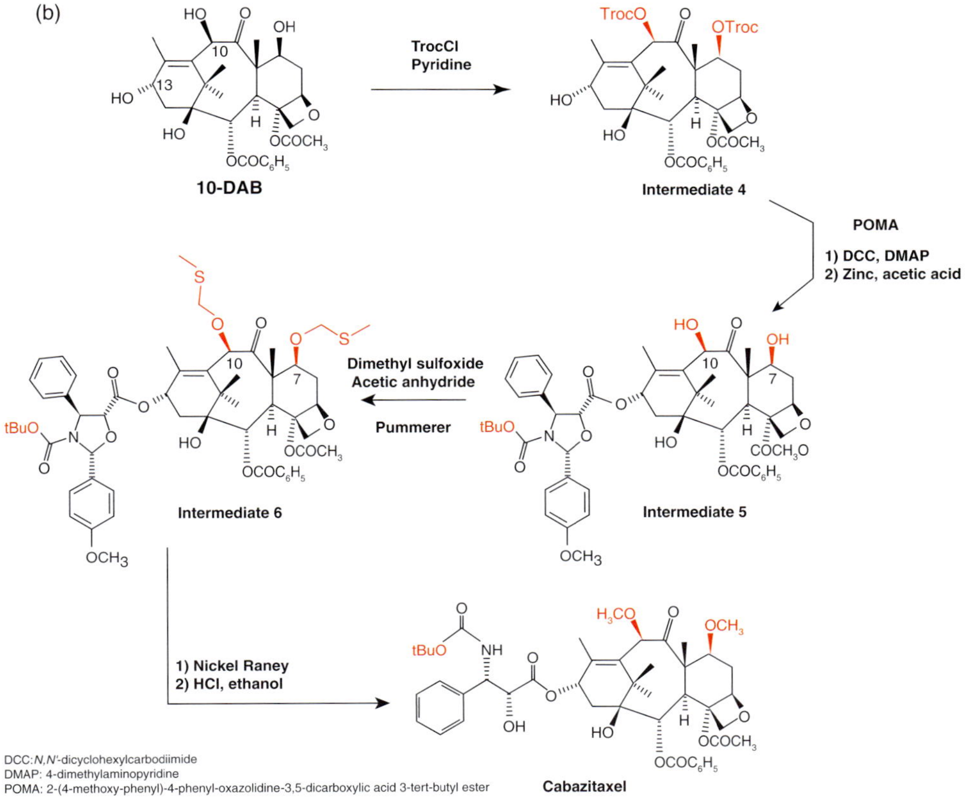

(b)

10-DAB

TrocCl
Pyridine

Intermediate 4

POMA
1) DCC, DMAP
2) Zinc, acetic acid

Intermediate 5

Dimethyl sulfoxide
Acetic anhydride
Pummerer

Intermediate 6

1) Nickel Raney
2) HCl, ethanol

Cabazitaxel

DCC: *N,N'*-dicyclohexylcarbodiimide
DMAP: 4-dimethylaminopyridine
POMA: 2-(4-methoxy-phenyl)-4-phenyl-oxazolidine-3,5-dicarboxylic acid 3-tert-butyl ester

Scheme 13.1 (*Continued*)

than the one at position C-13, methylation of intermediate **2** with sodium hydride and methyl iodide resulted in the dimethyl ether (intermediate **3**). Esterification of the hydroxy group at position C-13 with a protected form of the side chain 2-(4-methoxyphenyl)-4-phenyloxazolidine-3,5-dicarboxylic acid-3-*tert*-butyl ester (POMA) under standard conditions (*N,N'*-dicyclohexylcarbodiimide, 4-dimethylaminopyridine) [28], followed by cleavage of the *para*-methoxybenzylidene protecting group under acidic conditions, allowed completion of the synthesis of cabazitaxel.

Although this first synthetic scheme proved to be useful and efficient for the preparation of various regioselective C-7 and C-10 taxane analogues, it was not a dedicated straightforward synthesis for cabazitaxel. Therefore, an alternative synthesis was developed, minimizing the number of protection/deprotection steps and resulting in simultaneous methylation of the hydroxy functions at positions C-7 and C-10 (Scheme 13.1b). Under standard conditions, esterification of the POMA-protected side chain with 7,10-di-Troc-baccatin III (intermediate **4**) followed by cleavage of the Troc groups (2,2,2-trichloroethoxycarbonyl) with zinc in acetic acid produced the 7,10-dihydroxy taxoid (intermediate **5**). Pummerer reaction conditions (dimethyl sulfoxide, acetic anhydride) applied to intermediate **5** permitted the simultaneous functionalization of the C-7 and C-10 positions as methylthiomethyl ethers resulting in intermediate **6**. Reduction of the methylthioether groups of intermediate **6** with Raney nickel produced the dimethoxy analogue that was then deprotected on its side chain under acidic conditions, as previously described, to complete the alternative synthesis of cabazitaxel.

13.3 Cabazitaxel Preclinical and Clinical Development

13.3.1 Preclinical Development

Cabazitaxel was selected for preclinical testing based on its enhanced antiproliferative activity in chemotherapy-resistant cell lines compared with docetaxel. In addition, cabazitaxel was shown to promote tubulin assembly *in vitro* and to stabilize microtubules against cold-induced depolymerization as efficiently as docetaxel [30].

Using tumor cell lines with acquired resistance to doxorubicin, vincristine, vinblastine, paclitaxel, and docetaxel, resistance factors (calculated by dividing the IC_{50} in resistant cells by the IC_{50} in sensitive cells) ranged from 1.8 to 10 for cabazitaxel, compared with 4.8–59 for docetaxel [30]. In Caco-2 TC7 cells (a cell line that expresses high levels of the P-gp efflux pump), cabazitaxel was shown to be a highly permeable compound (as expected, based on its lipophilicity (log $P = 3.9$)) despite being a substrate of P-gp (unpublished observations).

Like docetaxel, cabazitaxel exhibits very limited solubility in aqueous solution, and was formulated using a docetaxel-like formulation containing ethanol and polysorbate 80. In murine and human tumor xenograft models, cabazitaxel exhibited a broad spectrum of antitumor activity, not only in docetaxel-sensitive tumors, but also in tumors with little or no sensitivity to chemotherapy, including taxanes [31, 32]. In docetaxel-sensitive tumors, cabazitaxel was found to exhibit a similar potency to docetaxel, inducing complete regressions in advanced stage disease leading to tumor-free survivors in 8/16 mouse tumor models, including human prostate DU145, murine colon C38, human colon HCT 116, murine pancreas P03, human pancreas MIAPaCa-2, human gastric N87, human breast Calc 18, and human head and neck SR 475 (Table 13.2).

The pharmacokinetics (PK) and tumor distribution of cabazitaxel were evaluated in mice bearing advanced stage mammary adenocarcinoma MA16/C [33, 34]. At the highest nontoxic dose (HNTD) of 40 mg/kg, drug uptake into the tumor was both rapid (t_{max} occurred 2 min postdosing) and sustained (concentration of cabazitaxel was 40-fold higher in the tumor versus plasma at 48 h postdosing). Exposure to cabazitaxel was 2.9 times higher in the tumor than in plasma (Figure 13.4). Perhaps more interestingly, both the tumor and plasma concentrations were higher than the cellular antiproliferative IC_{50} for up to 24 h in plasma and up to 96 h in the tumor [34].

Cabazitaxel was selected for further clinical evaluation based on its activity in a tumor model rendered resistant to docetaxel *in vivo* in an attempt to mimic

Table 13.2 Preclinical antitumor activity of cabazitaxel and docetaxel in mice bearing docetaxel-sensitive solid tumors.

Subcutaneous tumor[a)]	IV cabazitaxel			IV docetaxel		
	CR	TFS	SRI score[b)]	CR	TFS	SRI score[b)]
Advanced human prostate DU145	6/6	5/6	++++	nd	nd	nd
Early murine colon C51	–	–	+++	–	–	++++
Advanced murine colon C38	5/5	5/5	++++	0/5	–	++++
Advanced human colon HCT 116	7/7	2/7	++++	nd	nd	nd
Advanced human colon HT-29	6/6	–	+++	6/6	–	++++
Advanced murine pancreas P03	5/5	4/5	++++	nd	nd	nd
Advanced human pancreas MIA PaCa-2	6/6	6/6	++++	6/6	6/6	++++
Early murine breast MA16/C	–	–	++++	–	–	++++
Early murine breast MA17/A	–	–	++++	–	nd	nd
Early human breast Calc18	–	5/8	++++	–	nd	nd
Advanced human gastric N87	–	1/8	++++	–	1/8	++++
Advanced human lung NCI-H460	2/6	–	+++	nd	nd	nd
Advanced human lung A549	2/6	–	+++	0/5	–	++
Early murine B16 melanoma	–	–	++++	–	–	++
Advanced human head and neck SR475	6/6	6/6	++++	1/6	–	+++
Advanced human kidney Caki-1	5/6	–	++	2/5	–	++

CR, complete regression; IV, intravenous; nd, not determined in the same study; SC, subcutaneous; TFS, tumor-free survivors.

a) Advanced stage disease defined for median tumor burden >100 mg.

b) SRI (Southern Research Institute) score criteria: – (inactive) = log cell kill total <0.7; + = 0.7–1.2; ++ = 1.3–1.9; +++ = 2.0–2.8; ++++ (highly active) = >2.8.

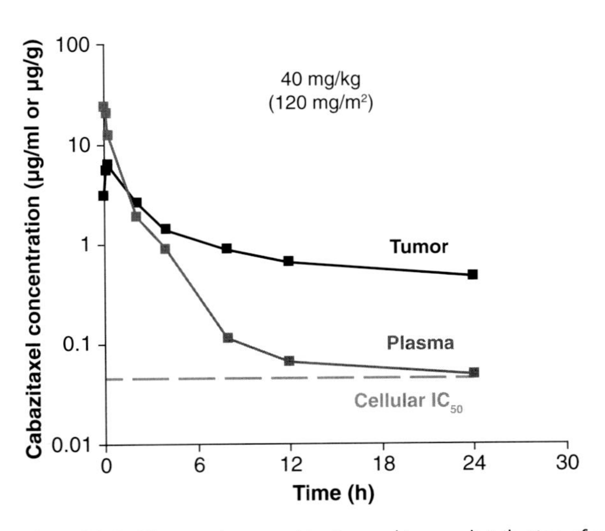

Figure 13.4 Plasma pharmacokinetics and tumor distribution of cabazitaxel in MA16/C-bearing mice.

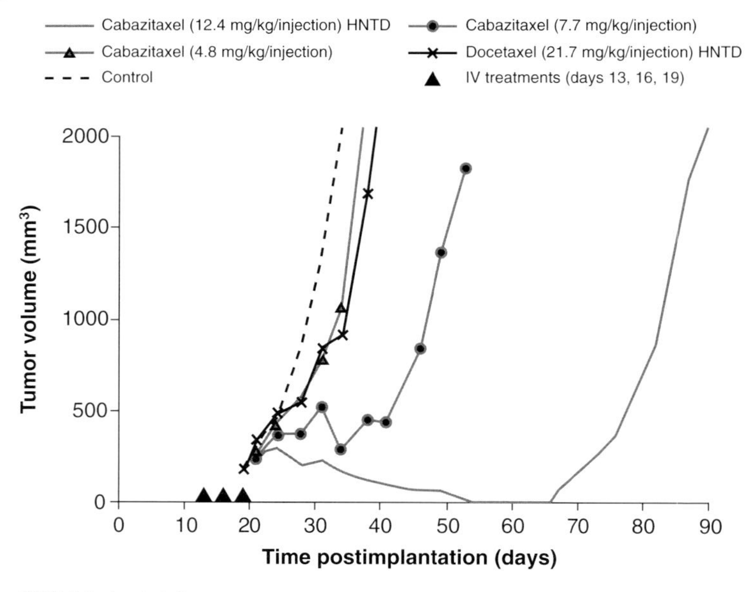

Figure 13.5 Antitumor activity of cabazitaxel in human breast UISO BCA-1 xenografts.

the clinical situation. Mice bearing docetaxel-sensitive B16 tumors were treated at the HNTD of docetaxel for 17 months to achieve full resistance to docetaxel [30]. In addition, cabazitaxel was more active than docetaxel in tumor models that were less sensitive or insensitive to docetaxel, such as murine P388 leukemia, human gastric GXF-209, murine lung 3LL, and human breast carcinoma UISO BCA-1. The latter HER2-positive breast tumor was obtained from a patient never treated with taxanes [35]. Further, docetaxel at its HNTD of 21.7 mg/kg per injection was not able to delay UISO BCA-1 tumor growth whereas cabazitaxel induced a significant delay in tumor growth (75 days) at its HNTD of 12.4 mg/kg per injection and also at the dose below the HNTD (7.7 mg/kg per injection) (Figure 13.5).

Another feature that distinguishes cabazitaxel from docetaxel is the ability of cabazitaxel to penetrate the blood–brain barrier in rodents [36]. In addition, antitumor activity of cabazitaxel has been observed in mice bearing intracranial glioblastoma xenografts [37].

13.3.2 Clinical Studies

The safety, efficacy, and PK of cabazitaxel have been evaluated in a series of studies involving patients with a number of advanced solid tumors. A selection of these studies is summarized in Table 13.3.

Table 13.3 Summary of selected cabazitaxel clinical studies.

Study	Tumor type (no. of patients)	Treatment	Key results
Phase I [21]	Advanced solid tumors previously treated with <2 chemotherapy regimens ($n = 25$)	CBZ 10–25 mg/m^2 q3w	RD: 20 mg/m^2 q3w DLTs: hematologic toxicity and diarrhea
Phase I [38, 39]	Advanced solid tumors previously treated with chemotherapy ($n = 21$)	CBZ 10–30 mg/m^2 q3w	RD: 25 mg/m^2 q3w DLTs: hematologic toxicity and diarrhea
Phase I [40]	Advanced solid tumors previously treated with chemotherapy ($n = 31$[a])	CBZ 1.5–12 mg/m^2 weekly (4/5 weeks)	RD: 10 mg/m^2 weekly DLTs: diarrhea
Phase I/II [23]	Metastatic breast cancer previously treated with taxane therapy ($n = 33$)	CBZ (20 mg/m^2) on day 1 + CAP (825 mg/m^2) bid on days 1–12 q3w	MTD: CBZ 20 mg/m^2 plus capecitabine 1000 mg/m^2
Phase II [22]	Metastatic breast cancer previously treated with taxane therapy ($n = 71$)	CBZ 20 mg/m^2 (cycle 1) and 25 mg/m^2 from cycle 2 in the absence of cycle 1 toxicity; q3w	Efficacy: CR ($n = 2$); PR ($n = 8$); SD ($n = 18$) Safety: grade 3/4 neutropenia 73%; febrile neutropenia 3%; neutropenia infection 4%
Phase III (TROPIC; NCT00417079) [24][1)]	Metastatic CRPC previously treated with docetaxel ($n = 755$)	CBZ 25 mg/m^2 q3w + prednisone 10 mg/day *or* mitoxantrone 12 mg/m^2 q3w + prednisone 10 mg/day	Efficacy: median OS 15.1 months (CBZ) versus 12.7 months (mitoxantrone); hazard ratio of death for CBZ relative to mitoxantrone 0.70 (95% CI: 0.59–0.83; $p < 0.0001$) Safety: grade 3/4 neutropenia CBZ 82%, mitoxantrone 58%; febrile neutropenia CBZ 7.5%, mitoxantrone 1.3%

(*continued*)

Table 13.3 (*Continued*)

Study	Tumor type (no. of patients)	Treatment	Key results
Phase III (PROSELICA; NCT01308580)[2)]	Metastatic CRPC	CBZ 20 mg/m^2 q3w + prednisone 10 mg/day *or* CBZ 25 mg/m^2 q3w + prednisone 10 mg/day	Study ongoing
Phase III (FIRSTANA; NCT01308567)[3)]	Metastatic CRPC chemonaive	CBZ 20 mg/m^2 q3w + prednisone 10 mg/day *or* CBZ 25 mg/m^2 q3w + prednisone 10 mg/day *or* docetaxel 75 mg/m^2 q3w + prednisone 10 mg/day	Study ongoing

bid, twice daily; CAP, capecitabine; CBZ, cabazitaxel; CI, confidence interval; CR, complete response; CRPC, castration-resistant prostate cancer; DLT, dose-limiting toxicity; mg/m^2, milligrams per square meter of body surface area; MTD, maximum tolerated dose; PR, partial response; q3w, every 3 weeks; RD, recommended dose; SD, stable disease.
a) Unpublished observations.

13.3.2.1 Phase I and II Studies

Phase I/II studies including patients with a variety of solid tumors indicated that cabazitaxel had an acceptable safety profile and also, similar to other taxanes, evidence of antitumor activity. Two dose-ranging phase I studies investigated cabazitaxel administered as a 1 h infusion every 3 weeks. In one of these studies [21], neutropenia was identified as main dose-limiting toxicity and the recommended dose of cabazitaxel was 20 mg/m^2. Objective clinical responses included partial responses (PR) in two patients with metastatic prostate cancer, including one with docetaxel-refractory disease, and 12 patients had stable disease (SD). In the other phase I study, neutropenia was also the primary dose-limiting toxicity [38, 39]; however, the recommended dose of cabazitaxel was identified as 25 mg/m^2. Among the 21 patients who participated, one achieved an unconfirmed PR (lung cancer) and six had SD.

Another phase I study investigated a weekly dosing schedule of cabazitaxel in 31 patients with advanced solid tumors ([40]; unpublished observations). Diarrhea was the main dose-limiting toxicity and the recommended dose for weekly dosing studies was 10 mg/m^2 administered for 4 out of 5 weeks. Two patients with breast cancer achieved PR and 13 patients had SD.

A phase II study in patients with metastatic breast cancer resistant to prior taxane therapy reported two complete responses (CR) and eight PR among the

71 patients who received treatment with cabazitaxel; a further 18 patients had SD for at least 3 months [22]. Median time to tumor progression was 2.7 months and median overall survival was 12.3 months. A subsequent phase I/II study evaluated cabazitaxel in combination with capecitabine (**9** in Figure 13.2) in patients with metastatic breast cancer whose disease had progressed after taxane therapy [23]. The recommended doses were cabazitaxel 20 mg/m^2 every 3 weeks plus capecitabine 1000 mg/m^2 twice daily from day 1 to day 14. PK analysis revealed no apparent drug–drug interaction. Promising clinical activity was observed with 2 CR, 5 PR, and 20 SD among the 33 patients. The overall response rate was 23.8%. The safety profile was consistent with what would be expected with the combination of a taxane plus capecitabine. At the recommended dose (received by 21 patients), the main grade 3–4 adverse events were neutropenia (57%), asthenia (10%), dyspnea (10%), hand–foot syndrome (10%), anorexia (5%), and febrile neutropenia (5%).

13.3.2.2 Clinical Pharmacokinetics

The PK profile of cabazitaxel is similar to that of docetaxel. Cabazitaxel exhibits dose proportionality across a dose range of 10–25 mg/m^2 [21]. Like docetaxel, the elimination profile of cabazitaxel is triphasic; however, the terminal phase $t_{1/2}$ is longer and the plasma clearance (CL) is higher than that of docetaxel. In addition, the mean volume of distribution at steady state (V_{ss}) of cabazitaxel is substantially greater than that of docetaxel.

A population PK model for cabazitaxel was developed and validated using data obtained from 170 patients (unpublished observations) with advanced solid tumors included in five phase I–III studies [21, 22, 24, 38, 40]. In agreement with data previously reported in a single phase I study [21], the PK profile of cabazitaxel was consistent with a three-compartment model characterized by rapid initial and intermediate phases (population half-lives = 4.4 min and 1.6 h, respectively) and a long terminal phase (half-life = 95.1 h). Cabazitaxel exhibited a very large V_{ss} (population PK estimate 4870 l; 2640 l/m^2 for a median body surface area (BSA) of 1.84 m^2) and a relatively high plasma CL (population PK estimate 48.5 l/h; 26.4 $l/h/m^2$ for a median BSA of 1.84 m^2). The model showed that the impact of intrinsic and extrinsic factors on the PK behavior of cabazitaxel was limited to BSA, with no effect of gender, age, race, and mild to moderate renal impairment observed. The PK data did not suggest a need for dose adjustment in these special populations. In addition, the concomitant administration of the weak CYP3A inducers prednisone or prednisolone (**6** and **7** in Figure 13.2) in the phase III study ([1]; unpublished observations) or the concomitant administration of capecitabine [23] did not modify the PK profile of cabazitaxel.

1) ClinicalTrials.gov. XRP6258 plus prednisone compared to mitoxantrone plus prednisone in hormone refractory metastatic prostate cancer (TROPIC). NCT00417079. Available at http://clinicaltrials.gov/ct2/results?term=00417079.

Another phase I study investigated the disposition of [^{14}C]-cabazitaxel administered at a dose of 25 mg/m^2 [41]. In plasma, the parent drug was the main circulating compound, representing approximately 70% of the radioactivity area under the curve (AUC). No relevant metabolites were observed in plasma (i.e., AUC metabolite $\leq$5% of the parent drug AUC), indicating that cabazitaxel is the only entity responsible for the pharmacological activity in humans. Approximately 80% of the dose was recovered in the excreta within 2 weeks. Cabazitaxel was largely excreted in the feces (76% of the dose) as numerous metabolites. The urinary route contributed markedly less to the overall excretion (3.7% of the dose with 2.3% excreted as unchanged drug). These results indicate that cabazitaxel is extensively metabolized in the liver. The main metabolites corresponded to combined mono- or di-*O*-demethyl derivatives on the taxane ring with hydroxyl or cyclized derivatives on the lateral chain. Docetaxel (di-*O*-demethyl cabazitaxel) was only detected as traces in plasma and excreta.

13.3.2.3 **Phase III Trial**

Based on clinical activity observed in patients with tumors resistant to taxanes including patients with prostate cancer in the phase I trial [20] and its manageable safety profile, cabazitaxel was further evaluated in a large, multinational, randomized, controlled trial, known as TROPIC (NCT00417079).[1)] This study was conducted in 755 patients with mCRPC who had disease progression following previous docetaxel-based therapy. TROPIC compared the efficacy of cabazitaxel with the active agent mitoxantrone (**8** in Figure 13.2). Cabazitaxel was administered intravenously every 3 weeks at a dose of 25 mg/m^2, with the comparator group receiving intravenous mitoxantrone at a dose of 12 mg/m^2 every 3 weeks. Patients in both groups received oral prednisone (**6** in Figure 13.2) 10 mg/day.

Patients who received cabazitaxel had a 30% reduction in the risk of death compared with those who received mitoxantrone (hazard ratio 0.70 (95% confidence interval (CI): 0.59; 0.83); $p < 0.0001$) [24]. Median overall survival was 15.1 months (95% CI: 14.1; 16.3) for cabazitaxel versus 12.7 months (95% CI: 11.6; 13.7) for mitoxantrone. Cabazitaxel was the first drug to demonstrate a significant improvement in survival in patients with mCRPC who had progressed following previous docetaxel-based therapy.

Other clinical end points measured in the TROPIC trial (progression-free survival, tumor response rate, prostate-specific antigen response rate, and time to tumor progression) were also improved following treatment with cabazitaxel compared with mitoxantrone (Table 13.4).

With regard to side effects, more patients in the cabazitaxel group experienced neutropenia of at least grade 3 severity (82% for cabazitaxel; 58% for mitoxantrone). Febrile neutropenia (FN) was reported in 7.5% of the cabazitaxel patients versus 1.3% of the mitoxantrone patients. The incidence of grade $\geq$3 diarrhea was also higher in the cabazitaxel group (6.2% versus 0.3%). Proactive management of these potential side effects of cabazitaxel treatment is highly recommended. Neutropenia may be effectively managed with the

Table 13.4 Summary of efficacy results in the TROPIC trial[a][42].

End point	Mitoxantrone ($n = 377$)	Cabazitaxel ($n = 378$)	HR (95% CI)	p-Value
Median OS (months)	12.7	15.1	0.70 (0.59–0.83)	<0.0001
Median PFS (months)	1.4	2.8	0.74 (0.64–0.86)	<0.0001
Tumor response rate (%)[b]	4.4	14.4	—	0.0005
PSA response rate (%)[c]	17.8	39.2	—	0.0002
Pain response rate (%)[d]	7.7	9.2	—	0.63
Median TTP (months)	5.4	8.8	0.61 (0.49–0.76)	<0.0001
Median time to PSA progression (months)	3.1	6.4	0.75 (0.63–0.90)	0.001
Median time to pain progression (months)	Not reached	11.1	0.91 (0.69–1.19)	0.52

CI, confidence interval; HR, hazard ratio; OS, overall survival; PFS, progression-free survival; PSA, prostate-specific antigen; TTP, time to tumor progression. Reproduced from Ref. [42] with permission of Future Medicine Ltd.

a) From final analysis, cutoff date September 25, 2009 [18].
b) Number of evaluable patients: 204 (mitoxantrone); 201 (cabazitaxel).
c) Number of evaluable patients: 325 (mitoxantrone); 329 (cabazitaxel).
d) Number of evaluable patients: 168 (mitoxantrone); 174 (cabazitaxel).

prophylactic use of granulocyte colony-stimulating factor (G-CSF), in particular in patients with high-risk clinical features (including those aged >65 years and those with advanced disease, comorbidities, prior episodes of FN, extensive prior radiotherapy, etc.). Primary G-CSF prophylaxis was not permitted in the TROPIC trial.

Based on the positive results from the TROPIC trial, cabazitaxel has been approved by the US Food and Drug Administration, the European Medicines Agency, and other national health authorities worldwide for the treatment of humans with mHRPC previously treated with a docetaxel-containing treatment regimen.

13.3.3
Other Ongoing Trials

Among other strategies available to alleviate the risk of neutropenic complications with cabazitaxel treatment is the implementation of a dose reduction. This strategy is being formally investigated in an ongoing phase III trial, PROSELICA,[2] which is comparing the standard 25 mg/m^2 dose with a reduced dose of 20 mg/m^2. Another ongoing phase III trial is evaluating these two doses of cabazitaxel versus docetaxel

2) ClinicalTrials.gov. Cabazitaxel at 20 mg/m^2 compared to 25 mg/m^2 with prednisone for the treatment of metastatic castration resistant prostate cancer (PROSELICA). NCT01308580. Available at http://clinicaltrials.gov/ct2/results?term=NCT01308580.

in patients with mCRPC who have not previously received chemotherapy.[3)] Other early-phase clinical trials are investigating cabazitaxel in combination with various chemotherapy agents and hormonal therapies.

13.4 Summary

Cabazitaxel is a novel semisynthetic taxane that promotes tubulin assembly and stabilizes microtubules as efficiently as docetaxel. Cabazitaxel is structurally distinct from docetaxel due to the presence of two methoxy groups at positions C-7 and C-10. Two chemical syntheses for cabazitaxel have been developed that involve modification of positions C-7 and C-10 in the naturally occurring 10-DAB precursor molecule and esterification of a POMA moiety at position C-13.

The selection of cabazitaxel for clinical development was based on its superior antiproliferative activity compared with docetaxel when tested against chemotherapy-resistant tumor cell lines as well as its broad spectrum of *in vivo* antitumor activity. The activity of cabazitaxel has been demonstrated in docetaxel-sensitive tumors including prostate, colon, lung, pancreas, head and neck, gastric, skin, and kidney. Cabazitaxel also has activity in tumor models in which docetaxel was either poorly active or inactive, including B16/TXT melanoma, a tumor model with *in vivo* acquired resistance to docetaxel. Further, unlike docetaxel, cabazitaxel is able to cross the blood–brain barrier, and displays better antitumor activity than docetaxel against intracranial glioblastomas. The PK profile of cabazitaxel is similar to that of docetaxel; both molecules show a triphasic elimination profile, although the terminal phase of cabazitaxel is longer than that of docetaxel. The plasma clearance of cabazitaxel is also higher than that of docetaxel.

The clinical development of cabazitaxel is being conducted worldwide and is focused on solid tumors. Based on the results of studies that have been completed, cabazitaxel has a manageable safety profile consistent with that seen with other taxanes. The clinical activity of cabazitaxel was observed in phase I studies. Proof of concept was first achieved in a phase II study with responses obtained in patients with metastatic breast tumors resistant to previous docetaxel therapy. Clinical activity was then confirmed in the pivotal phase III study in mCRPC patients previously treated with docetaxel, where cabazitaxel in combination with prednisone demonstrated a statistically significant overall survival benefit when compared with mitoxantrone plus prednisone. Cabazitaxel in combination with prednisone is currently approved in the United States, the European Union, Canada, Switzerland, and several other countries in Latin America, Asia, and the Middle East for the treatment of patients with mHRPC previously treated with a docetaxel-containing treatment regimen.

3) ClinicalTrials.gov. Cabazitaxel versus docetaxel both with prednisone in patients with metastatic castration resistant prostate cancer (FIRSTANA). NCT01308567. Available at http://clinicaltrials.gov/ct2/results?term=01308567.

Acknowledgments

The authors gratefully acknowledge François Lavelle, Alain Commerçon, Marie-Christine Bissery, Cécile Combeau, Jean-François Riou, and Jean-Dominique Bourzat for their contribution to the discovery of cabazitaxel, and Michèle Besenval, Sunil Gupta, Sylvie Assadourian, Emmanuelle Magherini, Gerard Sanderink, Eric Beys, Véronique Benning, Yves Archimbaud, Serge Sable, Laurence Ridoux, Olivier Pasquier, and Marie-Helene Pascual for their contribution to the preclinical and clinical development of cabazitaxel. Editorial assistance for preparing this chapter was supported by Sanofi.

References

1 Fischer, J. and Ganellin, C.R. (eds) (2006) *Analogue-Based Drug Discovery*, Wiley-VCH Verlag GmbH, Weinheim.

2 Fischer, J. and Ganellin, C.R. (eds) (2010) *Analogue-Based Drug Discovery II*, Wiley-VCH Verlag GmbH, Weinheim.

3 Erhardt, P.W. and El-Dakdouki, M. (2010) Paclitaxel and epothilone analogues, anticancer drugs, in *Analogue-Based Drug Discovery II* (eds J. Fischer and C.R. Ganellin), Wiley-VCH Verlag GmbH, Weinheim, pp. 243–268.

4 Abal, M., Andreu, J.M., and Barasoain, I. (2003) Taxanes: microtubule and centrosome targets, and cell cycle dependent mechanisms of action. *Curr. Cancer Drug Targets*, **3**, 193–203.

5 Jordan, M.A. and Wilson, L. (2004) Microtubules as a target for anticancer drugs. *Nat. Rev. Cancer*, **4**, 253–265.

6 Schiff, P.B., Fant, J., and Horwitz, S.B. (1979) Promotion of microtubule assembly *in vitro* by taxol. *Nature*, **277**, 665–667.

7 Perez, E.A. (2009) Microtubule inhibitors: differentiating tubulin-inhibiting agents based on mechanisms of action, clinical activity, and resistance. *Mol. Cancer Ther.*, **8**, 2086–2095.

8 Wani, M., Taylor, H., Wall, M., Coggon, P., and McPhail, A. (1971) Plant antitumor agents. VI. The isolation and structure of taxol, a novel antileukemic and antitumor agent from *Taxus brevifolia*. *J. Am. Chem. Soc.*, **93**, 2325–2327.

9 Holton, R.A., Somoza, C., Kim, H.-B., Liang, F., Biediger, R.J., Boatman, P.D., Shindo, M., Smith, C.C., and Kim, S. (1994) First total synthesis of taxol. 1. Functionalization of the B ring. *J. Am. Chem. Soc.*, **116**, 1597–1598.

10 Holton, R.A., Somoza, C., Kim, H.-B., Liang, F., Biediger, R.J., Boatman, P.D., Shindo, M., Smith, C.C., and Kim, S. (1994) First total synthesis of taxol. 2. Completion of the C and D rings. *J. Am. Chem. Soc.*, **116**, 1599–1600.

11 Nicolaou, K.C., Yang, Z., Liu, J.J., Ueno, H., Nantermet, P.G., Guy, R.K., Claiborne, C.F., Renaud, J., Couladouros, E.A., Paulvannan, K. *et al.* (1994) Total synthesis of taxol. *Nature*, **367**, 630–634.

12 Denis, J.N., Greene, A.E., Guenard, D., Gueritte-Voegelein, F., Mangatal, L., and Potier, P. (1988) Highly efficient, practical approach to natural taxol. *J. Am. Chem. Soc.*, **110**, 5917.

13 Holton, R.A., Biediger, R.J., and Boatman, P.D. (1995) *Taxol: Science and Applications* (ed. M. Suffness), CRC Press, Boca Raton, FL, pp. 97–121.

14 Venkat, K. (1998) Paclitaxel production through plant cell culture: an exciting approach to harnessing biodiversity. *Pure Appl. Chem.*, **70**, 2127.

15 Clarke, S.J. and Rivory, L.P. (1999) Clinical pharmacokinetics of docetaxel. *Clin. Pharmacokinet.*, **36**, 99–114.

16 Chien, A.J. and Moasser, M.M. (2008) Cellular mechanisms of resistance to anthracyclines and taxanes in cancer: intrinsic and acquired. *Semin. Oncol.*, **35** (2 Suppl. 2), S1–S14.

17 Fojo, T. and Menefee, M. (2007) Mechanisms of multidrug resistance: the potential role of microtubule stabilizing agents. *Ann. Oncol.*, **18** (Suppl. 5), v3–v8.

18 Baas, P., Szczesna, A., Albert, I., Milanowski, J., Juhász, E., Sztancsik, Z. *et al.* (2008) Phase I/II study of a 3 weekly oral taxane (DJ-927) in patients with recurrent, advanced non-small cell lung cancer. *J. Thorac. Oncol.*, **3**, 745–750.

19 Roche, M., Kyriakou, H., and Seiden, M. (2006) Drug evaluation: tesetaxel – an oral semisynthetic taxane derivative. *Curr. Opin. Invest. Drugs*, **7**, 1092–1099.

20 Saif, M.W., Sarantopoulos, J., Patnaik, A., Tolcher, A.W., Takimoto, C., and Beeram, M. (2011) Tesetaxel, a new oral taxane, in combination with capecitabine: a phase I, dose-escalation study in patients with advanced solid tumors. *Cancer Chemother. Pharmacol.*, **68** (6), 1565–1573.

21 Mita, A.C., Denis, L.J., Rowinsky, E.K., Debono, J.S., Goetz, A.D., Ochoa, L., Forouzesh, B., Beeram, M., Patnaik, A., Molpus, K., Semiond, D., Besenval, M., and Tolcher, A.W. (2009) Phase I and pharmacokinetic study of XRP6258 (RPR 116258A), a novel taxane, administered as a 1-hour infusion every 3 weeks in patients with advanced solid tumors. *Clin. Cancer Res.*, **15**, 723–730.

22 Pivot, X., Koralewski, P., Hidalgo, J.L., Chan, A., Gonçalves, A., Schwartsmann, G., Assadourian, S., and Lotz, J.P. (2008) A multicenter phase II study of XRP6258 administered as a 1-h i.v. infusion every 3 weeks in taxane-resistant metastatic breast cancer patients. *Ann. Oncol.*, **19**, 1547–1552.

23 Villanueva, C., Awada, A., Campone, M., Machiels, J.P., Besse, T., Magherini, E., Dubin, F., Semiond, D., and Pivot, X. (2011) A multicentre dose-escalating study of cabazitaxel (XRP6258) in combination with capecitabine in patients with metastatic breast cancer progressing after anthracycline and taxane treatment: a phase I/II study. *Eur. J. Cancer*, **47**, 1037–1045.

24 de Bono, J.S., Oudard, S., Ozguroglu, M., Hansen, S., Machiels, J.-P., Kocak, I., Gravis, G., Bodrogi, I., Mackenzie, M.J., Shen, L., Roessner, M., Gupta, S., and Sartor, A.O. (the TROPIC Investigators) (2010) Prednisone plus cabazitaxel or mitoxantrone for metastatic castration-resistant prostate cancer progressing after docetaxel treatment: a randomised open-label trial. *Lancet*, **376**1147–1154.

25 Bourzat, J.D., Bouchard, H., Commerçon, A., Bissery, M.C., Combeau, C., Vrignaud, P., Riou, J.F., and Lavelle, F. (1994) Preparation and biological evaluation of new docetaxel analogs modified at the 3′ position of the side chain. Proceedings of 16th International Cancer Congress, vol. 4, pp. 2751–2755.

26 Bourzat, J.D., Lavelle, F., and Commerçon, A. (1995) Synthesis and biological activity of *para*-substituted 3′-phenyl docetaxel analogs. *Bioorg. Med. Chem. Lett.*, **5**, 809–814.

27 Georg, G.I., Harriman, G.C.B., Hepperle, M., and Himes, R.H. (1994) Heteroaromatic taxol analogs: the chemistry and biological activities of 3′-furyl and 3′-pyridyl substituted taxanes. *Bioorg. Med. Chem. Lett.*, **4**, 1381–1384.

28 Pulicani, J.-P., Bézard, D., Bourzat, J.-D., Bouchard, H., Zucco, M., Deprez, D., and Commerçon, A. (1994) Direct access to 2-debenzoyl taxoids by electrochemistry, synthesis of 2-modified docetaxel analogs. *Tetrahedron Lett.*, **35**, 9717–9720.

29 Bouchard, H., Pulicani, J.-P., Vuilhorgne, M., Bourzat, J.D., and Commerçon, A. (1994) Improved access to 19-nor-7β,8β-methylene-taxoids and formation of a 7-membered C-ring analog of docetaxel by electrochemistry. *Tetrahedron Lett.*, **35**, 9713–9716.

30 Bissery, M.C., Bouchard, H., Riou, J.F., Vrignaud, P., Combeau, C., Bourzat, J.D. *et al.* (2000) Preclinical evaluation of TXD258, a new taxoid. *Proc. Am. Assoc. Cancer Res.*, **41**, abstract no. 1364.

31 Aller, A.W., Kraus, L.A., and Bissery, M.C. (2000) *In vitro* activity of TXD258 in chemotherapeutic resistant tumor cell lines. *Proc. Am. Assoc. Cancer Res.*, **41**, abstract no. 1923.

32 Vrignaud, P., Lejeune, P., Chaplin, D., Lavelle, F., and Bissery, M.C. (2000) *In vivo* efficacy of TXD258, a new taxoid, against human tumor xenografts. *Proc.*

Am. Assoc. Cancer Res., **41**, abstract no. 1365.

33 Corbett, T.H., Griswold, D.P., Jr., Roberts, B.J., Peckham, J.C., and Schabel, F.M., Jr. (1978) Biology and therapeutic response of a mouse mammary adenocarcinoma (16/C) and its potential as a model for surgical adjuvant chemotherapy. *Cancer Treat. Rep.*, **62**, 1471–1499.

34 Archimbaud, Y., Gires, P., Pellerin, R., Ridoux, L., Vrignaud, P., Bissery, M.C., Semiond, D., and Marietta, M. (2000) Pharmacokinetics and tissue distribution of a new taxoid antitumor agent, TXD258, in tumor-bearing mice. *Proc. Am. Assoc. Cancer Res.*, **41**, abstract no.1375.

35 Mehta, R.R., Bratescu, L., Graves, J.M., Hart, G.D., Shilkaitis, A., Green, A. *et al.* (1992) Human breast carcinoma cell lines: ultrastructural, genotypic, and immunocytochemical characterization. *Anticancer Res.*, **12**, 683–692.

36 Cisternino, S., Bourasset, F., Archimbaud, Y., Sémiond, D., Sanderink, G., and Scherrmann, J.M. (2003) Nonlinear accumulation in the brain of the new taxoid TXD258 following saturation of P-glycoprotein at the blood–brain barrier in mice and rats. *Br. J. Pharmacol.*, **138**, 1367–1375.

37 Dykes, D.J., Sarsat, J.P., and Bissery, M.C. (2000) Efficacy evaluation of TXD258, a taxoid compound, against orthotopic and subcutaneous glioblastomas. *Proc. Am. Assoc. Cancer Res.*, **41**, abstract no. 1916.

38 Lorthoraly, A., Pierga, J.Y., Delva, R., Girre, V., Gamelin, E., Terpereau, A., Crespel, G., Pouillard, P., Fontaine, H., Semiond, D., Perard, D., Besenval, M., and Dieras, V. (2000) Phase I and pharmacokinetics study of RPR116258A given as 1-hour infusion in patients with advanced solid tumors. *Clin. Cancer Res.*, **6** (Suppl.), abstract no. 569.

39 Dieras, V, Lortholary, A, Laurence, V, Delva, R, Girre, V, Livartowski, A, Assadourian, S, Semiond, D, and Pierga, J.Y. (2011) Cabazitaxel as a 1-hour infusion every 3 weeks in patients with advanced solid tumours: a phase 1 and pharmacokinetic study. Accepted for publication to the European Journal of Cancer.

40 Fumoleau, P, Trigo, J, Campone, M, Baselga, J, Sistac, F, Giminez, P, Manos, L, Fontaine, H, Semiond, D, Sanderink, G, Perard, D, and Besenval, M. (2001) Phase I and pharmacokinetic study of RPR 116258A given as a weekly 1-hour infusion at day 1, day 8, day 15, day 22 every 5 weeks in patients with advanced solid tumors. *Clin. Cancer Res.*, **7** (Suppl.), Abstract no. 282.

41 Ridoux, L, Semiond, D, Vincent, C, Fontaine, H, Mauriac, C, Sanderink, G, Oprea, C, and Clive, S. (2012.) A phase I open-label study investigating the disposition of [^{14}C] cabazitaxel in patients with advanced solid tumors. Annual Meeting of the American Association of Cancer Research, abstract no. 749.

42 Oudard, S. (2011) TROPIC: phase III trial of cabazitaxel for the treatment of metastatic castration-resistant prostate cancer. *Future Oncol.*, **7**, 497–506.

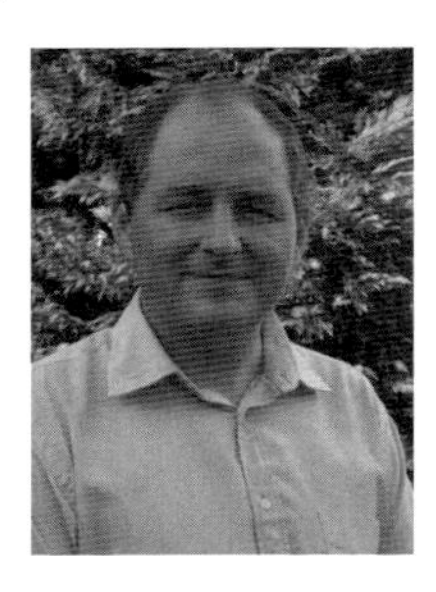

Hervé Bouchard completed his Ph.D. on natural product synthesis under the supervision of Professor J.-Y. Lallemand at the University Pierre et Marie Curie, Paris, in 1990 before conducting postdoctoral research on the total synthesis of reserpine in the laboratory of Professor S. Hanessian. In 1991, Dr. Bouchard joined the Medicinal Chemistry Department of Rhône-Poulenc Rorer (Vitry, France). He initiated total and hemisynthesis studies of natural products in oncology, antibiotic and antidiabetic therapeutic areas, and contributed to the discovery of several new chemical entities. These efforts led to the development of two new taxanes, namely, larotaxel (RPR109881) and cabazitaxel (RPR116258), which resulted in the recent approval by FDA and EMA of cabazitaxel in metastatic castration-resistant prostate cancer. After driving research activities in combinatorial chemistry, CB1 antagonism, and kinase inhibition pathways in oncology, Dr. Bouchard's current interests are focussed on immunoconjugate biotherapeutics.

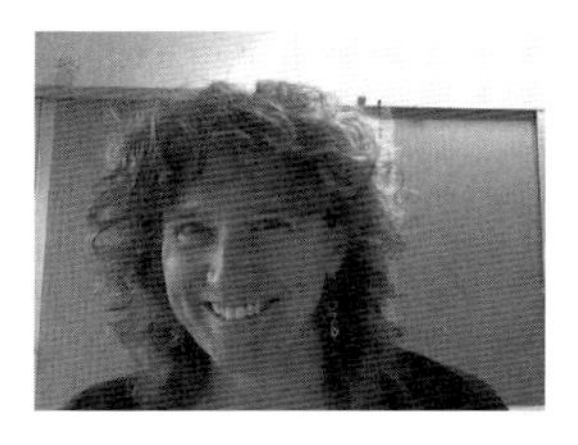

Marie-Laure Risse obtained her medical degree from Paris VI University (Paris, France) before completing postgraduate courses in clinical oncology (Paris VI University), palliative care and chemotherapy (both Gustave Roussy Institute, Villejuif, France), and HIV infection (Paris VI University). She was Resident at the Gustave Roussy Institute for 1 year (1996–1997) before taking up a position as Oncology Clinical Project Leader in the Department of Clinical Development and Medical Communication at Rhône-Poulenc Rorer French affiliate (later Aventis Pharma). Dr. Risse became Clinical Study Director in 2002 (Aventis) and then Clinical Research Director in 2008 (Sanofi-Aventis) in Research and Development. Her current position is Cabazitaxel Medical Lead in the Global Oncology Division at Sanofi.

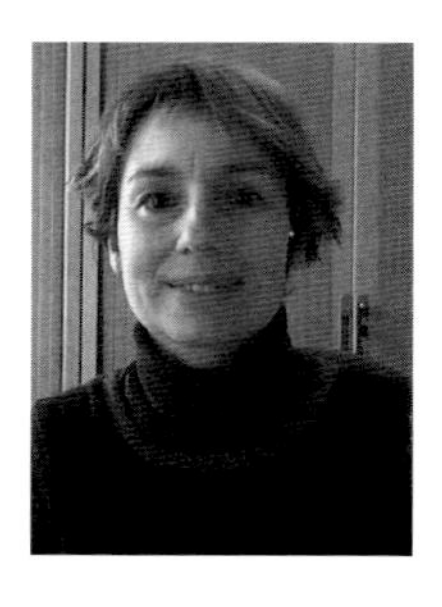

Dorothée Semiond received two master's degrees, one in Analytical Chemistry (Claude Bernard University, Lyon, France) and the other in Clinical Pharmacokinetics (Institute of Pharmaceutical and Biological Sciences of Lyon (ISPBL), Lyon, France), and completed her Ph.D. at the University of Pharmacy in Paris under the supervision of Dr. J.M. Schermann on the subject of "Add on of pharmacokinetic modeling in the development of new taxoids." She also received her Pharm.D. degree from the Institute of Pharmaceutical and Biological Sciences of Lyon (ISPBL). From 1996 to 2006, Dr. Semiond served as a clinical pharmacokineticist and drug disposition project team representative at Rhône-Poulenc Rorer (later Aventis Pharma, then Sanofi-Aventis), and from 2006 to 2010 she managed the Pharmacokinetic Unit at Sanofi-Aventis. Since 1997, Dr. Semiond has served as the clinical pharmacokineticist and project team representative for drug disposition in the development of two novel taxanes larotaxel (RPR109881) and cabazitaxel (RPR116258). Dr. Semiond is currently the dedicated project expert for drug disposition in the Department of Disposition, Safety and Animal Research at Sanofi, where she focuses on oncology projects. She has authored 8 papers and 20 congress abstracts.

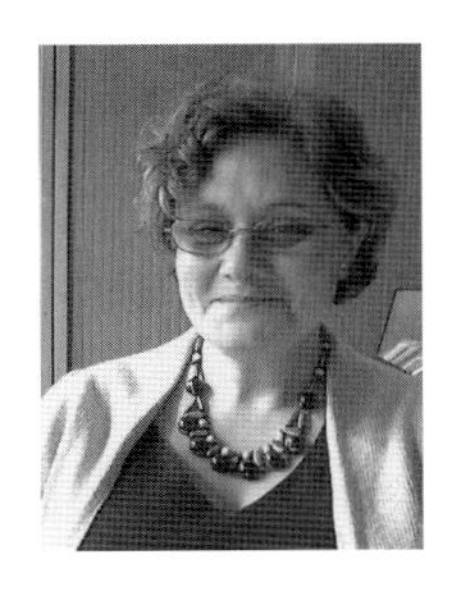

Patricia Vrignaud received her Ph.D. in Nutrition and Metabolism from Bordeaux I University. Her thesis "Growth rates of chemically induced sarcomas in mice: influence of age, sex and number of primotransplants" was written under the directorship of Dr. M. Dénéchaud. Following her Ph.D., Dr. Vrignaud worked as a Research Scientist at the Fondation Bergonié (Cancer Hospital), Bordeaux, where she studied the pharmacokinetics and metabolism of anthracyclines and the cellular pharmacology of anthracyclines and multidrug resistance. From 1991 to 2002, she served as Head of the Laboratory in Experimental Therapeutics in Oncology at Rhône-Poulenc Rorer. She then went on to become the Head of Section evaluating anticancer agents in experimental models at Aventis Pharma (later Sanofi-Aventis), where she participated in the registration processes for docetaxel and irinotecan and served as the preclinical lead for cabazitaxel. Dr. Vrignaud is currently the Head of Late Development – discovery liaison in Translational & Experimental Medicine at Sanofi. She has authored 46 papers, 20 patents, and 155 congress abstracts.

14
Discovery of Boceprevir and Narlaprevir: A Case Study for Role of Structure-Based Drug Design

Srikanth Venkatraman, Andrew Prongay, and George F. Njoroge

List of Abbreviations

Boc	*tert*-butyl carbamate
FDA	Food and Drug Administration
HCV	hepatitis C virus
HNE	human neutrophil elastase
NS3	nonstructural protein 3
SAR	structure–activity relationship
SVR	sustained virologic response

The hepatitis C epidemic rightly termed as a silent killer has attracted major attention in recent years. The identification of hepatitis C virus (HCV) by Choo *et al.* as the primary causative agent for non-A, non-B hepatitis resulted in explosive growth in the number of publication describing the viral life cycle and new targets for drug intervention [1, 2]. HCV is a positive strand RNA virus of the *Flaviviridae* family, whose members include dengue, west Nile, and Japanese encephalitis. Unscreened blood transfusions in the 1960s and 1970s resulted in many new infections [3]. A vast majority of these infections turn chronic resulting in liver cirrhosis and hepatocellular carcinoma [4]. The slow progression of the disease and lack of symptoms has made early detection difficult. HCV infections are the primary causes for late-stage liver transplantations in the United States. Recent advances in detection techniques allow early diagnosis of patients by screening for HCV antibodies. Prior to the development of Victrelis (boceprevir) and Incivek (telaprevir), the standard of care for treatment was a combination of peg-interferon and ribavirin [5]. This combination though effective in genotype 2 is suboptimal for treatment of genotype 1. Only approximately 40% of genotype 1-treated patients achieve sustained virologic response (SVR) defined as undetectable viral RNA after 6 months of completion of therapy [6]. Recent advances in virology have identified many proteins vital for

Analogue-based Drug Discovery III, First Edition. Edited by János Fischer, C. Robin Ganellin, and David P. Rotella.
© 2013 Wiley-VCH Verlag GmbH & Co. KGaA. Published 2013 by Wiley-VCH Verlag GmbH & Co. KGaA.

HCV viral replication [7, 8]. Development of inhibitors targeting these enzymes could potentially develop new direct-acting antiviral.

HCV is a bloodborne pathogen, which primarily infects hepatocytes. Most of these infections turn chronic. After infecting hepatocytes, the virus codes a single polypeptide of ~3000 amino acids that contains all the core and functional proteins. This polypeptide containing proteins C-E1-E2-P7-NS2-NS3-NS4A-NS4B-NS5A-NS5B undergoes a *cis*-cleavage at the NS3-NS4A junction followed by *trans*-cleavage at NS4A-NS4B, NS4B-NS5A, and NS5A-NS5B junctions catalyzed by a serine enzyme NS3 protease. This central role of NS3 protease in the life cycle of the enzyme makes it an important target for drug intervention.

HCV NS3 protease is a serine enzyme belonging to the chymotrypsin superfamily [9–12]. Its functionality is formed by the N-terminal third of the NS3 bifunctional protein. The N-terminal 181 residues fold into two β-barrel subdomains. The active site of the enzyme is located on the surface and is a shallow, featureless cleft that is solvent exposed. The catalytic triad (His57, Asp81, and Ser139) is located between the two β-barrel subdomains. There is a zinc ion at a distance of ~20 Å from the catalytic site that is coordinated by Cys97, Cys99, Cys145, and a water molecule that is hydrogen bonded to His149. It plays a critical role in maintaining structural stability and integrity of the protein. The substrate of the protease is long and recognizes the enzyme with a series of hydrogen bonds. The P_1 and P1′ residues of the natural substrate of NS3 protease are highly conserved [13–15]. Cysteine is retained at the P1 position in all three *trans*-cleavage sites (NS4A/NS4B, NS4B/NS5A, and NS5A/NS5B) and is replaced by threonine in *cis*-cleavage event (NS3/NS4A).

NS4A, a 54 amino acid cofactor, enhances catalytic activity and the stability of the protease. This protein binds to NS3 with residues 21–32 forming a β-strand that is situated between the first (A0) and second (A1) strands of the N-terminal β-barrel subdomain and with the main chain amide and carbonyl groups of these three chains sharing hydrogen bonds. The binding of the NS4A cofactor organizes the catalytic triad in a preferred conformation by orienting His57 to facilitate deprotonation of Ser139 and hydrogen bond to Asp81. Thus, in the absence of NS4A cofactor the enzymatic activity of the protease is greatly diminished making its binding a prerequisite for efficient catalytic turnover.

The quintessential role of HCV NS3 protease in the life cycle of the virus makes it an attractive target for drug intervention. We initiated our search for inhibitors by screening compound libraries to identify potential leads. It was very disheartening to find that even with new advances in high-throughput screening and evaluation of many compound libraries, we could not identify any viable lead. We therefore decided to pursue a structure-based drug design. This required the development of a continuous spectrophotometric assay [16] to facilitate assessing the kinetic parameters of slow tight binding inhibitors [17]. An undecapeptide **1** with a ketoamide electrophilic trap was identified that inhibited the enzyme with a $K_i^* = 1.9\,\text{nM}$ (Figure 14.1). With this as our starting point, we explored various modifications to engineer desirable pharmaceutical properties. Our initial goal for the modification of **1** was to reduce its molecular weight and identify the minimal fragment that

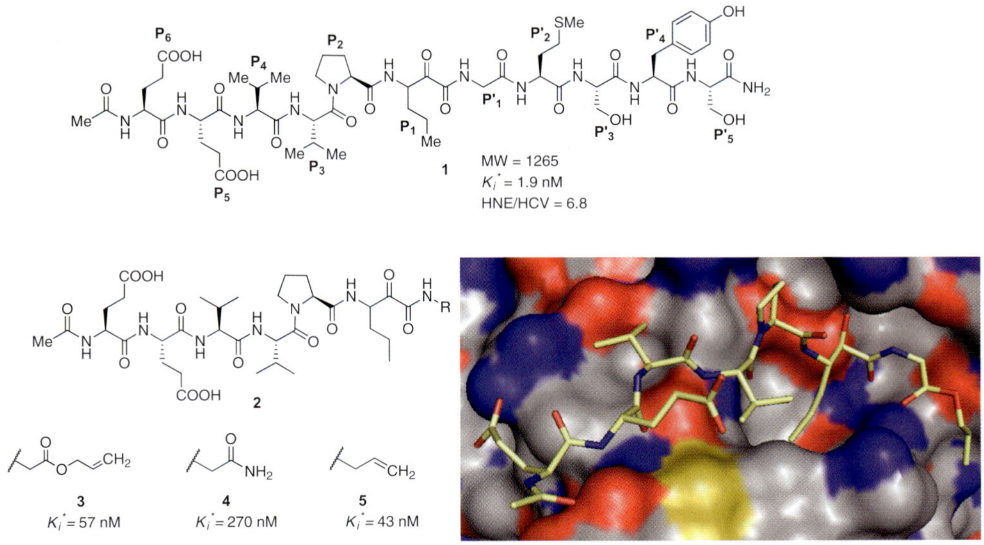

Figure 14.1 X-ray structure of undecapeptide **1** bound to HCV NS3 protease.

retained potent binding. It was also decided to replace various proteinogenic amino acids with modified synthetic amino acids to enhance metabolic stability and improve ligand efficiency.

Synthesized compounds were evaluated in a continuous spectrophotometric assay for the inhibition of hydrolysis of chromogenic ester from the acetyl-DTEDVVP(norvaline)-*O*-phenylazophenol substrate. Progression curves were fit into a two-step slow tight binding model and a composite inhibition constant K_i^* was derived, which allowing rank ordering of compounds. Compounds that displayed acceptable binding were evaluated in a replicon-based cell assay. Key compounds that had excellent enzyme inhibition and acceptable cellular activity were dosed in rats in a rapid rat assay. After a single oral dose, blood was periodically withdrawn and concentration of the parent compound was analyzed in the plasma generating AUC for exposure and other pharmacokinetic parameters.

Some interesting compounds were soaked with HCV NS3 protease and bound structure was solved by X-ray diffraction. The crystals of the HCV NS3 protease domain (residues 1–181) complexed with a peptide containing the NS4A sequences spanning residues 21–39 were crystallized by vapor diffusion using sodium chloride as the precipitant. The structures of the inhibitor compounds were obtained by soaking the crystals in a solution of the inhibitor at 10–100 μM concentration overnight at 12 °C. The crystals were transferred to a cryoprotectant solution containing sucrose prior to super cooling in liquid nitrogen. The diffraction data were collected as previously described [18].

Thus, replacement of P1′–P5′ segment of inhibitor **1** with glycine allyl ester resulted in compound **2** with a $K_i^* = 57\,\text{nM}$ (Figure 14.1). Similarly, introduction of glycine primary amide and allyl amide in the place of P1′–P5′ was also well tolerated resulting in analogues **4** ($K_i^* = 270\,nM$) and **5** ($K_i^* = 43\,nM$). Even though these modifications resulted in analogues with diminished potency compared to **1**, it was reassuring to note that the compounds were still potent allowing us to make a decision to limit our future analogues at P2′, thus reducing molecular weights.

The X-ray structure of **3** bound to NS3 protease revealed the propyl chain of P1 norvaline that was buried into the S1 pocket. However, the side chain did not completely fill the S1 pocket and the van der Waals contacts were not optimized. As seen in Figure 14.1, the pucker of the P2 proline ring was oriented toward the solvent and away from the protein surface resulting in a suboptimal interaction. It was also clear that the remaining binding sites were shallow and other residues made only partial contact to the protease. We decided to reduce polarity of analogues of type 2 by capping our inhibitors at the P3 position removing acidic amino acids at P5 and P6. We hypothesized that this transformation would facilitate absorption and permeability into cells of resulting analogues (Figure 14.2).

Boc-capped P3 truncated inhibitor **6** had modest activity in inhibition of HCV NS3 protease. Even though this activity was much reduced compared to inhibitors spanning from P6 to P2′, it was clear that one could retain potency with truncated inhibitors. The X-ray structure of **6** bound to the protease revealed various sites for modification to improve activity. From the structure, it was once again clear that the P1 norvaline occupied the S1 pocket effectively, albeit incompletely. The P2′ allyl ester made lipophilic interaction with the butyl side chain of Lys136. This stabilized

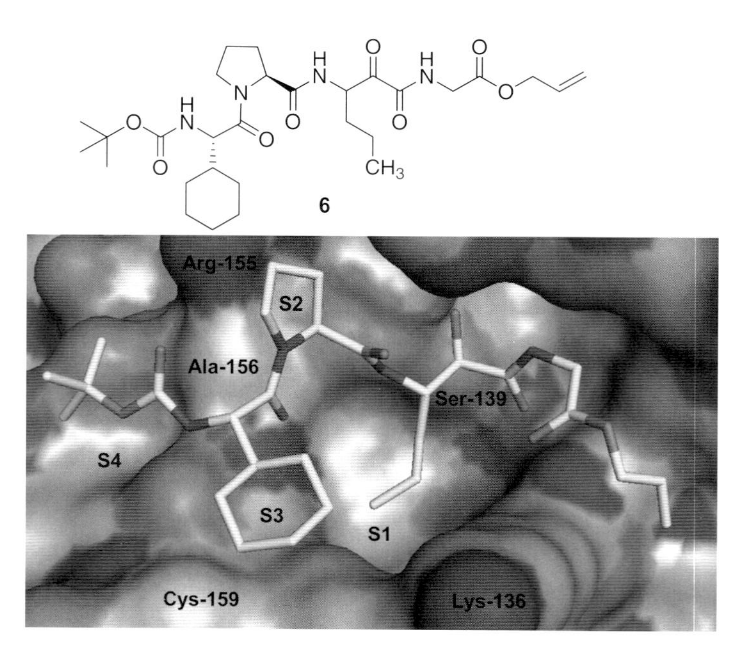

Figure 14.2 X-ray structure of P3–P1′ truncated analogue **6** in the active site of HCV NS3.

the side chain of Lys136 in an extended conformation as the P2′ allyl and P1 norvaline side chains packed against it. The binding of the allyl group projected toward a pocket that could potentially provide additional binding energy. As with compound **3**, the pucker of the P2 proline projects the Cγ atom toward the solvent, leaving the S2 pocket incompletely filled. The His57 and Arg155 side chains formed a U-shaped wall on either side of the proline ring. The P3 cyclohexylglycine made surface contact as its side chain laid above the shallow S3 pocket with its Cβ, Cδ1, and Cδ2 atoms projecting closest to the pocket. The closest contact is between Cδ2 and Cys159Sγ at ~3.3Å, while Cδ1 and Cδ2 are each ~3.9 Å from Ile132Cβ. These contacts are the result of the side chains of Cys159 and Ile132 adopting alternate rotamer positions to optimize the van der Waals interactions. The *tert*-butyl group of the Boc cap occupied the S4 pocket, which had undergone a conformational change with the rotation of R123 and Asp168 side chains. One *tert*-butyl methyl group projects toward the bottom of the pocket resulting in a fairly snug packing.

To improve potency and depeptidize inhibitor **6**, various modifications were evaluated based on the structural information. It was clear from the X-ray structure that the P1 norvaline and P3 cyclohexylglycine were in close proximity. We therefore envisioned syntheses of P1–P3 macrocylic inhibitors that linked these groups by a suitable linker. Similarly, the proximity of P2 proline to the P4 Boc group resulted in novel ideas of linking these groups to synthesize many P2–P4 macrocylic inhibitors. It was also clear from the X-ray structure that the P2 proline made inefficient contact at the S2 site. We therefore decided to evaluate many modifications at proline from the 3, 4, and 5 positions to maximize interactions that could be beneficial to binding. Therefore, a large number of modified proline derivatives were synthesized and incorporated into **6**. We also decided to modify the P2′ allyl ester in an effort to gain improvement in binding. The results of these modifications are discussed below (Figure 14.3).

The incorporation of 4-*tert*-butoxy proline at P2 and phenylglycine at P2′ resulted in marked improvement in binding (**7**, $K_i^* = 19$ nM) and HNE/HCV selectivity (HNE/HCV = 161) [19]. Inhibitor **7** also showed cellular activity in a replicon-based assay [20] ($EC_{90} = 2000$ nM). Introduction of bicyclic P2 (3a*R*,4*S*,6a*R*)-2,2-dimethylhexahydro-2*H*-furo[2,3-*c*]pyrrole-4-carboxylic acid resulted in analogue **8** with $K_i^* = 5$ nM and $EC_{90} = 400$ nM. Similarly, replacement of P2 proline with (1*R*,2*S*,5*S*)-6,6-dimethyl-3-azabicyclo[3.1.0]hexane-2-carboxylic acid [21] resulted in analogue **9** ($K_i^* = 10$ nM, HNE/HCV = 964, $EC_{90} = 400$ nM). It was clear that modification of P2 proline had a positive impact on binding and cellular activity. The introduction of modified proline analogues reduced molecular weight of resultant inhibitors compared to the undecapeptide **1**, retained enzyme inhibition, imparted cellular activity, and improved metabolic stability. Rat pharmacokinetic studies of **9** showed modest oral exposure with an AUC = 1.1 μM h when dosed at 10 mg/kg and a low bioavailability of 6%. The X-ray structure of **9** bound to the enzyme revealed that the P1′–P2′ glycine–phenylglycine amide made a "C-clamp" structure around Lys136 restricting its mobility. The aryl group of phenylglycine made van der Waals contact with the protruding amino butyl chain contributing to enhanced

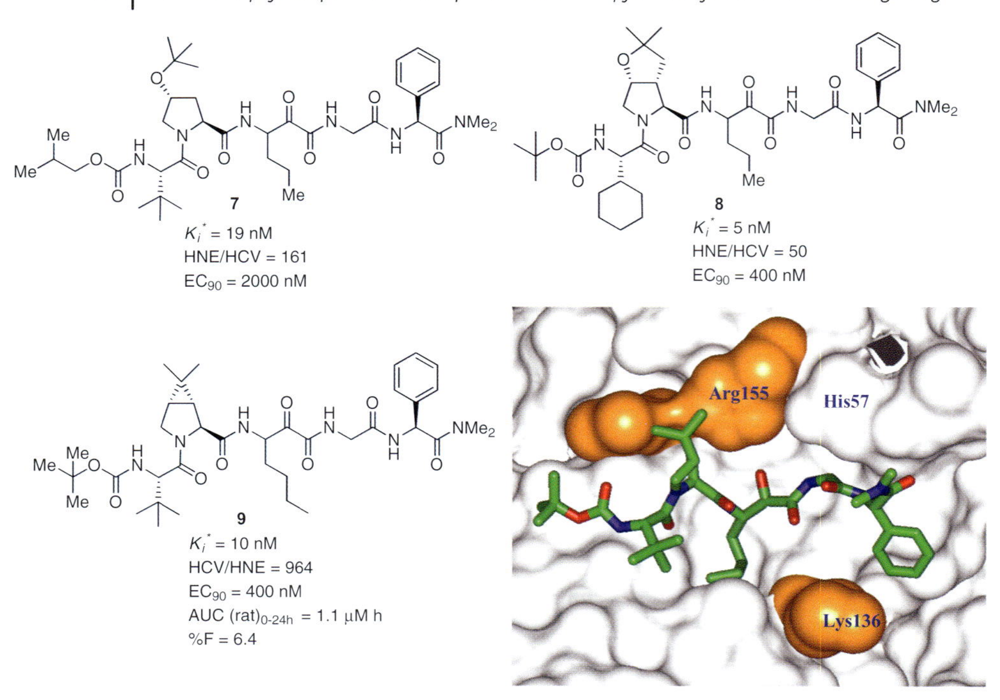

Figure 14.3 X-ray structure of norleucine derivative **9** bound to HCV protease. Key interactions to Arg155 and Lys136.

binding. As with compound **6**, this position of the Lys136 side chain provided an additional surface in the S1 pocket for the P1 side chain to pack against. The additional methylene group of the P1 norleucine side chain extends deeper into the S1 pocket nearly filling it completely. In contrast to the cyclohexyl P3 group of compound **6**, the P3 *tert*-butyl projects down into the S3 dimple, making close contacts and more completely filling the space. The methyl group Cγ3 packs at distances of 3.7, 4.0, and 4.3 Å from Cys159Sγ, Ala157Cβ, and Ile132Cδ1, respectively, while Cys159Sγ is 4.1 Å from the methyl group Cγ2. Unlike the pucker of the proline ring, the dimethylcyclopropyl ring of the proline analogue projects toward the Arg155 side chain, fitting snugly against the amidino group of the arginine side chain. With the Nη2 of Arg155 at 3.6 Å from the Cζ1 of P2 and Nη1 of Arg155 at 3.4 Å from Cζ2, and the Cβ at distances of 3.3 and 3.4 Å from His57Nε2 and Cε1, the S2 pocket is more snugly filled than with leucine or proline at P2. As a result of this packing, the side chain of His57 is swung in toward the protein surface ("In" position). The amidino group of Arg155 was also rotated to make room for the *gem*-dimethyls and remove steric clash between these groups.

The incorporation of modified proline resulted in analogues with desirable binding and cellular activity. However, these analogues spanning from P3 to P2′ were poorly absorbed and displayed low bioavailability. We therefore investigated syntheses of macrocyclic compounds (Figure 14.4).

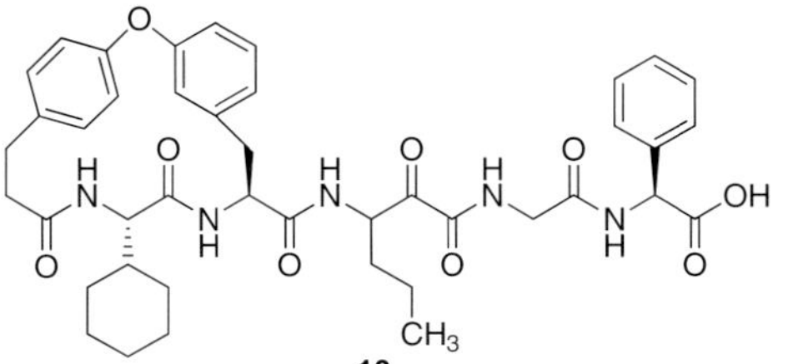

10
K_i^*=110 nM

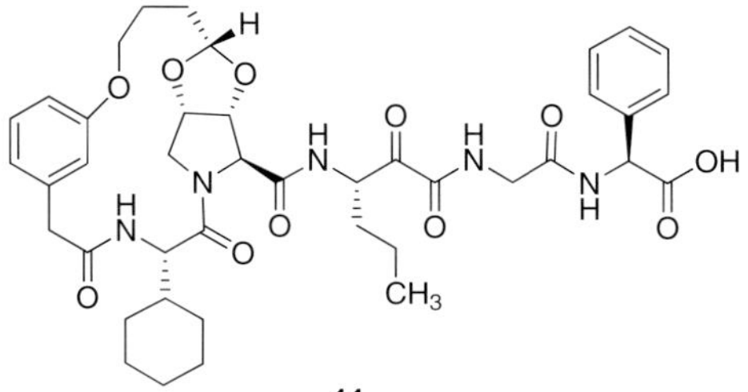

11
K_i^* = 38 nM

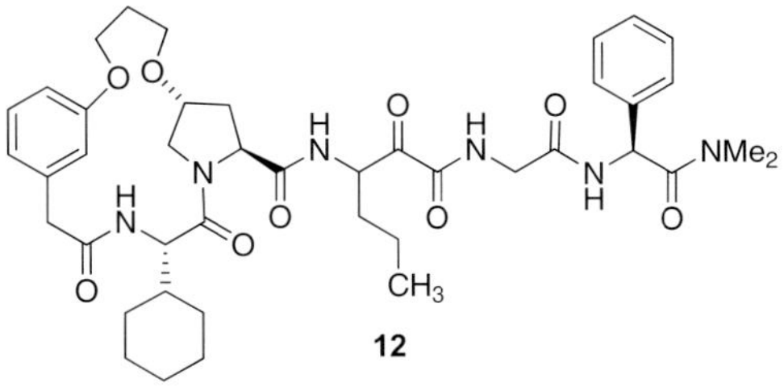

12
K_i^* = 8 nM
HCV/HNE = 46
EC_{90} = 1500 nM
AUC rat $_{0\text{-}24h}$ =1.5 μM h
%F =3

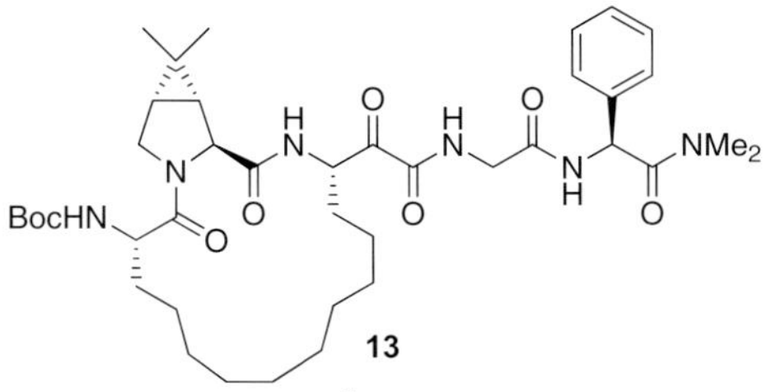

13
K_i^* = 6 nM
HCV/HNE = 780
EC_{90} = 600 nM

Figure 14.4

Biaryl P2–P4 macrocyclic inhibitor **10** derived from phenylalanine P2 and P4 phenyl propionic acid was one of the first macrocyclic compounds potent in inhibition of the HCV protease assay with a $K_i^* = 110\,\text{nM}$ [22]. However, this compound did not show any cellular activity. From previous SAR studies in the acyclic analogues, we had established that P2 proline compounds demonstrated good cellular potency. We therefore synthesized other macrocycles containing P2 proline modifications. This resulted in compounds such as the acetal analogue **11** that had a potent inhibition of $K_i^* = 38\,\text{nM}$, a threefold improved binding compared to biaryl analogue **10** [23]. Similarly, 4-hydroxyproline-derived macrocyclic analogue **12** displayed excellent enzyme inhibition ($K_i^* = 8\,\text{nM}$) and replicon-based cellular activity ($EC_{90} = 1.5\,\mu\text{M}$) [24]. We also synthesized P1–P3 macrocylic inhibitors of type **13**. These compounds were more potent than the P2–P4 analogues and had better cellular potency. Thus, the 16-membered P1–P3 macrocyclic analogue **13** had excellent binding $K_i^* = 6\,\text{nM}$ with acceptable cellular activity of $EC_{90} = 600\,\text{nM}$ [25]. Both P2–P4 and P1–P3 macrocyclic analogues were well tolerated and improved enzyme potency in some cases compared to the linear analogues. However, these compounds did not have markedly improved pharmacokinetics compared to acyclic derivatives. Macrocycle **12** was only partially absorbed in rats with a bioavailability of 3% that was no better than derivative **8**. These compounds were also poorly absorbed in monkeys and dogs without any plasma exposure.

It was clear from these studies that potent inhibitors of NS3 protease could be synthesized that also showed acceptable cellular activity in the replicon-based cellular assay. This was itself a substantial progress compared to the initial lead **1** that lacked any of these desired properties. From a point of inhibitor design, the structure-based hypothesis was successfully utilized for design and refinement resulting in analogues that differed structurally from the initial lead with many drug-like properties. However, to develop a drug candidate, incorporation of acceptable pharmacokinetics is paramount. Thus, we decided to focus on further modifying analogues of type **9**.

It was clear that inhibitors spanning from P3 to P2′ contained many amide bonds with multiple hydrogen bond donors and acceptors. We reasoned that the poor bioavailability of these analogues was due to high molecular weights and peptidic nature. At this point, we decided to truncate the molecules by reducing the number of amide bonds. Concurrently, we also explored different P1, P3, and capping residues to improve ligand efficiency (Figure 14.5).

Replacement of dimethylcarboxamide of P2 phenylglycine with a methyl group resulted in analogue **14** ($K_i^* = 55$ nM, AUC = 2.66 μM h), with improved exposure in rats compared to compounds of type **9**. It was very encouraging to notice that removal of a single amide group had profound impact on rat PK. Further truncation at P1′ with allyl amide resulted in analogue **15** that had excellent oral exposure in rats with AUC = 26 μM h when dosed at 10 mg/kg. The introduction of P1′ primary amide group resulted in compound **16** with a plasma exposure of 2.52 μM h.

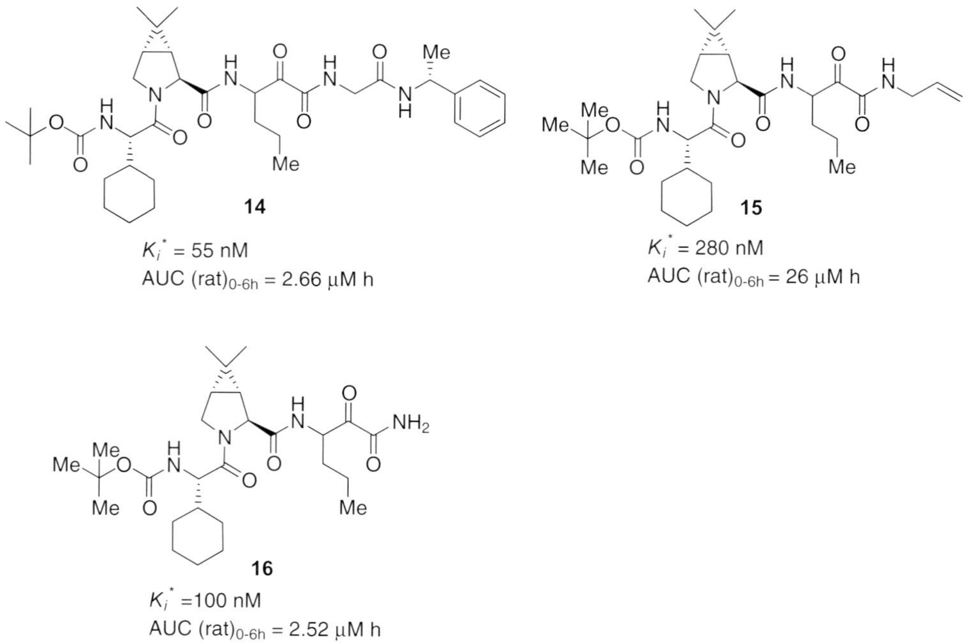

14
K_i^* = 55 nM
AUC $(rat)_{0\text{-}6h}$ = 2.66 μM h

15
K_i^* = 280 nM
AUC $(rat)_{0\text{-}6h}$ = 26 μM h

16
K_i^* =100 nM
AUC $(rat)_{0\text{-}6h}$ = 2.52 μM h

Figure 14.5

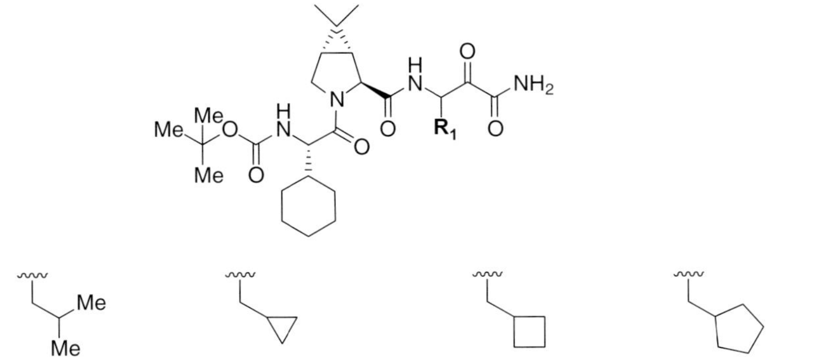

Me Me O H N N H N NH2 O O O R1 O Me O

Me Me

17
K_i^* = 400 nM
HNE/HCV = 9

18
K_i^* = 25 nM
HNE/HCV = 23
EC_{90} = 400 nM
AUC (rat) =1.3 μM h
%F=3

19
K_i^* = 8 nM
HNE/HCV = 138
EC_{90} = 700 nM
AUC (rat)=1.5 μM h
%F=28

20
K_i^* = 150 nM
HNE/HCV = 370

Figure 14.6

It was clear that improvement in plasma exposure could be achieved by truncation, but it was achieved at the expense of potency. With the knowledge of improving exposure by truncating analogues at the P1′ position, we focused our attention in modification of P1 residue to improve potency.

We synthesized a series of small cyclic P1 alanine amino acids and incorporated them into the inhibitors (Figure 14.6). Thus, replacement of norvaline in **16** with isoleucine resulted in compound **17** ($K_i^* = 400\,nM$), a fourfold loss in potency. However, incorporation of cyclopropyl alanine at this site was well tolerated resulting in **18** ($K_i^* = 25\,nM$, $EC_{90} = 400\,nM$) with a fourfold improvement in binding and good cellular activity compared to **17**. Homologation of cyclopropyl alanine to cyclobutyl alanine resulted in compound **19** with further improved potency ($K_i^* = 8\,nM$) and comparable cellular activity to **18**. The cyclobutyl analogue **19** had acceptable oral exposure and bioavailability warranting further investigation in this series. Structurally, the cyclopropyl alanine side chain resembled a branched norvaline side chain that filled the S1 pocket and introduced rotational and packing constraints. Similarly, cyclobutyl alanine side chain resembled a branched norleucine side chain that almost completely filled the S1 pocket and introduced further rotational and packing constraints. These constraints resulted in Ile132 rotating to make room for the cyclobutyl ring, while Lys136 rotates to make van der Waals contacts between its side chain and the cyclobutyl ring. The rotation of Lys136 to this new orientation is facilitated by the absence of the P1′ and P2′ moieties of previous compounds.

We further explored the modification of P1 cyclic alanine-derived compounds of type **18** and **19** by changing P3 amino acid and P3 cap. The SAR of these modifications are summarized in the cyclobutyl series in Figure 14.7.

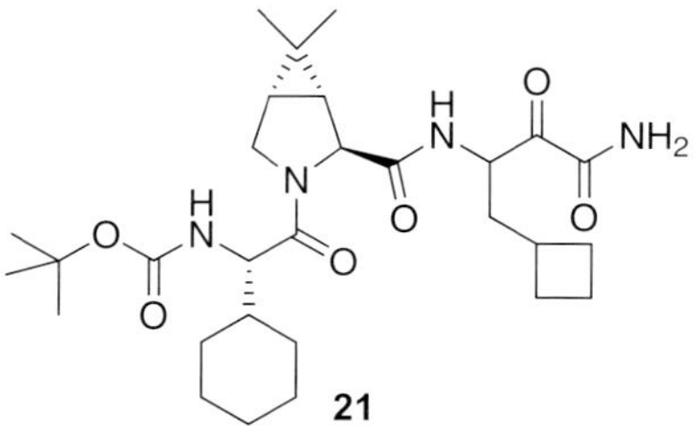

21
$K_i^* = 8$ nM
HNE/HCV= 138

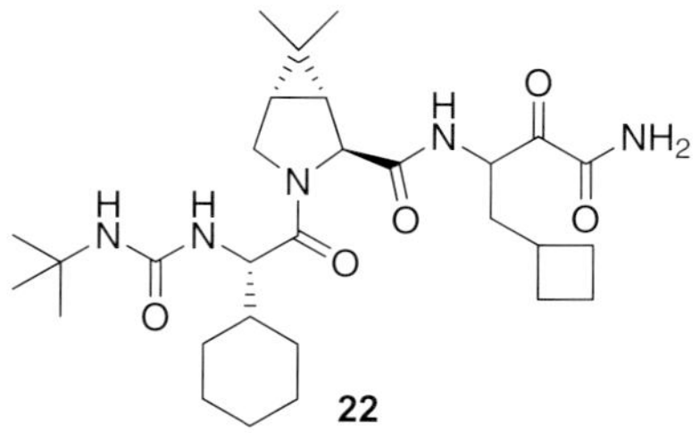

22
$K_i^* = 50$ nM
HNE/HCV= 90

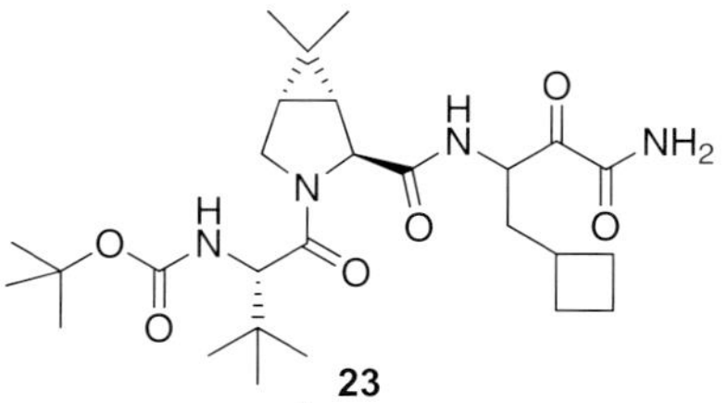

23
$K_i^* = 76$ nM
HNE/HCV= 684

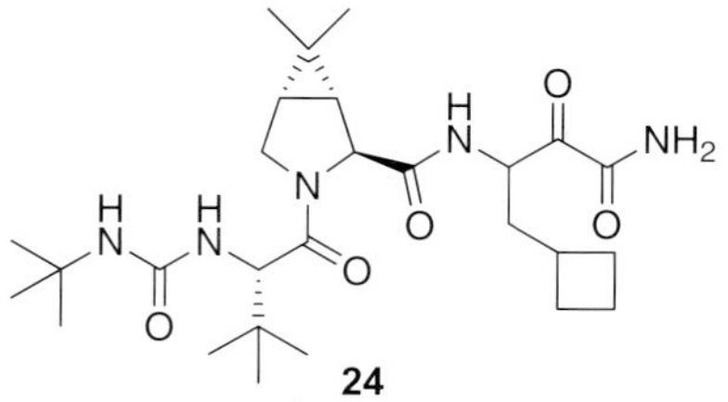

24
$K_i^* = 14$ nM
HNE/HCV= 2200
$EC_{90} = 350$ nM

Figure 14.7

The replacement of P3 cyclohexylglycine (**21**, $K_i^* = 8.0$ nM) with P3 *tert*-butylglycine (**23**, $K_i^* = 76$ nM) resulted in a marked loss in enzyme activity. However, this modification improved HNE/HCV selectivity (138 versus 684). Similarly, the replacement of the Boc group in analogue **21** with *tert*-butyl urea **22** resulted in a loss in enzyme activity as well as HNE/HCV selectivity. Even though both of these modifications independently were detrimental to potency and selectivity, in combination they proved to be very beneficial. The *tert*-butyl urea analogue of **23** resulted in **24** (boceprevir) with a $K_i^* = 14$ nM and HNE/HCV selectivity of 2200. Boceprevir (**24**) had good activity in the replicon-based cellular assay ($EC_{90} = 350$ nM) [26, 18]. Based on these and additional studies [27], it was progressed to clinical trials [28–30]. It was approved for treatment of genotype 1-infected patients by the FDA in May 2011 and is marketed with the trade name Victrelis.

We later initiated a backup program with the goal of identifying a more potent compound with improved PK in monkeys. For ease of development, we decided to develop a backup candidate that was single diastereomer at P1. To achieve these lofty goals, we once again visited the X-ray structure of inhibitors bound to protease to capitalize on additional interactions. It was clear from our previous studies that P1′ secondary amide analogues displayed better pharmacokinetics than primary ketoamide (example **15**). We therefore decided to retain allyl amide at P1′ in our initial screen of second-generation compounds.

As part of SAR investigation at the P4 region in the discovery of boceprevir, we replaced the *tert*-butyl urea cap of **24** with various carbamate and urea caps. Of

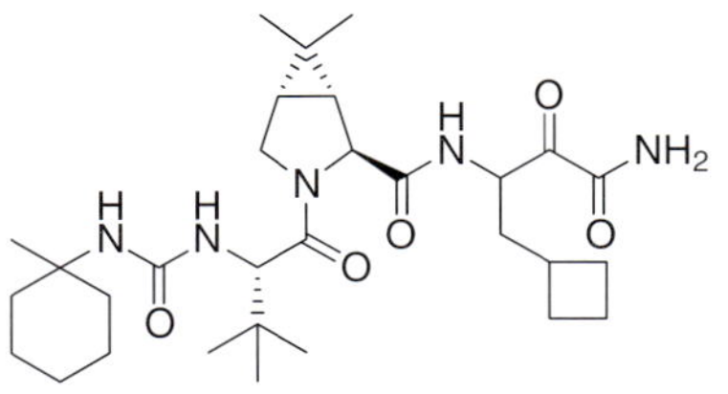

25
$K_i^* = 8$ nM
$EC_{90} = 100$ nM

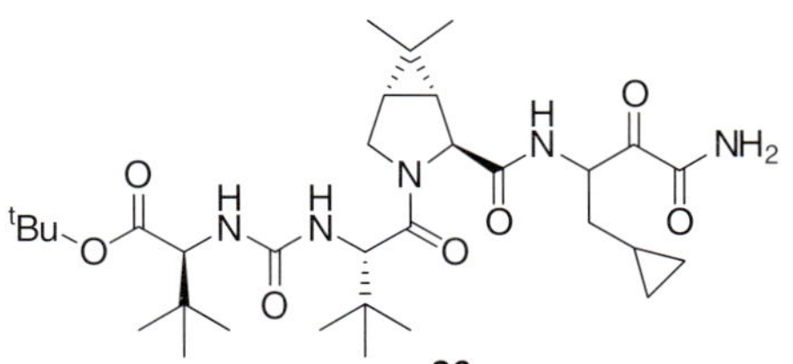

26
$K_i^* = 6$ nM
$EC_{90} = 200$ nM

Figure 14.8

these modifications, two classes of compounds, represented by **25** and **26**, demonstrated marginal improvement in cellular activity (Figure 14.8).

The incorporation of methylcyclohexyl urea cap at P3 in **24** resulted in analogue **25** ($K_i^* = 8$ nM; $EC_{90} = 100$ nM), a threefold improvement in cellular activity compared to boceprevir. Similarly, introduction of *tert*-butyl glycine *tert*-butyl ester cap in **24** yielded compound **26** ($K_i^* = 6$ nM; $EC_{90} = 200$ nM). Improved cellular activities of these analogues clearly showed that modifications at P4 could be beneficial in improving cellular potencies. We therefore further modified these analogues by introducing other functionalities in place of the methyl group in **25** and the ester moiety in **26**. After many modifications, four new series of analogues were identified that had improved cellular activities (Figure 14.9).

The incorporation of a *tert*-butyl sulfone group in the place of the methyl substituent on the P4 cap in **25** resulted in compound **27** with excellent enzyme binding and cellular potency ($K_i^* = 4$ nM; $EC_{90} = 100$ nM) [31]. However, it was poorly absorbed in rats with low plasma exposure. Analysis of X-ray structure of compounds of type **27** bound to the enzyme showed that the sulfone group was

27
$K_i^* = 4$nM
$EC_{90} = 100$nM
AUC $(Rat)_{0\text{-}6h} = 0.002$ µM h
AUC $(Mky)_{0\text{-}24h} = 3.18$ µM h

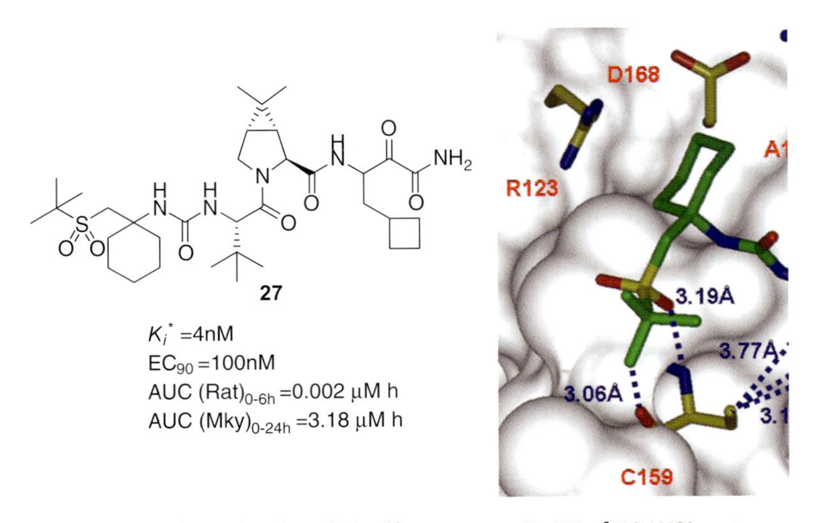

Figure 14.9 Hydrogen bonding of P4 sulfone oxygen to Cys159 of HCV NS3 protease.

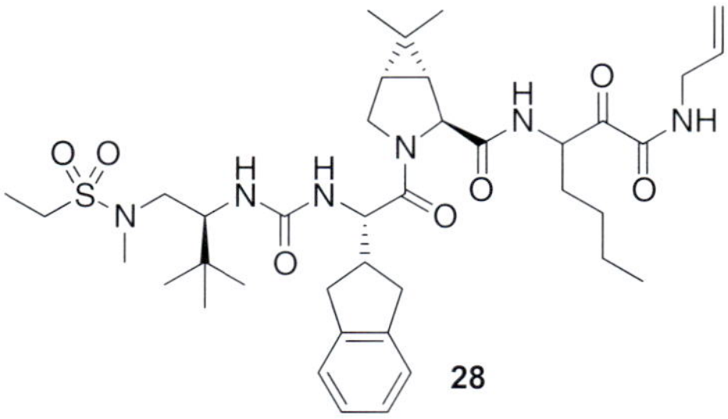

28

$K_i^* = 6$ nM
$EC_{90} = 60$ nM
AUC $(Rat)_{0\text{-}6h} = 1.2$ μM h
AUC $(Mky)_{0\text{-}24h} = 0.69$ μM h

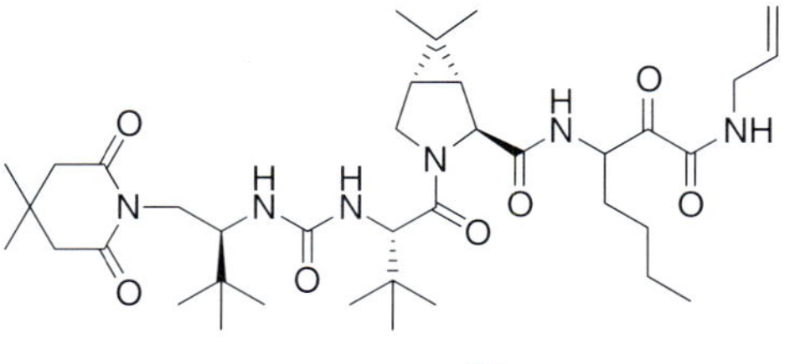

29

$K_i^* = 4$ nM
$EC_{90} = 45$ nM
AUC $(Rat)_{0\text{-}6h} = 1.58$ μM h
AUC $(Mky)_{0\text{-}24h} = 0.1$ μM h

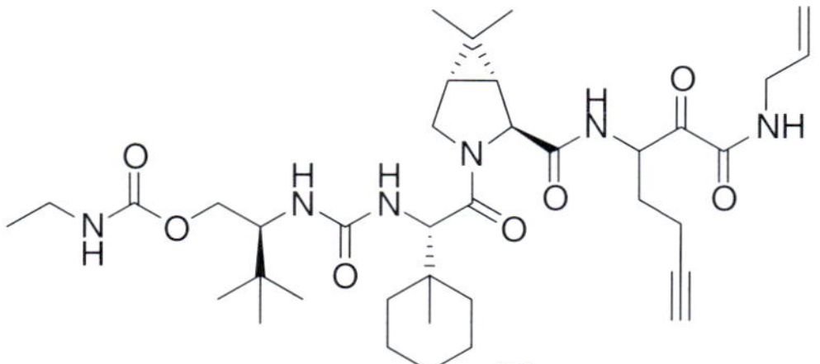

30

$K_i^* = 9$ nM
$EC_{90} = 150$ nM

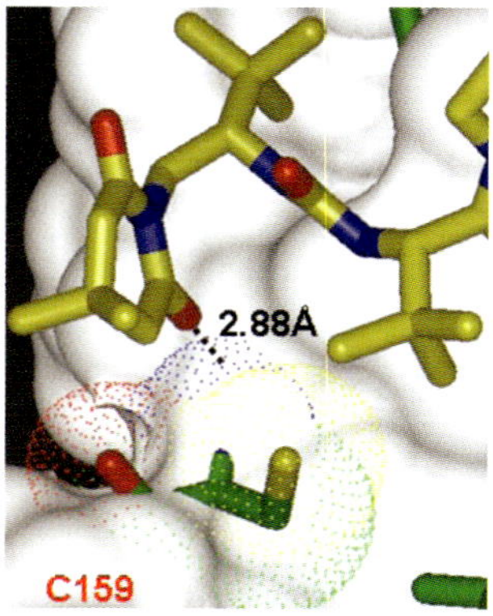

2.88Å
C159

Figure 14.10 X-ray structure of interaction between P4 imide and Cys159.

involved in a hydrogen bond interaction with the backbone amide nitrogen of Cys159. Interestingly, the structural constraints to minimize the binding energy placed one of the terminal *tert*-butyl methyl groups at a very close distance (∼3.1 Å) to the backbone carbonyl oxygen of Cys159. This close contact allows the *tert*-butyl group to remain in a *gauche* dihedral orientation with the sulfone oxygens. Similarly, modifications in the P4 *tert*-butyl glycine series also resulted in identification of many potent analogues that capitalized on this interaction with Cys159 (Figure 14.10).

Replacement of the ester at P4 in analogue of type **26** with a reverse sulfonamide group resulted in compound **28** [32] ($K_i^* = 6$ nM; $EC_{90} = 60$ nM), a sevenfold improvement in cellular activity compared to **24**. Similarly, introduction of dimethylcyclohexyl imide cap and reverse carbamate resulted in compounds of type **29** [33] ($EC_{90} = 45$ nM) and **30** ($EC_{90} = 150$ nM) with up to 10-fold improvement in cellular potency. Once again, the P4 functionalities were within hydrogen bonding distance to Cys159 amide nitrogen on the enzyme. It was very interesting to note that these compounds were allyl amides at P1′ and retained majority of the activity that of the primary ketoamide. We next designed new secondary amide analogues in the P4 spirocyclohexyl series of inhibitors **27** (Figure 14.11).

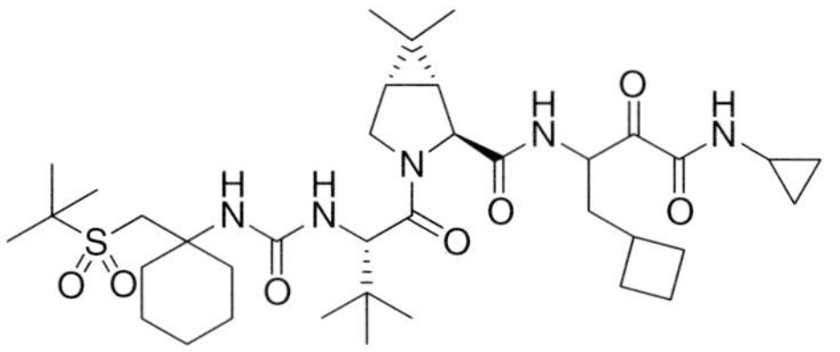

31
$K_i^* = 20nM$
HNE/HCV = 1600
$EC_{90} = 250$ nM
AUC $(Rat)_{0\text{-}6h} = 2.8$ μM h

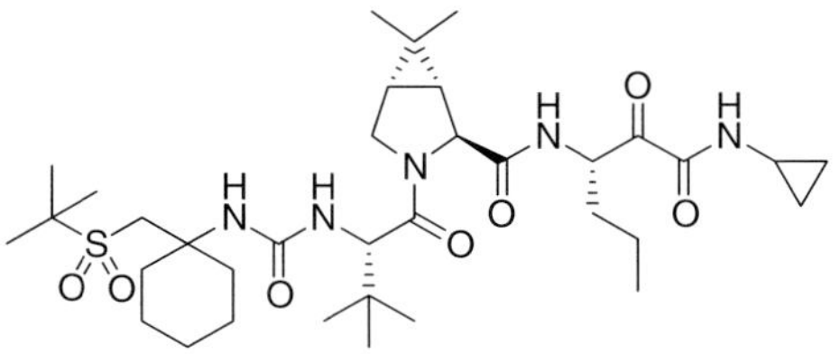

32
$K_i^* = 8$ nM
HNE/HCV = 8
$EC_{90} = 40$ nM
AUC $(Rat)_{0\text{-}24h} = 7.9$ μM h
AUC $(Mky)_{0\text{-}24h} = 1.1$ μM h

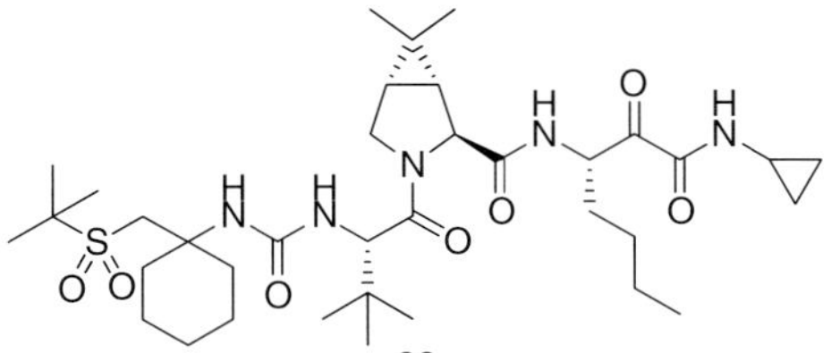

33
$K_i^* = 6$ nM
HNE/HCV= 600
$EC_{90} = 40$ nM
AUC $(Rat)_{0\text{-}24h} = 6.5$ μM h (F=46%)
AUC $(Mky)_{0\text{-}24h} = 1.1$ μM h (F=46%)

Figure 14.11

Modification of P1′ primary ketoamide in **27** with a cyclopropyl amide resulted in inhibitor **31** with poorer binding and cellular activity ($K_i^* = 20$ nM; $EC_{90} = 250$ nM) compared to **27**. However, it had good oral exposure in rats with AUC = 2.8 μM h, when dosed at 10 mg/kg. From our previous SAR studies in the identification of boceprevir, it was clear that P1 cyclobutyl alanine was less tolerated in the P1′ secondary amide series. P1 norvaline and norleucine were more preferred. We therefore synthesized analogues **32** and **33** containing P1 norvaline and norleucine moieties. In line with our expectations, compound **32** had excellent binding ($K_i^* = 8.0$ nM) and improved cellular activity ($EC_{90} = 40$ nM). This cellular activity was about 10-fold better than boceprevir. In addition, the norvaline derivative had good PK in rats. It had a good oral exposure of 7.9 μM h when dosed at 10 mg/kg in rats and 1.1 μM h in monkeys at 3 mg/kg. The incorporation of P1 norleucine resulted in inhibitor **33** that had similar characteristics to norvaline analogues, with a much improved HNE/HCV selectivity. Thus, compound **33** had an enzyme inhibition $K_i^* = 6$ nM and a cellular potency $EC_{90} = 40$ nM. It was selective against HNE with a HNE/HCV = 600 and well absorbed in animals. In rats, compound **33** had a good bioavailability ($F = 46\%$) and an exposure of 6.5 μM h when dosed at 10 mg/kg. It had a much improved PK in monkeys compared to boceprevir with an AUC = 1.1 μM h at 3 mg/kg and oral bioavailability of 46%. Based on these desirable properties, compound **33** (narlaprevir) [34] was chosen for further investigation and progressed to clinical trials.

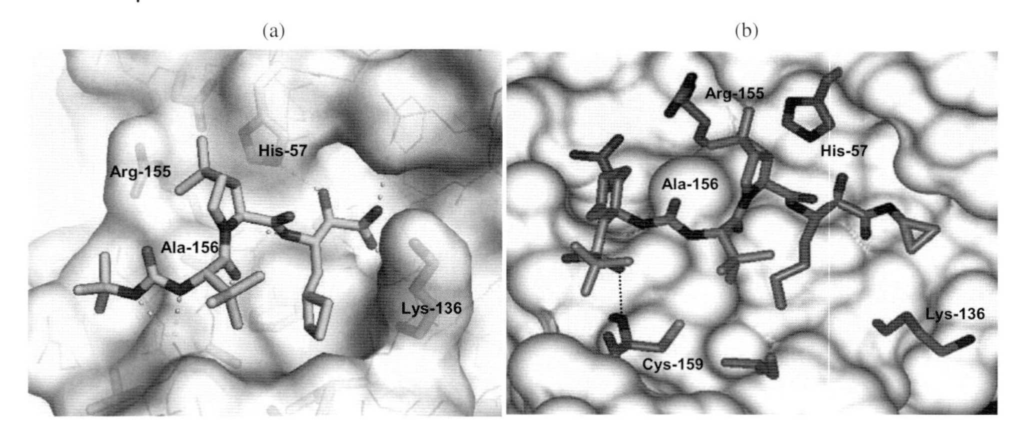

Figure 14.12 X-ray structures of boceprevir (**24**) (a) and narlaprevir (**33**) (b) bound to HCV protease.

Figure 14.12 shows the X-ray structures of boceprevir (**24**) and narlaprevir (**33**) bound to the active site of the HCV NS3 protease. Ser139 makes a covalent interaction with the ketoamide group in both compounds. While the absence of a prime side moiety in boceprevir allows the side chain of Lys136 to pack against the P1 cyclobutyl ring, thereby resulting in snug van der Waals interactions throughout the S1 pocket, the P1′ cyclopropyl cap causes the Lys136 side chain to rotate away from the S1 pocket. In addition, the more flexible linear chain of the P1 norleucine versus the constrained cyclobutyl ring pack in such a way that the Ile132 side chain adopts different rotamers in the two structures. While this alters the surface of the S1–S3 pockets somewhat, the P3 *tert*-butyl group binds in the same orientation in both structures. The P2 dimethylcyclopropyl-derived proline makes the same key interactions with the S2 pocket in both structures. The side chains of His57, Asp81, and Arg155 are in the same positions in both structures and make identical contacts with P2. Interestingly, the S4 pocket undergoes little change with the presence of the cyclohexyl ring – only the Arg123 side chain is different in the two structures. The reason is presumably that the binding orientation of the *tert*-butyl group of boceprevir has pushed the side chain of Asp168 into a rotamer position that enlarges the pocket. This new position of Asp168 upon binding either of these compounds combined with the rotations of Arg155 and His57 results in the formation of an ion-pair/H-bonding network that extends from His57–Asp81–Arg155–Asp168–Arg123. These side chains do not project face to face, but are aligned side by side. Interestingly, the binding of the P4 cyclohexyl ring in narlaprevir brings Arg123 in a bit closer to Asp168 as the readjusted pocket is tightened around the ring.

In addition to the previously described lipophilic interactions, the main chain atoms of boceprevir and narlaprevir make key hydrogen bonding interactions to the enzyme (Figure 14.13). The P1 ketoamide nitrogen donated a hydrogen bond to the side chain oxygen of Gln41, while the ketoamide oxygen projected into the oxyanion hole and accepted hydrogen bonds from the amide nitrogens of Ser139

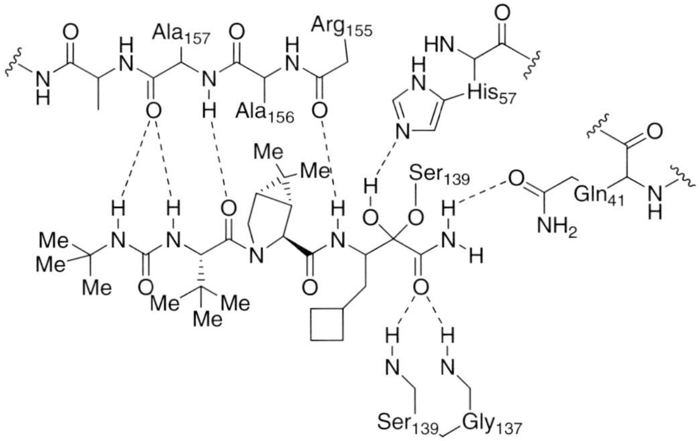

Figure 14.13 Hydrogen bonding network of boceprevir with protease backbone.

and Gly137. Similarly, the amide nitrogen of the P1 moiety donated a hydrogen bond to the carbonyl oxygen of Arg155. The P3 urea nitrogen made a pair of hydrogen bonds to the backbone carbonyl oxygen of Ala157. These interactions make the binding of boceprevir potent and selective. In addition to these hydrogen bonds, narlaprevir also made an additional hydrogen bond with the oxygen of the P4 sulfone that is in hydrogen bonding distance to the nitrogen of Cys159.

Computational analysis estimated the contribution of various ligand components toward the overall binding of the inhibitor to the enzyme. It revealed substantial proportions of binding correlates well with the contact surface area. About 50% of the surface area of boceprevir made contact to the enzyme contributing 10^5 orders of magnitude toward the binding potency. The remaining potency was achieved through hydrogen bonds and covalent interactions.

The use of structure-based design facilitated our understanding of binding interactions of inhibitors to the protease. It allowed new modifications to be conceived and synthesized. Not all these modifications resulted in improvement in activity. There were many instances into which the modeled compound fit very well in the active site but resulted in analogues with much diminished activity. Figure 14.14

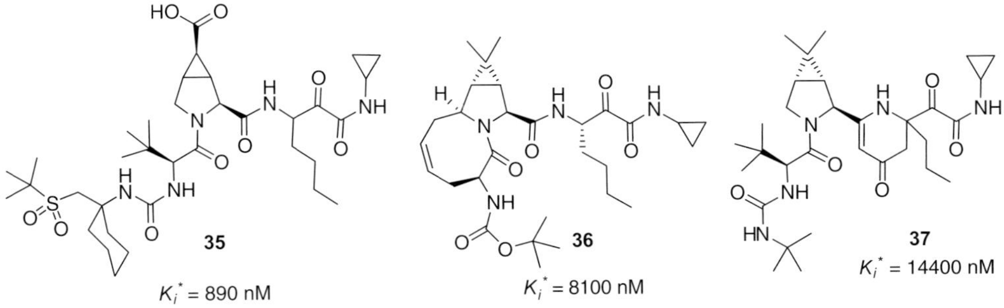

Figure 14.14

outlines three examples of these modifications that were acceptable by modeling, but had poor activity.

As previously mentioned, the X-ray structure of boceprevir indicated the methyl of the P2 proline group interacted with Arg155. Based on this and related compounds, we synthesized analogues of type **35** that contained a carboxylic acid on the proline. We modeled this analogue to make an ionic interaction with Arg155 and thereby improve potency. However, this effort did not bear fruit because the side chain of arginine was flexible and solvent exposed allowing it to occupy alternate rotamers. Other attempts to capture this interaction proved equally futile. We also explored many novel ideas to depeptidize the inhibitors in the acyclic series. Analogues **36** and **37** are representative compounds that modeled very well in the structure of the enzyme. Bicyclic analogues of **36** were synthesized in different ring sizes. These analogues were considerably less potent with analogue **36** having a $K_i^* = 8100\,\text{nM}$. We could not completely rationalize this loss based on structure. Similarly, modeled analogue **37** made an excellent fit to the protease active site based on the structure of the enzyme. However, the synthesis of this analogue resulted in compound that lost significant activity with a $K_i^* = 14\,400\,\text{nM}$. The loss in activity may possibly be due to the quaternization of P1, which hinders nucleophilic attack of serine to the ketoamide.

In the absence of a viable lead for modification, we embarked on a structure-based design to develop novel inhibitors for the HCV NS3 protease. The starting lead **1** was initially truncated at P1′ with an allyl group to identify compounds that retained most of the activity of **1**. From the X-ray structure of truncated compounds **5** and **6**, we identified various sites for modification that could potentially improve activity and depeptidize resultant analogues. Capping of inhibitors at P3 followed by modification at P2 prolines resulted in the discovery of novel analogues that were very potent in the enzyme and cellular assay. (1*R*,2*S*,5*S*)-6,6-Dimethyl-3-azabicyclo[3.1.0]hexane-2-carboxylic acid moiety was identified as an excellent P2 residue that allowed generation of potent compounds of type **9** spanning from P3 to P2′. These compounds though very potent in *in vitro* assays had poor PK in animals. Various depeptidization strategies were explored to improve PK in animals. P2–P4 and P1–P3 macrocyclic inhibitors were synthesized and evaluated resulting in many potent compounds. These analogues though retained and improved potency in some cases did not improve PK in animals.

In an effort to improve PK, we further truncated analogues to identify a primary ketoamide derivative **16** that retained significant activity of the initial leads. SAR studies on primary ketoamide compound **16** at the P1, P3, and P3 capping site resulted in the identification of cyclobutyl alanine, *tert*-butyl glycine, and *tert*-butyl urea as desirable moieties. This led to the discovery of boceprevir **24**, the first direct-acting HCV NS3 protease approved by FDA for the treatment of genotype 1 infections.

Toward the identification of a backup compound, we revisited the X-ray structure of inhibitors bound to the protease and identified modifications at P3 capping resulted in analogues with improved cellular activity. Four series of P3 modifications were discovered that yielded compounds with up to 10-fold improvement in cellular potencies. A *tert*-butyl sulfone group interacted with Cys159 was discovered resulting in analogue **33** (narlaprevir) that had excellent potency in enzyme and cellular assay. It was progressed to clinical trials.

The role of structure in modification of HCV NS3 protease inhibitors from **1** to boceprevir and narlaprevir is that of a successful journey. Based on the structure of inhibitors bound to the enzyme, new designs to depeptidize analogues and improve potency were framed. Many of these ideas resulted in compounds with improved activity, while others resulted in loss in potency. Structure-based design in combination with structure–activity relationship is a powerful tool to design inhibitors for enzymes where initial leads are not readily available. It is a tool that can facilitate improvement in enzyme activity of inhibitors allowing researchers to capitalize novel interactions with the protein. However, optimization of other properties such as cellular potency, PK, and selectivity needed for a successful drug development still requires traditional medicinal chemistry approaches such as SAR investigation.

References

1 Choo, Q.L., Kuo, G., Weiner, A.J., Overby, L.R., Bradley, D.W., and Houghton, M. (1989) Isolation of a cDNA clone derived from a blood-borne non-A, non-B viral hepatitis genome. *Science*, **244**, 359–362.

2 Kuo, G., Choo, Q.L., Alter, H.J., Gitnick, G.L., Redeker, A.G., Purcell, R.H., Miyamura, T., Dienstag, J.L., Alter, M.J., Stevens, C.E., Tegtmeier, G.E., Bonino, F., Colombo, M., Lee, W.-S., Kuo, C., Berger, K., Shuster, J.R., Overby, L.R., Bradley, W., and Houghton, M. (1989) An assay for circulating antibodies to a major etiologic virus of human non-A, non-B hepatitis. *Science*, **244**, 362–364.

3 Brown, R.S., Jr. and Gaglio, P. (2003) Scope of worldwide hepatitis C problem. *Liver Transpl.*, **9** (11), S10–S13.

4 Freeman, A.J., Dore, G.J., Law, M.G., Thorpe, M., Overbeck, J.V., Llyods, A.R., Marinos, G., and Kaldor, J.M. (2001) Estimating progression to cirrhosis in chronic hepatitis C infection. *Hepatology*, **34**, 809–816.

5 Zeuzem, S., Feinman, S.V., Rasenack, J., Heathcote, E.J., Lai, M.-Y., Gane, E., O'Grady, J., Reichen, J., Diago, M., Lin, A., Hoffman, J., and Brunda, M.J. (2000) Peginterferon alfa-2a in patients with chronic hepatitis C. *N. Engl. J. Med.*, **343** (23), 1666–1172.

6 Manns, M.P., McHutchison, J.G., Gordon, S.C., Rustgi, V.K., Shiffman, M., Reindollar, R., Goodman, Z.D., Koury, K., Ling, M.-H., and Albrecht, J.K. (International Hepatitis Interventional Therapy Group) (2001) Peginterferon alfa-2b plus ribavirin compared with interferon alfa-2b plus ribavirin for initial treatment of chronic hepatitis C: a randomized trial. *Lancet*, **358**, 958–965.

7 Bartenschlager, R. (1999) The NS3/4A proteinase of the hepatitis C virus: unraveling structure and function of an unusual enzyme and a prime target for antiviral therapy. *J. Virol. Hepat.*, **6**, 165–181.

8 Bartenschlager, R., Ahlborn-Laake, L., Mous, J., and Jacobsen, H. (1993) Nonstructural protein 3 of the hepatitis C virus encodes a serine-type proteinase required for cleavage at the NS3/4 and NS4/5 junctions. *J. Virol.*, **67**, 3835–3844.

9 Yan, Y., Li, Y., Munshi, S., Sardana, V., Cole, J.L., Sardana, M., Steinkuehler, C., Tomei, L., De-Francesco, R., Kuo, L.C., and Chen, Z. (1998) Complex of NS3 protease and NS4A peptide of BK strain hepatitis C virus: a 2.2 Å resolution structure in a hexagonal crystal form. *Protein Sci.*, **7**, 837–847.

10 Love, R.A., Parge, H.E., Wickersham, J.A., Hostomsky, Z., Habuka, N., Moomaw, E.W., Adachi, T., and Hostomska, Z. (1996) The crystal structure of hepatitis C virus NS3 proteinase reveals a trypsin-like fold and a structural zinc binding site. *Cell*, **87**, 331–342.

11 Kim, J.L., Morgenstern, K.A., Griffith, J. P., Dweyer, M.D., Thomson, J.A., Murcko, M.A., Lin, C., and Caron, P.R. (1998) Hepatitis C virus NS3 RNA helicase domain with a bound oligonucleotide: the crystal structure provides insights into the mode of unwinding. *Structure*, **6**, 89–100.

12 Kwong, A.D., Kim, J.L., Rao, G., Lipovsek, D., and Raybuck, S.A. (1998) Hepatitis C virus NS3/4A protease. *Antiviral Res.*, **40**, 1–18.

13 Steinkuhler, C., Urbani, A., Tomei, L., Biasiol, G., Sandana, M., Bianchi, E., Pessi, A., and DeFrancesco, R. (1996) Activity of purified hepatitis C virus protease NS3 on peptide substrates. *J. Virol.*, **70**, 6694–6700.

14 Urbani, A., Bianchi, E., Narjes, F., Tramontano, A., De Francesco, R., Steinkuhler, C., and Pessi, A. (1997) Substrate specificity of the hepatitis C virus serine protease NS3. *J. Biol. Chem.*, **272**, 9204–9209.

15 Kolykhalov, A.A., Agapov, E.V., and Rice, C.M. (1994) Specificity of the hepatitis C virus NS3 serine protease: effects of substitutions at the 3/4A, 4A/4B, 4B/5A, and 5A/5B cleavage sites on polyprotein processing. *J. Virol.*, **68**, 7525–7533.

16 Zhang, R., Beyer, B.M., Durkin, J., Ingram, R., Njoroge, F.G., Windsor, W.T., and Malcolm, B.A. (1999) A continuous spectrophotometric assay for the hepatitis C virus serine protease. *Anal. Biochem.*, **270**, 268–275.

17 Morrison, J.F. and Walsh, C. (1988) The behavior and significance of slow binding enzyme inhibitors, in *Advances in Enzymology*, vol. 61 (ed. A. Meister), John Wiley & Sons, Inc., New York, pp. 201–301.

18 Prongay, A.J., Guo, Z., Yao, N., Pichardo, J., Fischmann, T., Strickland, C., Myers, J., Jr., Weber, P.C., Beyer, B.M., Ingram, R., Hong, Z., Prosise, W.W., Ramanathan, L., Taremi, S.S., Yarosh-Tomaine, T., Zhang, R., Senior, M., Yang, R.S., Malcolm, B., Arasappan, A., Bennett, F., Bogen, S.L., Chen, K., Jao, E., Liu, Y.-T., Lovey, R.G., Saksena, A.K., Venkatraman, S., Girijavallabhan, V., Njoroge, F.G., and Madison, V. (2007) Discovery of the HCV NS3/4A protease inhibitor (1*R*,5*S*)-*N*-[3-amino-1-(cyclobutylmethyl)-2,3-dioxopropyl]-3-[2(*S*)-[[[(1,1-dimethylethyl) amino]carbonyl]amino]-3,3-dimethyl-1-oxobutyl]-6,6-dimethyl-3-azabicyclo[3.1.0] hexan-2(*S*)-carboxamide (Sch 503034). Key steps in structure-based optimization. *J. Med. Chem.*, **50**, 2310–2318.

19 Bogen, S.L., Arasappan, A., Bennett, F., Chen, K., Jao, E., Liu, Y.-T., Lovey, R.G., Venkatraman, S., Pan, W., Parekh, T., Pike, R.E., Ruan, S., Liu, R., Baroudy, B., Agrawal, S., Chase, R., Ingravallo, P., Pichardo, J., Prongay, A., Brisson, J.-M., Hsieh, T.Y., Cheng, K.-C., Kemp, S.J., Levy, O.E., Lim-Wilby, M., Tamura, S.Y., Saksena, A.K., Girijavallabhan, V., and Njoroge, F.G. (2006) Discovery of SCH446211 (SCH6): a new ketoamide inhibitor of the HCV NS3 serine protease and HCV subgenomic RNA replication. *J. Med. Chem.*, **49**, 2750–2757.

20 Lohmann, V., Körner, F., Koch, J.-O., Herian, U., Theilmann, L., and Bartenschlager, R. (1999) Replication of subgenomic hepatitis C virus RNAs in a hepatoma cell line. *Science*, **285**, 110–113.

21 Mamai, A., Zhang, R., Natarajan, A., and Madalengoitia, J.S. (2001) Poly-L-proline type-II peptide mimics based on the 3-azabicyclo[3.1.0]hexane system. *J. Org. Chem.*, **66**, 455–460.

22 Venkatraman, S., Njoroge, F.G., Girijavallabhan, V.M., Madison, V.S., Yao, N.H., Prongay, A.J., Butkiewicz, N., and Pichardo, J. (2005) Design and synthesis of depeptidized macrocyclic inhibitors of hepatitis C NS3-4A protease using structure-based drug design. *J. Med Chem.*, **48**, 5088–5091.

23 Chen, K.X., Njoroge, F.G., Vibulbhan, B., Prongay, A., Pichardo, J., Madison, V., Buevich, A., and Chan, T.-M. (2005) Proline-based macrocyclic inhibitors of the hepatitis C virus: stereoselective synthesis and biological activity. *Angew. Chem., Int. Ed.*, **44**, 7024–7028.

24 Chen, K., Njoroge, F.G., Arasappan, A., Venkatraman, S., Vibulbhan, B., Yang, W., Parekh, T.N., Pichardo, J., Prongay, A., Cheng, K.-C., Butkiewicz, N., Yao, N., Madison, V., and Girijavallabhan, V. (2006) Novel potent hepatitis C virus NS3 serine protease inhibitors derived from proline-based macrocycle. *J. Med. Chem.*, **49**, 995–1005.

25 Venkatraman, S., Velazquez, F., Wu, W., Blackman, M., Chen, K.X., Bogen, S., Nair, L., Tong, X., Chase, R., Hart, A., Agrawal, S., Pichardo, J., Cheng, K.-C., Girijavallabhan, V., Piwinski, J., Shih, N. Y., and Njoroge, F.G. (2009) Discovery and structure–activity relationship of P1–P3 ketoamide derived macrocyclic inhibitors of hepatitis C virus NS3 protease. *J. Med. Chem.*, **52**, 336–346.

26 Venkatraman, S., Bogen, S.L., Arasappan, A., Bennett, F., Chen, K., Jao, E., Liu, Y.-T., Lovey, R., Hendrata, S., Huang, Y., Pan, W., Parekh, T., Pinto, P., Popov, V., Pike, R., Ruan, S., Santhanam, B., Vibulbhan, B., Wu, W., Yang, W., Kong, J., Liang, X., Wong, J., Liu, R., Butkiewicz, N., Chase, R., Hart, A., Agarwal, S., Ingravallo, P., Pichardo, J., Kong, R., Baroudy, B., Malcolm, B., Guo, Z., Prongay, A., Madision, B.L., Cui, X., Cheng, K.-C., Hsieh, T.Y., Brisson, J.-M., Prelusky, D., Kormacher, W., White, R., Bogonowich-Knipp, S., Pavlovsky, A., Prudence, B., Saksena, A.K., Ganguly, A., Piwinski, J., Girijavallabhan, V., and Njoroge, F.G. (2006) Discovery of (1*R*,5*S*)-*N*-[3-amino-1-(cyclobutylmethyl)-2-3-dioxopropyl]-3-[2(*S*)-[[[(1,1-dimethylethyl)-amino]carbonyl]amio]-3,3-dimethyl-1-oxobutyl]-6,6-dimethyl-3-azabicyclo[3.1.0]hexan-2(*S*)-carboxamide (SCH 503034), a selective, potent, orally bioavailable, hepatitis C virus NS3 protease inhibitor: a potential therapeutic agent for the treatment of hepatitis C infection. *J. Med. Chem.*, **49**, 6074–6086.

27 Cheng, K.-C., Li, C., Liu, T., Wang, G., Hsieh, Y., Pavlovsky, A., Broske, L., Prelusky, D., Chen, J., Liu, R., Uss, A.S., White, R.E., Gupta, S., and Njoroge, F.G. (2009) Use of preclinical *in vitro* and *in vivo* pharmacokinetics for selection of potent hepatitis C protease inhibitor, boceprevir for clinical development. *Lett. Drug Des. Discov.*, **6**, 312–218.

28 Kwo, P.Y., Lawitz, E.J., McCone, J., Schiff, E.R., Vierling, J.M., Pound, D., Davis, M. N., Galati, J.S., Gordon, S.C., Ravendhran, N., Rossaro, L., Anderson, F.H., Jacobson, I.M., Rubin, R., Koury, K., Pedicone, L.D., Brass, C.A., Chaudhri, E., and Albrecht, J.K. (the SPRINT-1 Investigators) (2010) Efficacy of boceprevir, an NS3 protease inhibitor, in combination with peginterferon alfa-2b and ribavirin in treatment-naive patients with genotype 1 hepatitis C infection (SPRINT-1): an open-label, randomised, multicentre phase 2 trial. *Lancet*, **376**, 705–716.

29 Poordad, F., McCone JJr., J., Bacon, B.R., Bruno, S., Manns, M.P., Sulkowski, M.S., Jacobson, I.M., Reddy, K.R., Goodman, Z.D., Boparai, N., DiNubile, M.J., Sniukiene, V., Brass, C.A., Albrecht, J.K., and Bronowicki, J.-P. (the SPRINT-2 Investigators) (2011) Boceprevir for untreated chronic HCV genotype 1 infection. *N. Engl. J. Med.*, **364** (13), 1195–1206.

30 Bacon, B., Gordon, S.C., Lawitz, E., Marcellin, P., Vierling, J.M., Zeuzem, S., Poordad, F., Goodman, Z.D., Sings, H.L., Boparai, N., Burroughs, M., Brass, C.A., Albrecht, J.K., and Esteban, R. (the HCV RESPOND-2 Investigators) (2011) Boceprevir for previously treated chronic HCV genotype 1 infection. *N. Engl. J. Med.*, **364** (13), 1207–1217.

31 Bennett, F., Huang, Y., Hendrata, S., Lovey, R., Bogen, S., Pan, W., Guo, Z., Prongay, A., Chen, K.X., Arasappan, A., Venkatraman, S., Velazquez, F., Nair, L., Sannigrahi, M., Tong, X., Pichardo, J., Cheng, K.-C., Girijavallabhan, V.M., Saksena, A.K., and Njoroge, F.G. (2010) The introduction of P4 substituted 1-methylcyclohexyl groups into Boceprevir®: a change in direction in the search for a second generation HCV NS3 protease. *Bioorg. Med. Chem. Lett.*, **20**, 2617–2621.

32 Venkatraman, S., Blackman, M., Wu, W., Nair, L., Arasappan, A., Padilla, A., Bogen, S., Bennett, F., Chen, K., Pichardo, J., Tong, X., Prongay, A., Cheng, K.-C., Girijavallabhan, V., and Njoroge, F.G. (2009) Discovery of novel P3 sulfonamide-capped inhibitors of HCV NS3 protease.

Inhibitors with improved cellular potencies. *Bioorg. Med. Chem.*, **17**, 4486–449.

33 Arasappan, A, Padilla, A.I., Jao, E., Bennett, F., Bogen, S., Chen, K.X., Pike, R.E., Sannigrahi, M., Soares, J., Venkatraman, S., Vibulbhan, B., Saksena, A.K., Girijavallabhan, V., Tong, X., Cheng, K.C., and Njoroge, F.G. (2009) Discovery of novel P4 modified analogues with improved potency and pharmacokinetic profile. *J. Med. Chem.*, **52**, 2806–2817.

34 Arasappan, A., Bennett, F., Bogen, S., Venkatraman, S., Blackman, M., Chen, K. X., Hendrata, S., Huang, Y., Huelgas, R.M., Nair, L., Padilla, A.I., Pan, W., Pike, R., Pinto, P., Ruan, S., Sannigrahi, M., Velazquez, F., Vibulbhan, B, Wu, W., Yang, W., Saksena, A.K., Girijavallabhan, V., Shih, N.-Y., Kong, J., Meng, T., Jin, Y., Wong, J., McNamara, P., Prongay, A., Madison, V., Piwinski, J.J., Cheng, K.C., Morrison, R., Malcolm, B., Tong, X., Ralston, R., and Njoroge, F.G. (2010) Discovery of narlaprevir (SCH 900518): a potent, second generation HCV NS3 protease inhibitor. *ACS Med. Chem. Lett.*, **1**, 64–69.

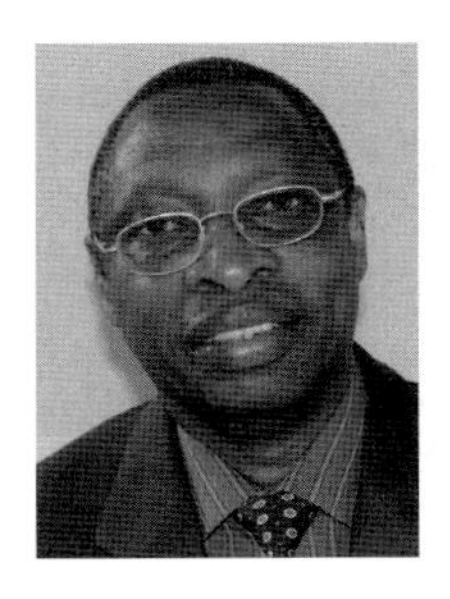

George F. Njoroge obtained his B.S. degree in Chemistry from University of Nairobi, Kenya, in 1979 and Ph.D. in Organic Chemistry from Case Western Reserve University (CWRU) in 1985. He was a postdoctoral fellow in the Institute of Pathology at CWRU working with Professor Vincent Monnier. He joined the former Schering-Plough (now Merck) as a Senior Research Scientist and rose through the ranks to the position of Director of Medicinal Chemistry. He is currently a Senior Research Fellow at Eli Lilly and Company.

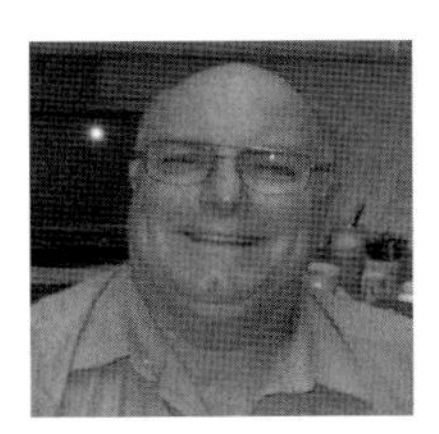

Andrew J. Prongay was born and raised in New Jersey. He earned a B.S. degree in Biology in 1982 from Cooks College, Rutgers University, New Brunswick, New Jersey. He earned a Ph.D. in Biological Chemistry in 1989 from The University of Michigan, Ann Arbor, Michigan, in the laboratory of Professor Charles H. Williams, Jr. He was a Scholar of the American Foundation for AIDS Research and performed postdoctoral studies in the laboratory of Professor Michael Rossmann of the Biology Department at Purdue University, West Lafayette, Indiana. In 1993, he began his industrial career that included research efforts in "protein science" and "structural chemistry".

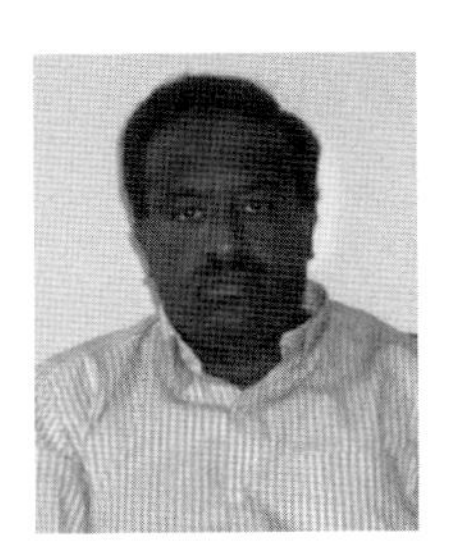

Srikanth Venkatraman obtained his B.Sc. degree in Chemistry from the University of Madras, India, and M.Sc. degree from the Indian Institute of Technology, Chennai. He later joined University of Pittsburgh and worked on azoles and azole natural products working with Dr. Peter Wipf to earn his Ph.D. After working for 2 years with Dr. Scott E. Denmark at the University of Illinois at Urbana Champaign, he joined Schering-Plough now Merck. He has extensively worked in many antiviral projects relating to hepatitis C.

15
A New-Generation Uric Acid Production Inhibitor: Febuxostat

Ken Okamoto, Shiro Kondo, and Takeshi Nishino

List of Abbreviations

AMP	adenosine monophosphate
ADP	adenosine diphosphate
ATP	adenosine triphosphate
FAD	flavin adenine dinucleotide
GMP	guanosine monophosphate
GDP	guanosine diphosphate
GTP	guanosine triphosphate
HGPRT	hypoxanthine guanine phosphoribosyltransferase
IMP	inosine monophosphate
NAD	nicotinamide adenine dinucleotide
PDB ID	protein data bank identification code
XDH	xanthine dehydrogenase
XO	xanthine oxidase
XOR	xanthine oxidoreductase

15.1
Introduction

Purine bases, which are components of nucleic acids and nucleotides, are catabolized in tissues and ultimately excreted into the urine as uric acid in humans. Xanthine oxidoreductase (XOR) catalyzes the last two steps in the purine catabolic pathway, that is, the oxidations of hypoxanthine to xanthine and xanthine to uric acid (Figure 15.1). Gout is a disease in which crystals of uric acid collect in tissues, causing painful inflammation. The factors that lead to gout are not fully understood, but include high levels of uric acid in the blood. As XOR inhibitors significantly lower uric acid production and concentration in the blood, they can be used to treat gout. Based on this strategy, Elion and coworkers of Burroughs Wellcome developed an XOR inhibitor, allopurinol (Figure 15.2), as a therapeutic drug for

Analogue-based Drug Discovery III, First Edition. Edited by János Fischer, C. Robin Ganellin, and David P. Rotella.
© 2013 Wiley-VCH Verlag GmbH & Co. KGaA. Published 2013 by Wiley-VCH Verlag GmbH & Co. KGaA.

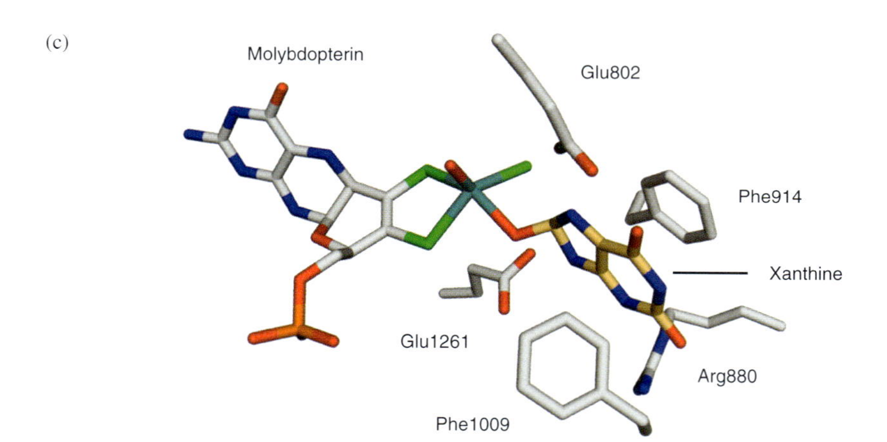

Figure 15.1 Catalytic roles of XOR in purine metabolism. (a) XOR catalyzes two steps of reaction (red arrows), that is, hypoxanthine to xanthine and xanthine to uric acid. Hypoxanthine is the metabolic product of inosine monophosphate (IMP) and adenine nucleotides (AMP, ADP, and ATP). Xanthine is also formed from guanine in the catabolism of guanine nucleotides (GMP, GDP, and GTP). (b) Proposed reaction mechanism of the molybdenum cofactor with xanthine as a substrate. Nucleophilic attack of Mo(VI)–O^- occurs at the C8 atom of xanthine to form the reaction intermediate (Mo(IV)–O–C) as illustrated. The two electrons are transferred to the other redox centers (the iron sulfur clusters and FAD) accompanied by breakdown of the reaction intermediate by hydrolysis with water to give urate. (c) The crystal structure of the reaction intermediate formed by the reduced Mo(IV) bound with excess urate under anaerobic conditions (PDB ID: 3AMZ).

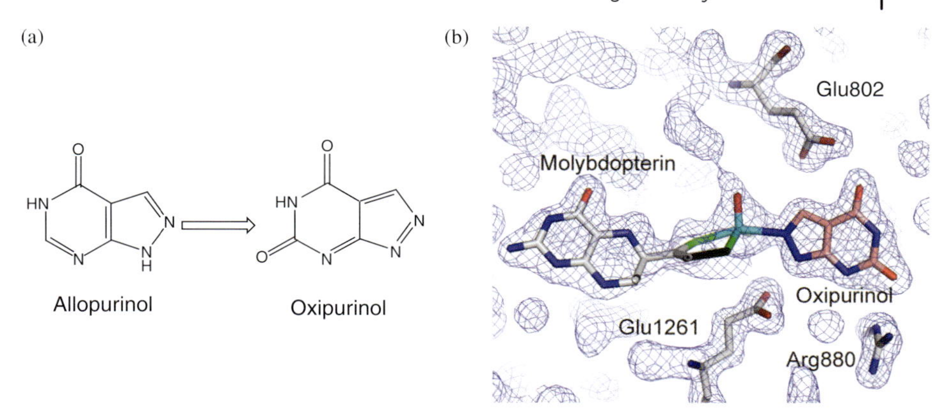

Figure 15.2 Inhibition of XOR by allopurinol. (a) Allopurinol is hydroxylated by XOR to give oxipurinol (alloxanthine). (b) The crystal structure of oxypurinol bound to the reduced Mo(IV) (PDB ID: 3BDJ). Two glutamines (Glu802 and Glu1261) and Arg880 form hydrogen bonds with oxipurinol, similarly to the urate-bound form (Figure 15.1).

gout [1]. It has been on the market for over 40 years, and the efficacy of XOR inhibition for treatment of gout is well established. However, in some cases allopurinol causes serious adverse effects [2, 3], and so new uric acid inhibitors have been sought to replace it. Many XOR inhibitors have been reported [4], but none of them has been found to be superior to allopurinol with regard to efficacy and safety; consequently, allopurinol is still the only XOR inhibitor in clinical use. Although allopurinol was first reported to be a competitive inhibitor [5], further characterization showed that it is a kind of suicide inhibitor, as described below, and this seems to be one of the reasons why many inhibitors having apparently higher affinity than allopurinol do not show greater efficacy than allopurinol. In recent years, however, Japanese pharmaceutical companies have developed several very effective inhibitors [6–9], including febuxostat, and these have attracted great interest as candidate therapeutic agents [10, 11]. Clinical trials indicate that febuxostat is superior to allopurinol in lowering uric acid production. By means of enzymatic, spectroscopic, and structural–biological analyses of the inhibition mechanism, the present authors have shown that febuxostat binds tightly to both the oxidized and reduced forms of XOR in a highly structure-specific manner [7].

15.2 Xanthine Oxidoreductase – Target Protein for Gout Treatment

Mammalian xanthine oxidoreductase is a homodimeric enzyme with a molecular mass of 290 kDa; each subunit contains one molybdenum cofactor, two [2Fe–2S] centers, and one FAD center [12]. It catalyzes the oxidative hydroxylation of purine substrates that takes place at the molybdenum center. The electrons are then transferred via the two [2Fe–2S] centers to the FAD center, where reduction of the physiological electron acceptor, NAD^+ or O_2, occurs. Mammalian XORs exist as two forms of the same gene product: xanthine dehydrogenase (XDH) and xanthine oxidase (XO). XDH prefers NAD^+ as an electron acceptor, whereas XO prefers molecular oxygen. In normal cells, XOR exists as its XDH form, but can be converted to XO reversibly by formation of disulfide bridges or irreversibly by limited proteolysis [12]. XO generates reactive oxygen species (H_2O_2 and O_2^-), which are associated with various diseases, such as reperfusion injury [13]. As XOR is the only enzyme that produces uric acid and patients with XO deficiency do not show serious disease symptoms [14], XOR is an excellent target for designing drugs to control uric acid production.

The active center of XOR for the production of uric acid is molybdopterin, where the pterin molecule is complexed with a molybdenum atom. X-ray crystallographic studies have revealed the structure in the vicinity of the cofactor [9, 15, 16]. Molybdopterin binds in a narrow groove formed by two phenylalanines, two glutamates, an arginine, and a threonine residue (Figure 15.1). Five atoms coordinate to the molybdenum atom: a water-exchangeable hydroxo ligand (—OH), a sulfide (=S) and two dithiolene sulfurs (—S) linked to the pterin moiety at equatorial positions, and the oxo (=O) group at an apical position [9]. The active site residues and the coordinating atoms in XOR are completely conserved among species from bacteria to humans [17]. The water-exchangeable oxygen atom is transferred from the molybdenum atom to the substrate as a hydroxyl group and then the active center is regenerated from oxygen derived from a water molecule during catalysis (Figure 15.1b). Two glutamic acids and an arginine form hydrogen bonds with substrate xanthine (Figure 15.1c).

15.3
Mechanism of XOR Inhibition by Allopurinol

Allopurinol is an isomer of hypoxanthine, in which the N7 nitrogen is replaced with carbon and the C8 carbon is replaced with nitrogen (Figure 15.2). The mechanism of XOR inhibition by allopurinol is complex, and allopurinol proved to be a more potent inhibitor than had originally been expected [18–20]. Allopurinol is converted into oxipurinol (4,6-dihydroxypyrazolopyrimidine) (Figure 15.2) by XOR and oxipurinol covalently binds to the reduced molybdenum (Mo^{4+}) (Figure 15.2); this is analogous to the binding mode of the reduced molybdenum with urate (Figure 15.1c) [16]. Formation of this oxipurinol–molybdenum complex is the reason for the inhibition by allopurinol. But, Mo^{4+} is gradually oxidized to Mo^{6+} with a half-life of 300 min at 25 °C [20] and the covalent bond of molybdenum with oxipurinol is broken. Different from the case of febuxostat, described later, the interaction of oxipurinol and oxidized XOR is weak in the absence of the covalent bond, and oxipurinol acts only as a weak competitive inhibitor with a K_i value of about 1.7×10^{-6} M [5]. Thus, the inhibition by allopurinol strongly depends on the oxidation or reduction state of the enzyme, and this may be the reason why allopurinol must be administered frequently (three times a day) to be effective, that is, to maintain a sufficient level of the oxipurinol-reduced molybdenum complex in the body.

15.4 Development of Nonpurine Analogue Inhibitor of XOR: Febuxostat

Analysis of the structure–activity relationship of various drug candidates suggested that a purine structure was not necessary for inhibitory activity [21–25], and that a five-membered heterocycle with a phenyl ring would be a suitable inhibitor template, as shown in Figure 15.3. Several scaffolds matching this template were synthesized and 2-phenyl-4-methyl-5-thiazolecarboxylic acid was found to have weak inhibitory activity with an IC_{50} value of 700 nM. This compound was selected as a lead compound. Preliminary modification of the lead compound revealed that the introduction of an electron-withdrawing substituent and hydrogen bond acceptor such as NO_2 or CF_3 at the 3-position of the phenyl ring or an electron-donating substituent such as OR or COOH at the 4-position led to an increase of the inhibitory activity. The NO_2-substituted derivative at high blood concentration showed prolonged hypouricemic action, so lead optimization was carried out using mainly nitro derivatives. The above substituent effects could also be seen in disubstituted compounds containing NO_2 at the 3-position of the phenyl ring and an alkoxy or alkylamino group at the 4-position of the thiazole ring. Ten or more compounds showed potent inhibitory activity with IC_{50} values of about 1 nM, and they reduced serum uric acid levels more effectively than did allopurinol in mice. However, almost all of the nitro derivatives showed mutagenic activity in the Ames test, even at low concentrations, as expected. Attempts to replace the nitro group with other electron-withdrawing substituents at the 3-position resulted in identification of the

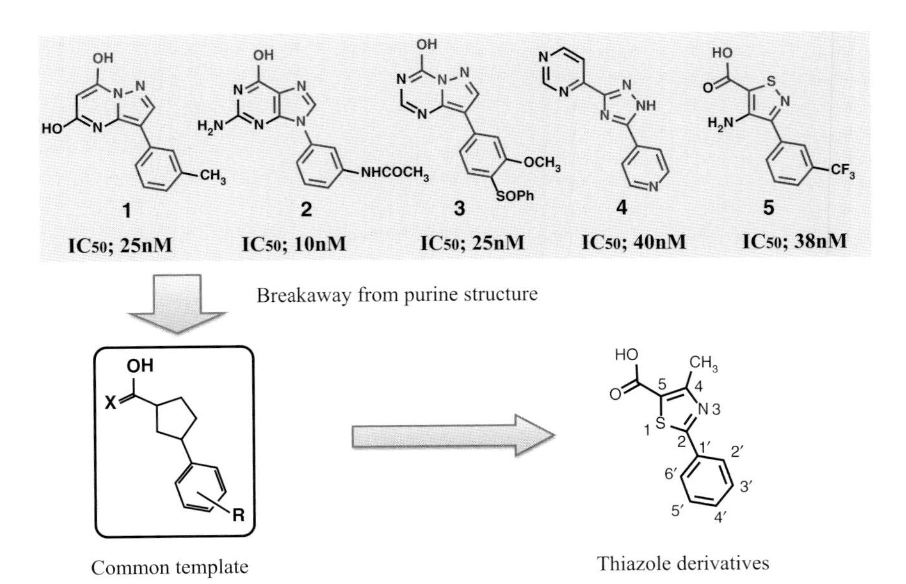

Figure 15.3 Lead compound of febuxostat. *Top*: Chemical structures and the IC_{50} values of various inhibitors reported in the literature [20–24]. *Bottom*: Lead compound for development of higher affinity inhibitors.

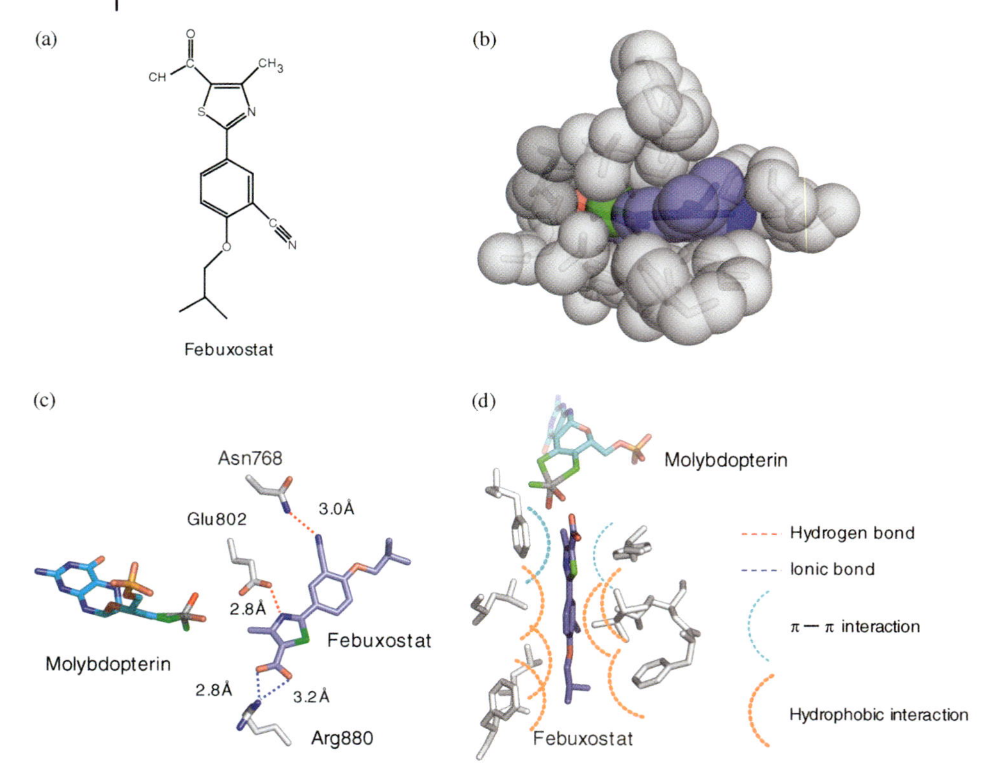

Figure 15.4 (a) Crystal structure of the complex of bovine XOR and febuxostat (PDB ID; 1N5X). (b) Amino acid residues of XOR located close to febuxostat are drawn using the van der Waals radius. (c) Hydrogen bonds are drawn with dotted red lines. Ionic bonds are drawn with dotted blue lines. Distances are taken from unpublished data of febuxostat-bound bovine XOR at 2.1 Å resolution. (d) Possible π–π interactions of amino acids with febuxostat are indicated with dotted blue lines and possible hydrophobic interactions with dotted orange lines.

cyano group as the best substituent among those examined. Finally, 2-(3-cyano-4-isobutoxyphenyl)-4-methyl-5-thiazolecarboxylic acid (febuxostat) (Figure 15.4a) was selected as a candidate for clinical development. The suitability of these substituents at the 3- and 4-positions is clearly supported by the structure of febuxostat-bound bovine XOR, as described below [7].

15.5 Mechanism of XOR Inhibition by Febuxostat

Febuxostat contains a thiazole ring with a methyl group at the 4-position and a benzene ring with a CN group at the 3-position (Figure 15.4a). These two rings can rotate freely. The structural similarity with purine is low, and the molecular weight is much larger than that of purine. The crystal structure of the complex of milk XOR with febuxostat shows features that account for the tight binding of febuxostat [7]. Febuxostat fits well into the substrate binding channel of XOR, and no open space remains in the channel after binding (Figure 15.4b). In contrast to allopurinol, febuxostat does not form a covalent bond with molybdenum. However, although no covalent bond is formed between the enzyme and the inhibitor, multiple weak interactions such as ionic and hydrogen bonds, π–π interactions between the thiazole ring and nearby phenylalanine residues, van der Waals interactions, and hydrophobic interactions were found in the structure (Figure 15.4c and d). The combination of these interactions results in tight binding; the dissociation constant determined for the desulfo form was $2 \pm 0.03 \times 10^{-9}$ M, and for the active form, the corresponding number was too low to allow accurate measurements [7]. Moreover, the fit of febuxostat to the enzyme's active site structure is enhanced by rotation of the region between the thiazole ring and the benzene ring. Thus, febuxostat efficiently matches the structure of the substrate binding region of the enzyme. A hydrogen bonding interaction of the CN group of the inhibitor with an asparagine residue of the enzyme should be noted. In the crystal structure, the side chain amide of Asn768 and the cyano group of 3-position are 2.9 Å apart, forming a hydrogen bond (Figure 15.4c). Although this asparagine residue (Asn768 in the bovine enzyme) is located too far from the active center for direct involvement in purine substrate recognition or catalytic activity, the CN group of febuxostat is necessary for potent enzyme inhibitory activity. When the 3-cyano moiety of febuxostat was replaced by hydrogen, the binding affinity was significantly decreased (S. Kondo, unpublished data). In contrast, when the cyano group of the inhibitor was substituted with a nitro ligand, which is also capable of accepting a hydrogen bond, the resulting derivative showed a binding affinity very similar to that of febuxostat. A bulky hydrophobic moiety at the 4-position is also essential for tight binding. The 4-isobutoxy group is surrounded by hydrophobic amino acids, with distances ranging from 3.7 to 4.2 Å (Figure 15.4d). Although some of these crystallographically determined values are too large to be consistent with a role of direct van der Waals binding, they construct a suitable pocket for bulky hydrophobic moieties, which might interact with the 4-isobutoxy tail.

The catalytic reaction of XOR involves a ping-pong mechanism alternating between Mo^{6+} and Mo^{4+} states, and the inhibition constants for the two states are different, so that febuxostat exhibits mixed-type inhibition in a Lineweaver–Burk plot [7]. However, the inhibition constants are extremely low in both cases, $K_i = 1.2 \times 10^{-10}$ M and $K_i = 9 \times 10^{-10}$ M for the oxidized and reduced forms of molybdenum, respectively. Thus, unlike allopurinol, the inhibitory activity of febuxostat is not much influenced by the valency of molybdenum. This indicates that febuxostat can bind to the enzyme irrespective of its redox state. That is to say, febuxostat binds stably to XOR throughout the *in vivo* lifetime of XOR (about 36 h from synthesis to degradation). It was expected from these crystallographic and enzymological analyses that a low administration frequency and low dose of febuxostat would be suitable for the treatment of gout. Indeed, clinical studies conducted in the United States and Japan supported this prediction (as described below).

Allopurinol contains a purine-like structure, and might cause adverse effects by interacting with purine metabolic enzymes other than XOR. Both allopurinol and oxypurinol are structurally similar to purines. As a result, they are substrates for certain purine and pyrimidine metabolic enzymes, such as hypoxanthineguanine phosphoribosyltransferase, or orotate phosphoribosyltransferase (HGPRT), which convert them to the corresponding ribonucleotides, that is, allopurinol-1′-ribonucleotide, oxypurinol-1′-ribonucleotide, and oxypurinol-7′-ribonucleotide [26–29]. These ribonucleotides are quite potent inhibitors of the pyrimidine biosynthesis enzyme orotidine-5′-monophosphate decarboxylase, with K_i values of 10^{-10} M order of magnitude [30–32]. On the other hand, febuxostat does not have a structural similarity to purine, and does not inhibit enzymes such as guanine deaminase, purine nucleoside phosphorylase, and HGPRT at concentrations lower than 10^{-4} M [33].

15.6
Excretion of XOR Inhibitors

Oxipurinol, an oxidation product of allopurinol, is excreted from the kidney into the urine, as is uric acid [34], so patients with renal dysfunction tend to have delayed excretion of oxipurinol as well as a high blood concentration of oxipurinol. An increased blood concentration of oxipurinol is correlated with the occurrence of adverse side effects; therefore, the administration of allopurinol must be adjusted with respect to the level of kidney function of the patients [2]. In contrast to allopurinol, febuxostat has multiple excretion routes, being excreted into urine and feces in a well-balanced manner after conjugation with glucuronic acid in the liver. Therefore, it was expected that febuxostat could be administered to patients who have a mild to moderate decrease in kidney function without the need to adjust the dose. Clinical trials confirmed that febuxostat could be used safely in patients with renal impairment [35–37].

15.7
Results of Clinical Trials of Febuxostat in Patients with Hyperuricemia and Gout

In a phase III placebo-controlled double-blind comparative study conducted among Japanese patients with hyperuricemia (including gout patients), administration of 20 or 40 mg of febuxostat once a day reduced serum uric acid concentration to below the target value of 6.0 mg/dl [38]. The ratio of patients who achieved a uric acid concentration of lower than 6 mg/dl (i.e., the achievement ratio) was 47 or 83% for patients who received 20 or 40 mg of febuxostat, respectively [39]. Notably, the results in the group given 40 mg of febuxostat, in terms of both the ratio of change in serum uric acid concentration and the achievement rate of serum uric acid concentration below 6 mg/dl, were significantly superior to those in the group given 200 mg allopurinol [40]. Moreover, in a phase III allopurinol-controlled clinical trial conducted in the United States, the ratio of patients achieving uric acid concentrations below 6 mg/dl was significantly higher in the 80 or 120 mg febuxostat group, as compared with the 300 mg allopurinol group [10]. There were no severe adverse effects that developed into clinically significant problems in either of the febuxostat groups, and there was no dose-dependent increase of adverse effects.

15.8 Summary

Febuxostat binds tightly to XOR, the target enzyme, via multiple weak interactions. The inhibition mechanism of febuxostat is completely different from that of allopurinol; in particular, its inhibitory effect on XOR remains almost constant over the *in vivo* lifetime of the XOR molecule, and it does not inhibit other enzymes involved in nucleic acid metabolism. In these respects, febuxostat is a more effective inhibitor of uric acid production than allopurinol, and its safety and efficacy for treatment of hyperuricemia (including gout) have been confirmed in phase III clinical trials.

15.9 Added in proof

Febuxostat inhibits bovine XOR with a Ki in the picomolar-order, but it is a much weaker inhibitor of Rhodobacter capsulatus XOR with a high Ki value (17.5 mM), even though the three-dimensional structures of the substrate-binding pockets are well-conserved and both enzymes permit the inhibitor to be accommodated in the active site as indicated by computational docking studies [41]. Molecular dynamics simulations indicate that differences in mobility of hydrophobic residues that do not directly interact with the substrate account for establishing a pocket well suited to accommodate bulky hydrophobic moieties of febuxostat.

References

1 Elion, G.B. (1966) Enzymatic and metabolic studies with allopurinol. *Ann. Rheum. Dis.*, **25**, 608–614.

2 Hande, K.R., Noone, R.M., and Stone, W. J. (1984) Severe allopurinol toxicity. Description and guidelines for prevention in patients with renal insufficiency. *Am. J. Med.*, **76**, 47–56.

3 Singer, S., Elion, G.B., and Hitchings, G. H. (1966) Resistance to inhibitors of dihydrofolate reductase in strains of *Lactobacillus casei* and *Proteus vulgaris*. *J. Gen. Microbiol.*, **42**, 185–196.

4 Borges, F., Fernandes, E., and Roleira, F. (2002) Progress towards the discovery of xanthine oxidase inhibitors. *Curr. Med. Chem.*, **9**, 195–217.

5 Elion, G.B., Kovensky, A., and Hitchings, G.H. (1966) Metabolic studies of allopurinol, an inhibitor of xanthine oxidase. *Biochem. Pharmacol.*, **15**, 863–880.

6 Okamoto, K. and Nishino, T. (1995) Mechanism of inhibition of xanthine oxidase with a new tight binding inhibitor. *J. Biol. Chem.*, **270**, 7816–7821.

7 Okamoto, K., Eger, B.T., Nishino, T., Kondo, S., Pai, E.F., and Nishino, T. (2003) An extremely potent inhibitor of xanthine oxidoreductase. Crystal structure of the enzyme–inhibitor complex and mechanism of inhibition. *J. Biol. Chem.*, **278**, 1848–1855.

8 Fukunari, A., Okamoto, K., Nishino, T., Eger, B.T., Pai, E.F., Kamezawa, M., Yamada, I., and Kato, N. (2004) Y-700 [1-[3-cyano-4-(2,2-dimethylpropoxy)phenyl]-1*H*-pyrazole-4-carboxylic acid]: a potent xanthine oxidoreductase inhibitor with hepatic excretion. *J. Pharmacol. Exp. Ther.*, **311**, 519–528.

9 Okamoto, K., Matsumoto, K., Hille, R., Eger, B.T., Pai, E.F., and Nishino, T. (2004) The crystal structure of xanthine oxidoreductase during catalysis: implications for reaction mechanism and enzyme inhibition. *Proc. Natl. Acad. Sci. USA*, **101**, 7931–7936.

10 Becker, M.A., Schumacher, H.R., Jr., Wortmann, R.L., MacDonald, P.A., Eustace, D., Palo, W.A., Streit, J., and Joseph-Ridge, N. (2005) Febuxostat compared with allopurinol in patients with hyperuricemia and gout. *N. Engl. J. Med.*, **353**, 2450–2461.

11 Bruce, S.P. (2006) Febuxostat: a selective xanthine oxidase inhibitor for the treatment of hyperuricemia and gout. *Ann. Pharmacother.*, **40**, 2187–2194.

12 Nishino, T., Okamoto, K., Eger, B.T., Pai, E.F., and Nishino, T. (2008) Mammalian xanthine oxidoreductase – mechanism of transition from xanthine dehydrogenase to xanthine oxidase. *FEBS J.*, **275** (13), 3278–3289.

13 Nishino, T. (1994) The conversion of xanthine dehydrogenase to xanthine oxidase and the role of the enzyme in reperfusion injury. *J. Biochem.*, **116** (1), 1–6.

14 Simmonds, H.A., Reiter, S., and Nishino, T. (1995) Hereditary xanthinuria, in *The Metabolic and Molecular Basis of Inherited Disease*, 7th edn, vol. **II** (eds C.R. Scriver, A.L. Beaudet, W.S. Sly, and D. Valle), McGraw-Hill, New York, pp. 1781–1797.

15 Enroth, C., Eger, B.T., Okamoto, K., Nishino, T., Nishino, T., and Pai, E.F. (2000) Crystal structures of bovine milk xanthine dehydrogenase and xanthine oxidase: structure-based mechanism of conversion. *Proc. Natl. Acad. Sci. USA*, **97** (20), 10723–10728.

16 Okamoto, K., Kawaguchi, Y., Eger, B.T., Pai, E.F., and Nishino, T. (2010) Crystal structures of urate bound form of xanthine oxidoreductase: substrate orientation and structure of the key reaction intermediate. *J. Am. Chem. Soc.*, **132** (48), 17080–17083.

17 Hille, R. (1996) The mononuclear molybdenum enzymes. *Chem. Rev.*, **96** (7), 2757–2816.

18 Spector, T. and Johns, D.G. (1968) Oxidation of 4-hydroxypyrazolo(3,4-*d*) pyrimidine by xanthine oxidase, the route of electron transfer from substrate to acceptor dyes. *Biochem. Biophys. Res. Commun.*, **32** (6), 1039–1044.

19 Spector, T. and Johns, D.G. (1970) 4-Hydroxypyrazolo(3,4-*d*)pyrimidine as a substrate for xanthine oxidase: loss of conventional substrate activity with catalytic cycling of the enzyme. *Biochem. Biophys. Res. Commun.*, **38** (4), 583–589.

20 Massey, V., Komai, H., Palmer, G., and Elion, G.B. (1970) The existence of nonfunctional active sites in milk xanthine oxidase: reaction with functional active site inhibitors. *Vitam. Horm.*, **28**, 505–531.

21 Springer, R.H., Dimmitt, M.K., Novinson, T., O'Brien, D.E., Robins, R. K., Simon, L.N., and Miller, J.P. (1976) Synthesis and enzymic activity of some novel xanthine oxidase inhibitors. *J. Med. Chem.*, **19**, 291–296.

22 Silipo, C. and Hansch, C. (1976) Correlation analysis of Baker's studies on enzyme inhibition. *J. Med. Chem.*, **19**, 62–71.

23 Fujii, S., Kawamura, H., Kiyokawa, H., and Yamada, S. (2012) Pyrazolotriazine compounds. EP 269859, JP 89079184, US Patent 4,824,834.

24 Baldwin, J.J., Kasinger, P.A., Novello, F.C., and Sprague, J.M. (1975) 4-Trifluoromethylimidazoles and 5-(4-pyridyl)-1,2,4-triazoles, new classes of xanthine oxidase inhibitors. *J. Med. Chem.*, **18**, 895–900.

25 Wortmann, R.L., Ridolfo, A.S., Lightfoot, R. W., Jr., and Fox, I.H. (1985)

Antihyperuricemic properties of amflutizole in gout. *J. Rheum.*, **12**, 540–543.

26 Reiter, S., Loffler, W., Grobner, W., and Zollner, N. (1986) Urinary oxipurinol-1-riboside excretion and allopurinol-induced oroticaciduria. *Adv. Exp. Med. Biol.*, **195** (Part A), 453–460.

27 Simmonds, H.A., Reiter, S., Davies, P.M., and Cameron, J.S. (1991) Orotidine accumulation in human erythrocytes during allopurinol therapy: association with high urinary oxypurinol-7-riboside concentrations in renal failure and in the Lesch–Nyhan syndrome. *Clin. Sci.*, **80**, 191–197.

28 Nelson, D.J. and Elion, G.B. (1984) Metabolic studies of high doses of allopurinol in humans. *Adv. Exp. Med. Biol.*, **165**Pt (A), 167–170.

29 Krenitsky, T.A., Elion, G.B., Strelitz, R. A., and Hitchings, G.H. (1967) Ribonucleosides of allopurinol and oxoallopurinol. Isolation from human urine, enzymatic synthesis, and characterization. *J. Biol. Chem.*, **242**, 2675–2682.

30 Kelley, W.N. and Beardmore, T.D. (1970) Allopurinol: alteration in pyrimidine metabolism in man. *Science*, **169**, 388–390.

31 Fyfe, J.A., Miller, R.L., and Krenitsky, T.A. (1973) Kinetic properties and inhibition of orotidine 5′-phosphate decarboxylase. Effects of some allopurinol metabolites on the enzyme. *J. Biol. Chem.*, **248**, 3801–3809.

32 Brown, G.K. and O'Sullivan, W.J. (1977) Inhibition of human erythrocyte orotidylate decarboxylase. *Biochem. Pharmacol.*, **26**, 1947–1950.

33 Takano, Y., Hase-Aoki, K., Horiuchi, H., Zhao, L., Kasahara, Y., Kondo, S., and Becker, M.A. (2005) Selectivity of febuxostat, a novel non-purine inhibitor of xanthine oxidase/xanthine dehydrogenase. *Life Sci.*, **76**, 1835–1847.

34 Elion, G.B., Yu, T.F., Gutman, A.B., and Hitchings, G.H. (1968) Renal clearance of oxipurinol, the chief metabolite of allopurinol. *Am. J. Med.*, **45**, 69–77.

35 Hoshide, S., Takahashi, Y., Ishikawa, T., Kubo, J., Tsuchimoto, M., Komoriya, K., Ohno, I., and Hosoya, T. (2004) PK/PD and safety of a single dose of TMX-67 (febuxostat) in subjects with mild and moderate renal impairment. *Nucleosides Nucleotides Nucleic Acids*, **23**, 1117–1118.

36 Mayer, M.D., Khosravan, R., Vernillet, L., Wu, J.T., Joseph-Ridge, N., and Mulford, D.J. (2005) Pharmacokinetics and pharmacodynamics of febuxostat, a new non-purine selective inhibitor of xanthine oxidase in subjects with renal impairment. *Am. J. Ther.*, **12**, 22–34.

37 Becker, M.A., Schumacher, H.R., Espinoza, L.R., Wells, A.F., MacDonald, P., Lloyd, E., and Lademacher, C. (2010) The urate-lowering efficacy and safety of febuxostat in the treatment of the hyperuricemia of gout: the CONFIRMS trial. *Arthritis Res. Ther.*, **12** (2), R63.

38 Shoji, A., Yamanaka, H., and Kamatani, N. (2004) A retrospective study of the relationship between serum urate level and recurrent attacks of gouty arthritis: evidence for reduction of recurrent gouty arthritis with antihyperuricemic therapy. *Arthritis Rheum.*, **51**, 321–325.

39 Naoyuki, K., Shin, F., Toshikazu, H., Tatsuo, H., Kenjiro, K., Toshitaka, N., Takanori, U., Tetsuya. Y., Hisashi, Y., and Yuji, M. (2011) Placebo-controlled double-blind dose-response study of the non-purine-selective xanthine oxidase inhibitor febuxostat (TMX-67) in patients with hyperuricemia (including gout patients) in japan: late phase 2 clinical study. *J. Clin. Rheumatol.* **17**(Suppl 2), S35–43.

40 Kamatani, N., Fujimori, S., Hada, T., Hosoya, T., Kohri, K., Nakamura, T., Ueda, T., Yamamoto, T., Yamanaka, H., and Matsuzawa, Y. (2011) An allopurinol-controlled, randomized, double-dummy, double-blind, parallel between-group, comparative study of febuxostat (TMX-67), a non-purine-selective inhibitor of xanthine oxidase, in patients with hyperuricemia including those with gout in Japan: phase 3 clinical study. *J. Clin Rheumatol.* **17**(Suppl 2), S13–18.

41 Kikuchi, H., Fujisaki, H., Furuta, T., Okamoto, K., Leimkühler, S., and Nishino, T. (2012) Different inhibitory potency of febuxostat towards mammalian and bacterial xanthine oxidoreductases: insight from molecular dynamics. *Sci Rep.* **2**, 331.

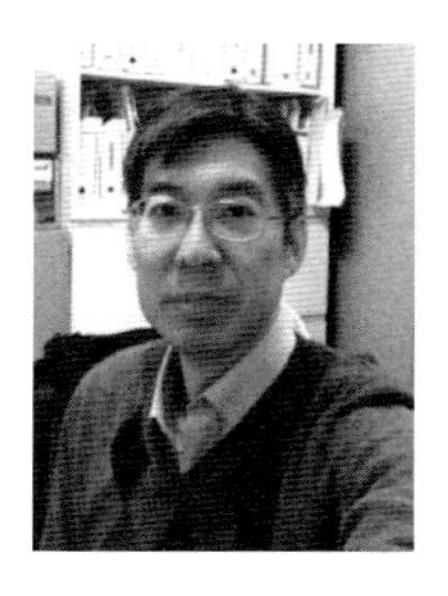

Ken Okamoto studied medicine at Yamanashi Medical College, receiving an M.D. in 1990. He studied biochemistry at Yokohama City University, receiving a Ph.D. in 1994 under Professor Takeshi Nishino, and was a Research Associate at Nippon Medical School with Professor Taro Okazaki and Takeshi Nishino in 1994. In 2000 and 2001, he learned X-ray crystallography at the University of Toronto under Professor Emil Pai. In 2005, he was an Associate Professor at Department of Biochemistry and Molecular Biology at Nippon Medical School.

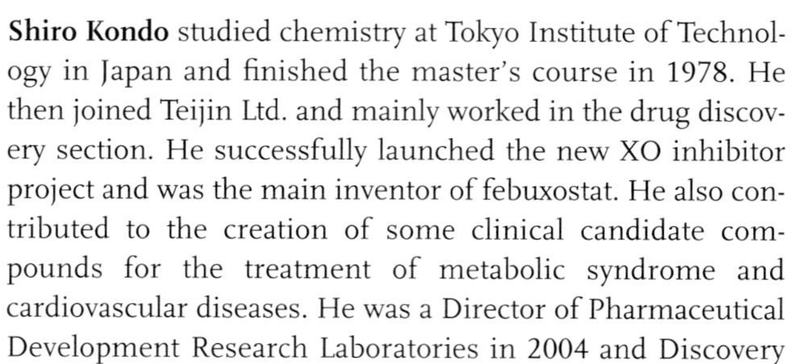

Shiro Kondo studied chemistry at Tokyo Institute of Technology in Japan and finished the master's course in 1978. He then joined Teijin Ltd. and mainly worked in the drug discovery section. He successfully launched the new XO inhibitor project and was the main inventor of febuxostat. He also contributed to the creation of some clinical candidate compounds for the treatment of metabolic syndrome and cardiovascular diseases. He was a Director of Pharmaceutical Development Research Laboratories in 2004 and Discovery Research Laboratories in 2006. He was awarded the title of Fellow of Teijin Ltd. in 2009 and is currently Head of the Kondo Research Laboratory of Teijin.

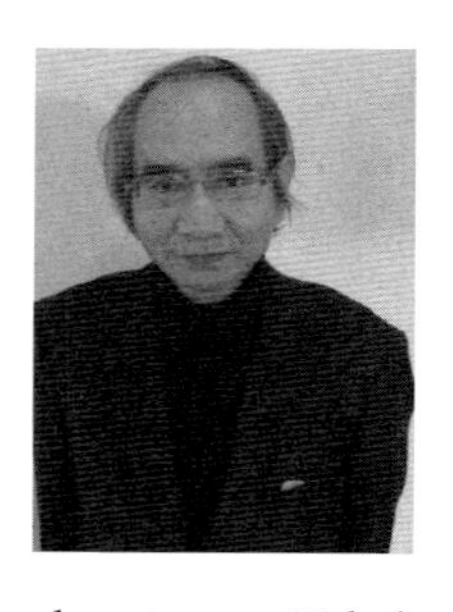

Takeshi Nishino studied medicine at Yokohama City University School of Medicine receiving an M.D. in 1970 and then studied biochemistry at Department of Biochemistry, Graduate School of Yokohama City University, under Professor Keizo Tsushima receiving Ph.D. in 1975. He was a Postdoctoral Fellow in 1976–1978 at Department of Biological Chemistry of The University of Michigan, Ann Arbor, with Professor Vincent Massey. He was an Assistant Professor and then an Associate Professor at Department of Biochemistry at Yokohama City University School of Medicine in 1976–1991. In 1992, he moved to Department of Biochemistry and Molecular Biology at Nippon Medical School in Tokyo, where he was appointed Professor and Chairman and then Professor Emeritus of Nippon Medical School in 2009. He was appointed the Distinguished Visiting Scholar of Biochemistry in University of California, Riverside, in 2009–2010. In 2011, he was appointed Specially Employed Professor of The Graduate School of Agricultural and Life Science at The University of Tokyo. He has been studying the various aspects of xanthine oxidoreductase and its related enzymes and has authored over 150 scientific publications. He was the Vice President of the Japanese Biochemical Society Meeting and was the Chairman of the International Symposium on Flavins and Flavoproteins in 2005.

Index

Analogue-based Drug Discovery III, First Edition. Edited by János Fischer, C. Robin Ganellin, and David P. Rotella.
© 2013 Wiley-VCH Verlag GmbH & Co. KGaA. Published 2013 by Wiley-VCH Verlag GmbH & Co. KGaA.